Emerging Topics in Statistics and Biostatistics

More information about this series at http://www.springer.com/series/16213

Indranil Ghosh • N. Balakrishnan
Hon Keung Tony Ng
Editors

Advances in Statistics - Theory and Applications

Honoring the Contributions of Barry C. Arnold in Statistical Science

Springer

Editors
Indranil Ghosh
Department of Mathematics and Statistics
University of North Carolina Wilmington
Wilmington, NC, USA

N. Balakrishnan
Department of Mathematics and Statistics
McMaster University
Hamilton, ON, Canada

Hon Keung Tony Ng
Department of Statistical Science
Southern Methodist University
Dallas, TX, USA

ISSN 2524-7735 ISSN 2524-7743 (electronic)
Emerging Topics in Statistics and Biostatistics
ISBN 978-3-030-62902-1 ISBN 978-3-030-62900-7 (eBook)
https://doi.org/10.1007/978-3-030-62900-7

This Springer imprint is published by the registered company Springer Nature Switzerland AG
The registered company address is: Gewerbestrasse 11, 6330 Cham, Switzerland

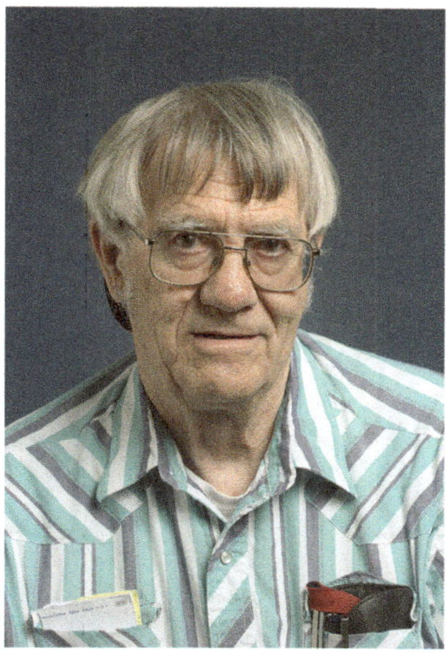

Barry C. Arnold

Life and Works of Barry C. Arnold

Barry C. Arnold was born on December 6, 1939, in the London borough of Lewisham to Charles and Irene Arnold. He was the second child born to his parents with his sister, Nina Arnold, born earlier on January 24, 1938. After their house was bombed by the Germans, they were evacuated from London and then lived in Herne Bay, Barrie, and Blackpool before settling in Caterham, Surrey, a few miles south of London. In April 1952, the family emigrated to Canada. After attending St. Laurent High School, Barry joined the Engineering Program at McGill University in 1956. When the family moved to Hamilton in 1958, he transferred to McMaster University and graduated in 1961 with a Bachelor's degree in mathematics (statistics). Barry subsequently entered the graduate program in statistics at the Stanford University, the school that he selected because not only was it highly recommended but it also had some palm trees on campus. This was a good choice as Stanford had an all-star faculty that included Ted Anderson, Herman Chernoff, Kai Lai Chung, Shanti Gupta, M. V. Johns, Sam Karlin, Ingram Olkin, Rupert Miller, Lincoln Moses, Emmanuel Parzen, Charles Stein, Herbert Solomon, and Pat Suppes. His classmates here were a pretty impressive group, too, which included Norm Breslow, Morris Eaton, Brad Efron, Leon Gleser, Burt Holland, Myles Hollander, Jay Kadane, Carl Morris, Jim Press, Richard Royall, Steve Samuels, Galen Shorack, Muni Srivastava, David Sylwester, Grace Wahba, and Jim Zidek. Barry graduated from Stanford in 1965 after writing a doctoral dissertation under the guidance of Pat Suppes. Another event of importance that occurred while Barry was at Stanford was that he got married to Carole Revelle in September 1964. From Stanford, Barry went to the Iowa State University and joined the faculty with a joint appointment in the Departments of Mathematics and Statistics. There, he had good friends and plenty of intellectual stimulation from many statisticians of repute including Ted Bancroft, H. A. David, H. T. David, Wayne Fuller, Dick Groeneveld, Chien-Pai Han, Dean Isaacson, B. K. Kale, Oscar Kempthorne, Bill Kennedy, Glen Meeden, Ed Pollak, Joe Sedransk, and Vince Sposito. During 1968–1969, Barry was a visiting professor at the Colegio de Postgraduados in Chapingo, Mexico, lecturing in pretty bad Spanish. During 1974–1975, he went on an AID assignment, working with the Ministry of Agriculture in

Lima, Peru. Although he was not successful in selling sampling methods there, he did improve his Spanish! In 1979, Barry hung up his snow shovel, donated his winter coat to the Salvation Army, and moved to Riverside, California, to join Jim Press (whom he knew from Stanford) and his department there. He has been there since. He spent two years (1982–1984) back in Mexico as the Director of the University of California Education Abroad Program. Barry Arnold has served the Department of Statistics at the University of California, Riverside, as Chair for a number of years. In addition, he has provided distinguished service to the statistical community at large by his activities in various capacities for professional societies such as the American Statistical Association and the Institute of Mathematical Statistics. He has participated in numerous national and international conferences and delivered many invited and plenary lectures. He has provided valuable service to several research journals in various capacities including as associate editor of Journal of Multivariate Analysis and Journal of the American Statistical Association and Communications in Statistics, editor-in-chief of Journal of Multivariate Analysis, and managing editor of The Annals of Statistics. Barry Arnold has been elected a Fellow of the American Statistical Association and the Institute of Mathematical Statistics, and a member of the International Statistical Institute. He has had a long list of stimulating coworkers and coauthors. Particularly noteworthy are Enrique Castillo and Jose Maria Sarabia (both at the University of Cantabria, Santander, Spain), H. N. Nagaraja (The Ohio State University, Columbus, Ohio, USA), and N. Balakrishnan (McMaster University, Hamilton, Ontario, Canada). Numerous visits to Santander, Hamilton, and Texcoco, Mexico (where Barry has worked with Jose Villasenor and Humberto Vaquera) have provided him with many pleasant productive interludes. In addition, he has been a frequent visitor to India in particular to Kolkata working with Ashis Sengupta, but also, over the years, attending conferences in many other parts of the country. His passport documents several visits to Portugal (working with Carlos Coelho), to Taiwan (working with Su-Fen Yang), and to Chile (working with Hector Gomez and colleagues at the University of Antofagasta). He has never been to a foreign country he did not like, and so he rarely turns down any invitation! Over the past 55 years, Barry Arnold, through his tremendous research in many different areas of statistics, and especially in distribution theory and ordered data, has greatly influenced the trend of research in these areas and has provided inspiration and encouragement to many young researchers. It is our wish and sincere hope that he will continue his contributions to the field with added vigor, interest, and energy!

Publications of Barry C. Arnold

Books

1. Arnold, B. C. (1983). Pareto Distributions, (Vol. I). International Co-operative Publishing House, Burtonsville, MD.
2. Arnold, B. C., Castillo, E., & Sarabia, J. M. (1987). Lecture notes in statistics. Springer-Verlag, Berlin.
3. Arnold, B. C., & Balakrishnan, N. (1989). Relations, Bounds and Approximations for Order Statistics, Lecture Notes in Statistics - 53, Springer-Verlag, New York.
4. Arnold, B. C., Balakrishnan, N., & Nagaraja, H. N. (1992). A First Course in Order Statistics, John Wiley & Sons, New York.
5. Arnold, B. C., Castillo, E., & Sarabia, J. M. (1993). Conditionally Specified Distributions. Lecture Notes in Statistics, (Vol. 73), Springer-Verlag, New York.
6. Arnold, B. C., Balakrishnan, N., & Nagaraja, H. N. (1998). Records. Wiley, New York.
7. Arnold, B. C., Castillo, E., & Sarabia, J. M. (1999). Conditional specification of statistical models. Springer Science & Business Media.
8. Arnold, B. C., Balakrishnan, N., & Nagaraja, H. N. (2008). A first course in order statistics. Society for Industrial and Applied Mathematics.
9. Marshall, A. W., Olkin, I., & Arnold, B.C. (2011). Inequalities: Theory of Majorization and its Applications, 2nd Edition, Springer, New York.
10. Arnold, B. C. (2012). Majorization and the Lorenz order: A brief introduction (Vol. 43). Springer Science & Business Media.
11. Arnold, B. C. (2015). Pareto Distributions, 2nd Edition. Chapman and Hall / CRC, London.
12. Arnold, B. C., & Sarabia, J. M. (2018). Majorization and the Lorenz order with applications in applied mathematics and economics. Springer International Publishing.
13. Coelho, C. A., & Arnold, B. C. (2019). Finite Form Representations for Meijer G and Fox H Functions: Applied to Multivariate Likelihood Ratio Tests Using Mathematica®, MAXIMA and R. Springer International Publishing.

Books Edited

1. Arnold, B. C., Gather, U., & Bendre, S.M. (Eds.). (2008). Advances in Statistics: B.K. Kale Felicitation Volume. Macmillan Publishers India, Delhi.
2. Arnold, B. C., Balakrishnan, N., Alegria, J. M. S., & Minguez, R. (Eds.). (2009). Advances in mathematical and statistical modeling. Springer Science & Business Media.

Papers

1. Arnold, B. C. (1967). A generalized urn scheme for simple learning with a continuum of responses. Journal of Mathematical Psychology, 4(2), 301–315.
2. Arnold, B. C. (1967). Response distribution for the continuous-time N-element pattern model. Journal of Mathematical Psychology, 4(3), 489–500.
3. Arnold, B. C. (1967). A note on multivariate distributions with specified marginals. Journal of the American Statistical Association, 62(320), 1460–1461.
4. Arnold, B. C. (1968). A modification of a result due to Moran. Journal of Applied Probability, 5(1), 220–223.
5. Arnold, B. C. (1968). Parameter estimation for a multivariate exponential distribution. Journal of the American Statistical Association, 63(323), 848–852.
6. Arnold, B. C. (1970). Inadmissibility of the usual scale estimate for a shifted exponential distribution. Journal of the American Statistical Association, 65(331), 1260–1264.
7. Arnold, B. C. (1970). An alternative derivation of a result due to Srivastava and Bancroft. Journal of the Royal Statistical Society: Series B, 32(2), 265–267.
8. Arnold, B. C. (1970). Hypothesis testing incorporating a preliminary test of significance. Journal of the American Statistical Association, 65(332), 1590–1596.
9. Arnold, B. C. (1971). Letter: Zero correlation and independence. The American Statistician, 26(4), p. 34.
10. Arnold, B. C. (1972). Some examples of minimum variance unbiased estimates. The American Statistician, 26(4), 34–36.
11. Arnold, B. C. (1972). The waiting time until first duplication. Journal of Applied Probability, 9(4), 841–846.
12. Arnold, B. C. (1973). Some characterizations of the exponential distribution by geometric compounding. SIAM Journal on Applied Mathematics, 24(2), 242–244.

13. Arnold, B. C. (1973). Response distributions for a generalized urn scheme under noncontingent reinforcement. Journal of Mathematical Psychology, 10(2), 232–239.
14. Arnold, B. C. (1973). Independence of squared order statistics. Communications in Statistics, 2(4), 357–362.
15. Arnold, B. C. (1974). On estimates of the smaller of two ordered normal means which incorporate a preliminary test of significance. Utilitas Mathematica 5, 65–74.
16. Arnold, B. C. (1974). Schwarz, regression, and extreme deviance. The American Statistician, 28(1), 22–23.
17. Arnold, B. C., & Groeneveld, R. A. (1974). Bounds for deviations between sample and population statistics. Biometrika, 61, 387–389.
18. Arnold, B. C. (1975). A characterization of the exponential distribution by multivariate geometric compounding. Sankhya: Series A, 37(1), 164–173.
19. Arnold, B. C. (1975). Multivariate exponential distributions based on hierarchical successive damage. Journal of Applied Probability, 12(1), 142–147.
20. Arnold, B. C. (1975). Significant category clustering in free recall. Psychometrika, 40(4), 579–581.
21. Arnold, B. C., & Meeden, G. (1975). Characterization of distributions by sets of moments of order statistics. The Annals of Statistics, 754–758.
22. Arnold, B. C., & Arroyo, R. (1975). Estadistica Experimental, Curso Basico. Multilithed for Biometry Office, Peruvian Ministry of Food.
23. Pollak, E., & Arnold, B. C. (1975). On sojourn times at particular gene frequencies. Genetics Research, 25(2), 89–94.
24. Arnold, B. C. (1976). Background variables as predictors of package scores. National Assessment of Education Progress, Denver, CO.
25. Arnold, B. C. (1976). On fitting assessment package scores with a binomial error model. National Assessment of Educational Progress, Denver, CO.
26. Arnold, B. C., & Isaacson, D. (1976). On solutions to $\min(X, Y) \stackrel{d}{=} aX$ and $\min(X, Y) \stackrel{d}{=} aX \stackrel{d}{=} bY$, Zeitschrift Wahrscheinlichkeitstheorie verwandte Gebiete, 35, 115–119.
27. Arnold, B. C., & Ghosh, M. (1976). A characterization of geometric distributions by distributional properties of order statistics. Scandinavian Actuarial Journal, 1976(4), 232–234.
28. Arnold, B. C., & Meeden, G. (1976). A characterization of the uniform distribution based on summation modulo one with application to fractional backlogs. Australian Journal of Statistics, 18(3), 173–175.
29. Arnold, B. C., & Leonor, L. (1976). A stochastic mechanism leading to asymptotically Paretian distributions. Proceedings of the Business and Economic Statistics Section of the ASA, 208–210.
30. Arnold, B. C. (1977). Disenos Experimentales : Conceptos y Aplicaciones. 240 pages. Multilithed for Biometry Office, Peruvian Ministry of Food.
31. Arnold, B. C. (1977). Recurrence relations between expectations of functions of order statistics. Scandinavian Actuarial Journal, 1977(3), 169–174.

32. Arnold, B. C., & Leonor, L. (1977). On generalized Pareto distributions with application to income data. International Studies in Economics, Monograph No. 10, 48 pages, Department of Economics, Iowa State University, Ames, IA.
33. Pollak, E., & Arnold, B.C. (1977). Distributions of times spent in various states in some absorbing processes arising in genetics. Proceedings of the Washington State University Conference on Biomathematics and Biostatistics, 145–169. May, 1974 Pullman, WA.
34. Arnold, B. C. (1978). On characterization and decomposition of Cauchy random variables. Proceedings of the 3rd. National Symposium on Probability and Statistics, Sao Paulo, Brazil, 139–141.
35. Arnold, B. C. (1978). Two modifications of Goodman's technique for improving estimates. Trabajos de Estadistica Y de Investigacion Operativa, 29(3), 61–70.
36. Arnold, B. C. (1978). Some elementary variations of the Lyapunov inequality. SIAM Journal of Applied Mathematics 35(1),117–118.
37. Arnold, B. C., & Groeneveld, R. A. (1978). Bounds on deviations of estimates arising in finite population regression models. Communications in Statistics—Theory and Methods, 7(12), 1173–1179.
38. Arnold, B. C., & Isaacson, D. L. (1978). On normal characterizations by the distribution of linear forms, assuming finite variance. Stochastic Processes and Applications 7(2), 227–230.
39. Isaacson, D., & Arnold, B. C. (1978). Strong ergodicity for continuous-time Markov chains. Journal of Applied Probability, 15(4), 699–706.
40. Arnold, B. C. (1979). Non-uniform decompositions of uniform random variables under summation modulo m. Bollettino Unione Matematica Italiana, 5(16-A), 100–102.
41. Arnold, B. C. (1979). Some characterizations of the Cauchy distribution. Australian Journal of Statistics, 21(2), 166–169.
42. Arnold, B. C., & Groeneveld, R. A. (1979). Bounds on expectations of linear systematic statistics based on dependent samples. The Annals of Statistics, 7(1), 220–223.
43. Huang, J. S., Arnold, B. C., & Ghosh, M. (1979). On characterizations of the uniform distribution based on identically distributed spacings. Sankhya: Series B, 41 (1/2), 109–115.
44. Meeden, G., & Arnold, B. C. (1979). The admissibility of a preliminary test estimator when the loss incorporates a complexity cost. Journal of the American Statistical Association, 74(368), 872–874.
45. Arnold, B. C. (1980). Distribution-free bounds on the mean of the maximum of a dependent sample. SIAM Journal on Applied Mathematics, 38(1), 163–167.
46. Arnold, B. C. (1980). Two characterizations of the geometric distribution. Journal of Applied Probability, 17(2), 570–573.
47. Arnold, B. C., & Groeneveld, R. A. (1980). Some properties of the arcsine distribution. Journal of the American Statistical Association, 75(369), 173–175.

48. Arnold, B. C., & Groeneveld, R. A. (1981). Maximal deviation between sample and population means in finite populations. Journal of the American Statistical Association, 76(374), 443–445.
49. Arnold, B. C., & Groeneveld, R. A. (1981). On excess life in certain renewal processes. Journal of Applied Probability, 18(2), 378–389.
50. Scott, M., Arnold, B. C., & Isaacson, D. L. (1982). Strong ergodicity for continuous-time, non-homogeneous Markov chains. Journal of Applied Probability, 19(3), 692–694.
51. Arnold, B. C., & Angus, J. E. (1983). Some limiting distributions associated with sequences of multinomial trials. Naval Research Logistics Quarterly, 30(1), 1–11.
52. Arnold, B. C., & Brockett, P. L. (1983). When does the βth percentile residual life function determine the distribution? Operations Research, 31(2), 391–396.
53. Arnold, B. C., & Brockett, P. L. (1983). Identifiability for dependent multiple decrement/competing risk models. Scandinavian Actuarial Journal, 1983(2), 117–127.
54. Arnold, B. C., & Press, S. J. (1983). Bayesian inference for Pareto populations. Journal of Econometrics, 21(3), 287–306.
55. Arnold, B. C., Becker, A., Gather, U., & Zahedi, H. (1984). On the Markov property of order statistics. Journal of Statistical Planning and Inference, 9(2), 147–154.
56. Arnold, B. C., Brockett, P. L., Torrez, W., & Wright, A. L. (1984). On the inconsistency of Bayesian non-parametric estimators in competing risks/multiple decrement models. Insurance: Mathematics and Economics, 3(1), 49–55.
57. Groeneveld, R. A., & Arnold, B. C. (1984). Limit laws in the best of $2n - 1$ Bernoulli trials. Naval Research Logistics Quarterly, 31(2), 275–281.
58. Arnold, B. C. (1985). Entry on Pareto distributions. Encyclopedia of Statistical Sciences, Kotz and Johnson (eds.), 6, 568–574, Wiley, New York.
59. Arnold, B. C. (1985). p-Norm bounds on the expectation of the maximum of a possibly dependent sample. Journal of Multivariate Analysis, 17(3), 316–332.
60. Arnold, B. C. (1986). A class of hyperbolic Lorenz curves. Sankhya: Series B, 48(3), 427–436.
61. Arnold, B. C. (1986). Some waiting time problems. Pakistan Journal of Statistics, 2, 39–45.
62. Arnold, B. C., & Press, S. J. (1986). Bayesian analysis of censored and grouped data from Pareto populations. Bayesian Inference and Decision Techniques (P. Goel and A. Zellner eds.).
63. Arnold, B. C., Robertson, C. A., & Yeh, H. C. (1986). Some properties of a Pareto-type distribution. Sankhya: Series A, 48(3), 404–408.
64. Arnold, B. C., & Villaseñor, J. A. (1986). Lorenz ordering of means and medians. Statistics & Probability Letters, 4(1), 47–49.
65. Arnold, B. C. (1987). Bivariate distributions with Pareto conditionals. Statistics & Probability Letters, 5(4), 263–266.

66. Arnold, B. C., Robertson, C. A., Brockett, P. L., & Shu, B. Y. (1987). Generating ordered families of Lorenz curves by strongly unimodal distributions. Journal of Business & Economic Statistics, 5(2), 305–308.
67. Strauss, D., & Arnold, B. C. (1987). The rating of players in racquetball tournaments. Journal of the Royal Statistical Society: Series C, 36(2), 163–173.
68. Arnold, B. C. (1988). A logistic process constructed using geometric minimization. Statistics & Probability Letters, 7(3), 253–257.
69. Arnold, B. C. (1988). Bounds on the expected maximum. Communications in Statistics—Theory and Methods, 17(7), 2135–2150.
70. Arnold, B. C., & Beaver, R. J. (1988). Estimation of the number of classes in a population. Biometrical Journal, 30(4), 413–424.
71. Arnold, B. C., & Brockett, P. L. (1988). Variance bounds using a theorem of Polya. Statistics & Probability Letters, 6(5), 321–326.
72. Arnold, B. C., & Pourahmadi, M. (1988). Conditional characterizations of multivariate distributions. Metrika, 35(1), 99–108.
73. Arnold, B. C., & Strauss, D. (1988). Bivariate distributions with exponential conditionals. Journal of the American Statistical Association, 83(402), 522–527.
74. Arnold, B. C., & Zahedi, H. (1988). On multivariate mean remaining life functions. Journal of Multivariate Analysis, 25(1), 1–9.
75. Shanmugam, R., & Arnold, B. C. (1988). Characterizations Based on Conditional Distributions Given the Minimum Value in the Sample. Sankhya: Series A, 50(3), 452–459.
76. Yeh, H. C., Arnold, B. C., & Robertson, C. A. (1988). Pareto processes. Journal of Applied Probability, 25(2), 291–301.
77. Arnold, B. C., & Hallett, J. T. (1989). A characterization of the Pareto process among stationary stochastic processes of the form $X_n = c \min(X_{n-1}, Y_n)$. Statistics & Probability Letters, 8(4), 377–380.
78. Arnold, B. C., & Press, S. J. (1989). Bayesian estimation and prediction for Pareto data. Journal of the American Statistical Association, 84(408), 1079–1084.
79. Arnold, B. C., & Press, S. J. (1989). Compatible conditional distributions. Journal of the American Statistical Association, 84(405), 152–156.
80. Arnold, B. C., Reneau, D. M., & Samaniego, F. J. (1989). New moment-identities based on the integrated survival function. IEEE Transactions on Reliability, 38(3), 358–361.
81. Arnold, B. C., & Robertson, C. A. (1989). Autoregressive logistic processes. Journal of Applied Probability, 26(3), 524–531.
82. Villaseñor, J., & Arnold, B. C. (1989). Elliptical Lorenz curves. Journal of Econometrics, 40(2), 327–338.
83. Arnold, B. C. (1990). A flexible family of multivariate Pareto distributions. Journal of Statistical Planning and Inference, 24(2), 249–258.
84. Arnold, B. C. (1990). The Lorenz order and the effects of taxation policies. Bulletin of Economic Research, 42(4), 249–264.

85. Arnold, B. C., & Groeneveld, R. A. (1990). Sequential sampling estimation for finite populations of $N = nr$ objects. Biometrical Journal, 32(2), 143–153.
86. Arnold, B. C., & Norton, R. M. (1990). On Cauchy-Like Distributions. Sankhya: Series A, 52(3), 371–375.
87. Anderson, D. N., & Arnold, B. C. (1991). Centered distributions with Cauchy conditionals. Communications in Statistics—Theory and Methods, 20(9), 2881–2889.
88. Arnold, B. C. (1991). Dependence in conditionally specified distributions. Topics in Statistical Dependence, IMS Lecture Notes/Monograph Series 16,13–18.
89. Arnold, B. C. (1991). Preservation and attenuation of inequality as measured by the Lorenz order. Lecture Notes-Monograph Series, 25–37.
90. Arnold, B. C., & Brockett, P. L. (1992). On distributions whose component ratios are Cauchy. The American Statistician, 46(1), 25–26.
91. Arnold, B. C., & Nagaraja, H. N. (1991). Lorenz ordering of exponential order statistics. Statistics & Probability Letters, 11(6), 485–490.
92. Arnold, B. C., & Nagaraja, H. N. (1991). On some properties of bivariate weighted distributions. Communications in Statistics—Theory and Methods, 20(5–6), 1853–1860.
93. Arnold, B. C., & Strauss, D. (1991). Pseudolikelihood estimation: some examples. Sankhya: Series B, 53(2), 233–243.
94. Arnold, B. C., & Strauss, D. J. (1991). Bivariate distributions with conditionals in prescribed exponential families. Journal of the Royal Statistical Society: Series B, 53(2), 365–375.
95. Arnold, B. C., & Villaseñor, J. A. (1991). Lorenz ordering of order statistics. Lecture Notes-Monograph Series, 38–47.
96. Arnold, B. C. (1992). Discussion of Order Statistics from Discrete Distributions. Statistics, 23, 209–211.
97. Arnold, B. C. (1992). Logistic and semi-logistic processes. Journal of Computational and Applied Mathematics, 40(2), 139–149.
98. Arnold, B. C. (1992). Multivariate logistic distributions. In: Handbook of the Logistic Distribution, N. Balakrishnan (eds.), Chapter 11, 237–261, Marcel Dekker, New York.
99. Arnold, B. C., Castillo, E. & Sarabia, J. M. (1992). Classical and Bayesian analysis of fatigue strength data. IABSE Reports, 66, 89–97.
100. Arnold, B. C., & Groeneveld, R. A. (1992). Skewness and kurtosis orderings: an introduction. Lecture Notes-Monograph Series, 22, 17–24.
101. Anderson, D. N., & Arnold., B. C. (1993). Non-parametric estimation of Lorenz curves. International Journal of Mathematical and Statistical Sciences 2, 57–72.
102. Arnold, B. C. (1993). Logistic processes involving Markovian minimization. Communications in Statistics—Theory and Methods, 22(6), 1699–1707.
103. Arnold, B. C., Beaver, R. J., Groeneveld, R. A., & Meeker, W. Q. (1993). The nontruncated marginal of a truncated bivariate normal distribution. Psychometrika, 58(3), 471–488.

104. Arnold, B. C., Castillo, E., & Sarabia, J. M. (1993) Conditionally specified models: structure and inference. In: Multivariate Analysis: Future Directions 2, C.M. Cuadras and C.R. Rao (eds.), 441–450, Amsterdam, North-Holland.
105. Arnold, B. C., Castillo, E., & Sarabia, J. M. (1993). Conjugate exponential family priors for exponential family likelihoods. Statistics, 25(1), 71–77.
106. Arnold, B. C., Castillo, E., & Sarabia, J. M. (1993). Multivariate distributions with generalized Pareto conditionals. Statistics & Probability Letters, 17(5), 361–368.
107. Anderson, D. N., & Arnold, B. C. (1993). Linnik distributions and processes. Journal of Applied Probability, 30(2), 330–340.
108. Arnold, B. C. (1994). Bayesian inference for conditionally specified models. Proceedings of the Section on Bayesian Statistical Science, Annual Meeting of the American Statistical Association, 165–168.
109. Arnold, B. C. (1994). Bhattacharyya's normal conditionals distribution. In: Essays on Probability and Statistics, Festschrift in honour of Professor Anil Kumar Bhattacharyya, S.P. Mukherjee, A. Chaudhuri and S.K. Basu (eds.), 1–13.
110. Arnold, B. C. (1994). Extremal Sojourn Times for Markov Chains. NIST special publication, 19–19.
111. Arnold, B. C. (1994). What price convenience? Parisankhyan Samikkha 1, 35–41.
112. Arnold, B. C. (1994). Where's the lack of memory? Computational Statistics and Data Analysis 18(2), 243–246.
113. Arnold, B. C., Castillo, E., & Sarabia, J. M. (1994). A conditional characterization of the multivariate normal distribution. Statistics & Probability Letters, 19(4), 313–315.
114. Arnold, B. C., Castillo, E., & Sarabia, J. M. (1994). Conditional characterization of the Mardia multivariate Pareto distribution. Pakistan Journal of Statistics, 10, 143–145.
115. Arnold, B. C., Castillo, E., & Sarabia, J. M. (1994). Multivariate normality via conditional specification. Statistics & Probability Letters, 20(5), 353–354.
116. Arnold, B. C., & Gokhale, D. V. (1994). On uniform marginal representation of contingency tables. Statistics & Probability Letters, 21(4), 311–316.
117. Villaseñor, J. A., & Arnold, B. C. (1994). El hombre mas alto del mundo. Memoria del IX Foro Nactional de Estadistica. Universidad Autonoma de Coahuila, Saltillo Coahuila, Mexico. September 26–30, 113–115.
118. Arnold, B. C. (1995). Conditional survival models. In: Recent Advances in Life-Testing and reliability, a volume in Honor of Alonzo Clifford Cohen, Jr., N. Balakrishnan (ed.), 589–601, CRC Press, Boca Raton.
119. Arnold, B. C., Castillo, E., & Sarabia, J. M. (1995). General conditional specification models. Communications in Statistics—Theory and Methods, 24(1), 1–11.
120. Arnold, B. C., & Enrique Castillo, J. M. S. (1995). Distribution with Conditionals in the Pickands-deHaan. IAPQR transactions, 20, 27–36.

121. Arnold, B. C., & Groeneveld, R. A. (1995). Measuring skewness with respect to the mode. The American Statistician, 49(1), 34–38.
122. Arnold, B. C., & Huang, J. S. (1995). Characterizations. Chapter 12 In: The Exponential Distribution: Theory, Methods and Applications, N. Balakrishnan and A.P. Basu (eds.), 185–203, Gordon and Breach, Philadelphia/ Newark.
123. Arnold, B. C., & Villasenor, J. (1995). The tallest man in the world. In: Statistical Theory and Applications: Papers in honor of Herbert A. David. H.N. Nagaraja, P.K. Sen, and D.F. Morrison (eds.), 81–88, Springer-Verlag, New York.
124. Anderson, D. N., & Arnold, B. C. (1996). Modeling gas release event behavior in hazardous waste tanks. Environmental and Ecological Statistics, 3(4), 281–290.
125. Arnold, B. C. (1996). Marginally and conditionally specified multivariate survival models: a Survey. Chapter 12 in Statistics of Quality, S. Ghosh, W.R. Schucany and W.B. Smith (eds.), Vol. 153, 233–252, Marcel Dekker, New York.
126. Arnold, B. C., Castillo, E., & Sarabia, J. M. (1996). Comparisons of means using conditionally conjugate priors. Journal of the Indian Society of Agricultural Statistics 49, 319–334.
127. Arnold, B. C., & Wesolowski, J. (1996). Multivariate distributions with Gaussian conditional structure. In: Stochastic Processes and Functional Analysis, J.A. Goldstein, N.E. Gresky, and J.J. Uhl, Jr. (eds.), 45–59.
128. Arnold, B. C., & Villaseñor, J. A. (1996). Normal attraction of records: variations on the theme. Journal of Statistical Research 30(2), 1–10.
129. Arnold, B. C., Castillo, E., & Sarabia, J. M. (1996). Modeling the fatigue life of longitudinal elements. Naval Research Logistics (NRL), 43(6), 885–895.
130. Arnold, B. C., Castillo, E., & Sarabia, J. M. (1996). Priors with convenient posteriors. Statistics: A Journal of Theoretical and Applied Statistics, 28(4), 347–354.
131. Arnold, B. C., Castillo, E., & Sarabia, J. M. (1996). Specification of distributions by combinations of marginal and conditional distributions. Statistics & Probability Letters, 26(2), 153–157.
132. Arnold, B. C., & Kim, Y. H. (1996). Conditional proportional hazards models. In: Lifetime Data: Models in Reliability and Survival Analysis, N.P. Jewell, A.C. Kimber, M.L.T. Lee, and G.A. Whitmore (eds.). Kluwer Academic, Dordrecht, Netherlands, pp. 21–28.
133. Arnold, B. C. (1997). Characterizations involving conditional specification. Journal of Statistical Planning and Inference, 63(2), 117–131.
134. Arnold, B. C. (1997). Specification of bivariate distributions. Encyclopedia of Statistical Sciences, S. Kotz, C.B. Read and D.L. Banks (eds.), 61–63, Wiley, New York.
135. Arnold, B. C., & Villaseñor, J. A. (1997). Gumbel records and Related Characterizations. In: Advances in the Theory and Practice of Statistics: A Volume in Honor of Samuel Kotz, N.L. Johnson and N. Balakrishnan (eds.), 441–453, Wiley, New York.

136. Arnold, B. C., & Villaseñor, J. A. (1997). Variance estimation with diffuse prior information. Statistics & Probability Letters, 33(1), 35–39.
137. Arnold, B. C. (1998). Castillo-Galambos Functional Equation. In: Encyclopedia of Statistical Sciences, S. Kotz, et al. (eds.) Third update volume, John Wiley, New York.
138. Arnold, B. C., Castillo, E., & Sarabia, J. M. (1998). Bayesian analysis for classical distributions using conditionally specified priors. Sankhya: Series B, 60(2), 228–245.
139. Arnold, B. C., Castillo, E., & Sarabia, J. M. (1998). Some alternative bivariate Gumbel models. Environmetrics, 9(6), 599–616.
140. Arnold, B. C., Castillo, E., & Sarabia, J. M. (1998). The use of conditionally conjugate priors in the study of ratios of gamma scale parameters. Computational Statistics & Data Analysis, 27(2), 125–139.
141. Arnold, B. C., & Gokhale, D. V. (1998). Distributions most nearly compatible with given families of conditional distributions. Test, 7(2), 377–390.
142. Arnold, B. C., & Shavelle, R. M. (1998). Joint confidence sets for the mean and variance of a normal distribution. The American Statistician, 52(2), 133–140.
143. Arnold, B. C., & Villaseñor, J. A. (1998). Lorenz ordering of order statistics and record values. In: Handbook of Statistics, C.R. Rao and N. Balakrishnan (eds.), Vol.16, 75–87, Elsevier, North-Holland, Amsterdam.
144. Sifuentes, M. C., Villaseñor, J. A., & Arnold, B. C. (1998). A distributional study of lifetime data from longitudinal specimens. Perfiles. Universidad Autonoma de Cahuila, Saltillo Coahuila, Mexico. May-June, August-September 1998, 32–48.
145. Arnold, B. C. (1999). The asymptotic distributions of sums of records. Extremes, 1(3), 351–363.
146. Arnold, B. C. (1999). Variations on a Bhattacharya theme. Calcutta Statistical Association Bulletin 49, 193–194.
147. Arnold, B. C., & Gokhale, D.V. (1999). Remarks on incompatible conditional distributions. Journal of the Indian Statistical Association, 37, 121–140.
148. Kim, Y., & Arnold, B. C. (1999). Parameter estimation under generalized ranked set sampling. Statistics & Probability Letters, 42(4), 353–360.
149. Kim, Y., & Arnold, B. C. (1999). Estimation of a distribution function under generalized ranked set sampling. Communications in Statistics-Simulation and Computation, 28(3), 657–666.
150. Arnold, B. C., & Beaver, R. J. (2000). Hidden truncation models. Sankhya: Series A, 62(1), 23–35.
151. Arnold, B. C., & Beaver, R. J. (2000). Some skewed multivariate distributions. American Journal of Mathematical and Management Sciences, 20(1–2), 27–38.
152. Arnold, B. C., & Beaver, R. J. (2000). The skew-Cauchy distribution. Statistics & Probability Letters, 49(3), 285–290.
153. Arnold, B. C., & Gokhale, D. V. (2000). Near compatibility of conditional densities. Journal of the Indian Statistical Association, 38, 155–170.

154. Arnold, B. C., & Joe, H. (2000). Variability ordering of functions. Internat. J. Math. Stat. Sci. 9, 179–189.
155. Sifuentes, M. C., Alva, J. A. V., & Arnold, B. C. (2000). A parametric regression model for possibly censored lifetime data. Agrociencia, 34(4), 453–465.
156. Arnold, B. C. (2001). Beads, bags, bayes, and the fundamental problem of sampling theory. Communications in Statistics—Theory and Methods, 30(8–9), 1963–1967.
157. Arnold, B. C. (2001). Conditional Specification In: A Estatistica em Movimento, Actas do VIII Congresso Annual da Sociedade Portuguesa de Estatistica. M.M. Neves, J. Cadima, M.J. Martins, F. Rosado (eds.), October 4–7, 2001, 3–13.
158. Arnold, B. C. (2001). Nonparametric Statistics: Records. International Encyclopedia of the Social and Behavioral Sciences, 10681–10685.
159. Arnold, B. C. (2001). Pareto Processes. In: Handbook of Statistics, D.N. Shanbhag and C.R. Rao (eds.), Vol. 19, 1–33, Elsevier, North-Holland, Amsterdam.
160. Arnold, B. C., Castillo, E., & Sarabia, J. M. (2001). A multivariate version of Stein's identity with applications to moment calculations and estimation of conditionally specified distributions. Communications in Statistics—Theory and Methods, 30(12), 2517–2542.
161. Arnold, B. C., Castillo, E., & Sarabia, J. M. (2001). Bivariate Distributions Compatible or Nearly Compatible with Given Conditional Information. In: Probability and Statistical Models with Applications, C. A. Charalambides, M.V. Koutras, N. Balakrishnan (eds.), Ch. 13, 225–237, Chapman and Hall/CRC Press, Boca-Raton, Florida.
162. Arnold, B. C., Castillo, E., & Sarabia, J. M. (2001). Conditionally specified distributions: an introduction (with comments and a rejoinder by the authors). Statistical Science, 16(3), 249–274.
163. Arnold, B. C., Castillo, E., & Sarabia, J. M. (2001). Quantification of incompatibility of conditional and marginal information. Communications in Statistics—Theory and Methods, 30(3), 381–395.
164. Sifuentes, M. C., Villaseñor Alva, J. A., & Arnold, B. C. (2001). Modeling the lifetime of longitudinal elements. Communications in Statistics-Simulation and Computation, 30(4), 717–741.
165. Arnold, B. C., Castillo, E., & Sarabia, J. M. (2001–2002). Multivariate Models involving Conditional Specification. (Invited paper) Journal of the Indian Society for Probability and Statistics, 6, 97–121
166. Arnold, B. C., & Beaver, R. J. (2002). Multivariate survival models incorporating hidden truncation. Distributions with given marginal and statistical modeling, 9–19, Kluwer Acad. Publ., Dordrecht.
167. Arnold, B. C., & Beaver, R. J. (2002). Parametric Inference with Generalized Rank Set Data. Uncertainty and Optimality. 293–318. World Scientific Publishing, River Edge, New Jersey.

168. Arnold, B. C., Beaver, R. J., Azzalini, A., Balakrishnan, N., Bhaumik, A., Dey, D. K., Cuadras, C. M., & Sarabia, J. M. (2002). Skewed multivariate models related to hidden truncation and/or selective reporting. Test, 11(1), 7–54.
169. Arnold, B. C., Castillo, E., & Sarabia, J. M. (2002). Bayesian Inference Using conditionally specified Priors. Handbook of Applied Econometrics and Statistical Inference, A. Ullah, A.T.K. Wan, A. Chaturvedi (eds.), 1–26, Marcel Dekker, New York.
170. Arnold, B. C., Castillo, E., & Sarabia, J. M. (2002). Compatibility and near compatibility in multiple assessment of Bayesian networks. Journal of Propagations in Probability and Statistics 2: 161–176.
171. Arnold, B. C., Castillo, E., & Sarabia, J. M. (2002). Conditionally specified multivariate skewed distributions. Selected articles from San Antonio conference in honor of C.R. Rao (San Antonio, TX 2000). Sankhya Series A, 64 (2), 206–226.
172. Arnold, B. C., Castillo, E., & Sarabia, J. M. (2002). Exact and near compatibility of discrete conditional distributions. Computational Statistics & Data Analysis, 40(2), 231–252.
173. Arnold, B. C., Castillo, E., & Sarabia, J. M. (2002). Goodness-of-Fit tests based on record data and generalized ranked set data. In: Goodness-of-Fit Tests and Model Validity. C. Huber-Carol, N. Balakrishnan, M.S. Nikulin, M. Mesbah (eds.), 143–157, Birkhauser, Boston.
174. Arnold, B. C., & Robertson, C. A. (2002). The conditional distribution of X given $X = Y$ can be almost anything! In: Advances on Theoretical and Methodological Aspects of Probability and Statistics, N. Balakrishnan (eds.), 75–81,Taylor and Francis, Philadelphia.
175. Arnold, B. C. (2003). Back to bayesics. Journal of Statistical Planning and Inference, 109(1–2), 179–187.
176. Arnold, B. C., & Gokhale, D. V. (2003). Distributions in given parametric families most nearly compatible with given conditional information. In: Statistical Methods and Practice: Recent Advances, N. Balakrishnan, N. Kannan and M.R. Srinivasan (eds.), 29–45, Narosa Publishing House, New Delhi.
177. Arnold, B. C., & Beaver, R. J. (2004). Alternative construction of skewed multivariate distributions. Acta et Commentationes Universitatis Tartuensis de Mathematica, 8, 1–9.
178. Arnold, B. C., & Beaver, R. J. (2004). Elliptical models subject to hidden truncation or selective sampling. In: Skew Elliptical Distributions their applications. M.G. Genton, (Eds.), 101–112, Chapman and Hall, Boca Raton.
179. Arnold, B. C., & Beaver, R. J. (2004). Some additive component skewness models. Journal of Probability and Statistical Science, 2, 139–147.
180. Arnold, B. C., Castillo, E., & Sarabia, J. M. (2004). Compatibility of partial or complete conditional probability specifications. Journal of Statistical Planning and Inference, 123(1), 133–159.

181. Arnold, B. C., Castillo, E., & Sarabia, J. M. (2004). Distributions with beta conditionals In: Handbook of Beta Distributions and it Applications. A.K. Gupta and S. Nadarajah, (eds.), 255–282, Marcel Dekker, New York.
182. Arnold, B. C., Castillo, E., Sarabia, J. M., & González-Vega, L. (2004). Multiple modes in densities with normal conditionals. Statistics & Probability Letters, 49, 355–363.
183. Arnold, B. C., & Lin, G. D. (2004). Characterizations of the skew-normal and generalized chi distributions. Sankhya: Series A, 66(4), 593–606.
184. Arnold, B. C. (2005). Characterizations of multivariate distributions involving conditional specification and/or hidden truncation. In: Advances in Models, Characterizations and Applications, N. Balakrishnan, O. Gebizlioglu and I. Bayramoglu, (eds.), 161–176, CRC Press, Boca-Raton, Florida.
185. Arnold, B. C. (2005). Inequality measures for multivariate distributions. Metron, 63(3), 317–327.
186. Arnold, B.C. (2005). Procrustean strategies for incompatible conditional and marginal information. Calcutta Statistical Association Bulletin, 56, 221–224.
187. Arnold, B. C., Castillo, E., & Sarabia, J. M. (2005). Distributions with conditionals in truncated weighted families. Statistics, 39(2), 133–147.
188. Arnold, B. C., & Villaseñor, J. A. (2005). On the value of imprecise prior information. Communications in Statistics—Theory and Methods, 34(4), 807–822.
189. Arnold, B. C., Castillo, E., & Sarabia, J. M. (2006). Families of multivariate distributions involving the Rosenblatt construction. Journal of the American Statistical Association, 101(476), 1652–1662.
190. Arnold, B. C., & SenGupta, A. (2006). Probability distributions and statistical inference for axial data. Environmental and Ecological Statistics, 13(3), 271–285.
191. Arnold, B. C., & SenGupta, A. (2006). Recent advances in the analyses of directional data in ecological and environmental sciences. Environmental and Ecological Statistics, 13, 253–256
192. Arnold, B. C. (2007). Comments on: Progressive censoring methodology: An appraisal. Test, 16, 268–270.
193. Arnold, B. C. (2007). Further variations on the skew normal theme. In; Statistical Techniques in Life-Testing, Reliability, Sampling Theory and Quality Control. B.N. Pandey, (Ed.), 21–26, Narosa Publishing House, New Delhi.
194. Arnold, B. C. (2007). Majorization: Here, there and everywhere. Statistical Science, 22(3), 407–413.
195. Arnold, B. C., & Beaver, R. J. (2007). Skewing around: relationships among classes of skewed distributions. Methodology and Computing in Applied Probability, 9(2), 153–162.
196. Arnold, B. C., Castillo, E., & Sarabia, J. M. (2007). Distributions with generalized skewed conditionals and mixtures of such distributions. Communications in Statistics—Theory and Methods, 36(8), 1493–1503.

197. Arnold, B. C., Castillo, E., & Sarabia, J. M. (2007). Variations on the classical multivariate normal theme. Journal of Statistical Planning and Inference, 137(11), 3249–3260.
198. Arnold, B.C., & Villaseñor, J.A. (2007). Progress on sums of records. In: Recent Developments in Ordered Random Variables, 155–169, Nova Scientific Publishers, New York.
199. Villaseñor, J. A., & Arnold, B. C. (2007). On limit laws for sums of Pfeifer records. Extremes, 10(4), 235–248.
200. Arnold, B. C. (2008). Enrique Castillo's contributions to conditional specification. In Advances in Mathematical and Statistical Modeling., B.C. Arnold, N. Balakrishnan, J.M. Sarabia and R. Minguez, (Eds.), 4–19. Birkhauser, Boston.
201. Arnold, B. C. (2008). Pareto and generalized Pareto distributions. In: Modeling Income Distributions and Lorenz Curves: D. Chotikapanich, (ed.), 119–145, Springer, New York.
202. Arnold, B. C. (2008). The Lorenz curve: Evergreen after 100 years. In Advances on Income Inequality and Concentration Measures. G. Betti and A Lemmi, (eds.), 12–24, Routledge, New York.
203. Arnold, B. C., Castillo, E., & Sarabia, J. M. (2008). Bivariate distributions characterized by one family of conditionals and conditional percentile or mode functions. Journal of Multivariate Analysis, 99(7), 1383–1392.
204. Arnold, B. C., Castillo, E., & Sarabia, J. M. (2008). Multivariate distributions defined in terms of contours. Journal of Statistical Planning and Inference, 138(12), 4158–4171.
205. Arnold, B. C., Castillo, E., & Sarabia, J. M. (2008). Some characterizations involving uniform and powers of uniform random variables. Statistics, 42(6), 527–534.
206. Arnold, B. C., Gokhale, D.V. (2008). Estimation of strata sizes from aggregate information. In Advances in Statistics: B.K. Kale Felicitation Volume. B.C. Arnold, U. Gather and S.M. Bendre, Eds. Macmillan Publishers India, Delhi. 3–11.
207. Bairamov, I., & Arnold, B. C. (2008). On the residual life lengths of the remaining components in an $n-k+1$ out of n system. Statistics & Probability Letters, 78(8), 945–952.
208. Jones, M. C., & Arnold, B. C. (2008). Distributions that are both log-symmetric and R-symmetric. Electronic Journal of Statistics, 2, 1300–1308.
209. Arnold, B. C. (2009). Flexible univariate and multivariate models based on hidden truncation. Journal of Statistical Planning and Inference, 139(11), 3741–3749.
210. Arnold, B. C. (2009). Prior elicitation for a binomial proportion. Pakistan Journal of Statistics, 25(4), 419–425.
211. Arnold, B. C., Castillo, E., & Sarabia, J. M. (2009). Multivariate order statistics via multivariate concomitants. Journal of Multivariate Analysis, 100(5), 946–951.

212. Arnold, B. C., Castillo, E., & Sarabia, J. M. (2009). On multivariate order statistics. Application to ranked set sampling. Computational Statistics & Data Analysis, 53(12), 4555–4569.
213. Arnold, B. C., & Gómez, H. W. (2009). Hidden truncation and additive components: Two alternative skewing paradigms. Calcutta Statistical Association Bulletin, 61(1–4), 17–32.
214. Arnold, B. C., Gómez, H. W., & Salinas, H. S. (2009). On multiple constraint skewed models. Statistics, 43(3), 279–293.
215. Arnold, B. C., & SenGupta, A. (2009). Flexible bivariate circular models. In: Advances in Multivariate Statistical Methods. A. SenGupta, (eds.), 95–106, World Scientific Press, Singapore.
216. Arnold, B. C., & Seshadri, V. (2009). Some New Independence Properties of the Inverse Gaussian Law. Sankhya: Series A, 71(1), 94–108.
217. Lesch, S. M., Arnold, B. C., & Jeske, D. R. (2009). Simple and accurate approximations for computing covariance matrices of gamma and Weibull order statistics. Communications in Statistics-Simulation and Computation, 38(3), 590–609.
218. Filus, J. K., Filus, L. Z., & Arnold, B. C. (2009). Families of multivariate distributions involving triangular transformations. Communications in Statistics—Theory and Methods, 39(1), 107–116.
219. Arnold, B. C. (2010). Admissible estimation of a multivariate normal mean. Journal of Statistical Research, 44(1), 129.
220. Arnold, B. C., & Ghosh, I. (2010). Inference for Pareto data subject to hidden truncation. Journal of the Indian Society for Probability and Statistics, 12, 1–16.
221. Coelho, C. A., Arnold, B. C., & Marques, F. J. (2010). Near-exact distributions for certain likelihood ratio test statistics. Journal of Statistical Theory and Practice, 4(4), 711–725.
222. Gutierrez, E., Villaseñor, J. A., Panteleeva, O. V., & Arnold, B. C. (2010). Tests of hypotheses for exchangeable variables. Far East Journal of Theoretical Statistics. 33, 147–162.
223. Saldaña-Zepeda, D. P., Vaquera-Huerta, H., & Arnold, B. C. (2010). A goodness of fit test for the Pareto distribution in the presence of type II censoring, based on the cumulative hazard function. Computational Statistics & Data Analysis, 54(4), 833–842.
224. Arnold, B. C. (2011). Inequality and majorization: Robin Hood in unexpected places. Calcutta Statistical Association Bulletin. 63. 71–80.
225. Arnold, B. C. (2011). The generalized Cantor distribution and its corresponding inverse distribution. Statistics & Probability Letters, 81(8), 1098–1103.
226. Arnold, B. C., & Ng, H. K. T. (2011). Flexible bivariate beta distributions. Journal of Multivariate Analysis, 102(8), 1194–1202.
227. Arnold, B. C., & SenGupta, A. (2011). Models for axial data. In: Advances in Directional and Linear Statistics. M.T. Wells and A. SenGupta, (Eds.) Physica Verlag, Heidelberg. 1–9.

228. Marques, F. J., Coelho, C. A., & Arnold, B. C. (2011). A general near-exact distribution theory for the most common likelihood ratio test statistics used in multivariate analysis. Test, 20(1), 180–203.
229. Arnold, B. C. (2012). On the Amato inequality index. Statistics & Probability Letters, 82(8), 1504–1506.
230. Arnold, B. C., & Villaseñor, J. A. (2012). Generalized order statistic processes and Pfeifer records. Statistics, 46(3), 373–385.
231. Joe, H., Seshadri, V., & Arnold, B. C. (2012). Multivariate inverse Gaussian and skew-normal densities. Statistics & Probability Letters, 82(12), 2244–2251.
232. Arnold, B. C., & Athreya, K. B. (2013). Power series with i.i.d. coefficients. Statistics & Probability Letters, 83(3), 923–929.
233. Arnold, B. C., Coelho, C. A., & Marques, F. J. (2013). The distribution of the product of powers of independent uniform random variables-a simple but useful tool to address and better understand the structure of some distributions. Journal of Multivariate Analysis, 113, 19–36.
234. Arnold, B. C., & Ghosh, I. (2013). Hidden Truncation in Multivariate Pareto Data. In Contemporary Topics in Mathematics and Statistics with Application, (Vol. 1), A. Adhikari, M. R . Adhikari, and Y. P. Chaubey, (eds.), 211–226, Asian Books, New Delhi.
235. Arnold, B. C., & Manjunath, B. G. (2013). Some remarks on normal conditionals and normal projections. In 18th European Young Statisticians Meeting, p. 56.
236. Arnold, B. C., & Villaseñor, J. A. (2013). Exponential characterizations motivated by the structure of order statistics in samples of size two. Statistics & Probability Letters, 83(2), 596–601.
237. Arnold, B. C., & Villaseñor, J. A. (2013). On orthogonality of $(X + Y)$ and $X/(X + Y)$ rather than independence. Statistics & Probability Letters, 83(2), 584–587.
238. Benjamin, S. M., Humberto, V. H., & Arnold, B. C. (2013). Use of the Dagum distribution for modeling tropospheric ozone levels. Journal Environmental Statistics, 5(6), 1–11.
239. Martínez-Flórez, G., Arnold, B. C., Bolfarine, H., & Gómez, H. W. (2013). The multivariate alpha-power model. Journal of Statistical Planning and Inference, 143(7), 1244–1255.
240. SenGupta, A., Kim, S., & Arnold, B. C. (2013). Inverse circular-circular regression. Journal of Multivariate Analysis, 119, 200–208.
241. Arnold, B.C. (2014). Bounds on Distributions Involving Partial, Marginal and Conditional Information: The Consequences of Incomplete Prior Specification. In Statistical Paradigms Recent Advances and Reconciliations. A. SenGupta, T. Samanta and A. Basu, (eds.), 39–52, World Scientific Publishing, Singapore.

242. Coelho, C. A., & Arnold, B. C. (2014). On the exact and near-exact distributions of the product of generalized Gamma random variables and the generalized variance. Communications in Statistics—Theory and Methods, 43(10–12), 2007–2033.
243. Arnold, B. C., & Gokhale, D.V. (2014). On segregation: Ordering and measuring. Sankhya B, 76, 141–166.
244. Arnold, B. C. (2014). Univariate and multivariate Pareto models. Journal of Statistical Distributions and Applications, 1(1), 11.
245. Yang, S. F., & Arnold, B. C. (2014). A simple approach for monitoring business service time variation. The Scientific World Journal, 2014.
246. Arnold, B. C., Gómez, H. W., & Olivares-Pacheco, J. F. (2014). Multiple constraint and truncated skew models. Statistics, 48(5), 971–982.
247. Arnold, B. C. (2015). On Zenga and Bonferroni curves. Metron, 73(1), 25–30.
248. Arnold, B. C., Gómez, H. W., & Salinas, H. S. (2015). A doubly skewed normal distribution. Statistics, 49(4), 842–858.
249. De La Huerta Contreras, V., Vaquera Huerta, H., & Arnold, B. C. (2015). A test for equality of variances with censored samples. Journal of Statistical Computation and Simulation, 85(3), 450–467.
250. Yang, S., Arnold, B. C. (2015). A Simple Approach for Monitoring Process Mean and Variance Simultaneously, in Frontiers in Statistical Quality Control 11, S. Knoth, W. Schmid (eds.), 135–150, Springer International Publishing, Switzerland.
251. Arnold, B. C., & Villaseñor, J. A. (2015). Orthogonal Spacings. Communications in Statistics–Theory and Methods, 44(19), 3998–4006.
252. Coelho, C. A., Arnold, B. C., & Marques, F. J. (2015). The exact and near-exact distributions of the main likelihood ratio test statistics used in the complex multivariate normal setting. Test, 24(2), 386–416.
253. Arnold, B. C., & Gokhale, D. V. (2015). Parametric constraints for generalized hyperexponential distributions. Journal of the Indian Statistical Association, 53(1–2), 1–9.
254. Arnold, B. C., & Villaseñor, J. A. (2015). Bias of the sample Lorenz curve. In: Ordered Data Analysis, Modeling and Health Research Methods, P.K. Choudhary, C.H. Nagaraja, and H.K.T. Ng (eds.), 3–15, Springer, Cham, Switzerland.
255. Kim, S., SenGupta, A., & Arnold, B. C. (2016). A multivariate circular distribution with applications to the protein structure prediction problem. Journal of Multivariate Analysis, 143, 374–382.
256. Gupta, R. C., & Arnold, B. C. (2016). Preservation of failure rate function shape in weighted distributions. AStA Advances in Statistical Analysis, 100(1), 1–20.
257. Arnold, B. C., & Gupta, R. C. (2016). Alternative approaches to conditional specification of bivariate distributions. Metron, 74(1), 21–36.
258. Yang, S. F., & Arnold, B. C. (2016). A new approach for monitoring process variance. Journal of Statistical Computation and Simulation, 86(14), 2749–2765.

259. Singpurwalla, N. D., Arnold, B. C., Gastwirth, J. L., Gordon, A. S., & Ng, H. K. T. (2016). Adversarial and amiable inference in medical diagnosis, reliability and survival analysis. International Statistical Review, 84(3), 390–412.
260. Yang, S. F., & Arnold, B. C. (2016). Monitoring process variance using an ARL-unbiased EWMA-p control chart. Quality and Reliability Engineering International, 32(3), 1227–1235.
261. Arnold, B. C., & Ghosh, I. (2017). Bivariate Beta and Kumaraswamy models developed using the Arnold-Ng bivariate beta distribution. REVSTAT, 15(2), 223–250.
262. Arnold, B. C., Ghosh, I., & Alzaatreh, A. (2017). Construction of bivariate and multivariate weighted distributions via conditioning. Communications in Statistics—Theory and Methods, 46(18), 8897–8912.
263. Arnold, B. C., & Ghosh, I. (2017). Some alternative bivariate Kumaraswamy models. Communications in Statistics—Theory and Methods, 46(18), 9335–9354.
264. Arnold, B. C., & Ghosh, I. (2017): Bivariate Kumaraswamy models involving use of Arnold-Ng copulas. Journal of Applied Statistical Science, 22, 37–60.
265. Arnold, B. C., & Gokhale, D. V. (2017). Lorenz order with common finite support. Metron, 75(2), 215–226.
266. Arnold, B. C., & Hamedani, G. G. (2017). Bivariate, multivariate, and matrix variate normal characterizations: A brief survey II. Communications in Statistics—Theory and Methods, 46(24), 11949–11971.
267. Gallardo, D. I., Gómez, Y. M., Arnold, B. C., & Gómez, H. W. (2017). The Pareto IV power series cure rate model with applications. SORT, 1(2), 297–318.
268. Gómez, Y. M., Gallardo, D. I., & Arnold, B. C. (2018). The power piecewise exponential model. Journal of Statistical Computation and Simulation, 88(5), 825–840.
269. Arnold, B. C., & Sarabia, J. M. (2018). Analytic expressions for multivariate Lorenz surfaces. Sankhya: Series A, 80(1), 84–111.
270. Arnold, B. C., Gómez, H. W., Varela, H., & Vidal, I. (2019). Univariate and bivariate models related to the generalized epsilon-skew-Cauchy distribution. Symmetry, 11(6), 794.
271. Arnold, B. C. (2020). Further Examples Related to the Identical Distribution of $X/(X+Y)$ and $Y/(X+Y)$. The American Statistician, 74(1), 93–97.

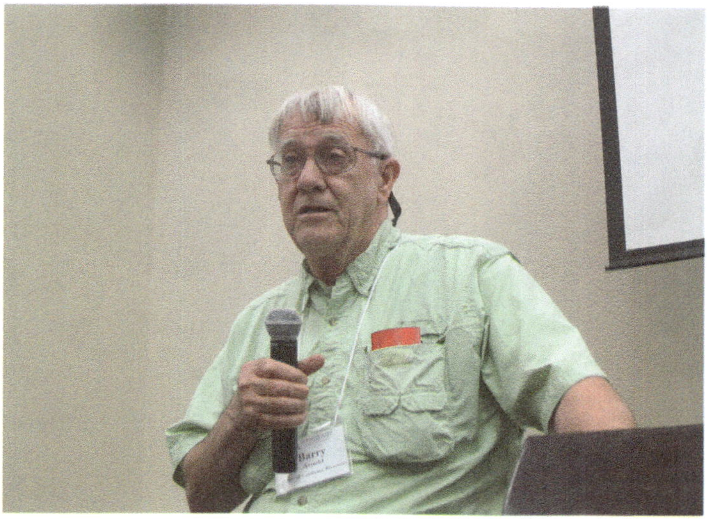

Barry C. Arnold at the Ordered Data Analysis, Models and Health Research Methods—An International Conference in Honor of H.N. Nagaraja for His 60th Birthday held at the University of Texas at Dallas, March 7–9, 2014, Richardson, Texas, USA

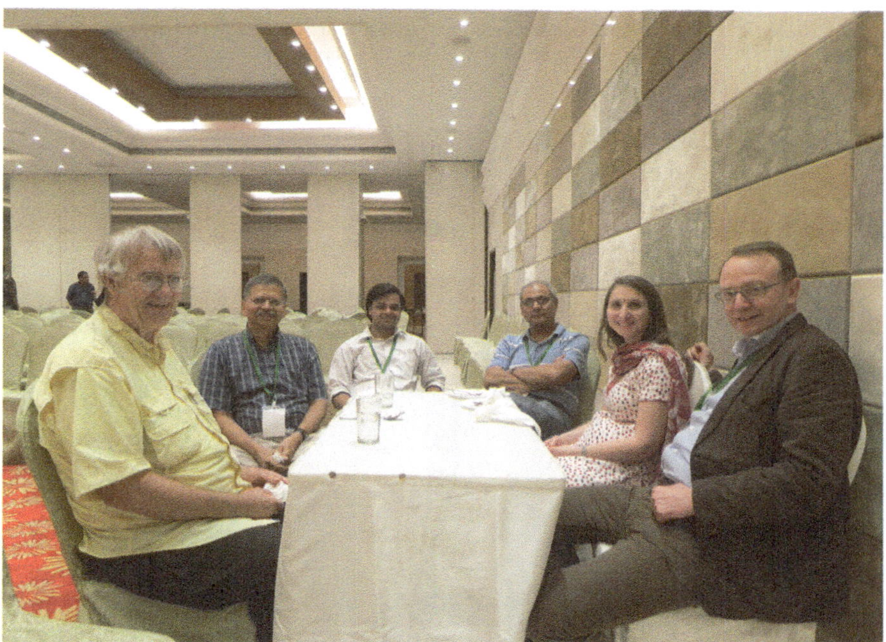

From left to right: Barry C. Arnold, H.N. Nagaraja, Suvra Pal, N. Balakrishnan, Katherine Davies, and Adelchi Azzalini at the IISA Conference 2013 in Chennai, India. Thanks are due to Dr. Charitra Nagaraja (Fordham University, New York) for kindly providing this photograph

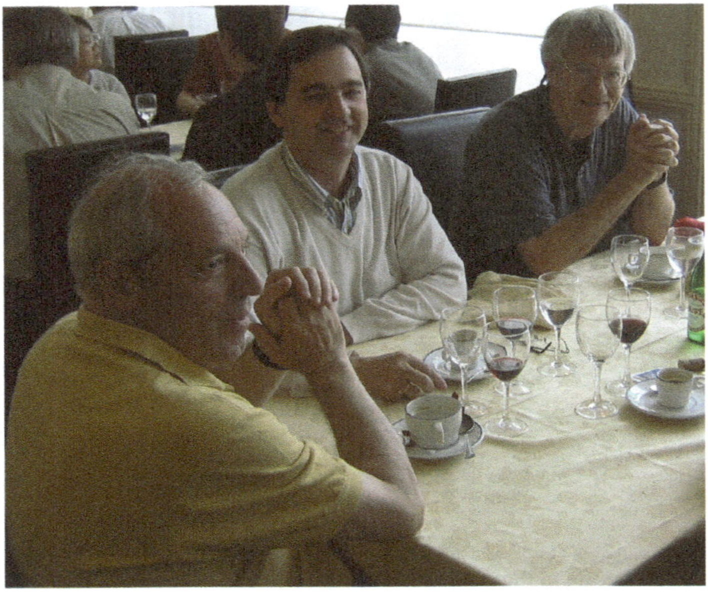

From left to right: Enrique Castillo, Jose Maria Sarabia, and Barry C. Arnold at the International Conference on Distribution Theory, Order Statistics and Inference in Honor of Barry C. Arnold, June 16–18, 2004, Spain. Thanks are due to Prof. José María Sarabia (University of Cantabria, Spain) for kindly providing this photograph

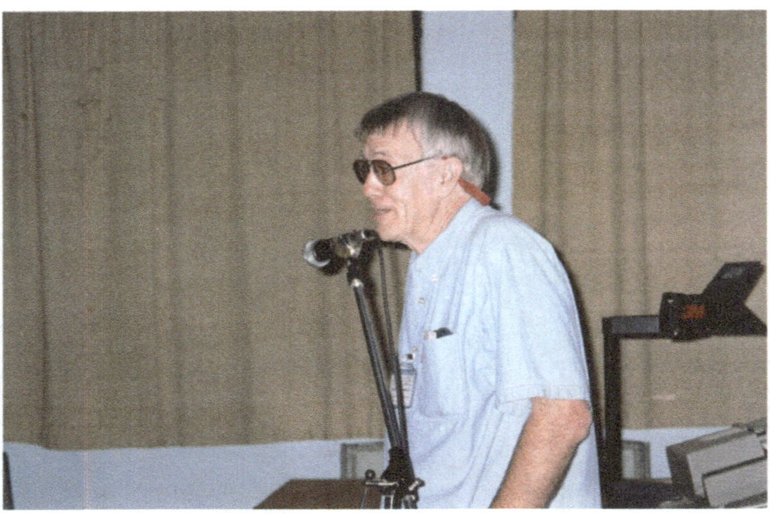

Barry C. Arnold at the International Conference on Order Statistics and Extreme Values: Theory and Applications held at the University of Mysore, December 16–18, 2000, India. Thanks are due to Dr. H.N. Nagaraja (The Ohio State University) for kindly providing this photograph

Preface

Barry C. Arnold, as many know well, has had an exemplary and distinguished academic career. He has an impressive list of journal publications and many books to his credit (the list presented later in the write-up about him will provide an ample testimony to this!). Over the years, Barry has interacted and collaborated with numerous researchers all over the world! We three (the Editors of this volume), and in fact many of the authors in this volume, have also been part of this band of researchers, for varying periods of time, of course! Needless to say, we have benefited from his wisdom and sound knowledge, his contagious enthusiasm for research, and the clever arguments that he provides during discussions. These have resulted in the form of many research articles and books (for one of us!).

A casual look through Barry's publications even his earliest work will reveal that, though he has very broad interests (NB: I remember him once telling me that any problem someone brings to him that perks his interest is worth spending time on!), he has spent considerable time and energy especially in the following areas of Statistics:

1. Ordered Data,
2. Distribution Theory: Univariate and Multivariate,
3. Characterization Problems,
4. Statistical Inference—Classical and Bayesian,
5. Inequalities and Majorization Problems,
6. Multivariate Analysis.

So, it is no wonder that a major part of his publications have also been on these areas. It is for this reason that, when we planned to bring out a volume for Barry on the occasion of his 80th birthday, we targeted these specific areas to attract articles from those with whom he has been associated with. We found it heartening that our initial invitations were enthusiastically accepted by almost all whom we approached and that, in our view, is a clear sign of how people view and respect Barry as an academic and as a friend!

We express our sincere thanks to all the authors for presenting their articles in a timely fashion and also for assisting us in the review work of articles of other authors that are present in this volume. We also pass on our great appreciation to Ms. Laura Aileen Briskman, Editor, Statistics, from Springer who took great interest in this project when we approached them, and helped us all the way till the final production of the volume. Thanks are also due to the Department of Statistics at the UC Riverside for providing the colorful portrait of Barry that is present in the first page, and to Dr. H.N. Nagaraja, Dr. Chaitra Nagaraja, and Dr. Jose Maria Sarabia, for sharing with us some pictures of Barry at different points of his life and career. For posterity, we have presented these pictures at the end of our writing about Barry which, we hope, will put a smile on his face (and also force him to think about when and where each is from!).

With great pleasure, we have prepared this volume to honor our friend, collaborator, and mentor, Barry C. Arnold, and it is our sincere hope that he will enjoy going over this volume as much as we enjoyed putting it together!

Wilmington, NC, USA — Indranil Ghosh
Hamilton, ON, Canada — N. Balakrishnan
Dallas, TX, USA — Hon Keung Tony Ng

Contents

Contributors

Rui P. Alberto Centro de Matemática e Aplicações, FCT NOVA, NOVA University of Lisbon, Lisbon, Portugal

Reinaldo B. Arellano-Valle Departamento de Estadística, Facultad de Matemática, Pontificia Universidad Católica de Chile, Santiago, Chile

N. Balakrishnan Department of Mathematics and Statistics, McMaster University, Hamilton, ON, Canada

Yong Bao Department of Economics, Krannert School of Management, Purdue University, West Lafayette, IN, USA

Andriëtte Bekker University of Pretoria, Pretoria, South Africa

Enrique Castillo University of Cantabria, Santander, Spain

Asis Kumar Chattopadhyay Department of Statistics, University of Calcutta, Kolkata, West Bengal, India

Carlos A. Coelho Departamento de Matemática and Centro de Matemática e Aplicações, FCT NOVA, NOVA University of Lisbon, Lisbon, Portugal

Vincenzo Coia Department of Statistics, University of British Columbia, Vancouver, BC, Canada

Ngoc Anh Dao Department of Statistics, Texas A&M University, College Station, TX, USA

Dipak K. Dey Department of Statistics, University of Connecticut, Storrs, CT, USA

Johan Ferreira University of Pretoria, Pretoria, South Africa

Marc G. Genton Statistics Program, King Abdullah University of Science and Technology, Thuwal, Saudi Arabia

Indranil Ghosh Department of Mathematics and Statistics, University of North Carolina Wilmington, Wilmington, NC, USA

Gyuhyeong Goh Department of Statistics, Kansas State University, Manhattan, KS, USA

E. González-Estrada Department of Statistics, Colegio de Postgraduados, México, México

Simone B. Harnik Departamento de Estatística, Instituto de Matemática e Estatística, Universidade de São Paulo, São Paulo, Brazil

Mu He Department of Mathematics and Statistics, McMaster University, Hamilton, ON, Canada

Harry Joe Department of Statistics, University of British Columbia, Vancouver, BC, Canada

Debasis Kundu Department of Mathematics and Statistics, Indian Institute of Technology, Kanpur, India

Boya Lai The City University of Hong Kong, Kowloon, Hong Kong

Xiaotian Liu Department of Economics, Krannert School of Management, Purdue University, West Lafayette, IN, USA

Filipe J. Marques Centro de Matemática e Aplicações (CMA), FCT, UNL and Departamento de Matemática, FCT, UNL, Lisbon, Portugal

Glen Meeden School of Statistics, University of Minnesota, Minneapolis, MN, USA

William Q. Meeker Department of Statistics, Iowa State University, Ames, IA, USA

Sharmishtha Mitra Department of Mathematics and Statistics, Indian Institute of Technology, Kanpur, India

Chaitra H. Nagaraja Fordham University, Strategy and Statistics Area, Gabelli School of Business, New York, NY, USA

Haikady N. Nagaraja The Ohio State University, Division of Biostatistics, College of Public Health, Columbus, OH, USA

Hon Keung Tony Ng Department of Statistical Science, Southern Methodist University, Dallas, TX, USA

Natalia Nolde Department of Statistics, University of British Columbia, Vancouver, BC, Canada

Ayan Pal Department of Mathematics and Statistics, Indian Institute of Technology, Kanpur, India

Lochana Kanishka Palayangoda Department of Statistical Science, Southern Methodist University, Dallas, TX, USA

Moumita Roy Department of Statistics, Midnapore College (Autonomous), Midnapore, West Bengal, India

Tomasz Rychlik Institute of Mathematics, Polish Academy of Sciences, Warsaw, Poland

Debashis Samanta Department of Mathematics and Statistics, Aliah University, Kolkata, West Bengal, India

José María Sarabia Department of Economics, University of Cantabria, Santander, Spain

Ashis SenGupta Applied Statistics Unit, Indian Statistical Institute, Kolkata, West Bengal, India

Nozer D. Singpurwalla The George Washington University, Washington, DC, USA

Michael Soma Department of Statistics, Iowa State University, Ames, IA, USA

Magdalena Szymkowiak Institute of Automation and Robotics, Poznan University of Technology, Poznań, Poland

Aman Ullah Department of Economics, University of California Riverside, CA, USA

J. A. Villaseñor Department of Statistics, Colegio de Postgraduados, México, México

Wei Zhang Department of Statistics, Iowa State University, Ames, IA, USA

About the Editors

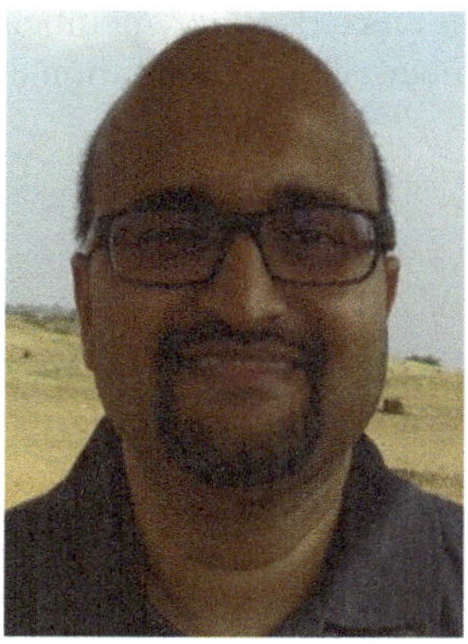

Indranil Ghosh is currently an Associate Professor of Statistics in the Department of Mathematics and Statistics at the University of North Carolina Wilmington. Currently, he is serving as a guest editor for a special issue of the journal Computational and Mathematical Methods published by John Wiley & Sons, on the editorial board of the Journal of Business Analytics published by Taylor & Francis, and an associate editor for the Journal of the Iranian Statistical Society. He is elected as the Chair-Elect 2021 of the Section on Risk Analysis of the American Statistical Association. He is an elected member of the International Statistical Institute.

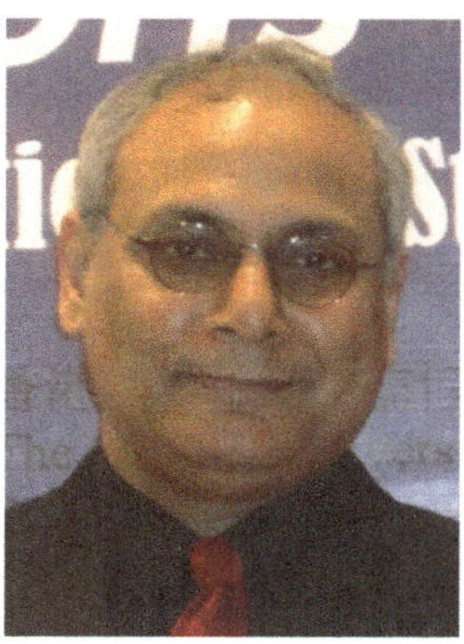

N. Balakrishnan Distinguished University Professor, is in the Department of Mathematics and Statistics, McMaster University, Hamilton, Ontario, Canada. Professor Balakrishnan is an internationally recognized expert on many areas of statistics, and especially on statistical distribution theory and ordered data analysis. He is currently the Editor-in-Chief of Communications in Statistics published by Taylor & Francis and was previously the Editor-in-Chief for the revised version of Encyclopedia of Statistical Sciences published by John Wiley & Sons. He is a Fellow of the American Statistical Association and a Fellow of the Institute of Mathematical Statistics, and in 2016, he received an Honorary Doctorate from The National and Kapodistrian University of Athens, Athens, Greece.

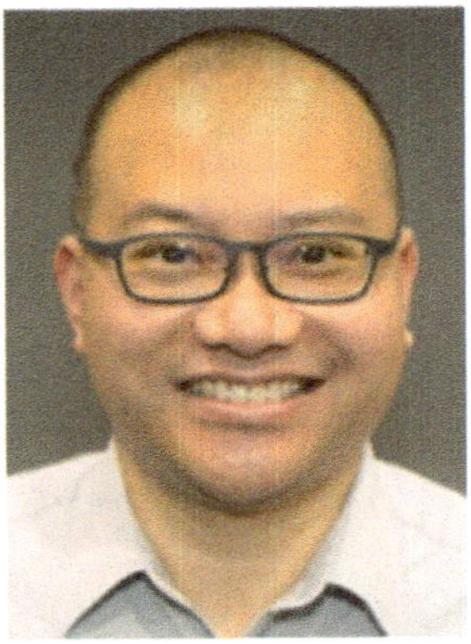

Hon Keung Tony Ng is currently a Professor of statistical science with the Southern Methodist University, Dallas, TX, USA. He is an associate editor of Communications in Statistics, Computational Statistics, IEEE Transactions on Reliability, Journal of Statistical Computation and Simulation, Naval Research Logistics, Sequential Analysis, and Statistics & Probability Letters. His research interests include reliability, censoring methodology, ordered data analysis, nonparametric methods, and statistical inference. He is the co-editor of Ordered Data Analysis, Modeling and Health Research Methods, Statistical Modeling for Degradation Data, and Statistical Quality Technologies—Theory and Practice published by Springer. He is a Fellow of the American Statistical Association, an elected senior member of IEEE, and an elected member of the International Statistical Institute.

Part I
Ordered Data Analysis

A Record-Based Transmuted Family of Distributions

N. Balakrishnan and M. He

Abstract Recently, much attention in distribution theory has focused on the family of transmuted distributions derived through a quadratic rank transmutation map. Its stochastic construction as a mixture, through the use of order statistics, facilitated a generalization of the original family of transmuted distributions. In this work, continuing on with a similar idea, we put forward a new family of transmuted distributions based on the theory of records and examine its hazard properties, and also discuss some special cases of interest.

1 Introduction

During the last two decades, many authors have put forward different methods and constructions to come up with "general" families of distributions that offer more flexibility while modeling statistical data than their classical counterparts. Among these are the following well-known and extensively studied families of distributions: families of skewed models (Azzalini and Capitanio 2013; Genton 2004), families with the addition of a parameter (Marshall and Olkin 1997, 2007), exponentiated families of distributions (see, for example, Gupta and Kundu (1999), Mudholkar and Srivastava (1993), and Mudholkar et al. (1995)), generalized forms of distributions (Hosking and Wallis 2005), beta-generated family of distributions (Eugene et al. 2002; Jones 2004), and the subsequent works of Arnold et al. (2006) who introduced a multivariate version of this family and of Ferreira and Steel (2006, 2007) who used it to construct skewed distributions, gamma-generated family of distributions (Balakrishnan and Ristić 2016; Zografos and Balakrishnan 2009), Kumaraswamy-generalized distributions (Jones 2009; Kumaraswamy 1980), general families of quantile models (Gilchrist 2000; Nair et al. 2013), and family of

N. Balakrishnan (✉) · M. He
Department of Mathematics and Statistics, McMaster University, Hamilton, ON, Canada
e-mail: bala@mcmaster.ca; hem11@math.mcmaster.ca

I. Ghosh et al. (eds.), *Advances in Statistics - Theory and Applications*, Emerging Topics in Statistics and Biostatistics, https://doi.org/10.1007/978-3-030-62900-7_1

transmuted distributions (see, for example, Shaw and Buckley (2007, 2009) and Granzotto et al. (2017)).

In this work, we focus specifically on the last one in the above list, namely, the family of transmuted distributions. After providing a brief description of this family as proposed by Shaw and Buckley (2007, 2009) and its alternative stochastic construction through order statistics as given by Granzotto et al. (2017), we introduce here a new family of transmuted distributions based on the theory of records. We then examine some general properties of this family of distributions, and also focus on some special cases based on uniform, exponential, linear-exponential, Weibull, normal, and logistic baseline distributions, which are all quite tractable.

2 Transmuted Distributions

Let X be a random variable with its support as S, an absolutely continuous probability density function (PDF) $g(x)$, and a cumulative distribution function (CDF) $G(x)$. We refer to this as the baseline distribution. It is important to mention here that the assumption of continuous distribution for the variable X is purely for convenience in the ensuing discussion. It will become evident in the subsequent sections that all the results developed here could easily be formulated for the discrete case as well, but we abstain from furnishing the corresponding details for the sake of brevity.

Based on the baseline distribution $G(x)$, Shaw and Buckley (2007, 2009) considered a transformation map to introduce a "quadratic rank transmuted distribution" of the form

$$F(x) = (1+\lambda)G(x) - \lambda G^2(x), \quad x \in S, \tag{1}$$

where $-1 \leq \lambda \leq 1$. With different choices of the baseline distribution $G(x)$ in (1), many authors have studied numerous special cases of this family. One may see, for example, Aryal and Tsokos (2009, 2011), Elbatal and Aryal (2013), Khan and King (2014), Tian et al. (2014), Granzotto and Louzada (2015), Al-Babtain et al. (2017), Fattah et al. (2017), Khan et al. (2017), Nofal et al. (2017), and Kemaloglu and Yilmaz (2017), to name a few. Kozubowski and Podgórski (2016) have shown interestingly that transmuted models are a special case of extremal distributions.

Now, let us suppose X_1 and X_2 are independent and identically distributed (I.I.D.) random variables with support S, PDF $g(x)$, and CDF $G(x)$. Let $X_{1:2} = \min(X_1, X_2)$ and $X_{2:2} = \max(X_1, X_2)$ denote the corresponding order statistics. Then, it is known that their PDFs are

$$g_{1:2}(x) = 2\{1 - G(x)\}g(x), \qquad g_{2:2}(x) = 2G(x)g(x), \quad x \in S, \tag{2}$$

and their CDFs are

$$G_{1:2}(x) = 1 - \{1 - G(x)\}^2 \qquad G_{2:2}(x) = \{G(x)\}^2, \quad x \in S, \tag{3}$$

respectively; see, for example, Arnold et al. (1992). Let us now define a new random variable Y with the following two-component mixture distribution function:

$$F_Y(x) = \pi G_{1:2}(x) + (1 - \pi)G_{2:2}(x), \quad x \in S,$$

where $\pi \in [0, 1]$ is the mixing probability. Upon substituting for $G_{1:2}(x)$ and $G_{2:2}(x)$ from (3), we get

$$\begin{aligned} F_Y(x) &= \pi[1 - \{1 - G(x)\}^2] + (1 - \pi)G^2(x) \\ &= 2\pi G(x) + (1 - 2\pi)G^2(x), \quad x \in S. \end{aligned} \tag{4}$$

From the mixture CDF form in (4), upon setting $\lambda = 2\pi - 1 \in [-1, 1]$, Granzotto et al. (2017) arrived at the transmuted CDF in (1) through this mixture stochastic representation. It should be noted that, while the pure mixture form in (4) would require the mixture probability 2π to be in [0, 1], the fact that $G(x) \geq G^2(x)$ for all $x \in S$ facilitates the extended parameter range for the model.

Granzotto et al. (2017) then extended this mixture representation to introduce a "cubic rank transmuted distribution" in the following manner. Let X_1, X_2, X_3 be I.I.D. random variables with support S, PDF $g(x)$, and CDF $G(x)$, and $X_{1:3} < X_{2:3} < X_{3:3}$ denote the corresponding order statistics. Then, it is known that their PDFs are

$$\begin{aligned} g_{1:3}(x) &= 3\{1 - G(x)\}^2 g(x), \\ g_{2:3}(x) &= 6G(x)\{1 - G(x)\}g(x), \\ g_{3:3}(x) &= 3G^2(x)g(x), \quad x \in S, \end{aligned} \tag{5}$$

and their CDFs are

$$\begin{aligned} G_{1:3}(x) &= 1 - \{1 - G(x)\}^3, \\ G_{2:3}(x) &= 3G^2(x)\{1 - G(x)\} + G^3(x), \\ G_{3:3}(x) &= G^3(x), \quad x \in S \end{aligned} \tag{6}$$

respectively; see Arnold et al. (1992). Then, Granzotto et al. (2017) considered the following three-component mixture distribution function:

$$F_Y(x) = \pi_1 G_{1:3}(x) + \pi_2 G_{2:3}(x) + \pi_3 G_{3:3}(x),$$

where $0 \leq \pi_1, \pi_2, \pi_3 \leq 1$, such that $\pi_1 + \pi_2 + \pi_3 = 1$, are the mixing probabilities. Upon substituting for $G_{1:3}(x)$, $G_{2:3}(x)$, $G_{3:3}(x)$ from (6), we get

$$F_Y(x) = 3\pi_1 G(x) + 3(\pi_2 - \pi_1)G^2(x) + (1 - 3\pi_2)G^3(x), \quad x \in S, \tag{7}$$

which Granzotto et al. (2017) reparametrized in the form

$$F_Y(x) = \lambda_1 G(x) + (\lambda_2 - \lambda_1)G^2(x) + (1 - \lambda_2)G^3(x), \quad x \in S. \tag{8}$$

Subsequently, many authors have discussed numerous special cases of this cubic transmuted family in (8) by using different choices of the baseline distribution G(x). Interested readers may see, for example, Rahman et al. (2018), Saraçoğlu and Taniş (2018), Celik (2018), Ogunde and Chukwu (2020) and Ogunde et al. (2020).

3 Record-Based Transmuted Distributions

In the preceding section, stochastic mixture representations were given for quadratic and cubic rank transmuted distributions based on order statistics. We now use the same principle, but based on the theory of record values to propose record-based transmuted families of distributions.

First, let us recall the definition of record values and their distributions. Let $X_1, X_2, \cdots$ be a sequence of I.I.D. random variables with absolutely continuous PDF $g(x)$ and CDF $G(x)$, and support S. Let $X_{U(1)} \equiv X_1, X_{U(2)} \cdots$ be the sequence of upper record values, where

$$U(1) = 1 \quad \text{with probability 1}, \tag{9}$$

and for $n > 1$,

$$U(n) = \min\{i : i > U(n-1), X_i > X_{U(n-1)}\}.$$

In the above, $\{U(n)\}_{n=1}^{\infty}$ are called upper record times, while $\{X_{U(n)}\}_{n=1}^{\infty}$ is the corresponding record sequence, whose distributional theory has been developed in great length; see, for example, Arnold et al. (1998) and Nevzorov (2001).

The marginal PDF of $X_{U(n)}$, the n-th upper record value, is known to be (see Arnold et al. (1998))

$$g_{U(n)}(x) = \frac{1}{(n-1)!}\{-\ln\left(1 - G(x)\right)\}^{n-1} g(x), \quad x \in S, \tag{10}$$

for $n = 1, 2, \cdots$. Evidently, $g_{U(1)} \equiv g(x)$, by definition. Moreover, the corresponding CDF is given by

$$G_{U(n)}(x) = 1 - \left(1 - G(x)\right) \sum_{i=0}^{n-1} \frac{1}{i!}\{-\ln\left(1 - G(x)\right)\}^i, \quad x \in S. \tag{11}$$

Now, analogous to the mixture representation for the quadratic rank transmuted distribution presented in the last section, let us consider a new random variable with the following two-component mixture density

$$\begin{aligned} f_{R_2}(x) &= \pi g_{U(1)}(x) + (1-\pi) g_{U(2)}(x) \\ &= \pi g(x) + (1-\pi)\{-\ln\big(1-G(x)\big)\}g(x) \\ &= g(x)[\pi + (1-\pi)\{-\ln\big(1-G(x)\big)\}], \quad x \in S, \end{aligned} \tag{12}$$

where $\pi \in [0, 1]$ is the mixing probability. The corresponding survival function (SF) follows readily from (11) as

$$\begin{aligned} \bar{F}_{R_2}(x) &= \pi\big(1-G(x)\big) + (1-\pi)\big(1-G(x)\big)[1+\{-\ln(1-G(x))\}] \\ &= \big(1-G(x)\big)[1+(1-\pi)\{-\ln\big(1-G(x)\big)\}], \quad x \in S. \end{aligned} \tag{13}$$

We shall refer to the family of distributions introduced in (12) (or (13)) as *record-based transmuted family of distributions of order* 2. The use of order 2 in the name refers to the fact that the family is constructed as a mixture of distributions of the first two upper record values from the distribution $G(x)$. As with the transmuted distributions discussed in the last section, $G(x)$ here is the baseline distribution.

Remark 1 Let $h_G(x) = \frac{g(x)}{1-G(x)}$ be the hazard function of the baseline distribution $G(x)$. Then, from (12) and (13), we readily find the hazard function of the distribution $F_{R_2}(x)$ to be

$$h_{F_{R_2}}(x) = h_G(x)\left[\frac{\pi + (1-\pi)\{-\ln\big(1-G(x)\big)\}}{1+(1-\pi)\{-\ln\big(1-G(x)\big)\}}\right], \quad x \in S. \tag{14}$$

From (14), we can readily observe the following three features of the record-based transmuted distributions:

1. Even if we start with a baseline distribution $G(x)$ that belongs to the proportional hazards family, such as exponential or Weibull, the corresponding record-based transmuted distribution of order 2 will not inherit that property;
2. Because the mixing probability parameter $\pi \in [0, 1]$, it is evident from (14) that $h_{F_{R_2}}(x) \le h_G(x)$. In other words, the transmutation process on the baseline distribution $G(x)$, through the use of first two record values, always has a dampening effect on the hazard function;
3. From (14), we observe that if the baseline distribution $G(x)$ is IFR (Increasing Failure Rate), then in order for the record transmuted distribution $F_{R_2}(x)$ to be IFR, it is sufficient to check whether the second term on the right-hand side of (14) is non-decreasing. In fact, with $\stackrel{\text{sgn}}{=}$ denoting that both sides of an equation have the same sign, we have

$$\frac{d}{dx}h_{F_{R_2}}(x) \overset{\text{sgn}}{=} \frac{d}{dx}\left[\frac{\pi + (1-\pi)\{-\ln(1-G(x))\}}{1+(1-\pi)\{-\ln(1-G(x))\}}\right] \overset{\text{sgn}}{=} (1-\pi)^2 h_G(x), \tag{15}$$

which is clearly positive. This proves that if the baseline distribution $G(x)$ is IFR, then so is the corresponding record-based transmuted distribution of order 2.

Remark 2 Though we have constructed in (13) a record-based transmuted distribution of order 2 by mixing the distributions of the first two upper record values, it is evident from the PDF and CDF of the n-th upper record value given in (10) and (11), respectively, a mixture of the distributions of the first n upper record values from $G(x)$ can be readily constructed to form the so-called *record-based transmuted family of distributions of order n*.

For example, analogous to the cubic ranked transmuted distribution in (7) as proposed by Granzotto et al. (2017), we construct the family of *record-based transmuted distributions* of order 3 through a mixture of the distributions of three upper record values with its PDF as follows:

$$\begin{aligned} f_{R_3}(x) &= \pi_1 g_{U(1)}(x) + \pi_2 g_{U(2)}(x) + (1-\pi_1-\pi_2) g_{U(3)}(x) \\ &= g(x)\left[\pi_1 + \pi_2\{-\ln(1-G(x))\} + \frac{1-\pi_1-\pi_2}{2}\{-\ln(1-G(x))\}^2\right], \quad x \in S, \end{aligned} \tag{16}$$

where $0 \le \pi_1, \pi_2 \le 1$, with $\pi_1 + \pi_2 \le 1$, are the mixing probabilities. The corresponding SF follows immediately from (11) as, for $x \in S$,

$$\begin{aligned} \bar{F}_{R_3}(x) &= (1-G(x))\Big[\pi_1 + \pi_2\Big(1 + \{-\ln(1-G(x))\}\Big) \\ &\quad + (1-\pi_1-\pi_2)\Big(1 + \{-\ln(1-G(x))\} + \frac{1}{2}\{-\ln(1-G(x))\}^2\Big)\Big] \\ &= (1-G(x))\Big[1 + (1-\pi_1)\{-\ln(1-G(x))\} \\ &\quad + \frac{1-\pi_1-\pi_2}{2}\{-\ln(1-G(x))\}^2\Big]. \end{aligned} \tag{17}$$

Remark 3 Here again, with $h_G(x)$ denoting the hazard function of the baseline distribution $G(x)$, we readily have the hazard function of the distribution $F_{R_3}(x)$ to be, for $x \in S$,

$$h_{F_{R_3}}(x) = h_G(x)\left[\frac{\pi_1 + \pi_2\{-\ln(1-G(x))\} + \frac{1-\pi_1-\pi_2}{2}\{-\ln(1-G(x))\}^2}{1 + (1-\pi_1)\{-\ln(1-G(x))\} + \frac{1-\pi_1-\pi_2}{2}\{-\ln(1-G(x))\}^2}\right]. \tag{18}$$

As stated in Remark 1, in this case as well, even if the baseline distribution $G(x)$ belongs to the proportional hazards family, the corresponding record-based transmuted distribution of order 3 will not inherit this property. Moreover, due to the facts that $\pi_1 \leq 1$ and $\pi_2 \leq 1 - \pi_1$, we simply realize that the second term on the RHS of (18) is at most 1, which yields $h_{F_{R_3}}(x) \leq h_G(x)$. This means that the transmutation process of order 3 on the baseline distribution $G(x)$ also has a dampening effect on the hazard function.

Remark 4 As a matter of fact, we can also compare the hazard functions $h_{F_{R_2}}(x)$ and $h_{F_{R_3}}(x)$ in (14) and (18), respectively, to examine the impact of increasing the order in the record transmutation process. For this purpose, let us first choose in (18) $\pi_1 = \pi, \pi_2 = 1 - \pi - a$ (so the first mixing probability in the two models are the same, while the second mixing probability in the second model is smaller), and set $y = -\ln\left(1 - G(x)\right) > 0$. Then, upon realizing that proving the inequality

$$\frac{\pi + (1-\pi)y}{1 + (1-\pi)y} > \frac{\pi + (1-\pi-a)y + \frac{a}{2}y^2}{1 + (1-\pi)y + \frac{a}{2}y^2}$$

is equivalent to showing that

$$ay + \frac{a}{2}(1-\pi)y^2 > 0,$$

which is obviously true, we see that the third order record transmutation has further decreased the hazard function, resulting in $h_G(x) > h_{F_{R_2}}(x) > h_{F_{R_3}}(x)$ for all $x \in S$.

Next, let us perturb the first mixing probability in (18) and set $\pi_1 = \pi - a$, $\pi_2 = 1 - \pi$ (so the second mixing probability in the two models are the same, while the first mixing probability in the second model is smaller), and set $y = -\ln\left(1 - G(x)\right) > 0$. Then, upon realizing that proving the inequality

$$\frac{\pi + (1-\pi)y}{1 + (1-\pi)y} > \frac{(\pi - a) + (1-\pi)y + \frac{a}{2}y^2}{1 + (1-\pi+a)y + \frac{a}{2}y^2}$$

is equivalent to showing that

$$a + \{1 - \pi(\pi - a)\}y + \frac{a}{2}(1-\pi)y^2 > 0,$$

which is obviously true, we observe that the third order record transmutation has once again decreased the hazard function, resulting in $h_G(x) > h_{F_{R_2}}(x) > h_{F_{R_3}}(x)$ for all $x \in S$.

It is important to mention, however, that this property need not be true in general. To see this, let us consider now the inequality

$$\frac{\pi + (1-\pi)y}{1+(1-\pi)y} > \frac{\pi_1 + \pi_2 y + \frac{1-\pi_1-\pi_2}{2}y^2}{1+(1-\pi_1)y + \frac{1-\pi_1-\pi_2}{2}y^2}.$$

Upon cross-multiplying and rearranging the terms, we see that proving the above inequality is equivalent to showing that

$$(\pi - \pi_1) + (1-\pi_1-\pi_2)y + (1-\pi)\left(\frac{1-\pi_1-\pi_2}{2}\right)y^2 > 0, \tag{19}$$

which clearly does not hold for all $y > 0$. In fact, it is evident that if $\pi_1 > \pi$ and y is small (close to 0), the quantity on the left side will be clearly negative!

Earlier in Remark 1, we noted that if the baseline distribution $G(x)$ is IFR, then so is the corresponding record-based transmuted distribution of order 2. We may now ask the question whether this is true for the record-based transmuted distribution of order 3 in (17). The answer, unfortunately, turns out to be negative. To see this, we observe from (18), after considerable algebraic simplification, that

$$\begin{aligned}
\frac{d}{dx}h_{F_{R_3}}(x) &\overset{\text{sgn}}{=} \Big[1+(1-\pi_1)\{-\ln\left(1-G(x)\right)\} + \frac{1-\pi_1-\pi_2}{2}\{-\ln\left(1-G(x)\right)\}^2\Big] \\
&\quad \times \left[\pi_2 + (1-\pi_1-\pi_2)\{-\ln\left(1-G(x)\right)\}\right] \\
&\quad - \left[\pi_1 + \pi_2\{-\ln\left(1-G(x)\right)\} + \frac{1-\pi_1-\pi_2}{2}\{-\ln\left(1-G(x)\right)\}^2\right] \\
&\quad \times \left[(1-\pi_1) + (1-\pi_1-\pi_2)\{-\ln\left(1-G(x)\right)\}\right] \\
&\overset{\text{sgn}}{=} \{\pi_2 - \pi_1(1-\pi_1)\} + (1-\pi_1)(1-\pi_1-\pi_2)\{-\ln\left(1-G(x)\right)\} \\
&\quad + \frac{1}{2}(1-\pi_1-\pi_2)^2\{-\ln\left(1-G(x)\right)\}^2.
\end{aligned} \tag{20}$$

From (20), we see that the first term on the right side will be negative if $\pi_2 < \pi_1(1-\pi_1)$ while the second and third terms can be made arbitrarily small by letting x close to 0. So, because $\frac{d}{dx}h_{F_{R_3}}(x)$ in (20) can be negative, we immediately conclude that the record-based transmuted distribution of order 3 in (17) need not be IFR in general. However, we do see that $\pi_2 \geq \pi_1(1-\pi_1)$ is indeed a sufficient condition for $F_{R_3}(x)$ to be IFR when the baseline distribution $G(x)$ is IFR.

4 Special Cases

First, it needs to be mentioned that the newly proposed record-based transmuted distributions in (13) and (17), for example, could prove useful in modeling lifetime data just as the corresponding transmuted distribution counterparts described in Sect. 2. Of course, the use of different baseline distributions would result in different families of record-based transmuted distributions. If one were to choose the baseline distribution $G(x)$ to be a member of the scale-family of distributions (say, scaled exponential distribution), then the record transmuted distribution in (13) would possess a scale parameter and an additional mixing parameter π to provide flexibility while modeling. In addition, it would also facilitate an easy interpretation in terms of the mixture of the two underlying random variables used in the stochastic representation in (13). Alternatively, the baseline distribution could also come from location-scale or log-location-scale families of distributions. We now present several examples here and briefly describe their properties and characteristics and for this purpose, without loss of any generality, we take the baseline distribution $G(x)$ to be the standard distribution without scale parameter.

4.1 *Record-Based Transmuted Uniform Distribution*

Let us start with the standard uniform distribution for the baseline distribution $G(x)$, i.e., $G(x) = x$, $0 < x < 1$. Then, from (12)–(14), we have

$$f_{R_2}^U(x) = \pi + (1-\pi)\{-\ln(1-x)\}, \quad 0 < x < 1, \tag{21}$$

$$F_{R_2}^U(x) = (1-x)[1 + (1-\pi)\{-\ln(1-x)\}], \quad 0 < x < 1, \tag{22}$$

and

$$h_{F_{R_2}^U}(x) = \frac{1}{1-x}\left[\frac{\pi + (1-\pi)\{-\ln(1-x)\}}{1 + (1-\pi)\{-\ln(1-x)\}}\right], \quad 0 < x < 1. \tag{23}$$

Clearly, the hazard function of the baseline distribution, $h_G(x) = \frac{1}{1-x}$, is increasing and so, according to Remark 1, the above record-based transmuted uniform distribution is IFR.

4.2 *Record-Based Transmuted Exponential Distribution*

Let us take the baseline distribution $G(x) = 1 - e^{-x}$, $x > 0$, corresponding to the standard exponential distribution. We then have from (12)–(14) the corresponding PDF, SF and hazard function to be

$$f_{R_2}^E(x) = e^{-x}\{\pi + (1-\pi)x\}, \quad x > 0, \pi \in [0, 1], \tag{24}$$

$$\bar{F}_{R_2}^E(x) = e^{-x}\{1 + (1-\pi)x\}, \quad x > 0, \pi \in [0, 1], \tag{25}$$

and

$$h_{F_{R_2}^E}(x) = \frac{\pi + (1-\pi)x}{1+(1-\pi)x}, \quad x > 0, \pi \in [0,1]. \tag{26}$$

The PDF in (24) is nothing but the Lindley distribution; see Lindley (1958). From the hazard function in (26), it can be verified that its derivative is

$$h'_{F_{R_2}^E}(x) = \left[\frac{1-\pi}{1+(1-\pi)x}\right]^2 > 0, \tag{27}$$

implying that the record-based transmuted exponential distribution in (24) belongs to the IFR class of distributions.

In Fig. 1, we have presented plots of the PDF in (24) and the hazard function in (26) for $\pi = 0.25, 0.5$, and 0.75. The fact that this distribution belongs to the IFR class of distributions, as commented in Remark 1, can be readily seen in this plot.

4.3 Record-Based Transmuted Linear-Exponential Distribution

Let us now consider the baseline distribution $G(x) = 1 - e^{-(\lambda x + \mu x^2/2)}$, $x > 0$, $\lambda, \mu > 0$, corresponding to the linear-exponential distribution; see Bain (1974) and Johnson et al. (1994) for details on its properties and reliability applications. We then have from (12)–(14) the corresponding PDF, SF, and hazard function to be

$$f_{R_2}^{LE}(x) = (\lambda + \mu x)e^{-(\lambda x + \mu x^2/2)}\left[\pi + (1-\pi)\left(\lambda x + \frac{\mu x^2}{2}\right)\right], \quad x > 0, \mu > 0, \lambda > 0, \tag{28}$$

$$\bar{F}_{R_2}^{LE}(x) = e^{-(\lambda x + \mu x^2/2)}\left[1 + (1-\pi)\left(\lambda x + \frac{\mu x^2}{2}\right)\right], \quad x > 0, \mu > 0, \lambda > 0, \tag{29}$$

and

$$h_{F_{R_2}^{LE}}(x) = (\lambda + \mu x)\left[\frac{\pi + (1-\pi)(\lambda x + \frac{\mu x^2}{2})}{1 + (1-\pi)(\lambda x + \frac{\mu x^2}{2})}\right], \quad x > 0, \mu > 0, \lambda > 0, \tag{30}$$

with $\pi \in [0, 1]$. From Remark 1, we know that the record-based transmuted linear-exponential distribution in (28) belongs to the IFR class of distributions as the baseline linear-exponential distribution is.

In Fig. 2, we have presented plots of the PDF in (28) and the hazard function in (30) for $\pi = 0.25, 0.5$, and 0.75, $\lambda = 0.5$, and $\mu = 1.0, 2.0$. From the plot of the hazard function, we can readily see that it is in agreement with the comment in

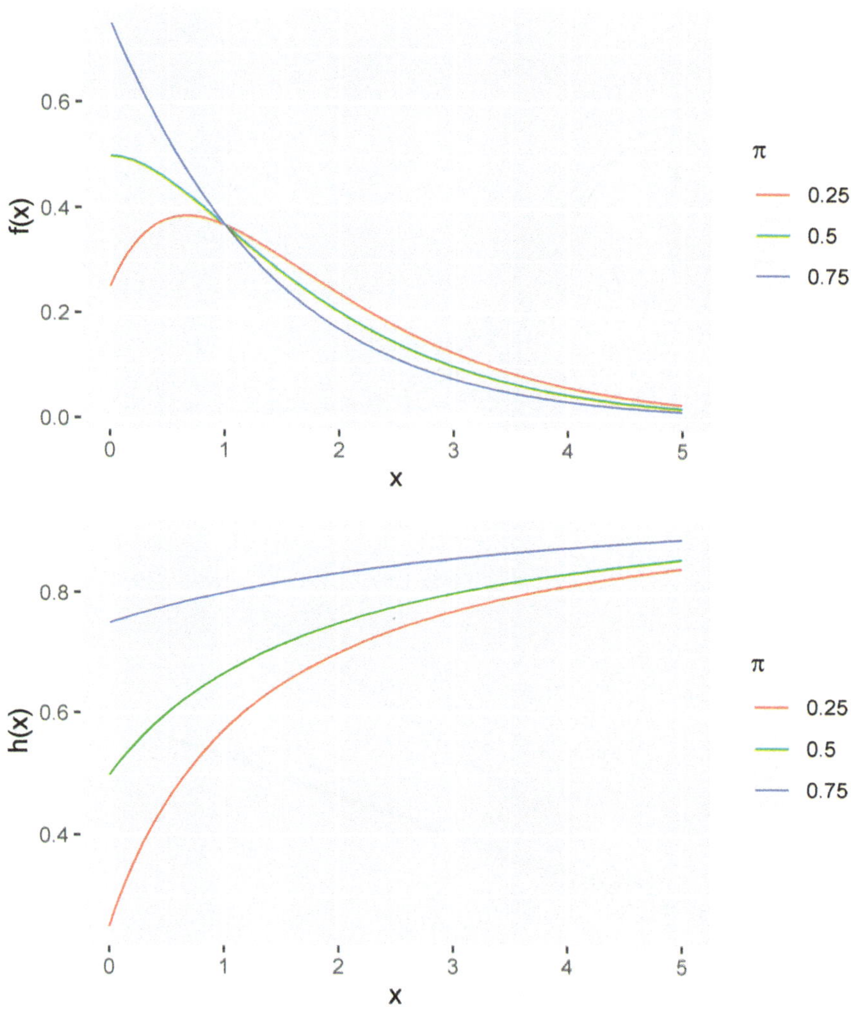

Fig. 1 Density and hazard functions of record-based transmuted exponential distribution

Remark 1 that this distribution belongs to the IFR class. In the plot, we have Group 1 ($\pi = 0.25, \mu = 1.0$), Group 2 ($\pi = 0.5, \mu = 1.0$), Group 3 ($\pi = 0.75, \mu = 1.0$), Group 4 ($\pi = 0.25, \mu = 2.0$), Group 5 ($\pi = 0.5, \mu = 2.0$), and Group 6 ($\pi = 0.75, \mu = 2.0$).

Finally, it should be mentioned that by adopting a lifetime distribution with a polynomial hazard function as the one considered by Krane (1963), for example, as the baseline distribution $G(x)$ in (28), we can propose a very general family of *record-based transmuted polynomial-exponential distribution*, and then study its properties and applications. Furthermore, upon letting the intercept parameter

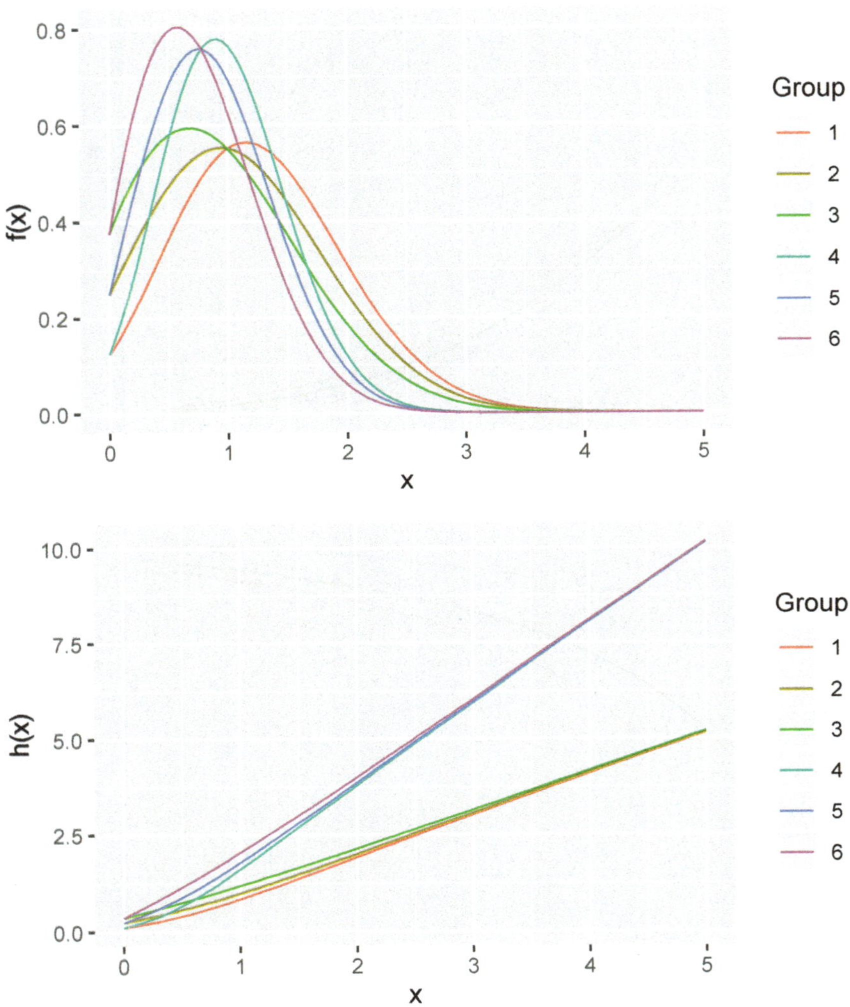

Fig. 2 Density and hazard functions of record-based transmuted linear-exponential distribution

$\lambda \to 0$ in the baseline distribution $G(x)$ used in (28), so that the linear-exponential distribution reduces in this case to the Rayleigh distribution (see Polovko (1968) and Johnson et al. (1994)), we will deduce the family of *record-based transmuted Rayleigh distributions*.

4.4 Record-Based Transmuted Weibull Distribution

Next, we consider the baseline distribution to be $G(x) = 1 - e^{-x^\alpha}$, $x > 0, \alpha > 0$, corresponding to the standard Weibull distribution with shape parameter $\alpha > 0$. It is well-known that this distribution is IFR when $\alpha > 1$, exponential with constant hazard function when $\alpha = 1$, and DFR (Decreasing Failure Rate) distribution when $0 < \alpha < 1$; one may refer to Johnson et al. (1994) and Murthy et al. (2004) for detailed reviews of various properties and developments on Weibull distribution.

With the choice of Weibull distribution as the baseline distribution $G(x)$, we have from (12)–(14) the corresponding PDF, SF, and hazard function to be

$$f_{R_2}^W(x) = \alpha x^{\alpha-1} e^{-x^\alpha}[\pi + (1-\pi)x^\alpha], \quad x > 0, \alpha > 0, \tag{31}$$

$$S_{R_2}^W(x) = e^{-x^\alpha}[1 + (1-\pi)x^\alpha], \quad x > 0, \alpha > 0, \tag{32}$$

and

$$h_{F_{R_2}^W}(x) = \alpha x^{\alpha-1}\left[\frac{\pi + (1-\pi)x^\alpha}{1 + (1-\pi)x^\alpha}\right] \quad x > 0, \alpha > 0, \tag{33}$$

with $\pi \in [0, 1]$. From the hazard function in (33), it can be verified that its derivative, for $x > 0$, is given by

$$h'_{F_{R_2}^W}(x) = \frac{\alpha(\alpha-1)x^{\alpha-2}[1 + (1-\pi)x^\alpha][\pi + (1-\pi)x^\alpha] + \alpha^2(1-\pi)^2 x^{2\alpha-2}}{[1 + (1-\pi)x^\alpha]^2}. \tag{34}$$

From (34), it is evident that $h'_{F_{R_2}^W}(x) > 0$ when $\alpha > 1$, implying that record-based transmuted Weibull distribution is IFR, which is in agreement with Remark 1. Next, when $\alpha = 1$, (34) simply reduces to (27) for the case of exponential distribution showing that the corresponding record-based transmuted exponential distribution is also IFR (see the comment in Sect. 4.2). Finally, for the case $0 < \alpha < 1$, the first term on RHS of (34) is negative while the second term is positive. A careful examination of (34) suggests that when $0 < \alpha \leq \frac{1}{2}$, $h'_{F_{R_2}^W}(x)$ is negative which implies that the corresponding record-based transmuted Weibull distribution is DFR just as the baseline Weibull distribution is. But, in the range $\frac{1}{2} < \alpha < 1$, it need not be DFR!

In Fig. 3, we have presented plots of the PDF in (31) and the hazard function in (33) for $\pi = 0.25, 0.5$, and 0.75, and $\alpha = 0.3, 0.75$, and 2.0, with Group 1 ($\pi = 0.25, \alpha = 0.3$), Group 2 ($\pi = 0.25, \alpha = 0.75$), Group 3 ($\pi = 0.25, \alpha = 2.0$), and so on, and Group 9 ($\pi = 0.75$, $\alpha = 2.0$) in the plot. This plot supports the observations made about the hazard characteristics of this distribution.

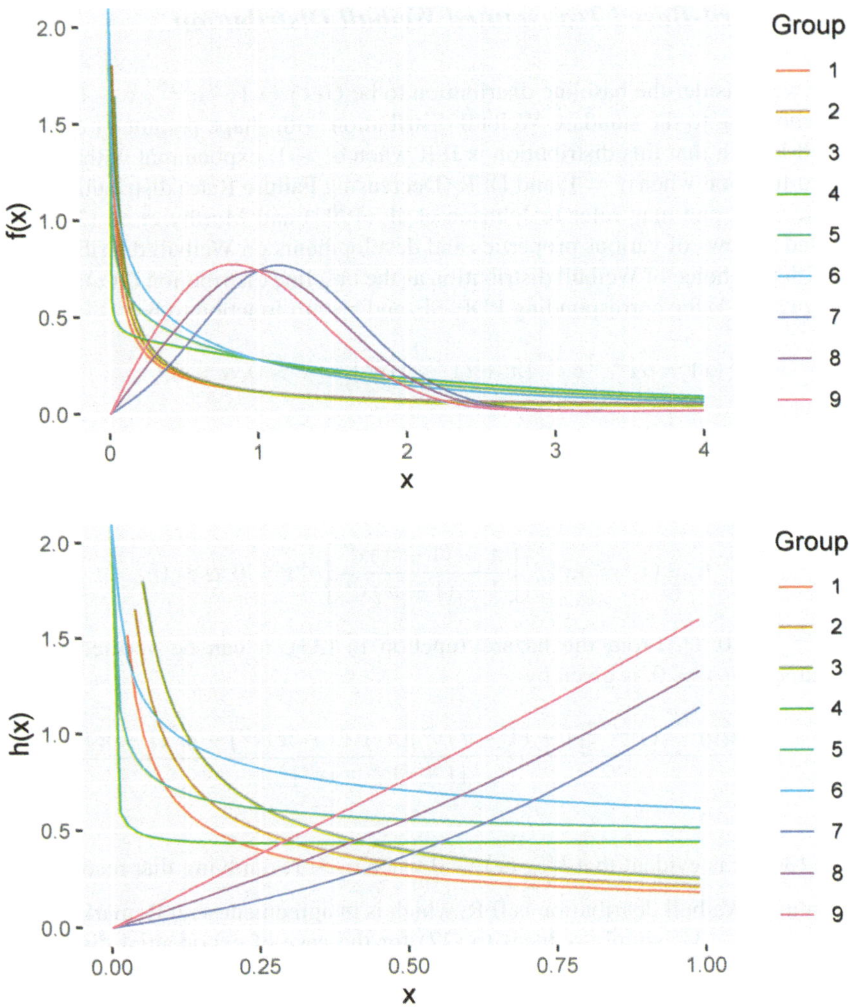

Fig. 3 Density and hazard functions of record-based transmuted Weibull distribution

4.5 Record-Based Transmuted Normal Distribution

Let us now take the baseline distribution to be standard normal, which is known to be IFR; see Johnson et al. (1994). In this case, we have from (12)–(14) the corresponding PDF, SF, and hazard function to be

$$f_{R_2}^{N}(x) = \phi(x)\big[\pi + (1-\pi)\{-\ln\big(1-\Phi(x)\big)\}\big], -\infty < x < \infty, \tag{35}$$

$$\bar{F}_{R_2}^N(x) = \left(1 - \Phi(x)\right)\left[1 + (1-\pi)\{-\ln\left(1-\Phi(x)\right)\}\right], -\infty < x < \infty, \tag{36}$$

and

$$h_{F_{R_2}^N}(x) = \frac{\phi(x)}{1-\Phi(x)}\left[\frac{\pi + (1-\pi)\{-\ln\left(1-\Phi(x)\right)\}}{1 + (1-\pi)\{-\ln\left(1-\Phi(x)\right)\}}\right], -\infty < x < \infty, \tag{37}$$

with $\pi \in [0, 1]$, where Φ and ϕ denote the standard normal CDF and PDF, respectively. From Remark 1, we know that the record-based transmuted normal distribution in (35) belongs to the IFR class of distributions.

In Fig. 4, we have presented plots of the PDF in (35) and the hazard function in (37) for $\pi = 0.25, 0.5$, and 0.75, which supports the observation made about the hazard function of this distribution.

4.6 Record-Based Transmuted Logistic Distribution

As a final case, let us take the baseline distribution to be standard logistic distribution with CDF $G(x) = \frac{1}{1+e^{-x}}$ and PDF $g(x) = \frac{e^{-x}}{(1+e^{-x})^2} = G(x)\left(1 - G(x)\right)$, for $-\infty < x < \infty$. Evidently, $h_G(x) = \frac{g(x)}{1-G(x)} = G(x)$ is monotone increasing, implying that the baseline logistic distribution is IFR. In this case, we have from (12)–(14) the corresponding PDF, SF, and hazard function to be

$$f_{R_2}^L(x) = g(x)[\pi + (1-\pi)\{-\ln\left(1-G(x)\right)\}], \quad -\infty < x < \infty, \tag{38}$$

$$\bar{F}_{R_2}^L(X) = \left(1 - G(x)\right)[1 + (1-\pi)\{-\ln\left(1-G(x)\right)\}], \quad -\infty < x < \infty, \tag{39}$$

and

$$h_{F_{R_2}^L}(x) = G(x)\left[\frac{\pi + (1-\pi)\{-\ln\left(1-G(x)\right)\}}{1 + (1-\pi)\{-\ln\left(1-G(x)\right)\}}\right], \quad -\infty < x < \infty, \tag{40}$$

with $\pi \in [0, 1]$. It is known from Remark 1 that the record-based transmuted logistic distribution in (38) belongs to the IFR class of distributions.

In Fig. 5, we have presented plots of the PDF in (38) and the hazard function in (40) for $\pi = 0.25, 0.5$, and 0.75. The plot of the hazard function once again supports the observations made about the hazard characteristic of this distribution.

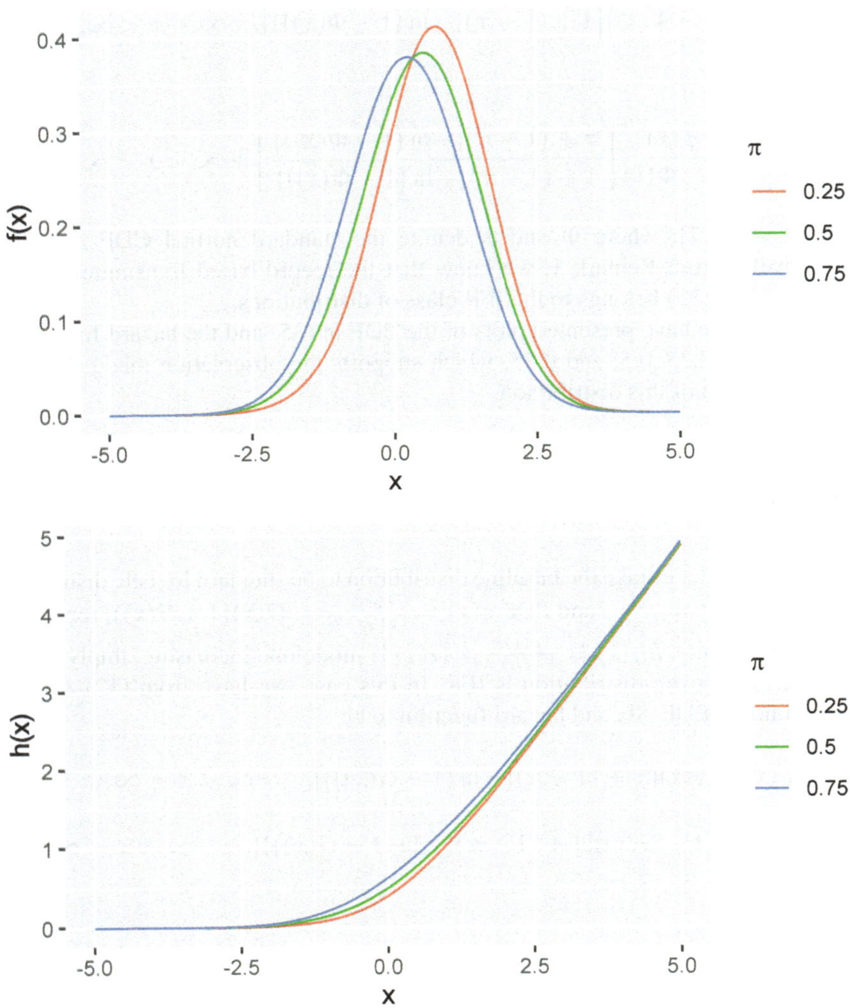

Fig. 4 Density and hazard functions of record-based transmuted normal distribution

5 Dual Record-Based Transmuted Distributions

In Sect. 3, to develop record-based transmuted distributions, we started with a sequence of upper record values. Instead, if we use lower record values, we will obtain a dual family of record-based transmuted distributions.

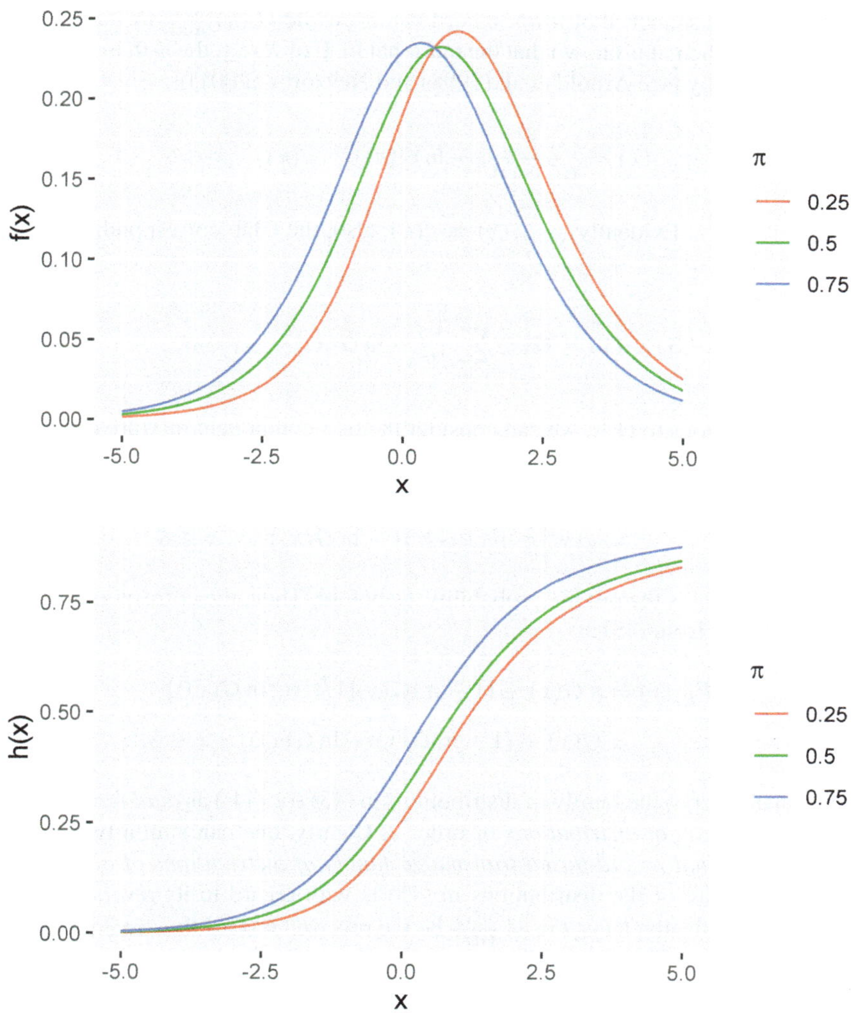

Fig. 5 Density and hazard functions of record-based transmuted logistic distribution

To be specific, let $\{X_i\}_{i=1}^{\infty}$ be a sequence of I.I.D. random variables from a continuous baseline distribution with PDF $g(x)$ and CDF $G(x)$, and support S. Then, the sequence $\{X_{L(n)}\}_{n=1}^{\infty}$, where

$$L(1) = 1 \quad \text{with probability } 1,$$

and for $n > 1$,

$$L(n) = \min\left\{i : i > L(n-1),\, X_i < X_{L(n-1)}\right\} \tag{41}$$

is said to be the sequence of lower record values, while $\{L(n)\}_{n=1}^{\infty}$ are called lower record times. Then, it is known that the marginal PDF of $X_{L(n)}$, the n-th lower record value, is given by (see Arnold et al. (1998) and Nevzorov (2001))

$$g_{L(n)}(x) = \frac{1}{(n-1)!}\big(-\ln G(x)\big)^{n-1} g(x), \quad x \in S, \tag{42}$$

for $n = 1, 2, \cdots$. Evidently, $g_{L(1)}(x) \equiv g(x)$; also, the CDF corresponding to (42) is

$$G_{L(n)}(x) = G(x) \sum_{i=0}^{n-1} \frac{1}{i!}\big(-\ln G(x)\big)^{i}, \quad x \in S. \tag{43}$$

Now, analogous to (12), we can consider the two-component mixture density

$$\begin{aligned} f^*_{R_2}(x) &= \pi g(x) + (1-\pi)\big(-\ln G(x)\big) g(x) \\ &= g(x)\big[\pi + (1-\pi)\big(-\ln G(x)\big)\big], \quad x \in S, \end{aligned} \tag{44}$$

where $\pi \in [0, 1]$ is the mixing probability, as before. Then, the corresponding CDF readily follows from (43) as

$$\begin{aligned} F^*_{R_2}(x) &= \pi G(x) + (1-\pi) G(x)[1 + (-\ln G(x))] \\ &= G(x) + (1-\pi) G(x)(-\ln G(x)), \quad x \in S. \end{aligned} \tag{45}$$

We shall refer to the family of distributions in (43) (or (44)) as *dual record-based transmuted family of distributions* of order 2. Clearly, one can similarly construct the family of *dual record-based transmuted family of distributions of order n*. An important feature of the distributions in (45) is with regard to its reversed hazard function. Specifically, let $r_G(x) = \frac{g(x)}{G(x)}$ be the reversed hazard function of baseline distribution $G(x)$. Then, from (44) and (45), we readily obtain the reversed hazard function of the distribution $F^*_{R_2}$ to be

$$r^*_{F_{R_2}}(x) = r_G(x) \left[\frac{\pi + (1-\pi)\big(-\ln G(x)\big)}{1 + (1-\pi)\big(-\ln G(x)\big)} \right], \quad x \in S, \tag{46}$$

with $\pi \in [0, 1]$. We then observe immediately the following features of the dual record-based transmuted distributions:

1. Even if we start with a baseline distribution $G(x)$ that belongs to the proportional reversed hazard family, such as Fréchet or inverse Weibull distribution, with CDF $e^{-x^{-\alpha}}$, $x > 0$, the corresponding dual record-based transmuted distribution of order 2 will not inherit that property;

2. Due to the fact that $\pi \in [0, 1]$, we observe immediately from (46) that $r_{F^*_{R_2}}(x) \leq r_G(x)$, implying that the transmutation process on the baseline distribution $G(x)$ has a dampening effect on its reversed hazard function.

We can similarly examine the family of *dual record-based transmuted family of distributions of order 3* and its characteristics and properties. But, we refrain from it here for the sake of brevity.

Remark 5 Due to the symmetry (around zero) of standard normal and standard logistic distributions, we readily see that the dual record-based transmuted families of distributions in these cases will simply be mirror images of the corresponding record-based transmuted families of distributions presented earlier in Sects. 4.5 and 4.6.

Remark 6 Recall that, in Remark 1, it has been shown that if the baseline distribution G is IFR, then so is the corresponding record-based transmuted distribution. In an analogous manner, it can be shown that if the baseline distribution G has a decreasing reversed hazard function, then so will the corresponding dual record-based transmutation distribution.

6 Concluding Remarks

The family of transmuted distributions was introduced by Shaw and Buckley (2007, 2009) through a quadratic rank transmutation map. Granzotto et al. (2017) showed that this family is in fact a mixture of distributions of minima and maxima from a sample of size 2 from the baseline distribution. They then used this mixture representation to introduce cubic rank transmuted distributions, generalizing the family of distributions by Shaw and Buckley (2007, 2009), by considering mixtures of distributions of order statistics from a sample size 3 from the baseline distribution. In this work, we have instead used the distributions of record values (both upper and lower) to put forward two new general families of distributions. We have then discussed some of its properties based on hazard and reversed hazard functions, and as to how they relate to proportional hazards and reversed hazards families of distributions. Some special cases based on the uniform, exponential, linear-exponential, Weibull, normal, logistic, and Fréchet distributions have also been discussed. It will be of great interest to develop efficient inferential methods for these families of distributions. We are currently working in this direction and hope to report the findings in a future paper.

Acknowledgments With great pleasure, NB dedicates this article to Barry, who has had an immense impact on his work and his life in general. He cannot think of a better topic than a combination of order statistics and record values, and a playful mathematical exercise as this one, as a dedication to Barry! The support from the Natural Sciences and Engineering Research Council of Canada, through an Individual Discovery Grant, is acknowledged by NB, while MH thanks McMaster University for providing support for his PhD study, under the supervision of Professor N. Balakrishnan.

References

Al-Babtain, A., Fattah, A. A., Ahmed, A. H. N., & Merovci, F. (2017). The Kumaraswamy-transmuted exponentiated modified Weibull distribution. *Communications in Statistics-Simulation and Computation, 46*(5), 3812–3832.

Arnold, B. C., Balakrishnan, N., & Nagaraja, H. N. (1992). *A first course in order statistics*. New York: Wiley.

Arnold, B. C., Balakrishnan, N., & Nagaraja, H. N. (1998). *Records*. New York: Wiley.

Arnold, B. C., Castillo, E., & Sarabia, J. M. (2006). Families of multivariate distributions involving the Rosenblatt construction. *Journal of the American Statistical Association, 101*(476), 1652–1662.

Aryal, G. R., & Tsokos, C. P. (2009). On the transmuted extreme value distribution with application. *Nonlinear Analysis: Theory, Methods & Applications, 71*(12), e1401–e1407.

Aryal, G. R., & Tsokos, C. P. (2011). Transmuted Weibull distribution: A generalization of the Weibull probability distribution. *European Journal of Pure and Applied Mathematics, 4*(2), 89–102.

Azzalini A., & Capitanio, A. (2013). *The skew-normal and related families*. Cambridge: Cambridge University Press.

Bain, L. J. (1974). Analysis for the linear failure-rate life-testing distribution. *Technometrics, 16*(4), 551–559.

Balakrishnan, N., & Ristić, M. M. (2016). Multivariate families of gamma-generated distributions with finite or infinite support above or below the diagonal. *Journal of Multivariate Analysis, 143*, 194–207.

Celik, N. (2018). Some cubic rank transmuted distributions. *Journal of Applied Mathematics, Statistics and Informatics, 14*(2), 27–43.

Elbatal, I., & Aryal, G. (2013). On the transmuted additive Weibull distribution. *Austrian Journal of Statistics, 42*(2), 117–132.

Eugene, N., Lee, C., & Famoye, F. (2002). Beta-normal distribution and its applications. *Communications in Statistics-Theory and Methods, 31*(4), 497–512.

Fattah, A. A., Nadarajah, S., & Ahmed, A. H. N. (2017). The exponentiated transmuted Weibull geometric distribution with application in survival analysis. *Communications in Statistics-Simulation and Computation, 46*(6), 4244–4263.

Ferreira, J. T. S., & Steel, M. F. J. (2006). A constructive representation of univariate skewed distributions. *Journal of the American Statistical Association, 101*(474), 823–829.

Ferreira, J. T. S., & Steel, M. F. J. (2007). Model comparison of coordinate-free multivariate skewed distributions with an application to stochastic frontiers. *Journal of Econometrics, 137*(2), 641–673.

Genton, M. G. (2004). *Skew-elliptical distributions and their applications: A journey beyond normality*. Boca Raton, FL: Chapman & Hall/CRC Press.

Gilchrist, W. (2000). *Statistical modelling with quantile functions*. Boca Raton, FL: Chapman & Hall/CRC Press.

Granzotto, D. C. T., & Louzada, F. (2015). The transmuted log-logistic distribution: Modeling, inference, and an application to a polled Tabapua race time up to first calving data. *Communications in Statistics-Theory and Methods, 44*(16), 3387–3402.

Granzotto, D. C. T., Louzada, F., & Balakrishnan, N. (2017). Cubic rank transmuted distributions: inferential issues and applications. *Journal of Statistical Computation and Simulation, 87*(14), 2760–2778.

Gupta, R. D., & Kundu, D. (1999). Theory & methods: Generalized exponential distributions. *Australian & New Zealand Journal of Statistics, 41*(2), 173–188.

Hosking, J. R. M., & Wallis, J. R. (2005). *Regional frequency analysis: An approach based on L-moments*. Cambridge: Cambridge University Press.

Johnson, N. L., Kotz, S., & Balakrishnan, N. (1994). *Continuous univariate distributions* (Vol. 1, 2nd ed.). New York: Wiley.

Jones, M. C. (2004). Families of distributions arising from distributions of order statistics. *Test, 13*(1), 1–43.
Jones, M. C. (2009). Kumaraswamy's distribution: A beta-type distribution with some tractability advantages. *Statistical Methodology, 6*(1), 70–81.
Kemaloglu, S. A., & Yilmaz, M. (2017). Transmuted two-parameter Lindley distribution. *Communications in Statistics-Theory and Methods, 46*(23), 11866–11879.
Khan, M. S., & King, R. (2014). A new class of transmuted inverse Weibull distribution for reliability analysis. *American Journal of Mathematical and Management Sciences, 33*(4), 261–286.
Khan, M. S., King, R., & Hudson, I. L. (2017). Transmuted generalized exponential distribution: A generalization of the exponential distribution with applications to survival data. *Communications in Statistics-Simulation and Computation, 46*(6), 4377–4398.
Kozubowski, T. J., & Podgórski, K. (2016). Transmuted distributions and random extrema. *Statistics & Probability Letters, 116*, 6–8.
Krane, S. A. (1963). Analysis of survival data by regression techniques. *Technometrics, 5*(2), 161–174.
Kumaraswamy, P. (1980). A generalized probability density function for double-bounded random processes. *Journal of Hydrology, 46*(1–2), 79–88.
Lindley, D. V. (1958). Fiducial distributions and Bayes' theorem. *Journal of the Royal Statistical Society. Series B, 20*, 102–107.
Marshall, A. W., & Olkin, I. (1997). A new method for adding a parameter to a family of distributions with application to the exponential and Weibull families. *Biometrika, 84*(3), 641–652.
Marshall, A. W., & Olkin, I. (2007). *Life distributions: Structure of nonparametric, semiparametric, and parametric families*. New York: Springer.
Mudholkar, G. S., & Srivastava, D. K. (1993). Exponentiated Weibull family for analyzing bathtub failure-rate data. *IEEE Transactions on Reliability, 42*(2), 299–302.
Mudholkar, G. S., Srivastava, D. K., & Freimer, M. (1995). The exponentiated Weibull family: A reanalysis of the bus-motor-failure data. *Technometrics, 37*(4), 436–445.
Murthy, D. P., Xie, M., & Jiang, R. (2004). *Weibull models*. Hoboken, NJ: Wiley.
Nair, N. U., Sankaran, P. G., & Balakrishnan, N. (2013). *Quantile-based reliability analysis*. Boston: Birkhäuser.
Nevzorov, V. B. (2001). *Records: Mathematical theory*. Providence, RI: American Mathematical Society.
Nofal, Z. M., Afify, A. Z., Yousof, H. M., & Cordeiro, G. M. (2017). The generalized transmuted-G family of distributions. *Communications in Statistics-Theory and Methods, 46*(8), 4119–4136.
Ogunde, A. A., & Chukwu, A. U. (2020). The characterization of the cubic rank inverse Weibull distribution. *Asian Research Journal of Mathematics, 16*, 20–33.
Ogunde, A. A., Olayode, F., & Adejumoke, A. (2020). Cubic transmuted Gompertz distribution: As a life time distribution. *Journal of Advances in Mathematics and Computer Science, 35*, 105–116.
Polovko, A. M. (1968). *Fundamentals of reliability theory*. New York: Academic Press.
Rahman, M. M., Al-Zahrani, B., & Shahbaz, M. Q. (2018). Cubic transmuted Pareto distribution. *Annals of Data Science, 7*, 1–18.
Saraçoğlu, B., & Taniş, C. (2018). A new statistical distribution: Cubic rank transmuted Kumaraswamy distribution and its properties. *Journal of the National Science Foundation of Sri Lanka, 46*(4), 505–518.
Shaw, W. T., & Buckley, I. R. (2007). The alchemy of probability distributions: Beyond Gram-Charlier & Cornish-Fisher expansions, and skew-normal or kurtotic-normal distributions. *UCL discovery repository*, pp. 1–16.
Shaw, W. T., & Buckley, I. R. (2009). The alchemy of probability distributions: beyond Gram-Charlier expansions, and a skew-kurtotic-normal distribution from a rank transmutation map. https://arxiv.org/abs/0901.0434

Tian, Y., Tian, M., & Zhu, Q. (2014). Transmuted linear exponential distribution: A new generalization of the linear exponential distribution. *Communications in Statistics-Simulation and Computation, 43*(10), 2661–2677.

Zografos, K., & Balakrishnan, N. (2009). On families of beta- and generalized gamma-generated distributions and associated inference. *Statistical Methodology, 6*(4), 344–362.

Large-Sample Properties of Jackknife Estimators of the Variance of a Sample Quantile

Haikady N. Nagaraja and Chaitra H. Nagaraja

Abstract We study for a finite d (≥ 1), the limit properties of the family of delete-d jackknife estimators of the variance of a sample quantile from a random sample of size n as $n \to \infty$. We consider central and intermediate sample quantiles and for the central case, we provide asymptotically unbiased delete-d jackknife estimators of its large-sample variance. In the intermediate case, the limit distribution of the delete-d jackknife estimator is free of d. For the sample median, the limit distributions of the delete-d jackknife estimators of its variance differ for sequences of odd and even values of $n - d$.

1 Introduction

Consider a continuous cumulative distribution function (cdf) F with inverse cdf F^{-1} and probability density function (pdf) f whose functional form is unknown. For a given $p \in (0, 1)$ suppose there exists an x_p such that $F(x_p) = p$ and $f(x_p) > 0$. Then, $x_p = F^{-1}(p)$ is the pth population quantile. Let $X_{k:n}$, $1 \leq k \leq n$, be the kth order statistic of a random sample of size n from F. When $k = [np] + 1$, and $[\cdot]$ is the greatest integer function, the sample quantile $X_{k:n}$ represents a commonly used distribution-free estimator of x_p. Numerous point and interval estimators of x_p based on selected sample quantiles exist in the literature; for a recent review, see Nagaraja and Nagaraja (2020).

It is well-known that whenever $f(x_p) > 0$ and $0 < p < 1$,

H. N. Nagaraja (✉)
The Ohio State University, Division of Biostatistics, College of Public Health, Columbus, OH, USA
e-mail: nagaraja.1@osu.edu

C. H. Nagaraja
Fordham University, Strategy and Statistics Area, Gabelli School of Business, New York, NY, USA
e-mail: cnagaraja@fordham.edu

I. Ghosh et al. (eds.), *Advances in Statistics - Theory and Applications*, Emerging Topics in Statistics and Biostatistics, https://doi.org/10.1007/978-3-030-62900-7_2

$$\sqrt{n}(X_{k:n} - x_p) \xrightarrow{D} N\left(0, \sigma_p^2\right), \tag{1}$$

where $\xrightarrow{D}$ indicates convergence in distribution and where

$$\sigma_p^2 = \frac{p(1-p)}{\{f(x_p)\}^2} \tag{2}$$

is positive and finite. See, for example, David and Nagaraja (2003, p. 288). When the mean of F is finite, $f(x_p) > 0$, and f' is bounded in a neighborhood of x_p, it follows from Theorem 6.1.1 of Reiss (1989, p. 207) that

$$nVar(X_{k:n}) \to \sigma_p^2. \tag{3}$$

The unknown parameter in σ_p^2 is $1/f(x_p)$, the derivative of $F^{-1}(p)$ with respect to p and is called the *quantile density function* (Parzen 1979). Thus, the problem of estimating the quantile density function at x_p is closely related to the distribution-free estimation of the large-sample variance of $X_{k:n}$.

Jackknife (JK) methodology, introduced by Quenouille (1949), provides an established approach for estimating an arbitrary distributional parameter and is shown to reduce bias in many cases. It has been successfully used to identify outliers (see, for example, Martin et al. 2010). However, for estimating σ_p^2 in (2) it has been shown that the delete-1 JK estimator is inconsistent for the sample median from even-sized samples and has a large bias (see, Efron 1982, p. 13, 16).

Martin (1990) has shown that the limit distribution of the delete-1 JK variance estimator of a central sample quantile (that is, $k = [np] + 1, 0 < p < 1$) is Weibull. Peng and Yang (2009) have extended his work to intermediate order statistics (that is, $k/n \to 0$ or 1). Assuming d is proportional to n as $n \to \infty$, Shao (1988) has established the consistency of the delete-d JK estimator in estimating σ_p^2 for a central quantile. But as the methodology depends on d and computational time increases quickly with d, small d values are desirable. With this in mind, we study the limit distribution of the delete-d JK estimator of the limiting variance of central and intermediate order statistics for a fixed and finite $d \geq 1$. For the sample median, we show that the limit distribution depends on whether $n - d$ approaches infinity through even or odd values.

Section 2 formally introduces two JK variance estimators and known limit results on spacings around a specified central or intermediate order statistic. Section 3 discusses the limit distribution of the commonly used delete-d JK estimators of the variance of $X_{k:n}$ for the central and upper intermediate cases for a finite d. Section 4 focuses on the limit distribution of the JK variance estimator of the sample median. Section 5 contains a short discussion of our results.

Now, some notation for quick reference. Equality in distribution, convergence in distribution, and convergence in probability will be denoted respectively by $\stackrel{D}{=}$, $\xrightarrow{D}$, and $\xrightarrow{P}$. For two sequences a_n and b_n, we write $a_n \approx b_n$ if $a_n/b_n \to 1$ as $n \to \infty$.

For two sequences of random variables (rvs) A_n and B_n, we write $A_n \stackrel{D}{\approx} B_n$ if $A_n/B_n \stackrel{P}{\to} 1$. A standard exponential rv will be denoted by Z or $Z_i, i \geq 1$. The sum of m independent standard exponential rvs is a $Gamma(\eta = m, \beta = 1)$ rv where η and β are, respectively, the shape and scale parameters. With $\eta = m/2$ and $\beta = 2$, we obtain a $\chi^2_{(m)}$ rv with m degrees of freedom. A Weibull distribution with shape parameter η and scale parameter β will be denoted by $Wei(\eta, \beta)$. A normal rv with mean μ and variance σ^2 is represented by $N(\mu, \sigma^2)$. A binomial rv with n trials and success probability p will be represented by $Bin(n, p)$ and its cdf is given by $F_B(\cdot; n, p)$.

We note that rvs $(\chi^2_{(2)}/2)^2$, $Wei(1, 1/2)$, and Z^2 are identically distributed with pdf

$$f(w) = \frac{1}{2\sqrt{w}} e^{-\sqrt{w}}, \; w \geq 0. \tag{4}$$

Furthermore, for an rv Y with finite variance $Var(Y)$,

$$Var(Y) = \frac{1}{2} E(Y_1 - Y_2)^2, \tag{5}$$

where Y_1 and Y_2 are independent copies of Y.

2 Preliminaries

We now introduce some known results on jackknife estimators and spacings of order statistics in a neighborhood.

2.1 *Jackknife Estimators of Variance of an Estimator*

Let θ be a (scalar) parameter and $\hat{\theta}_n$ be its estimator based on a random sample of size n. Define $\mathcal{S}_{n,n-d}$ to be the family of all $\binom{n}{d}$ subsets B with $n - d$ observations, obtained by dropping d observations from the sample. Let $\hat{\theta}_{n-d}(B)$ denote the estimator based on the subset $B \in \mathcal{S}_{n,n-d}$, and $\bar{\hat{\theta}}$ be the average of these $\binom{n}{d}$ estimators. Then $\bar{\hat{\theta}}$ is the JK estimator of θ that is associated with $\hat{\theta}_n$.

The classical delete-d JK estimator of the variance of $\sqrt{n}\hat{\theta}_n$ is (Shao and Tu 1995, p. 50–51)

$$V_n(d) = \frac{n-d}{d\binom{n}{d}} \sum_{B \in \mathcal{S}_{n,n-d}} \left(\hat{\theta}_{n-d}(B) - \bar{\hat{\theta}}\right)^2. \tag{6}$$

Shao and Wu (1989) propose another JK estimator

$$V_{2,n}(d) = \frac{n-d}{d\binom{n}{d}} \sum_{B \in \mathcal{S}_{n,n-d}} \left(\hat{\theta}_{n-d}(B) - \hat{\theta}_n\right)^2 = V_n(d) + \frac{n-d}{d}\left(\bar{\hat{\theta}} - \hat{\theta}_n\right)^2. \quad (7)$$

For us, $\theta = x_p$ and $\hat{\theta}_n$ is the sample quantile $X_{k:n}$ with $k = [np] + 1, 0 < p < 1$, for the central case and $p = k/n \to 1$ such that $(n - k) \to \infty$ for the upper intermediate case.

For $d = 1$ and $0 < p < 1$, Martin (1990) has shown that $V_n(1)$ can be expressed as

$$(n-1)\frac{(n-1-[(n-1)p])([(n-1)p]+1)}{n^2}\left(X_{([(n-1)p]+2):n} - X_{([(n-1)p]+1):n}\right)^2, \quad (8)$$

and that $nV_n(1)/\sigma_p^2 \xrightarrow{D} Wei(1, 1/2)$ (i.e., Z^2) with pdf given by (4).

2.2 *Joint Limit Distribution of Spacings in a Neighborhood*

All of the JK estimators of the limiting variance of $X_{k:n}$ are continuous functions of a finite number of spacings (that is, the difference between consecutive order statistics) in its neighborhood. Therefore, we need the joint limiting distribution of these spacings. It is given below, and is taken from Theorems 2a and 3 of Nagaraja et al. (2015). See the references therein for earlier work.

Lemma 1

(a) Let $k/n \to p \in (0, 1)$, and a and b be fixed positive integers. Assume $f(x_p)$ is positive and finite and f is continuous at x_p. Then

$$\left(nf(x_p)(X_{k+j:n} - X_{k+j-1:n}), -(a-1) \le j \le b\right) \xrightarrow{D} (Z_1, \ldots, Z_{a+b}).$$

(b) Let one of the three Von Mises conditions (von Mises 1936; David and Nagaraja 2003, p. 299–300) hold, and $n, k, n-k \to \infty$ such that $k/n = p_n \to 1$. Then,

$$\left(nf(x_{p_n})(X_{k+j:n} - X_{k+j-1:n}), -(a-1) \le j \le b\right) \xrightarrow{D} (Z_1, \ldots, Z_{a+b}).$$

In both cases, the Z's are independent and identically distributed (i.i.d.) standard exponential rvs.

3 Delete-*d* Jackknife Estimators of the Variance of $X_{k:n}$

We now present results on the limiting properties of the jackknife estimators of the variance for the central and intermediate cases.

3.1 *The Central Case*

For a central quantile x_p, we have $\hat{\theta}_n = X_{k:n}$ where $k = [np] + 1$, and for a chosen subset B of size $n-d$ in $\mathcal{S}_{n,n-d}$, $\hat{\theta}_{n-d}(B) = X_{s:n-d}(B)$, where $s = [(n-d)p]+1$. Then, conditioned on the observed order statistics $x_{1:n} < \cdots < x_{n:n}$ from the entire sample, $X_{s:n-d}(B)$ takes $d + 1$ distinct values $x_{s:n} < \cdots < x_{s+d:n}$ depending on the configuration of the d dropped order statistics.

Let $w_n(i)$ denote the proportion among $\binom{n}{d}$ subsamples that yield $X_{s:n-d}(B) = x_{s+i:n}$. Then,

$$w_n(i) = P(i \text{ values below } x_{s+i:n} \text{ and } (d-i) \text{ values above } x_{s+i:n} \text{ are dropped})$$

$$= \frac{\binom{i+s-1}{i}\binom{n-i-s}{d-i}}{\binom{n}{d}}, \quad 0 \le i \le d, \tag{9}$$

represents a hypergeometric probability. These weights have also been given by Shao (1988). With $\bar{\hat{\theta}}$ representing the weighted average of $X_{s+i:n}$, and $\hat{\theta}_n = X_{k:n}$, we obtain respectively from (6) and (7),

$$V_n(d) = \frac{n-d}{d} \sum_{i=0}^{d} w_n(i)(X_{s+i:n} - \bar{\hat{\theta}}\,)^2, \text{ and} \tag{10}$$

$$V_{2,n}(d) = \frac{n-d}{d} \sum_{i=0}^{d} w_n(i)(X_{s+i:n} - \hat{\theta}_n)^2. \tag{11}$$

The sum in (10) can be viewed as the variance of a discrete rv Y taking on the value $X_{s+i:n}$ with probability $w_n(i)$, for $i = 0, \ldots, d$. Using (5), this sum can be expressed as

$$\sum_{i=0}^{d} w_n(i)\left(X_{s+i:n} - \bar{\hat{\theta}}\right)^2 = \frac{1}{2}\sum_{i=0}^{d}\sum_{j=0}^{d} w_n(i)w_n(j)(X_{s+j:n} - X_{s+i:n})^2$$

$$= \sum_{i=0}^{d-1}\sum_{j=i+1}^{d} w_n(i)w_n(j)(X_{s+j:n} - X_{s+i:n})^2.$$

As $n \to \infty$, $s/n \to p$ and $w_n(i) \to \binom{d}{i}p^i(1-p)^{d-i}$. Also, from part (a) of Lemma 1, $\{nf(x_p)\}^2(X_{s+j:n} - X_{s+i:n})^2 \xrightarrow{D} \left(\sum_{l=i+1}^{j} Z_l\right)^2$, where the Z_l, $l \geq 1$, are i.i.d. standard exponential rvs. Now define

$$T_i = \sum_{l=0}^{i} Z_l, 0 \leq i \leq d, \text{ with } Z_0 \equiv 0, \tag{12}$$

and note that $\sum_{l=i+1}^{j} Z_l = T_j - T_i$. Thus, we have proved the following result.

Proposition 1 *For $0 < p < 1$, take $k = [np] + 1$, and assume that $0 < f(x_p) < \infty$, and f is continuous at x_p. Then the first delete-d JK estimator of the variance of $\sqrt{n}X_{k:n}$ in (6) can be expressed as*

$$V_n(d) = \frac{n-d}{d} \sum_{i=0}^{d} \sum_{j=i+1}^{d} w_n(i)w_n(j)(X_{s+j:n} - X_{s+i:n})^2; \tag{13}$$

and

$$n\{f(x_p)\}^2 V_n(d) \xrightarrow{D} \frac{1}{d} \sum_{i=0}^{d-1} \sum_{j=i+1}^{d} \binom{d}{i}\binom{d}{j} p^{i+j}(1-p)^{2d-i-j} \left(T_j - T_i\right)^2, \tag{14}$$

$$= \frac{1}{d} \sum_{i=0}^{d} \binom{d}{i} p^i(1-p)^{d-i} \left(T_i - \overline{T}\right)^2 \equiv V(d;p) \tag{15}$$

where $s = [(n-d)p] + 1$, the $w_n(i)$ are given in (9), T_i in (12), and $\overline{T}$ is the binomially weighted average of these T_i's.

Equivalence of the sums in (14) and (15) is established by appealing again to (5).

When $d = 1$, the expression for the limiting rv $V(d;p)$ simplifies to $p(1-p)Z^2$, and the above proposition essentially reduces to Theorem 2.1 of Martin (1990). This is a scaled Weibull rv (Z^2) whose pdf is given in (4) and is unbounded near 0.

For $d > 1$, obtaining a closed form for the limiting pdf is too cumbersome. Therefore, we simulate $V(d;p)$ starting with i.i.d. rvs $Z_1, \ldots, Z_d$ and approximate the pdf of $V(d;p)$. Figure 1 provides these approximations for selected p and d. It shows that the limiting pdf of the JK variance estimator is bounded for $d > 1$, is positively skewed, and the skewness decreases as d increases. For a fixed d, skewness decreases as p approaches 0.5. Further, the pdf of $V(d;p)$ is symmetric around $p = 0.5$.

Convergence in distribution, established above, does not ensure the convergence of moments. In particular, to provide an asymptotically unbiased estimator of σ_p^2 that is a function of $nV_n(d)$, we need to examine the limit behavior of the

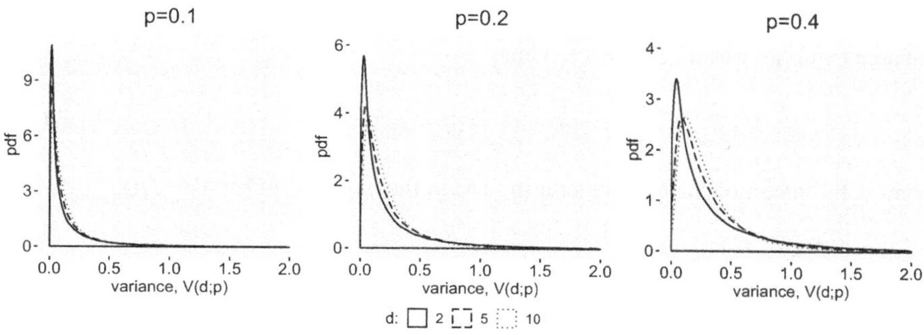

Fig. 1 Simulated pdfs of the limiting rv $V(d; p)$ for $d = 2, 5, 10$ and for $p = 0.1, 0.2$, and 0.4. (Smoothed density created from 100,000 simulations of V and uses a Gaussian kernel)

sequence $nE\{V_n(d)\}$. This can be done under additional smoothness conditions on the behavior of f around x_p, and is given below.

Proposition 2 *For $0 < p < 1$, take $k = [np] + 1$, assume that $0 < f(x_p) < \infty$, and that f has bounded derivative in a neighborhood of x_p. Further, assume that F has a finite mean. Then, as $n \to \infty$,*

$$n\{f(x_p)\}^2 E\{V_n(d)\} \to p(1-p)\left\{1 + \frac{E|Y_1 - Y_2|}{2dp(1-p)}\right\}, \tag{16}$$

where $V_n(d)$ is given by (13), and Y_1 and Y_2 are i.i.d. Bin(n, p) rvs.

Proof With the rv $V(d; p)$ given on the right side of (15), first we establish under our assumed conditions that $nE\{V_n(d)\} \to E\{V(d; p)\}$. Next, we show that $E\{V(d; p)\}$ has the form given in (16).

Under the finite mean and smoothness assumptions, it follows from Reiss (1989, p. 207) that for $s = [np] + O(n^{-1})$, $nE(X_{s:n} - x_p)^2 \to \sigma_p^2$. Thus, $nE(X_{s:n} - x_p)^2$ is a bounded sequence. Consider

$$\begin{aligned} E(X_{s+j:n} - X_{s+i:n})^2 &= E(X_{s+j:n} - x_p)^2 + E(X_{s+i:n} - x_p)^2 \\ &\quad - 2E(X_{s+i:n} - x_p)(X_{s+j:n} - x_p). \end{aligned}$$

Since $X_{s+i:n}$ and $X_{s+j:n}$ are associated rvs (Esary et al. 1967), the product moment is nonnegative (actually positive) and hence

$$E(X_{s+j:n} - X_{s+i:n})^2 \leq E(X_{s+j:n} - x_p)^2 + E(X_{s+i:n} - x_p)^2.$$

Since both terms on the right are bounded, each of the terms in the finite sum on the right in (13) is bounded as well. Consequently, $nE\{V_n(d)\}$ is a bounded sequence. This fact, along with the convergence in distribution proved in Proposition 1, establishes the moment convergence (see, e.g., Chung 1974, p. 95).

From (12) it follows that $T_j - T_i = \sum_{l=i+1}^{j} Z_l$ is a $Gamma(j-i, 1)$ rv with mean as well as variance $(j-i)$. Thus,

$$E\left(T_j - T_i\right)^2 = (j-i) + (j-i)^2, \quad 0 \le i < j \le d. \tag{17}$$

Hence, the mean of the double sum in (15) in the expression for $V(d;p)$,

$$\begin{aligned}
&\sum_{i=0}^{d-1}\sum_{j=i+1}^{d}\binom{d}{i}\binom{d}{j}p^{i+j}(1-p)^{2d-i-j}E\left(T_j - T_i\right)^2 \\
&= \sum_{i=0}^{d-1}\sum_{j=i+1}^{d}\binom{d}{i}\binom{d}{j}p^{i+j}(1-p)^{2d-i-j}\left\{(j-i)+(j-i)^2\right\} \\
&= \frac{1}{2}\sum_{i=0}^{d}\sum_{j=0}^{d}\binom{d}{i}\binom{d}{j}p^{i+j}(1-p)^{2d-i-j}|j-i| \\
&\quad + \frac{1}{2}\sum_{i=0}^{d}\sum_{j=0}^{d}\binom{d}{i}\binom{d}{j}p^{i+j}(1-p)^{2d-i-j}(j-i)^2.
\end{aligned} \tag{18}$$

Let Y be a $Bin(d, p)$ rv and Y_1 and Y_2 be independent copies of Y. The first term in (18) can be viewed as $\frac{1}{2}E|Y_1 - Y_2|$, and from (5), the second term represents $Var(Y) = dp(1-p)$. Hence, (14) leads us to conclude that

$$E(V(d;p)) = \frac{1}{d}\left\{\frac{1}{2}E|Y_1 - Y_2| + dp(1-p)\right\} = p(1-p)\left\{1 + \frac{E|Y_1 - Y_2|}{2dp(1-p)}\right\}.$$

□

Simple expressions are available for $E|Y_1 - Y_2|$, the mean of the sample range from a random sample of size 2 from a binomial distribution. From Siotani (1956), we conclude that

$$E|Y_1 - Y_2| = 2\sum_{i=0}^{d-1} F_B(i;d,p)(1 - F_B(i;d,p)). \tag{19}$$

The expression in (19) can be computed for any d and p.

Proposition 2 implies that

$$E(nV_n(d)) \approx \sigma_p^2\left\{1 + \frac{E|Y_1 - Y_2|}{2dp(1-p)}\right\}.$$

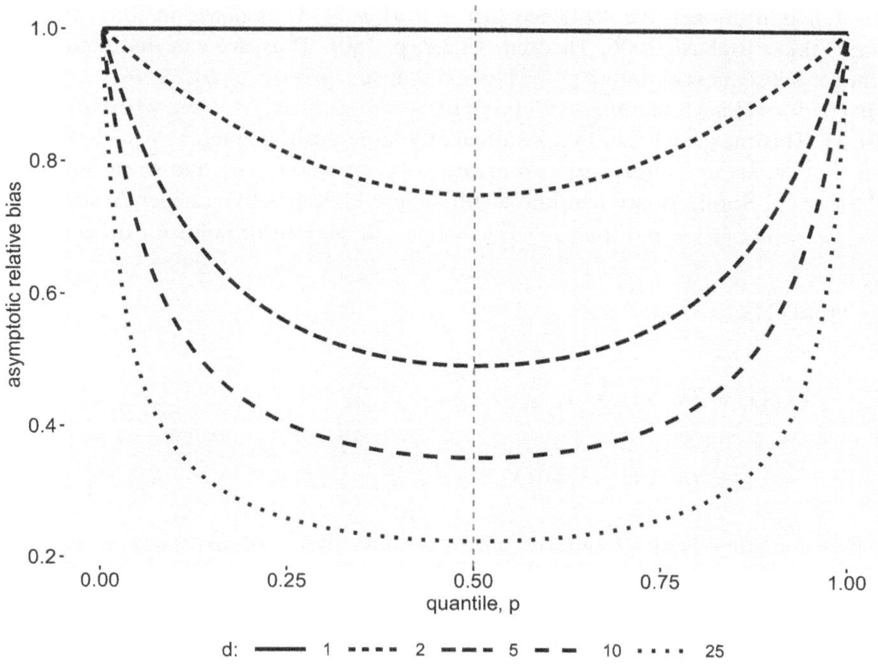

Fig. 2 The asymptotic relative bias of the d-delete JK estimator $nV_n(d)$ as an estimator of σ_p^2 for $0 < p < 1$ and selected $d \geq 1$

Hence the asymptotic relative bias of $nV_n(d)$ in estimating σ_p^2 is $E|Y_1 - Y_2|/(2dp(1-p))$. Figure 2 shows this quantity for selected $d \geq 1$ and $p \in (0, 1)$; we can see that the relative bias is symmetric around 0.5. When $d = 1$, $E|Y_1 - Y_2|$ simplifies to $2p(1-p)$ and hence the relative bias is constant at 1. For fixed p, the asymptotic relative bias decreases as d increases, and for fixed d, it decreases as p approaches 0.5.

While $nV_n(d)$ converges in distribution to a rv $V(d; p)$ that has a closed form representation (given in (14) or (15)), we now show that the limit distribution of $nV_{2,n}(d)$ does not exist when d is finite. For this first we show the following.

Lemma 2 *For any* $p \in (0, 1)$ *there exist distinct subsequences of positive integers* n *satisfying one of the following conditions: (i)* $[(n-1)p] = [np]$*; or (ii)* $[(n-1)p] = [np] - 1$.

Proof Suppose p is rational. Then there exist positive integers a and b such that $p = a/b$ or $a = bp$. Let $n = mb + 1$ where m is an arbitrary positive integer. Then $[np] = [mbp + p] = ma$ and $[(n-1)p] = [np - p] = [mbp] = ma$. So, (i) holds for $n = mb + 1$. Now with $n = mb$, we have $[np] = ma$ and $[(n-1)p] = [mbp - p] = [ma - 1] = ma - 1$; that is, (ii) holds.

If p is irrational, the sequence $\{np - [np], n \geq 1\}$ is dense in [0, 1] (Miller and Takloo-Bighash 2006, Theorem 12.2.2, p. 280). Thus, we can find increasing integer subsequences $\{m_{1,j}, j \geq 1\}$ such that $m_{1,j}p - [m_{1,j}p] \to \theta_1 > p$, and $\{m_{2,j}, j \geq 1\}$ such that $m_{2,j}p - [m_{2,j}p] \to \theta_2 < p$, as $j \to \infty$, where $\theta_1, \theta_2 \in (0, 1)$. This means we can find a sufficiently large positive integer N such that for all $j > N$, $m_{1,j}p > [m_{1,j}p] + p$ or $(m_{1,j} - 1)p > [m_{1,j}p]$, and so (i) holds for these $m_{1,j}$. Similarly, we can find a sufficiently large positive integer N such that $m_{2,j}p < [m_{2,j}p] + p$ or $(m_{2,j} - 1)p < [m_{2,j}p]$, and so (ii) holds for these $m_{2,j}$. □

From (11),

$$\begin{aligned} V_{2,n}(1) &= (n-1)\sum_{i=0}^{1} w_n(i)(X_{s+i:n} - X_{k:n})^2 \\ &= (n-1)\left\{w_n(0)(X_{s:n} - X_{k:n})^2 + w_n(1)(X_{s+1:n} - X_{k:n})^2\right\}, \qquad (20) \end{aligned}$$

where $s = [(n-1)p] + 1$ and $k = [np] + 1$. Of the two terms in the sum above, one always vanishes. Using Lemma 2, we conclude that there exist integer subsequences $m_{1,j}, j \geq 1$, such that

$$V_{2,m_{1,j}}(1) = (m_{1,j} - 1)w_{m_{1,j}}(1)(X_{[m_{1,j}p]+2:n} - X_{[m_{1,j}p]+1:n})^2,$$

and subsequences $m_{2,j}, j \geq 1$, such that

$$V_{2,m_{2,j}}(1) = (m_{2,j} - 1)w_{m_{2,j}}(0)(X_{[m_{2,j}p]+1:n} - X_{[m_{2,j}p]:n})^2.$$

We know that $w_n(i) \to p^i(1-p)^{1-i}$ as $n \to \infty$. Consequently, we conclude that, as $j \to \infty$,

$$m_{1,j}\{f(x_p)\}^2 V_{2,m_{1,j}}(1) \xrightarrow{D} pZ^2; \quad m_{2,j}\{f(x_p)\}^2 V_{2,m_{2,j}}(1) \xrightarrow{D} (1-p)Z^2.$$

Thus, the limit distributions are distinct unless $p = 0.5$. When $p = 0.5$, condition (i) of Lemma 2 holds when n is odd; when n is even, condition (ii) holds. Thus for both odd and even sequences the limit distributions coincide. Hence, we have proved the following result.

Proposition 3 *As in Proposition 1, take $0 < p < 1$, $k = [np] + 1$, and assume that $0 < f(x_p) < \infty$, and f is continuous at x_p. Consider the second delete-1 JK estimator of the variance of $\sqrt{n}X_{k:n}$, given by*

$$V_{2,n}(1) = (n-1)\sum_{i=0}^{1} w_n(i)(X_{s+i:n} - X_{k:n})^2,$$

where the $w_n(i)$ are defined in (9). The sequence $\{nV_{2,n}(1), n \geq 1\}$ does not converge in distribution if $p \neq 0.5$. When $p = 0.5$, however,

$$nV_{2,n}(1) \xrightarrow{D} \frac{1}{2\{f(x_{0.5})\}^2} Z^2. \tag{21}$$

Remarks

1. Non-existence of the limit distribution for $nV_{2,n}(d)$ for $p \neq 0.5$ can be established for $d > 1$ as well. The key point is that only one term among the $d+1$ terms constituting (11) vanishes and we can choose subsequences for which we can make a specified term vanish, resulting in different limit distributions.
2. When $p = 0.5$ we have shown that the limit distribution of $nV_{2,n}(1)$ exists and is given in (21). This limit distribution differs from that of $nV_n(1)$ (denoted as $V(1; 0.5)$) given in Proposition 1. In fact, the limit distributions of $2nV_n(1)$ and $nV_{2,n}(1)$ are identical.
3. When $p = 0.5$, x_p is the population median. The corresponding sample quantile is the sample median $\hat{\theta}_{n-d}$ that is computed differently for even and odd values of $(n - d)$. The limit distribution of $nV_n(d)$ given in Proposition 1 holds if $n - d$ remains odd (where the sample median of the subsample is a single order statistic), and does not hold if $n - d$ remains even as it approaches infinity. See Sect. 4 for a detailed discussion.

3.2 *Intermediate Case*

We focus on the upper intermediate case where $k = [np_n] + 1$ with $p_n \to 1$, but $(n - k) \approx n(1 - p_n) \to \infty$. A similar approach can be used for the lower intermediate case (i.e., $k/n \to 0$) and is not presented.

The expression for $V_n(d)$ remains the same as in the central case, as given in (13) of Proposition 1, and weights $w_n(i)$ given in (9), but with $s = [(n - d)p_n] + 1$.

We first examine the limit behavior of the weight $w_n(i)$ for $0 \leq i \leq d$. Upon simplification, we obtain

$$\begin{aligned} w_n(i) &= \frac{\binom{i+s-1}{i}\binom{n-i-s}{d-i}}{\binom{n}{d}} = \frac{d!}{i!(d-i)!} \times \prod_{l=1}^{i} \frac{i+s-l}{n+1-l} \times \prod_{l=1}^{d-i} \frac{n-s-d+l}{n-d+l} \\ &= \eta_1 \times \eta_2 \times \eta_3, \end{aligned} \tag{22}$$

where η_1 is free of n, η_2 is made up of i factors and is to be interpreted as 1 when $i = 0$, and η_3 consists of $(d - i)$ factors and is interpreted as 1 when $i = d$. Hence for all $i \geq 0$, η_2 approaches 1 since $s/n \to 1$. Each of the $(d - i)$ factors of η_3 approaches 0 as $(n - s)/n \to 0$. Thus, when we consider the product $w_n(i)w_n(j)$ appearing in (13) with $i < j$, we have $(2d - i - j)$ factors that approach 0. The number of such factors will be the smallest at 1 when $i = d - 1$, $j = i + 1 = d$. From (22) it follows that

$$w_n(d-1)w_n(d) = d\prod_{l=1}^{d-1}\left(\frac{d-1+s-l}{n+1-l}\right)\prod_{l=1}^{d}\left(\frac{d+s-l}{n+1-d}\right)\frac{n-s-d+1}{n-d+1}$$
$$\approx d \times 1 \times 1 \times \frac{(n-d)(1-p_n)}{n-d} \approx d(1-p_n),$$

where the asymptotic approximation holds since $s = [(n-d)p_n] + 1$ and $p_n \to 1$. From the representation for $V_n(d)$ given in (13) it follows that

$$\frac{n}{1-p_n}\{f(x_{p_n})\}^2 V_n(d) \overset{D}{\approx} \left\{nf(x_{p_n})(X_{s+d-1:n} - X_{s+d:n})\right\}^2.$$

Under the regularity conditions due to von Mises (1936), we can use part (b) of Lemma 1 to establish the following result.

Proposition 4 *Let one of the three Von Mises conditions hold, $n, k, n-k \to \infty$ such that $k/n = p_n \to 1$, and $x_{p_n} = F^{-1}(p_n)$. Then*

$$\frac{n}{1-p_n}\{f(x_{p_n})\}^2 V_n(d) \overset{D}{\to} Z^2 = Wei(1, 1/2).$$

The pdf of the limit distribution established above is given by (4) and is free of d; it matches the result for $d = 1$ in the central case. The limit distribution of $nV_n(1)$ in the intermediate case was established earlier by Peng and Yang (2009).

4 Delete-*d* Jackknife Estimator of the Variance of the Sample Median

Miller (1974) stated that Moses (in an unpublished note) was the first to observe the inconsistency of the delete-1 JK variance estimator of the sample median for even-sized samples. Efron (1982, Sec. 3.4, p. 16) has shown that, for even sample sizes, the limit distribution of $4n\{f(x_{0.5})\}^2 V_n(1)$ is $\{\chi^2_{(2)}/2\}^2$; the pdf of this rv is given by (4). The limit properties of $V_n(d)$ for a finite $d > 1$ and an even n, and for any finite $d \geq 1$ and an odd n, have not been examined. As we see below, the limit depends on whether $n - d$ remains odd or even.

When $n - d$ is odd, the sample median based on a subsample of size $n - d$ is a single order statistic of the form $X_{(n-d+1)/2:n-d}(B)$ where $B \in \mathcal{S}_{n,n-d}$ is a subset of size $n - d$ from $X_{1:n} < \cdots < X_{n:n}$. Thus, Proposition 1 applies.

When $n - d$ is even, the median of the subsample is the average of two central order statistics. Let $s = \frac{1}{2}(n-d)$ so that $n = 2s + d$. Then $\hat{\theta}_B =$

$(X_{s:n-d}(B) + X_{s+1:n-d}(B))/2$ is the median for the subsample generated by the subset B. Conditioned on the observed order statistics $x_{1:n} < \cdots < x_{n:n}$ of the entire sample, possible values of $\hat{\theta}_B$ are of the form $(x_{s+i:n} + x_{s+j:n})/2$ with $0 \le i < j \le d+1$. Let $w_n(i, j)$ denote the associated proportion of subsamples among $\binom{n}{n-d}$ such samples. This is a hypergeometric probability given by

$$w_n(i,j) = \frac{\binom{i+s-1}{s-1}\binom{j-i-1}{0}\binom{s+d-j}{s-1}}{\binom{2s+d}{2s}}, \quad 0 \le i < j \le d+1, \text{ and}$$

$$V_n(d) = \frac{n-d}{d} \sum_{i=0}^{d} \sum_{j=i+1}^{d+1} w_n(i,j) \left((X_{s+i:n} + X_{s+j:n})/2 - \bar{\hat{\theta}} \right)^2, \tag{23}$$

where the $w_n(i, j)$ are nonnegative and sum to 1, and $\bar{\hat{\theta}}$ is the weighted average of $(X_{s+i:n} + X_{s+j:n})/2$ values. The weights can be expressed as

$$\begin{aligned} w_n(i,j) = \frac{\binom{i+s-1}{i}\binom{s+d-j}{d+1-j}}{\binom{2s+d}{2s}} &= \frac{d!}{i!(d-j+1)!} \\ &\times \frac{\{(i+s-1)\cdots s\}\{(s+d-j)\cdots s\}}{(2s+d)\cdots(2s+1)}, \end{aligned} \tag{24}$$

where the product $\{(i+s-1)\cdots s\}$ in the numerator of the second factor is interpreted as 1 when $i = 0$, the product $\{(s+d-j)\cdots s\}$ is interpreted as 1 when $j = d+1$, and the numerator itself is 1 when $i = 0, j = d+1$. Further, only the second factor depends on $s = (n-d)/2$ and hence we investigate its limit behavior as $s \to \infty$. It has d factors in the denominator and $d + (i + 1 - j)$ factors in the numerator. Thus, the ratio goes to 0 as $s \to \infty$ if $j > i+1$ and to $(1/2)^d$ when $j = i+1$.

Consequently, we conclude using (24) that $w_n(i, j) \to 0$ if $j > i+1$, and $w_n(i, i+1) \to \binom{d}{i}\left(\frac{1}{2}\right)^d$ as $n \to \infty$. From (23) it now follows that the limit distribution of $nV_n(d)$ is the same as that of the sequence

$$\frac{n^2}{d} \sum_{i=0}^{d} \binom{d}{i} \left(\frac{1}{2}\right)^d \left((X_{s+i:n} + X_{s+i+1:n})/2 - \bar{\hat{\theta}} \right)^2.$$

In view of (5), the above expression can be seen as a function of a finite number of spacings in the neighborhood of a central order statistic. Define

$$T_i^* = \frac{T_i + T_{i+1}}{2} = \sum_{l=0}^{i} \frac{1}{2}(Z_l + Z_{l+1}),\ i = 0, \ldots, d,\ Z_0 \equiv 0, \tag{25}$$

where the T_i's are given by (12). Let $\overline{T}^*$ be the weighted average of the T_i^* with weights given by $Bin(d, 1/2)$ probabilities. Then, from part (a) of Lemma 1 it follows that

$$\{nf(x_{0.5})\}^2 \frac{1}{d} \sum_{i=0}^{d} \binom{d}{i} \left(\frac{1}{2}\right)^d \left(\frac{(X_{s+i:n} + X_{s+i+1:n})}{2} - \bar{\hat{\theta}}\right)^2$$

$$\xrightarrow{D} \frac{1}{d} \sum_{i=0}^{d} \binom{d}{i} \left(\frac{1}{2}\right)^d \left(T_i^* - \overline{T}^*\right)^2.$$

This discussion leads to the following.

Proposition 5 *Assume* $0 < f(x_{0.5}) < \infty$ *and* f *is continuous at* $x_{0.5}$*. Let the delete-d JK estimator of the variance of the sample median from a sample of size n, represented by (6) be denoted by* $V_n(d)$*.*

(a) If $n \to \infty$ *such that* $n - d$ *remains even,* $V_n(d)$ *has the form given in (23) with* $s = (n - d)/2$*, and*

$$n\{f(x_{0.5})\}^2 V_n(d) \xrightarrow{D} \frac{1}{d} \sum_{i=0}^{d} \binom{d}{i} \left(\frac{1}{2}\right)^d \left(T_i^* - \overline{T}^*\right)^2 \equiv V^*(d; 0.5), \quad (26)$$

where the T_i^* *are given in (25), and* $\overline{T}^*$ *is their binomially weighted average.*

(b) If $n - d$ *remains odd and* $n \to \infty$*,* $V_n(d)$ *has the form given in (13) with* $s = [(n - d)/2] + 1$*, and (from Proposition 1),*

$$n\{f(x_{0.5})\}^2 V_n(d) \xrightarrow{D} \frac{1}{d} \sum_{i=0}^{d} \binom{d}{i} \left(\frac{1}{2}\right)^d (T_i - \overline{T})^2 \equiv V(d; 0.5), \quad (27)$$

where the T_i *are given in (12), and* $\overline{T}$ *is their binomially weighted average.*

The rvs $V(d; 0.5)$ and $V^*(d; 0.5)$ given above are identical functions of different sets of rvs and thus it follows that the limit distribution of $nV_n(d)$ is different for even and odd values of $n-d$. Hence the sequence $\{nV_n(d), n \geq 1\}$ does not converge in distribution as $n \to \infty$.

We now illustrate the difference between the distributions of $V(d; 0.5)$ and $V^*(d; 0.5)$ for selected small d values.

With $d = 1$, upon simplification, it follows that

$$V(1; 0.5) \stackrel{D}{=} \frac{1}{4} Z_1^2 \equiv \frac{1}{4} W; \; V^*(1; 0.5) \stackrel{D}{=} \frac{1}{4} \left(\frac{Z_1 + Z_2}{2}\right)^2 \equiv \frac{1}{4} W^*.$$

The pdf of W, $f_W(w)$, is given by (4) and its cdf is given by

$$F_W(w) = 1 - e^{-\sqrt{w}}, w \geq 0. \tag{28}$$

The pdf and cdf of W^* are given respectively by

$$f_{W^*}(w) = 2e^{-2\sqrt{w}}; \text{ and } F^*_W(w) = 1 - e^{-2\sqrt{w}}\left(1 + 2\sqrt{w}\right), w \geq 0. \tag{29}$$

The pdf $f_W(w)$ is unbounded near 0 and has thicker tail than $f_{W^*}(w)$ on both ends of its support, $(0, \infty)$. The latter pdf is bounded, and dominates in the middle region $(0.128, 4.637)$ whose endpoints have been determined by solving $f_W(w) = f_{W^*}(w)$. The means of W and W^* are, respectively, 2 and 1.5, and the variances are 20 and 5.25. The means can be used to scale $nV_n(1)$ appropriately (n even or odd) to suggest an asymptotically unbiased estimate of the quantile density function $1/f(x_{0.5})$.

We can obtain an approximate 95% confidence interval for $1/f(x_{0.5})$ (or for $f(x_{0.5})$) using the percentiles of W or W^* that can be obtained from (28) and (29). The 2.5th and 97.5th percentiles of W are 0.0006 and 13.6078, and of W^* are 0.0147 and 7.761, respectively. When n is even (that is, $n - 1$ is odd), we use the former set of percentiles and when n is odd, we use the latter.

For $d > 1$, analytical expressions for the pdfs of $V(d; 0.5)$ and $V^*(d; 0.5)$ become too complex. We simulate these rvs starting with i.i.d. rvs $Z_1, \ldots, Z_d$ and find approximations to their pdfs for $d = 2$ and $d = 5$. They are reported in Fig. 3. The plot shows that for the chosen d values, the pdfs of $V(d; 0.5)$ and $V^*(d; 0.5)$ are both positively skewed, and both tails of the former are thicker than that of the latter. Further, the skewness decreases as d increases.

A closed form expression for $E\{V(d; 0.5)\}$ is available in Proposition 2, namely,

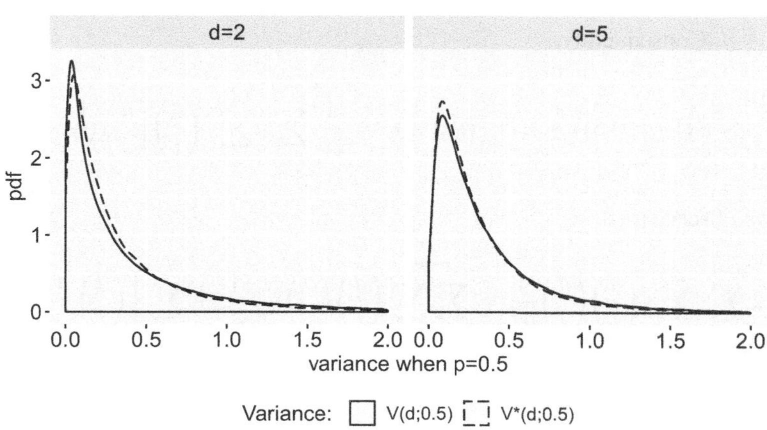

Fig. 3 Simulated pdfs of $V(d; 0.5)$ and $V^*(d; 0.5)$ for $d = 2$ and $d = 5$. (Smoothed density created from 100,000 simulations of V and V^* and uses a Gaussian kernel)

$$E\{V(d;0.5)\} = \frac{1}{4d}\{d + 2E|Y_1 - Y_2|\},$$

where Y_1 and Y_2 are i.i.d. $Bin(n, 1/2)$ rvs.

To derive an expression for $E\{V^*(d;0.5)\}$ we proceed as follows. As in Proposition 2, consider an alternative expression for $V^*(d;0.5)$ given by

$$\frac{1}{d}\sum_{i=0}^{d-1}\sum_{j=i+1}^{d}\binom{d}{i}\binom{d}{j}\left(\frac{1}{2}\right)^{2d}\left(T_j^* - T_i^*\right)^2, \tag{30}$$

where the T_i^* are defined in (25). Therefore,

$$\begin{aligned} E\left(T_j^* - T_i^*\right)^2 &= E\left\{\frac{1}{2}(Z_{i+1} + Z_{j+1}) + \sum_{l=i+2}^{j} Z_l\right\}^2 \\ &= Var\left\{\frac{1}{2}(Z_{i+1} + Z_{j+1}) + \sum_{l=i+2}^{j} Z_l\right\} \\ &\quad + \left\{\frac{1}{2}E(Z_{i+1} + Z_{j+1}) + \sum_{l=i+2}^{j} E(Z_l)\right\}^2 \\ &= \left(j - i - \frac{1}{2}\right) + (j-i)^2 = E(T_j - T_i)^2 - \frac{1}{2}, \end{aligned} \tag{31}$$

where the last equality follows from (17). The final form in (31) holds for all $0 \le i < j \le d$. Consequently,

$$E\{V(d;0.5)\} - E\{V^*(d;0.5)\} = \frac{1}{2d}\sum_{i=0}^{d-1}\sum_{j=i+1}^{d}\binom{d}{i}\binom{d}{j}\frac{1}{4^d}. \tag{32}$$

We now observe that

$$\begin{aligned} 2\sum_{i=0}^{d-1}\sum_{j=i+1}^{d}\binom{d}{i}\binom{d}{j}\frac{1}{4^d} &= \sum_{i=0}^{d}\sum_{j=0}^{d}\binom{d}{i}\binom{d}{j}\frac{1}{2^d}\frac{1}{2^d} - \sum_{i=0}^{d}\left\{\binom{d}{i}\frac{1}{2^d}\right\}^2 \\ &= 1 - \sum_{i=0}^{d}\left\{\binom{d}{i}\frac{1}{2^d}\right\}^2 = 1 - P(Y_1 = Y_2), \end{aligned}$$

where Y_1 and Y_2 are i.i.d. $Bin(d, 1/2)$ rvs. Upon using the above simplification, we conclude from (32) that

$$E\{V(d;0.5)\} - E\{V^*(d;0.5)\} = \frac{1}{4d}\{P(Y_1 \neq Y_2)\}. \tag{33}$$

Assuming the existence of the mean and that f' is bounded in a neighborhood of $x_{0.5}$, one can show that $E\{nV_n(d)\} \to E\{V^*(d;0.5)\}$ as $(n-d) \to \infty$ through even values. Details are omitted. For odd $(n-d)$ sequences, Proposition 2 holds with $p = 1/2$ and consequently $E\{nV_n(d)\} \to E\{V(d;0.5)\}$.

5 Concluding Remarks

We have developed asymptotic theory for the delete-d JK estimator of the variance for a sample quantile by viewing it as a function of spacings around the sample quantile, and obtained its limit distribution for all finite $d > 1$. Building upon this theory, we have examined the special case of the sample median. We have shown that the limit distribution of the JK estimators of the variance of a sample median for even and odd $(n-d)$ values are different and that the limiting mean is smaller for even values of $(n-d)$.

We also show that when d is finite, the commonly used JK variance estimator of a central sample quantile, $nV_n(d)$, and a variant, $nV_{2,n}(d)$, discussed in Shao and Wu (1989), can have different limit properties, and that the $nV_{2,n}(d)$ sequence may not have a limit distribution at all!

When d is finite, the delete-d JK estimator of the variance of a sample quantile is not consistent, and yields an asymptotically scale-biased estimator of σ_p^2, and of $\{1/f(x_p)\}^2$. But the bias can be corrected using a scale factor given by Proposition 2. In the case of the sample median, the bias correction factor is dependent on whether $(n-d)$ is odd or even. Our results are also useful in producing asymptotically distribution-free approximate $100(1-\alpha)\%$ confidence intervals for σ_p^2, the quantile density function $1/f(x_p)$, and also for the pdf $f(x_p)$.

This investigation improves over Martin's (1990) work for a central quantile, Peng and Yang's (2009) work for an intermediate quantile, and Efron's (1982) note on the sample median for even sample sizes.

Acknowledgments The authors thank the reviewer for the helpful comments. H.N. Nagaraja would also like to express his gratitude to Professor Barry Arnold for being an inspiring teacher, a great mentor, a conscientious collaborator, and a wonderful friend.

References

Chung, K. L. (1974). *A course in probability theory* (2nd edn). Academic Press: New York.
David, H. A., Nagaraja, H. N. (2003). *Order statistics* (3rd edn). Hoboken, NJ: Wiley.
Efron, B. (1982). *The jackknife, the bootstrap, and other resampling plans*. SIAM: Philadelphia.

Esary, J. D., Proschan, F., Walkup, D. W. (1967). Association of random variables. *Annals of Mathematical Statistics, 44*, 1466–1474.
Martin, M. A. (1990). On using the jackknife to estimate quantile variance. *The Canadian Journal of Statistics, 18*(2), 149–153.
Martin, M., Roberts, S., Zheng, L. (2010). Delete-2 and delete-3 jackknife procedures for unmasking in regression. *Australian and New Zealand Journal of Statistics, 52*(1), 45–60.
Miller, R. G. (1974). The jackknife: A review. *Biometrika, 61*, 1–15.
Miller, S. J., Takloo-Bighash, R. (2006). *An invitation to modern number theory*. Princeton University: Princeton.
Nagaraja, C. H., Nagaraja, H. N. (2020). Distribution-free approximate methods for constructing confidence intervals for quantiles. *International Statistical Review, 88*(1), 75–100.
Nagaraja, H. N., Bharath, K., Zhang, F. (2015). Spacings around an order statistic. *Annals of the Institute of Statistical Mathematics, 67*, 515–540.
Parzen, E. (1979). Nonparametric statistical modelling (with comments). *Journal of the American Statistical Association, 74*, 105–131.
Peng, L., Yang, J. (2009). Jackknife method for intermediate quantiles. *Journal of Statistical Planning and Inference, 139*, 2372–2381.
Quenouille, M. (1949). Approximate tests of correlation in time series. *Journal of the Royal Statistical Society, Series B, 11*(1), 68–84.
Reiss, R.-D. (1989). *Approximate distributions of order statistics*. Springer: Berlin.
Shao, J. (1988). Consistency of jackknife estimators of the variances of sample quantiles. *Communications in Statistics Theory and Methods, 17*(9), 3017–3028.
Shao, J., Tu, D. (1995). *The jackknife and bootstrap*. Springer: New York.
Shao, J., Wu, C. F. J. (1989). A general theory for jackknife variance estimation. *Annals of Mathematical Statistics, 17*, 1176–1197.
Siotani, M. (1956). Order statistics for discrete case with a numerical application to the binomial distribution. *Annals of the Institute of Statistical Mathematics, 8*, 95–104.
von Mises, R. (1936). La distribution de la plus grande *n* valeurs. *Reviews in Mathematical Union Interbalkanique, 1*, 141–160.

Properties of System Lifetime in the Classical Model with I.I.D. Exponential Component Lifetimes

Tomasz Rychlik and Magdalena Szymkowiak

Abstract We consider coherent and mixed systems composed of components with independent identically exponentially distributed lifetimes. We describe sufficient conditions assuring specific properties of the system lifetime density and failure rate functions expressed in terms of the system Samaniego signature. In particular, we determine conditions which guarantee monotonicity, unimodality, and strong unimodality of the density function, and monotonicity of the failure rate and mean residual life.

Mathematics Subject Classification Primary: 62N05, Secondary: 62G30

1 Introduction and Auxiliary Results

We assume that the component lifetimes $T_1, \dots, T_n$ of n-component system are I.I.D. exponential with common distribution function $F_\lambda(t) = 1 - \exp(-\lambda t)$, and density function $f_\lambda(t) = \lambda \exp(-\lambda t),\ t > 0$, for some positive λ. Let $T_{1:n}, \dots, T_{n:n}$ denote the respective order statistics which represent consecutive failure times of the components. If the system has a structure function $\varphi : \{0, 1\}^n \mapsto \{0, 1\}$, then the distribution function of the system lifetime T has the form

$$F_T(t) = \mathbb{P}(T \le t) = \sum_{r=1}^{n} s_r \mathbb{P}(T_{r:n} \le t), \tag{1}$$

T. Rychlik (✉)
Institute of Mathematics, Polish Academy of Sciences, Warsaw, Poland
e-mail: trychlik@impan.pl

M. Szymkowiak
Institute of Automation and Robotics, Poznan University of Technology, Poznań, Poland
e-mail: magdalena.szymkowiak@put.poznan.pl

I. Ghosh et al. (eds.), *Advances in Statistics - Theory and Applications*, Emerging Topics in Statistics and Biostatistics, https://doi.org/10.1007/978-3-030-62900-7_3

where $s_r = \mathbb{P}(T = T_{r:n})$, or equivalently

$$s_r = \frac{1}{\binom{n}{r-1}} \sum_{\sum_{j=1}^{n} x_j = n-r+1} \varphi(x_1, \dots x_n) - \frac{1}{\binom{n}{r}} \sum_{\sum_{j=1}^{n} x_j = n-r} \varphi(x_1, \dots x_n), \quad r = 1, \dots, n. \tag{2}$$

Representation (1) was established by Samaniego (1985), and formula (2) comes from Boland (2001). The vector $\mathbf{s} = (s_1, \dots, s_n)$ is called the Samaniego signature of the system. As follows from (2) it depends merely on the system structure, and is independent of the component lifetime distribution. Other variants of the system signatures and their significance in reliability engineering were extensively studied in Samaniego (2007). The coefficients of $\mathbf{s}$ are non-negative, sum to 1, and are rational with the denominators equal either to $n!$ or to its divisors. Special cases of the systems are so called k-out-of-n (more precisely k-out-of-n : F) systems, $k = 1, \dots, n$, which work till the kth consecutive component failure. Then $T = T_{k:n}$ and $\mathbf{s} = \mathbf{e}_k = (0, \dots, 0, 1, 0, \dots, 0)$ with 1 at the kth position. Note that by (1) the distribution of T is identical with the lifetime distribution of randomly chosen k-out-of-n system with respective probability s_k, $k = 1, \dots, n$. The observation was a stimulus for defining the mixed systems which were introduced in Boland and Samaniego (2004). The mixed system with n components is a randomly chosen k-out-of-n system with probability s_k, $k = 1, \dots, n$, where $s_1, \dots, s_n$ are arbitrary non-negative numbers such that $\sum_{r=1}^{n} s_r = 1$. Under our assumption the Samaniego representation (1) is valid for all coherent and mixed systems of sizes not greater than n.

Performance of coherent systems composed of elements with independent memoryless exponential lifetimes is one of the most classic problems in the reliability theory, and it was the topic of a number of papers. Here we mention only a few, recent ones. Many authors studied stochastic comparisons of particular system lifetimes with identical and nonidentical exponential component lifetimes with respect to various partial orderings. In particular, the parallel systems were analyzed in Dykstra et al. (1997), Wang (2015), Wang and Zhao (2016), and Cheng and Wang (2017). Various orders for 2-out-of-n systems, called also fail-safe systems, were considered by Zhao and Balakrishnan (2009, 2011), and Balakrishnan et al. (2015). Explicit expressions and bounds for the system reliability as well as other performance measures of system lifetimes were presented in Chaudhuri (2004), and Çekyay and Özekici (2015). Arulmozhi (2003), Wang (2012), and Gonzalez-Lopez et al. (2017) developed methods of estimating the exponential parameters of component lifetimes based on operating times of systems.

Our purpose is to describe probabilistic properties of mixed system lifetimes in the standard exponential model expressed in terms of the system signatures. Precisely, we present assumptions on the system signatures imposing unimodality, strong unimodality, and monotonicity of the failure rate and mean residual life of the system lifetime distribution. For completeness, we recall the definitions of these notions.

Definition 1 Let the distribution function F_X of a random variable X have a density function f_X which is positive inside its support interval $[a, b]$.

(a) X is unimodal if its density function f_X is either monotone in (a, b) or it is non-decreasing on $(a, m]$ and non-increasing on $[m, b)$ for some $a < m < b$.
(b) X is strongly unimodal if $\ln f_X$ is concave on (a, b).
(c) X has an increasing (decreasing) failure rate if the failure rate function $\lambda_X(t) = \frac{f_X(t)}{1-F_X(t)}$ is non-decreasing (non-increasing) on (a, b).
(d) X with a finite expectation has an increasing (decreasing) mean residual life if the mean residual life function $\mu_X(t) = \mathbb{E}(X - t|X > t)$ is non-decreasing (non-increasing) on (a, b).

Strong unimodality of X is a stronger condition than the classical unimodality. It means that the sum $X + Y$ is unimodal for every unimodal random variable Y independent of X. Its characterization by log-concavity of the density function was proven by Ibragimov (1956). Below we use standard acronyms IFR (DFR) and IMRL (DMRL) for the properties of increasing (decreasing) failure rate and mean residual life, respectively. It is well-known that IFR implies DMRL, and IMRL follows from DFR (see, e.g., Hollander and Proschan 1984). The other commonly known facts are unique characterizations of distributions by the failure rate and mean residual life functions. In particular, the scale members of the exponential distribution family are characterized by constant failure rate and mean residual life.

The paper is organized as follows. Below we gather some formulae and auxiliary lemmas useful in the proofs of our main results. In Sect. 2 we present conditions on the systems signatures which determine monotonicity, unimodality, and strong unimodality of density functions of system lifetimes. In Sects. 3 and 4 we describe analogous assumptions assuring monotonicity of respective failure rates and mean residual lifetimes, respectively. We also show that our conditions assuring strong unimodality, increasing failure rate, and decreasing mean residual life coincide, although they look different at the first glance.

Let

$$B_{r,n}(u) = \binom{n}{r} u^r (1-u)^{n-r}, \qquad 0 \le u \le 1,\ r = 0, \dots, n,$$

denote the family of Bernstein polynomials of degree n. It follows from the classical theory of order statistics (see, e.g., David and Nagaraja 2003, p. 9) that the lifetime distribution function of the r-out-of-n system whose components have I.I.D. exponential lifetimes is

$$F_{r:n}(t) = \sum_{i=r}^{n} B_{i,n}(F_\lambda(t)), \qquad 1 \le r \le n,\ t > 0.$$

The respective survival and density functions are

$$\bar{F}_{r:n}(t) = 1 - F_{r:n}(t) = \sum_{i=0}^{r-1} B_{i,n}(F_\lambda(t))), \tag{3}$$

$$f_{r:n}(t) = nB_{r-1,n-1}(F_\lambda(t))f_\lambda(t) = \lambda(n+1-r)B_{r-1,n}(F_\lambda(t)). \tag{4}$$

We also use a similar representation for the derivative of the density function

$$\begin{aligned} f'_{r:n}(t) &= n\lambda[B_{r-2,n-1}(F_\lambda(t)) - B_{r-1,n-1}(F_\lambda(t))]f_\lambda(t) \\ &= \lambda^2(n+1-r)(n+2-r)B_{r-2,n}(F_\lambda(t)) - \lambda^2(n+1-r)^2 B_{r-1,n}(F_\lambda(t)), \end{aligned}$$

under the convention that $B_{-1,n}(F_\lambda(t)) \equiv 0$. Due to representation (1), the respective formulae for general coherent and mixed system are given below.

$$F_T(t) = \sum_{r=1}^{n} s_r \sum_{i=r}^{n} B_{i,n}(F_\lambda(t)) = \sum_{r=1}^{n} \left(\sum_{i=1}^{r} s_i \right) B_{r,n}(F_\lambda(t)),$$

$$\bar{F}_T(t) = 1 - F_T(t) = \sum_{r=1}^{n} s_r \sum_{i=0}^{r-1} B_{i,n}(F_\lambda(t)) = \sum_{r=1}^{n} \left(\sum_{i=r}^{n} s_i \right) B_{r-1,n}(F_\lambda(t)),$$

$$f_T(t) = nf_\lambda(t) \sum_{r=1}^{n} s_r B_{r-1,n-1}(F_\lambda(t)) = \lambda \sum_{r=1}^{n} (n+1-r)s_r B_{r-1,n}(F_\lambda(t)), \tag{5}$$

$$f'_T(t) = \lambda^2 \sum_{r=1}^{n} (n+1-r)[(n-r)s_{r+1} - (n+1-r)s_r]B_{r-1,n}(F_\lambda(t)), \tag{6}$$

under the convention that $s_{n+1} = 0$.

The main tool of our analysis is the Samaniego representation of the system lifetime distribution (1), and the variation diminishing property of the Bernstein polynomials described in the following lemma.

Lemma 1 (cf Rychlik 2001, p. 66) *The number of zeros of a given nonzero linear combination*

$$B(u) = \sum_{i=0}^{n} a_i B_{i,n}(u), \qquad 0 < u < 1,$$

of Bernstein polynomials of a fixed degree n is not greater than the number of sign changes in the sequence $a_0, \ldots, a_n$. Moreover, the signs of B in the right neighborhood of 0 and the left neighborhood of 1 coincide with the signs of the first and last nonzero elements among $a_0, \ldots, a_n$, respectively.

The first statement was proved in Schoenberg (1959). The second one is trivial. We also apply the following elementary lemma.

Lemma 2 *For two non-negative integers $p < q$, take sequences $\alpha_p, \ldots, \alpha_q \in \mathbb{R}$, and $\beta_p, \ldots, \beta_q > 0$. The sequence of ratios $\frac{\alpha_r}{\beta_r}$, $r = p, \ldots, q$, is non-decreasing (non-increasing, decreasing, increasing, constant, respectively), iff either of sequences*

$$\frac{\sum_{i=p}^{r} \alpha_i}{\sum_{i=p}^{r} \beta_i}, \qquad \frac{\sum_{i=r}^{q} \alpha_i}{\sum_{i=r}^{q} \beta_i}, \qquad r = p, \ldots, q, \tag{7}$$

is non-decreasing (non-increasing, decreasing, increasing, constant, respectively).

Numbering the elements of sequences from $p > 1$ looks strange at a first glance, and does not provide any generalization. However, formulating the results in the present form simplifies arguments in our applications below. The proofs of all the statements are similar, and we only show that non-decreasing property of the latter sequence of partial sums in (7) follows from the non-decreasing property of the quotients of their consecutive summands, and vice versa.

Proof of Lemma 2 We easily show that inequality $\frac{\alpha_{q-1}}{\beta_{q-1}} \leq \frac{\alpha_q}{\beta_q}$ is equivalent to the relations

$$\frac{\alpha_{q-1}}{\beta_{q-1}} \leq \frac{\alpha_{q-1} + \alpha_q}{\beta_{q-1} + \beta_q} \leq \frac{\alpha_q}{\beta_q}.$$

We assume so now that

$$\frac{\alpha_r}{\beta_r} \leq \frac{\sum_{i=r+1}^{q} \alpha_i}{\sum_{i=r+1}^{q} \beta_i}$$

for some $r = p, \ldots, q-1$. By simple calculation we obtain two equivalent relations

$$\frac{\alpha_r}{\beta_r} \leq \frac{\sum_{i=r}^{q} \alpha_i}{\sum_{i=r}^{q} \beta_i} \leq \frac{\sum_{i=r+1}^{q} \alpha_i}{\sum_{i=r+1}^{q} \beta_i}.$$

The induction argument shows that conditions for the non-decreasing property of both sequences $\frac{\alpha_r}{\beta_r}$ and $\frac{\sum_{i=r}^{q} \alpha_i}{\sum_{i=r}^{q} \beta_i}$, $r = p, \ldots, q$, are equivalent. ∎

2 Density Function

We first study the shape of the density function of the system lifetime.

Theorem 1 *Assume that a mixed system has signature $\mathbf{s} = (s_1, \ldots, s_n)$, and its components have I.I.D. exponential lifetime distributions with some intensity parameter $\lambda > 0$. Let $1 \leq p \leq q \leq n$ denote the indices of the first and last strictly positive elements, respectively, of the system signature.*

(a) *Under either of conditions*

(i) $p = q = 1$,
(ii) $p = 1 < q \leq n$, *and sequence* $a_r = (n + 1 - r)s_r$, $r = 1, \ldots, q$, *is either a constant or non-increasing,*

the system lifetime density function (5) *is decreasing on its support* $\mathbb{R}_+$.

(b) *If either of the following conditions holds:*

(i) $p \geq 2$, $q = p, p + 1$,
(ii) $p = 1 < q \leq n$, *and* $a_r = (n + 1 - r)s_r$, $r = 1, \ldots, q$, *is non-constant, either non-decreasing or first non-decreasing and then non-increasing,*
(iii) $p \geq 2$, $q \geq p + 2$, *and sequence* $a_r = (n + 1 - r)s_r$, $r = p, \ldots, q$, *is unimodal (i.e., either a constant, or non-decreasing, or non-increasing, or first non-decreasing and then non-increasing),*

then density function (5) *is first increasing and then decreasing.*

Remark 1 The density function (4) of each order statistic is decreasing for sufficiently large arguments, because each $B_{i,n}$, $i = 0, \ldots, n - 1$, (except for the last one $B_{n,n}$) is decreasing on a left neighborhood of 1, and $F_\lambda(t)$ increases to 1 as $t \to +\infty$. Therefore the convex combination $f_T(t) = \sum_{r=1}^n s_r f_{r:n}(t)$ is decreasing for large t as well. This implies that the lifetime density function of any coherent or mixed system whose components have I.I.D. exponential lifetimes cannot be increasing. By the same reason, the bath-tub shape of the density functions (i.e., first decrease and then increase) is impossible.

Remark 2 Among all the density functions of order statistics, only that of the sample minimum does not vanish at 0. This implies that the systems with $s_1 = 0$ cannot have decreasing density functions on $\mathbb{R}_+$, because they have to increase in a right neighborhood of the origin. The strict inequality $s_1 > 0$ does not assure decrease of the density function, though. It suffices to check that the signature with $s_1 = 1 - s_2 < \frac{n-1}{2n-1}$, and $s_r = 0$, $r = 3, \ldots, n$, satisfies the assumptions of Theorem 1(b(ii)). On the other hand, assumptions of Theorem 1(b) guarantying unimodality admit $s_1 \geq 0$.

Remark 3 Relations $0 < s_p > s_m = 0 < s_q = 0$ for some $1 \leq p < m < q \leq n$ contradict the assumptions of Theorem 1, because sequence a_r, $r = p, \ldots, q$, with $a_p > a_m < a_q$ is neither monotone nor unimodal. Note that any coherent system signature cannot have zeros between nonzero elements (see, e.g., Ross et al. 1980, and D'Andrea and Sanctis 2015).

Proof of Theorem 1 Since the density functions (5) are differentiable, it suffices to analyze changes of sign of their derivatives using (6).

(a) (i) For $p = q = 1$ we simply get

$$f_T'(t) = f_{1:n}'(t) = -\lambda^2 n^2 B_{0,n}(F_\lambda(t)) < 0.$$

(ii) Take now $p = 1 < q \leq n$. When $q = 2$, we obtain

$$f_T'(t) = s_1 f_{1:n}'(t) + s_2 f_{2:n}'(t) = \lambda^2 n[(n-1)s_2 - ns_1]B_{0,n}(F_\lambda(t))$$
$$-\lambda^2(n-1)^2 s_2 B_{1,n}(F_\lambda(t)).$$

Noting that $F_\lambda(t)$ increases from 0 to 1 as t increases in $(0, +\infty)$, we can apply Lemma 1. If $ns_1 \geq (n-1)s_2 = (n-1)(1-s_1)$, the former term is non-positive, and the latter is negative, which together imply that f_T itself is decreasing. However, when $ns_1 < (n-1)s_2$ (i.e., $s_1 < \frac{n-1}{2n-1}$), the density function is first increasing, and then decreasing.
For $p = 1$ and $3 \leq q \leq n$, the density derivative has the form

$$f_T'(t) = \lambda^2 \sum_{r=1}^{q-1} (n+1-r)[(n-r)s_{r+1} - (n+1-r)s_r]B_{r-1,n}(F_\lambda(t))$$
$$-\lambda^2(n+1-q)^2 s_q B_{q-1,n}(F_\lambda(t)).$$

The last term is evidently negative. If the sequence $a_r = (n+1-r)s_r$, $r = 1, \ldots, q$, is non-increasing (it suffices that it is even constant), then the whole sum is non-positive. It follows that f_T is decreasing on $\mathbb{R}_+$. This completes the proof of part (a). Note that non-increase as well as initial non-increase and final non-decreases of the sequence results in initial positivity and ultimate negativity of the derivative. In this way we also obtain the conclusion of part (b) under respective assumption (ii).

(b) Now we consider $p \geq 2$ with various q.

(i) For $q = p, p+1$ we have

$$f_T'(t) = f_{p:n}'(t) = \lambda^2(n+1-p)(n+2-p)B_{p-2,n}(F_\lambda(t))$$
$$-\lambda^2(n+1-p)^2 B_{p-1,n}(F_\lambda(t))$$

and

$$\begin{aligned} f_T'(t) &= s_p f_{p:n}'(t) + s_{p+1} f_{p+1:n}'(t) \\ &= \lambda^2(n+1-p)(n+2-p)s_p B_{p-2,n}(F_\lambda(t)) \\ &\quad +\lambda^2(n+1-p)[(n-p)s_{p+1} - (n+1-p)s_p]B_{p-1,n}(F_\lambda(t)) \\ &\quad -\lambda^2(n-p)^2 s_{p+1} B_{p,n}(F_\lambda(t)), \end{aligned}$$

respectively, with $s_{p+1} = 1 - s_p$ in the latter formula. In the first case Lemma 1 immediately implies that $f_T'(t)$ is first positive, and then negative. The same conclusion we get in the latter one, because the coefficients in the first and the last terms are positive and negative, respectively, and the sign of the middle one does not affect the sign order $+-$ in the whole summation.

(iii) When $p \geq 2$ and $p+2 \leq q \leq n$,

$$f'_T(t) = \lambda^2(n+1-p)(n+2-p)s_p B_{p-2,n}(F_\lambda(t))$$
$$+\lambda^2 \sum_{r=p}^{q-1}(n+1-r)[(n-r)s_{r+1}-(n+1-r)s_r]B_{r-1,n}(F_\lambda(t))$$
$$-\lambda^2(n+1-q)^2 s_q B_{q-1,n}(F_\lambda(t)).$$

The coefficients of the first and the last summands are positive and negative, respectively. The sign order of the whole sequence of coefficients remains undisturbed if the coefficients of the middle sum either have the same sign, or there is only one sign change which changes from plus to minus. This is equivalent to unimodality of the sequence $a_r = (n+1-r)s_r$, $r = p, \ldots, q$.

■

Example 1 Consider the weakest possible conditions of Theorem 1(a) assuring decrease of the system lifetime density function. Namely, we assume that for some $1 \leq q \leq n$ sequence a_r, $r = 1, \ldots, q$, is constant. Conditions $ns_1 = (n-1)s_2 = \ldots = (n+1-q)s_q$ and $\sum_{r=1}^{q} s_r = 1$ imply that

$$s_r = \frac{1}{(n+1-r)\sum_{i=1}^{q}\frac{1}{n+1-i}}, \qquad r = 1, \ldots, q. \tag{8}$$

Observe that the sequence is increasing. Plugging (8) into (5), we obtain

$$f_t(t) = \frac{\lambda}{\sum_{i=1}^{q}\frac{1}{n+1-i}} \sum_{r=1}^{q} B_{r-1,n}(F_\lambda(t)).$$

The sum of Bernstein polynomials represents the survival function of the qth order statistic (cf. (3)). Consequently,

$$f_T(t) = \frac{\overline{F}_{q:n}(t)}{\mathbb{E}T_{q:n}}$$

is the equilibrium density function associated with the qth order statistic (see, e.g., Andrews and Andrews (1962), Nakamura (2009)). It is also called the density of the length-biased (or size-biased) of order 1 weighted distribution of the qth order statistic. This is clearly decreasing, because so is the reliability function. When $q = 1$, this is obviously the density function of the series system

$$f_T(t) = n\lambda \exp(-n\lambda t), \qquad t > 0.$$

For $q = n$ yields

$$f_T(t) = \frac{\lambda}{\sum_{i=1}^{n} \frac{1}{i}} \{1 - [1 - \exp(-\lambda t)]^n\}, \qquad t > 0.$$

We provide some examples of signatures (8) for $n = 5$ and $1 \le q \le 5$. They have the following forms $(1, 0, 0, 0, 0)$, $\left(\frac{4}{9}, \frac{5}{9}, 0, 0, 0\right)$, $\left(\frac{12}{47}, \frac{15}{47}, \frac{20}{47}, 0, 0\right)$, $\left(\frac{12}{77}, \frac{15}{77}, \frac{20}{77}, \frac{30}{77}, 0\right)$, and $\left(\frac{12}{137}, \frac{15}{137}, \frac{20}{137}, \frac{30}{137}, \frac{60}{137}\right)$.

Theorem 1 together with Remark 1 describe necessary conditions for getting unimodality of the system lifetime density function. Combining the respective assumptions we obtain the following conditions:

(a) $q = p, p+1$, i.e., all the p-out-of-n systems, $p = 1, \ldots, n$, and all the mixtures of p-out-of-n and $(p+1)$-out-of-n systems,
(b) $q \ge p+2$, and unimodality of the sequence $a_r = (n+1-r)s_r$, $r = p, \ldots, q$.

Below we present more restrictive assumptions guarantying strong unimodality of the respective density function.

Theorem 2 *Assume the model and notation of Theorem* 1.

(a) *If* $q = p$, *then* $f_T = f_{p:n}$ *is strongly unimodal.*
(b) *If* $q = p + 1$, *the density function* (5) *is strongly unimodal iff*

$$0 < s_p = 1 - s_{p+1} \le \frac{n-p}{n-p+1}, \qquad p = 1, \ldots, n-1. \tag{9}$$

(c) *If* $q \ge p + 2$ *and sequence*

$$b_r = (n-r)\left(\frac{s_{r+1}}{s_r} - 1\right), \qquad r = p, \ldots, q, \tag{10}$$

is non-increasing, then (5) *is strongly unimodal.*

Remark 4 Inequality (9) is equivalent to (10) in the case $q = p + 1$. We consider $q = p+1$ and $q > p+1$ cases separately because (9) gives necessary and sufficient conditions for strong unimodality whereas (10) provides only a sufficient condition.

Remark 5 Strong unimodality obviously implies classical unimodality. We can also check that the conditions of strong unimodality of Theorem 2 are more restrictive than the conditions of unimodality presented above. Although the distribution of a single order statistic is strongly unimodal, in the case of mixtures of adjacent order statistics which are unimodal (see Theorem 1(b(i)) we need extra conditions in order to obtain the strong unimodality (see Theorem 2(b)). We also show that non-increasing property of $b_r,\ r = p, \dots, q$, implies that of $a_r,\ r = p, \dots, q$. To prove the statement, we assume the former. It follows that either

$$\frac{a_{r+1} - a_r}{s_r} = \frac{(n-r)s_{r+1} - (n+1-r)s_r}{s_r}, \qquad r = p, \dots, q,$$

does not change the sign, or it is first positive, then possibly equals zero, and finally negative. Due to the fact that $\frac{a_{q+1}-a_q}{s_q} = -(n+1-q) < 0$, sequence $\frac{a_{r+1}-a_r}{s_r}$, and, in consequence, $a_{r+1} - a_r$ itself, $r = p, \dots, q-1$, is either still non-positive, or first positive, then possibly equals zero, and finally it becomes negative. Therefore we observe that sequence $a_r = (n+1-r)s_r,\ r = p, \dots, q$, is either non-increasing or unimodal.

Proof of Theorem 2 Due to the classic result of Ibragimov (1956), strong unimodality of the system lifetime distribution is equivalent to logarithmic concavity of the associated density function (5). In our proof we check if the ratio $\frac{f_T'(t)}{f_T(t)}$ is non-increasing on $\mathbb{R}_+$.

(a) For the series system $\ln f_{1:n}(t) = -n\lambda t,\ t > 0$, is obviously concave. For $p = q \geq 2$, we have from (5) and (6),

$$\begin{aligned}\frac{f_T'(t)}{f_T(t)} &= \lambda \frac{(n+1-p)(n+2-p)B_{p-2,n}(F_\lambda(t)) - (n+1-p)^2 B_{p-1,n}(F_\lambda(t))}{(n+1-p)B_{p-1,n}(F_\lambda(t))} \\ &= \lambda(n+2-p)\frac{B_{p-2,n}(F_\lambda(t))}{B_{p-1,n}(F_\lambda(t))} - \lambda(n+1-p) \\ &= \lambda(p-1)\left(\frac{1}{F_\lambda(t)} - 1\right) - \lambda(n+1-p) = \frac{\lambda(p-1)}{F_\lambda(t)} - \lambda n,\end{aligned}$$

which is clearly decreasing.

(b) Let $2 \leq q = p+1 \leq n$. For $p = 1$, we have

$$\begin{aligned}\frac{f_T'(t)}{f_T(t)} &= \lambda \frac{n[(n-1)(1-s_1) - ns_1]B_{0,n}(F_\lambda(t)) - (n-1)^2(1-s_1)B_{1,n}(F_\lambda(t))}{ns_1 B_{0,n}(F_\lambda(t)) + (n-1)(1-s_1)B_{1,n}(F_\lambda(t))} \\ &= \lambda \frac{[(n-1)(1-s_1) - ns_1][1 - F_\lambda(t)] - (n-1)^2(1-s_1)F_\lambda(t)}{s_1[1 - F_\lambda(t)] + (n-1)(1-s_1)F_\lambda(t)}.\end{aligned}$$

Since

$$\frac{d}{dx}\frac{a(1-x) - bx}{c(1-x) + dx} = \frac{-bc - ad}{[c(1-x) + dx]^2},$$

we deduce

$$\frac{d}{dt}\frac{f_T'(t)}{f_T(t)} = -\lambda\, f_\lambda(t)\frac{(n-1)(1-s_1)[(n-1)(1-s_1)+(n-1)s_1+ns_1]}{[s_1[1-F_\lambda(t)]+(n-1)(1-s_1)F_\lambda(t)]^2}.$$

Negativity of the right-hand side expression is ensured by positivity of the factors in the numerator. This is just our assumption.

Taking $p = q - 1 \geq 2$, we obtain

$$\begin{aligned}
\frac{f_T'(t)}{f_T(t)} &= \frac{\lambda(n+1-p)(n+2-p)s_p B_{p-2,n}(F_\lambda(t))}{(n+1-p)s_p B_{p-1,n}(F_\lambda(t))+(n-p)(1-s_p)B_{p,n}(F_\lambda(t))} \\
&\quad + \frac{\lambda(n+1-p)[n-p-(2n+1-2p)s_p]B_{p-1,n}(F_\lambda(t))}{(n+1-p)s_p B_{p-1,n}(F_\lambda(t))+(n-p)(1-s_p)B_{p,n}(F_\lambda(t))} \\
&\quad - \frac{\lambda(n-p)^2(1-s_p)B_{p,n}(F_\lambda(t))}{(n+1-p)s_p B_{p-1,n}(F_\lambda(t))+(n-p)(1-s_p)B_{p,n}(F_\lambda(t))} \\
&= \frac{\lambda(n+1-p)(n+2-p)s_p B_{p-2,n}(F_\lambda(t))}{(n+1-p)s_p B_{p-1,n}(F)+(n-p)(1-s_p)B_{p,n}(F_\lambda(t))} \\
&\quad + \frac{\lambda(n+1-p)[n-p-(n+1-p)s_p]B_{p-1,n}(F_\lambda(t))}{(n+1-p)s_p B_{p-1,n}(F)+(n-p)(1-s_p)B_{p,n}(F_\lambda(t))} - \lambda(n-p) \\
&= \lambda p\,\frac{(p-1)s_p[1-F_\lambda(t)]^2+[n-p-(n+1-p)s_p]F_\lambda(t)[1-F_\lambda(t)]}{p s_p F_\lambda(t)[1-F_\lambda(t)]+(n-p)(1-s_p)F_\lambda^2(t)} \\
&\quad -\lambda(n-p).
\end{aligned}$$

Dividing the numerator and denominator by $[1-F_\lambda(t)]^2$, and introducing a new variable $x = x(t) = \frac{F_\lambda(t)}{1-F_\lambda(t)} = \exp(\lambda t) - 1$ that is increasing and transforms $\mathbb{R}_+$ onto itself, we obtain

$$\frac{f_T'(t)}{f_T(t)}_{|x=\exp(\lambda t)-1} = \lambda p\,\frac{a+bx}{cx+dx^2} - \lambda(n-p), \tag{11}$$

where

$$\begin{aligned}
a &= (p-1)s_p > 0, \\
b &= n-p-(n+1-p)s_p \in [-1, n-p], \\
c &= p s_p > 0, \\
d &= (n-p)(1-s_p) > 0.
\end{aligned} \tag{12}$$

It suffices to check when the right-hand side of (11) is decreasing on the positive half-axis. It has the derivative

$$\frac{d}{dx}\left[\lambda p\,\frac{a+bx}{cx+dx^2}-\lambda(n-p)\right]=\lambda p\,\frac{-bdx^2-2adx-ac}{(cx+dx^2)^2}.$$

If $b \le 0$, the derivative is obviously negative for all $x > 0$. If $b > 0$, it is negative when x is close to 0, and positive for large x's. It follows that the former condition with b defined in (12) is the necessary and sufficient condition for log-concavity of f_T.

(c) Under the assumption given in (10),

$$b_r-1=\frac{(n-r)s_{r+1}-(n+1-r)s_r}{s_r}=\frac{a_{r+1}-a_r}{s_r},\qquad r=p,\ldots,q,$$

is non-increasing as well. It follows that for each real c sequence $b_r-1-\frac{c}{\lambda}$, $r=p,\ldots,q$, changes the sign once at most, and if so, it is first positive, and finally negative. The same concerns

$$\begin{aligned}d_c(r)&=(n+1-r)s_r\left(b_r-1-\frac{c}{\lambda}\right)\\&=(n{+}1{-}r)\left[(n{-}r)s_{r+1}{-}(n{+}1{-}r)s_r{-}\frac{c}{\lambda}\,s_r\right],\qquad r=p,\ldots,q.\end{aligned}$$

For a moment exclude the case $p=1$, and for a given $p\ge 2$ define functions

$$\begin{aligned}\Delta_c(t)&=\lambda^2(n{+}1{-}p)(n{+}2{-}p)s_pB_{p-2,n}(F_\lambda(t)){+}\lambda^2\sum_{r=p}^{q}d_c(r)B_{r-1,n}(F_\lambda(t))\\&=\lambda^2(n{+}1{-}p)(n{+}2{-}p)s_pB_{p-2,n}(F_\lambda(t))\\&\quad+\lambda^2\sum_{r=p}^{q}(n{+}1{-}r)[(n{-}r)s_r{-}(n{+}1{-}r)s_r]B_{r-1,n}(F_\lambda(t))\\&\quad-c\lambda\sum_{r=p}^{q}(n{+}1{-}r)s_rB_{r-1,n}(F_\lambda(t))\\&=f_T'(t){-}cf_T(t),\qquad t>0,\ c\in\mathbb{R}.\end{aligned}\tag{13}$$

Consider the signs of coefficients of the above linear combination of Bernstein polynomials given in (13). The first one appearing at the $(p-2)$nd polynomial is positive, and the next ones have at most one sign change from $+$ to $-$. It means that for every $c\in\mathbb{R}$ the sign order of the whole sequence is either $+$ or $+-$, and the property is inherited by $f_T'(t)-cf_T(t)$, $t>0$, due to Lemma 1. Consequently, $\frac{f_T'(t)}{f_T(t)}$ crosses an arbitrary horizontal level c at most once, and if so, it does from top down. This provides the conclusion that $\frac{f_T'(t)}{f_T(t)}$ is decreasing on $\mathbb{R}_+$ and its antiderivative $\ln f_T(t)$ is concave there, as desired.

For $p = 1$ the reasoning is similar. The only difference is that the first term with $(p-2)$nd polynomial does not appear in Eq. (13). ∎

3 Failure Rate

It is well-known that every k-out-of-n system composed of elements with I.I.D. IFR lifetime distributions has the IFR distribution as well (cf., e.g., Barlow and Proschan 1975, Chapter 4, Theorem 5.8, and Ross 2010, Example 9.24). This is obviously true if the component lifetimes are exponential in particular. If, moreover, this is a series system, its failure rate is constant, which means that the system lifetime distribution is also a member of the DFR family. The other systems are treated in the following theorem.

Theorem 3 *Assume that an n-component mixed system has signature $\mathbf{s} = (0, \ldots, 0, s_p, \ldots, s_q, 0, \ldots, 0)$ for some $1 \leq p < q \leq n$, and its components have I.I.D. exponential lifetimes with a common density function $f_\lambda(t) = \lambda \exp(-\lambda t)$, $t > 0$, for some $\lambda > 0$. If the sequence*

$$g_r = \frac{(n+1-r)s_r}{\sum_{i=r}^{q} s_i}, \qquad r = p, \ldots, q, \tag{14}$$

is non-decreasing (non-increasing, respectively), then the system lifetime has an IFR (DFR, respectively) distribution.

Remark 6 Sequence (14) is non-negative, and its extreme elements $g_p = (n+1-p)s_p$ and $g_q = n+1-q$ are strictly positive. Monotonicity of the sequence excludes possibility that there exists $p < r < q$ such that $s_r = g_r = 0$. This is a property of all coherent system signatures which may have some zeros at the beginning and the end, but they cannot have any zeros between positive elements.

Remark 7 Bieniek and Burkschat (2019) use monotonicity conditions with more general $\tilde{g}_r = \frac{\gamma_r s_r}{\sum_{i=r}^{q} s_i}$, where $\gamma_r > 0$ replacing the g_r in (14). They establish preservation of IFR and DFR properties by system lifetimes in the so-called failure dependent proportional hazard reliability model. In their model, consecutive failures of system components have distributions identical with generalized order statistics with positive parameters γ_r, and $\gamma_r = n+1-r$ in the classical I.I.D. case.

Corollary 1 *Under assumptions of Theorem 3 with $q = p+1$, condition $s_p = 1 - s_{p+1} \leq \frac{n-p}{n+1-p}$ is sufficient and necessary for the IFR property of the system lifetime. The inequality is reversed iff the system lifetime has a DFR distribution.*

Note that the conditions for strong unimodality and increasing failure rate for mixtures of two adjacent order statistics are identical. We further show that the same concerns the other systems.

Proof of Theorem 3 The proof is similar to that of Theorem 2. We focus on the assumption that (14) is non-decreasing. Then for every positive c the difference $g_r - \frac{c}{\lambda}$ as well as $\left(g_r - \frac{c}{\lambda}\right)\sum_{i=r}^{q} s_i = (n+1-r)s_r - \frac{c}{\lambda}\sum_{i=r}^{q} s_i$, $r = p, \ldots, q$, have either a fixed sign or change sign from + to −. Lemma 1 implies that

$$f_T(t) - c\overline{F}_T(t) = \lambda \sum_{r-p}^{q}\left[(n+1-r)s_r - \frac{c}{\lambda}\sum_{i=r}^{q} s_i\right] B_{r-1,n}(F_\lambda(t)), \qquad t > 0,$$

either does not change the sign or the sign does it once from + to −. The same conclusion concerns $\frac{f_T(t)}{\overline{F}_T(t)} - c = \lambda_T(t) - c$. Therefore $\lambda_T(t)$ itself is decreasing on $\mathbb{R}_+$. The proof that non-increase of (14) implies the DFR property of the system lifetime distribution is analogous. ■

Corollary 2 *Non-decreasing property of sequence* (14) *assuring increasing failure rate of the system lifetime coincides with non-increasing property of sequence* (10) *guarantying strong unimodality of the respective distribution.*

Proof Consider the sequences $\alpha_r = (n-r)s_{r+1} - (n+1-r)s_r$ and $\beta_r = s_r$, $r = p, \ldots, q$. Their partial sums are $\sum_{i=r}^{q} \alpha_i = -(n+1-r)s_r$ and $\sum_{i=r}^{q} \beta_i = \sum_{i=r}^{q} s_i$, $r = p, \ldots, q$. By Lemma 2, sequence

$$b_r - 1 = \frac{(n-r)s_{r+1} - (n+1-r)s_r}{s_r} = \frac{\alpha_r}{\beta_r}, \qquad r = p, \ldots, q,$$

does not increase iff so does

$$\frac{\sum_{i=r}^{q} \alpha_i}{\sum_{i=r}^{q} \beta_i} = -\frac{(n+1-r)s_r}{\sum_{i=r}^{q} s_i}, \qquad r = p, \ldots, q.$$

The latter simply means non-decreasing property for (14). ■

On the other hand, we have the following.

Proposition 1 *Strong unimodality of a life distribution implies non-decreasing property for its failure rate.*

Proof Log-concavity of a density function f implies that there exists a monotone right continuous version f' of its derivative. Moreover, we have

$$\frac{f'(t)}{f(t)} \geq \frac{f'(t+s)}{f(t+s)}$$

for all $t, s \geq 0$. Consequently,

$$\frac{f'(t)f(t+s) - f'(t+s)f(t)}{f^2(t+s)} = \frac{d}{dt}\,\frac{f(t)}{f(t+s)} \geq 0,$$

for every non-negative t and s. It follows that for every $s \geq 0$ function $t \mapsto \frac{f(t+s)}{f(t)}$ is non-increasing with respect to t. The inequality is inherited by

$$\int_0^\infty \frac{f(t+s)}{f(t)} ds = \int_t^\infty \frac{f(x)}{f(t)} dx = \frac{1-F(t)}{f(t)}.$$

It follows that $\lambda(t) = \frac{f(t)}{\overline{F}(t)}$, $t \geq 0$, is non-decreasing. ■

4 Mean Residual Lifetime

It is well-known that the IFR distributions have decreasing mean residual lifetime (see, e.g., Bryson and Siddiqui 1969; Hollander and Proschan 1984). In fact, the proof is analogous to that of Proposition 1. Similarly, the DFR property implies IMRL. Due to the results of the previous section, all the k-out-of-n systems and the mixtures with $q = p+1$ and $s_p = 1 - s_{p+1} \leq \frac{n-p}{n+1-p}$ have a DMRL distribution. Moreover, the series system and the mixed systems with $s_p = 1 - s_{p+1} \geq \frac{n-p}{n+1-p}$ have an IMRL distribution. Below we consider other mixed and coherent systems.

Theorem 4 *Assume the conditions and notation of Theorems 1–3, and introduce* $\overline{S}_r = \frac{1}{n+1-r}\sum_{j=r}^n s_j$, $r = 1, \ldots, n$, *denoting the averages of the last* $n+1-r$ *signature components. If a system has a signature* **s** *such that*

$$h_r = \frac{\sum_{i=r}^q \overline{S}_i}{\sum_{i=r}^q s_i}, \qquad r = p, \ldots, q, \tag{15}$$

is non-increasing, then the system lifetime has distribution with decreasing mean residual lifetime. If $p = 1$, *and* (15) *is non-decreasing, then the system has an IMRL distribution.*

Proof Applying (3) and (4), we conclude

$$\int_t^\infty B_{j,n}(F_\lambda(s))ds = \frac{1}{\lambda(n-j)} \sum_{i=0}^j B_{i,n}(F_\lambda(t))$$

for $j = 1, \ldots, n-1$. Accordingly, by (3) again, we get

$$\int_t^\infty \overline{F}_{r:n}(s)ds = \sum_{j=0}^{r-1} \int_t^\infty B_{j,n}(F_\lambda(s))ds = \frac{1}{\lambda}\sum_{j=0}^{r-1} \frac{1}{n-j} \sum_{i=0}^j B_{i,n}(F_\lambda(t))$$

$$= \frac{1}{\lambda}\sum_{j=0}^{r-1}\left(\sum_{i=j}^{r-1} \frac{1}{n-i}\right) B_{i,n}(F_\lambda(t)).$$

Finally,

$$\int_t^\infty \overline{F}_T(s)ds = \sum_{r=1}^n s_r \int_t^\infty \overline{F}_{r:n}(s)ds = \frac{1}{\lambda}\sum_{r=1}^n s_r \sum_{j=0}^{r-1}\left(\sum_{i=j}^{r-1}\frac{1}{n-i}\right) B_{i,n}(F_\lambda(t))$$

$$= \frac{1}{\lambda}\sum_{r=1}^n\left(\sum_{i=r}^n \frac{\sum_{j=i}^n s_j}{n+1-i}\right) B_{r-1,n}(F_\lambda(t)) = \frac{1}{\lambda}\sum_{r=1}^n\left(\sum_{i=r}^n \overline{S}_i\right) B_{r-1,n}(F_\lambda(t)).$$

The mean residual lifetime of the system has the form

$$\mu_T(t) = \mathbb{E}(T-t|T>t) = \frac{\int_t^\infty \overline{F}_T(s)ds}{\overline{F}_T(t)} = \frac{1}{\lambda}\frac{\sum_{r=1}^n \left(\sum_{i=r}^n \overline{S}_i\right) B_{r-1,n}(F_\lambda(t))}{\sum_{r=1}^n \left(\sum_{i=r}^n s_i\right) B_{r-1,n}(F_\lambda(t))}.$$

If $s_q > 0 = s_{q+1} = \ldots = s_n$ for some $q \le n-1$, we have $\sum_{i=r}^n s_i = \sum_{i=r}^n \overline{S}_i = 0,\ r = q+1, \ldots, n$. This justifies rewriting the above expression for the mean residual life

$$\mu_T(t) = \frac{1}{\lambda}\frac{\sum_{r=1}^q \left(\sum_{i=r}^q \overline{S}_i\right) B_{r-1,n}(F_\lambda(t))}{\sum_{r=1}^q \left(\sum_{i=r}^q s_i\right) B_{r-1,n}(F_\lambda(t))}.$$

Mimicking the reasoning used in the proofs of the previous theorems we arrive at the conclusions that if the sequence $h_r = \frac{\sum_{i=r}^q \overline{S}_i}{\sum_{i=r}^q s_i}$, $r = 1, \ldots, q$, is non-increasing, then the above MRL function is decreasing on $(0, \infty)$. Non-decreasing property of the sequence results in the IMRL property of the function. However, if $s_p > 0 = s_r,\ r = 1, \ldots, p-1$, for some $p \ge 2$, then $\sum_{i=r}^q s_i = 1$ and $\sum_{i=r}^q \overline{S}_i = \sum_{i=r}^p \frac{1}{n+1-r} + \sum_{r=p+1}^q \overline{S}_r$, $r = 1, \ldots, p$. It follows that the subsequence

$$\frac{\sum_{i=r}^q \overline{S}_i}{\sum_{i=r}^q s_i} = \sum_{i=r}^p \frac{1}{n+1-r} + \sum_{r=p+1}^q \overline{S}_r, \qquad r = 1, \ldots, p,$$

is strictly decreasing. If the subsequence $\frac{\sum_{i=r}^q \overline{S}_i}{\sum_{i=r}^q s_i}$, $r = p, \ldots, q$ is non-increasing as well, then the MRL function is decreasing. For increase of the function we need $p = 1$ and non-decrease of the sequence h_r for $r = 1, \ldots, q$. ■

Corollary 3 *The necessary condition for the DMRL property of the system lifetime distribution presented in Theorem* 4 *is identical with the conditions of Theorems* 2 *and* 3 *assuring strong unimodality and IFR property of the system lifetime.*

Proof Owing to Corollary 1, it suffices to verify that non-increase of (14) is equivalent to non-decrease of (15). Accordingly, we claim that

$$\frac{\sum_{i=r}^{q} s_i}{\sum_{i=r}^{q} \overline{S}_i}, \qquad r = p, \ldots, q,$$

is non-decreasing iff so is

$$\frac{(n+1-r)s_r}{\sum_{i=r}^{q} s_i} = \frac{s_r}{\overline{S}_r}, \qquad r = p, \ldots, q.$$

Defining $\alpha_r = s_r$ and $\beta_r = \overline{S}_r$, which implies $\frac{\alpha_r}{\beta_r} = \frac{(n+1-r)s_r}{\sum_{i=r}^{q} s_i}$ and $\frac{\sum_{i=r}^{q} \alpha_i}{\sum_{i=r}^{q} \beta_i} = \frac{\sum_{i=r}^{q} s_i}{\sum_{i=r}^{q} \overline{S}_i}$, $r = p, \ldots, q$, we merely refer to Lemma 2 in order to reach the final conclusion. ■.

Remark 8 The conclusion of Corollary 3 can be represented as equivalent to the following conditions.

(a) Sequence

$$\frac{1}{1-b_r} = \frac{s_r}{(n+1-r)s_r - (n-r)s_{r+1}}, \qquad r = p, \ldots, q,$$

is non-increasing.

(b) Sequence

$$\frac{\sum_{i=r}^{q} s_r}{\sum_{i=r}^{q} [(n+1-r)s_r - (n-r)s_{r+1}]} = \frac{\sum_{i=r}^{q} s_i}{(n+1-r)s_r} = \frac{\overline{S}_r}{s_r}, \qquad r = p, \ldots, q,$$

is non-increasing.

(c) Sequence

$$\frac{\sum_{i=r}^{q} \overline{S}_r}{\sum_{i=r}^{q} s_r}, \qquad r = p, \ldots, q,$$

is non-increasing.

Notice that the implications of (c), (b), and (a), in order, are conditions (C), (B), (A), given below.

(C)

$$\mu_T(t) = \frac{\int_t^{\infty} \overline{F}_T(u)du}{\overline{F}_T(t)}, \qquad t > 0,$$

is non-increasing,

(B)

$$\frac{\frac{d}{dt}\int_t^\infty \overline{F}_T(u)du}{\frac{d}{dt}\overline{F}_T(t)} = \frac{-\overline{F}_T(t)}{-f_T(t)}, \qquad t > 0,$$

is non-increasing, which means that $\lambda_T(t) = \frac{f_T(t)}{\overline{F}_T(t)}$, $t > 0$, is non-decreasing,

(A)

$$\frac{\frac{d^2}{dt^2}\int_t^\infty \overline{F}_T(u)du}{\frac{d^2}{dt^2}\overline{F}_T(t)} = \frac{f_T(t)}{-f_T'(t)}, \qquad t > 0,$$

is non-increasing, i.e., $\frac{d}{dt}\ln f_T(t) = \frac{f_T'(t)}{f_T(t)}$, $t > 0$, is non-increasing.

Clearly strong unimodality, IFR, and DMRL are not equivalent properties of the system lifetimes. However, we find the above observation interesting, although we do not have a reasonable justification for it.

Example 2 We consider the weakest conditions of Theorems 2–4 which assure strong unimodality, increasing failure rate, and decreasing mean residual life of the system lifetime distribution. As we checked above, all the k-out-of-n systems possess these properties. For $1 \le p < q \le n$ we here check which signatures $(0, \ldots, 0, s_p, \ldots, s_q, 0, \ldots, 0)$ assure constancy of sequences (10), (14), and (15). Theorem 3 asserts that a signature with constant value for the g_r in (14) represents the distribution with a constant failure rate, which is exponential. Analogous conclusion can be drawn from Theorem 4. We claim that the signatures with constant (10), (14), and (15) have the forms

$$s_r = \begin{cases} \binom{n-r}{q-r} / \binom{n+1-p}{q-p}, & r = p, \ldots, q, \\ 0, & r = 1, \ldots, p-1, q+1, \ldots, n. \end{cases} \tag{16}$$

We first verify that for $r = p, \ldots, q$ the following equalities hold:

$$s_r = \binom{n-r}{q-r} s_q, \tag{17}$$

$$\sum_{i=r}^{q} s_i = \binom{n+1-r}{q-r} s_q.$$

Both the equalities are trivially true for $r = q$. Assume that they hold for $p + 1 \le r + 1 \le q$, i.e.,

$$s_{r+1} = \binom{n-r-1}{q-r-1} s_q, \qquad \sum_{i=r+1}^{q} s_i = \binom{n-r}{q-r-1} s_q. \tag{18}$$

Relations $b_r = (n-r)\left(\frac{s_{r+1}}{s_r} - 1\right) = b_q = q - n$ imply $s_r = \frac{n-r}{q-r} s_{r+1}$, $r = p, \ldots, q-1$. Using (18) we determine

$$s_r = \frac{n-r}{q-r}\binom{n-r-1}{q-r-1} s_q = \binom{n-r}{q-r} s_q$$

and

$$\sum_{i=r}^{q} s_i = \binom{n-r}{q-r} s_q + \binom{n-r}{q-r-1} s_q = \binom{n+1-r}{q-r} s_q.$$

Condition

$$1 = \sum_{i=p}^{q} s_i = \binom{n+1-p}{q-p} s_q$$

allows us to determine $s_q = 1/\binom{n+1-p}{q-p}$, and, in combination with (17), provides the final claim (16).

From the equality $(n+1-r)s_r = (n+1-q)\sum_{i=r}^{q} s_r$ we obtain

$$\frac{f_T(t)}{\overline{F}_T(t)} = \frac{\sum_{r=p}^{q} \lambda(n+1-r)s_r B_{r-1,n}(F_\lambda(t))}{\sum_{r=p}^{q}\sum_{i=r}^{q} s_r B_{r-1,n}(F_\lambda(t))} = \lambda(n+1-q).$$

This means that the system with signature (16) has the same lifetime distribution as the series system with $n+1-q$ components. We also note that (16) satisfy $s_{r+1} = \frac{q-r}{n-r} s_r \le s_r$, with strict inequality for $q < n$. Non-increasing property of (16) contradicts the increasing property of (8). Signatures (16) specified for $n = 5$ with $q - p \ge 2$ have the forms $\left(\frac{3}{5}, \frac{3}{10}, \frac{1}{10}, 0, 0\right)$, $\left(0, \frac{1}{2}, \frac{1}{3}, \frac{1}{6}, 0\right)$, $\left(0, 0, \frac{1}{3}, \frac{1}{3}, \frac{1}{3}\right)$, $\left(\frac{2}{5}, \frac{3}{10}, \frac{1}{5}, \frac{1}{10}, 0\right)$, $\left(0, \frac{1}{4}, \frac{1}{4}, \frac{1}{4}, \frac{1}{4}\right)$, and $\left(\frac{1}{5}, \frac{1}{5}, \frac{1}{5}, \frac{1}{5}, \frac{1}{5}\right)$.

Example 3 There are many coherent systems which satisfy the conditions of Theorem 1 guarantying unimodality and decreasing properties of the density functions of their lifetimes. It is, though, difficult to find systems with signatures guarantying strong unimodality, IFR and DMRL properties, except for the classical k-out-of-n systems. One such example is the 5-component system with minimal path sets $\{1, 2, 3\}$ and $\{1, 4, 5\}$ (for the definition of the notion, see, e.g., Barlow and Proschan 1975, p. 9, Ross 2010, Subsection 9.2.1), and lifetime $T = \min\{T_1, \min\{T_2, T_3\}, \min\{T_4, T_5\}\}$. It has signature $\left(\frac{1}{5}, \frac{3}{5}, \frac{1}{5}, 0, 0\right)$ (cf. Navarro and Rubio 2010, Tables 1 and 2, system 10). The respective vector $a_r = (n+1-r)s_r$, $r = 1, 2, 3$, takes on values $a_1 = 1$, $a_2 = \frac{12}{5}$, $a_3 = \frac{3}{5}$, which guarantees unimodality of the system lifetime density function. It is also strongly unimodal, and the corresponding failure rate and mean residual life are increasing and decreasing, respectively, because sequence $b_r = (n-r)\left(\frac{s_{r+1}}{s_r} - 1\right)$, $r = 1, 2, 3$, with values $b_1 = 8$, $b_2 = b_3 = -2$ is non-increasing. Observe that the dual system with minimal path sets $\{1\}$, $\{2,4\}$, $\{2,5\}$, $\{3,4\}$, $\{3,5\}$ and signature $\left(0, 0, \frac{1}{5}, \frac{3}{5}, \frac{1}{5}\right)$ (see Navarro and Rubio 2010, Tables 1 and 2, system 172) satisfies $a_3 = \frac{3}{5}$, $a_4 = \frac{6}{5}$, $a_5 = \frac{1}{5}$ and $b_3 = 8$, $b_2 = -1$, $b_5 = 0$. It follows that its unimodality is guaranteed, but the other properties are not.

Example 4 We finally analyze a family of n-component systems, $n \geq 3$, with minimal path sets $P_1 = \{2, \ldots, n\}$, and $P_i = \{1, i\}$, $i = 2, \ldots, n$, (cf. Bieniek and Burkschat 2018, Example 3.1). They have signatures $(0, 1, 0)$, $\left(0, \frac{1}{2}, \frac{1}{2}, 0\right)$, and $\left(0, \frac{2}{n}, \frac{1}{n}, \ldots, \frac{1}{n}, \frac{2}{n}, 0\right)$, when $n = 3$, 4, and $n \geq 5$, respectively. Theorem 1(bi) and Theorem 2(a,b) assert that the system lifetime density functions in cases $n = 3$ and 4 are both increasing-decreasing and log-concave. For $n = 5$, sequence $a_r = (6-r)s_r$, $r = 2, 3, 4$, takes on values $\frac{8}{5}$, $\frac{3}{5}$, and $\frac{4}{5}$, which means that the assumptions of Theorem 1 do not guarantee unimodality of f_T. A similar conclusion is derived for $n \geq 6$, because $a_{n-3} = a_{n-1} = \frac{4}{n} > a_{n-2} = \frac{3}{n}$. It follows that the assumptions of Theorems 2, 3, and 4 do not ensure strong unimodality, increasing failure rate, and decreasing mean residual life, either.

It occurs that these properties are preserved for small system sizes, and disappear gradually as n increases. All of them hold for the systems with 5 and 6 components. In the cases $7 \leq n \leq 12$, only decreasing mean residual life remains valid, and the others are not. Eventually, for $n \geq 13$ the DMRL property vanishes as well. This is illustrated in Figs. 1, 2, and 3, where the graphs of density function f_T, derivative of its logarithm $(\ln f_T)'$, failure rate λ_T, and mean residual life μ_T functions are presented for $n = 5$, 9, and 15. We assumed here that the component lifetimes are standard exponential. In order to improve visuality of the results we rescaled the time replacing t running over the whole positive half-axis by $0 < u = -\ln(1-t) < 1$.

Note that for the systems of this type we do not observe the case when the strong unimodality property fails to hold, whereas IFR and DMRL properties still hold. This happens, e.g., for the 5-component system with minimal path sets $P_i = \{1, i+1\}$, $i = 1, \ldots, 4$, and signature $\left(\frac{1}{5}, \frac{1}{5}, \frac{1}{5}, \frac{2}{5}, 0\right)$ (see Fig. 4).

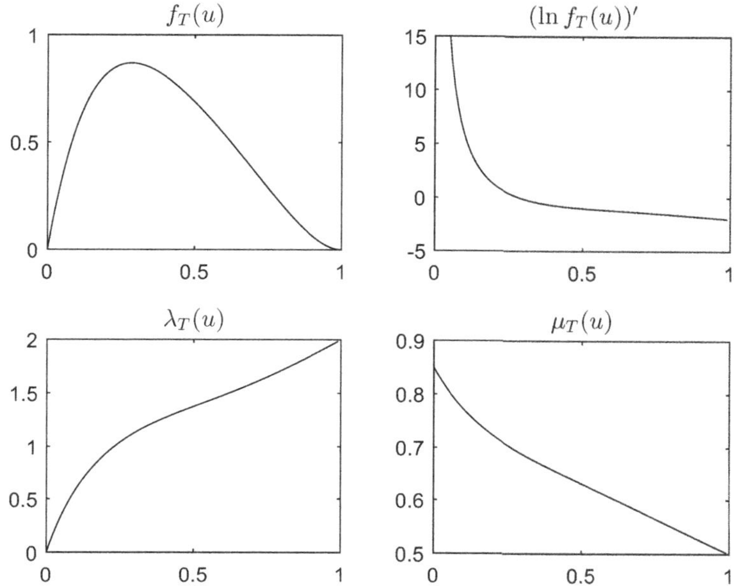

Fig. 1 Density function f_T, derivative of its logarithm $(\ln f_T)'$, failure rate λ_T, and mean residual life μ_T of the lifetime distribution of the system with signature $\left(0, \frac{2}{n}, \frac{1}{n}, \ldots, \frac{1}{n}, \frac{2}{n}, 0\right)$ and $n = 5$

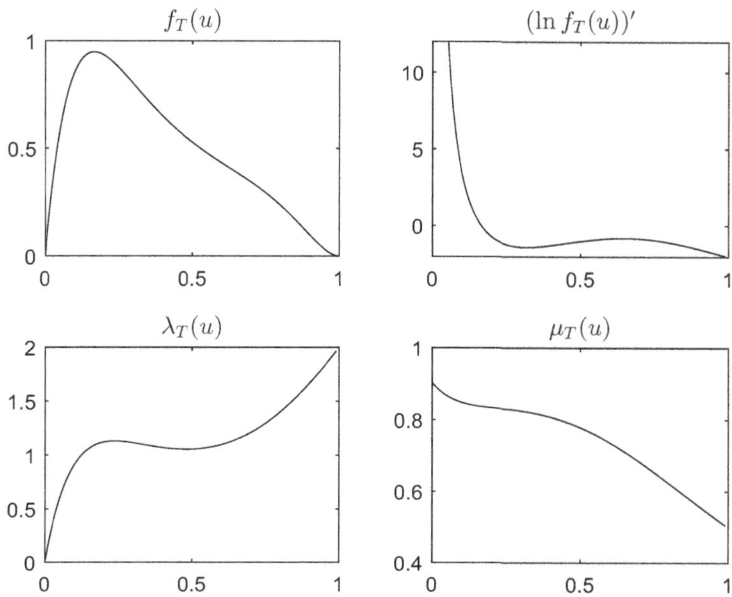

Fig. 2 Density function f_T, derivative of its logarithm $(\ln f_T)'$, failure rate λ_T, and mean residual life μ_T of the lifetime distribution of the system with signature $\left(0, \frac{2}{n}, \frac{1}{n}, \ldots, \frac{1}{n}, \frac{2}{n}, 0\right)$ and $n = 9$

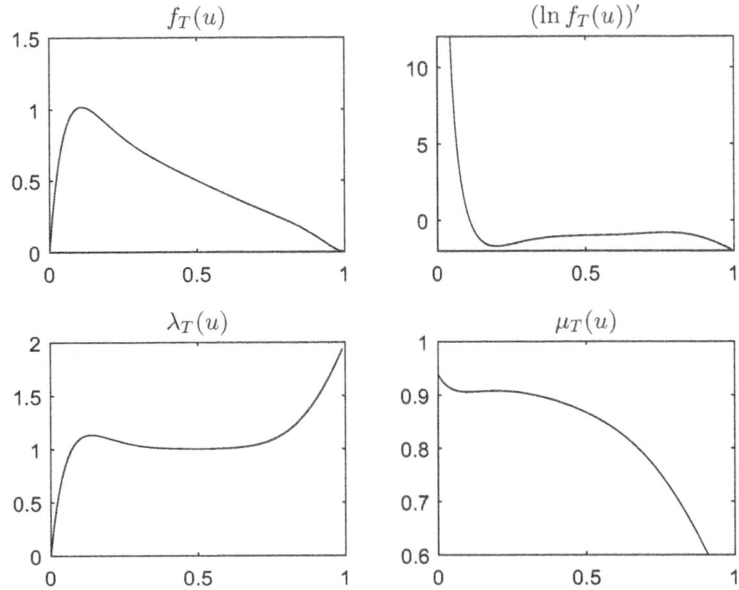

Fig. 3 Density function f_T, derivative of its logarithm $(\ln f_T)'$, failure rate λ_T, and mean residual life μ_T of the lifetime distribution of the system with signature $\left(0, \frac{2}{n}, \frac{1}{n}, \dots, \frac{1}{n}, \frac{2}{n}, 0\right)$ and $n = 15$

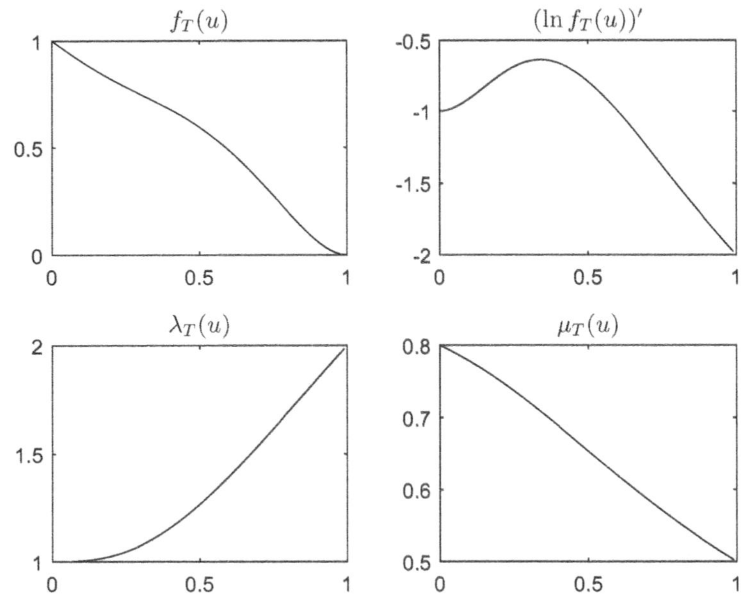

Fig. 4 Density function f_T, derivative of its logarithm $(\ln f_T)'$, failure rate λ_T, and mean residual life μ_T of the lifetime distribution of the system with signature $\left(\frac{1}{5}, \frac{1}{5}, \frac{1}{5}, \frac{2}{5}, 0\right)$

References

Andrews, F. C., & Andrews, A. C. (1962). The form of the equilibrium distribution function. *Transactions of the Kansas Academy of Science, 65*, 247–256.

Arulmozhi, G. (2003). Maximum likelihood estimation of exponential parameters of reliability systems. *Advanced Modeling and Optimization, 5*, 117–132.

Balakrishnan, N., Haidari, A., & Barmalzan, G. (2015). Improved ordering results for fail-safe systems with exponential components. *Communications in Statistics - Theory and Methods, 44*, 2010–2023.

Barlow, R. E., & Proschan, F. (1975). *Statistical theory of reliability and life-testing*. New York: Holt, Rinehart, and Winston.

Bieniek, M., & Burkschat, M. (2018). On unimodality of the lifetime distribution of coherent systems with failure-dependent component lifetimes. *Journal of Applied Probability, 55*, 473–487.

Bieniek, M., & Burkschat, M. (2019). Preservation of the increasing failure rate property for coherent systems under the failure-dependent proportional hazard rate model (submitted).

Boland, P. J. (2001). Signatures of indirect majority systems. *Journal of Applied Probability, 38*, 597–603.

Boland, P. J., & Samaniego, F. (2004). The signature of a coherent system and its applications in reliability. In Soyer, R., Mazzuchi, T., & Singpurwalla, N. D. (eds.). *Mathematical reliability: An expository perspective* (pp. 1–29). Boston: Kluwer Publishers.

Bryson, M. C., & Siddiqui, M. M. (1969). Some criteria for aging. J. Amer. Statist. Assoc. *64*, 1472–1483.

Çekyay, B., & Özekici, S. (2015). Reliability, MTTF and steady-state availability analysis of systems with exponential lifetimes. *Applied Mathematical Modelling, 39*, 284–296.

Chaudhuri, G. (2004). A lower confidence limit for reliability of a coherent system with independent exponential components. *Calcutta Statistical Association Bulletin, 55*, 119–127.

Cheng, B., & Wang J. (2017). Stochastic comparison of parallel systems with heterogeneous exponential components. *Journal of Applied Probability, 54*, 970–976.

D'Andrea, A., & De Sanctis, L. (2015). The Kruskal-Katona theorem and a characterization of system signatures. *Journal of Applied Probability, 52*, 508–518.

David, H. A., & Nagaraja, H. N. (2003). *Order statistics* (3rd ed.) Wiley Series in Probability and Statistics. Hoboken, NJ: Wiley-Interscience.

Dykstra, R., Kochar, S., & Rojo, J. (1997). Stochastic comparisons of parallel systems of heterogeneous exponential components. *Journal of Statistical Planning and Inference, 65*, 203–211.

Gonzalez-Lopez, V. A., Gholizadeh, R., & Galarza, C. E. (2017). E-Bayesian estimation for system reliability and availability analysis based on exponential distribution. *Communications in Statistics - Simulation and Computation, 46*, 6221–6241.

Hollander, M., & Proschan, F. (1984). Nonparametric concepts and methods in reliability. In Krishnaiah, P. R., & Sen, P. K. (eds.). *Nonparametric methods. Handbook of statistics* (Vol. 4, pp. 613–655). Amsterdam: North-Holland.

Ibragimov, I. A. (1956). On the composition of unimodal distributions. *Theory of Probability and Its Applications, 1*, 255–260.

Nakamura, T. K. (2009). Relativistic equilibrium distribution by relative entropy maximization. *Europhysics Letters Association, 88*(4). https://doi.org/10.1209/0295-5075/88/40009

Navarro, J., & Rubio, R. (2010). Computations of signatures of coherent systems with five components. *Communications in Statistics - Simulation and Computation, 39*, 68–84.

Ross, S. M. (2010). *Introduction to probability models* (10th ed.). Amsterdam: Elsevier.

Ross, S. M., Shahshahani, M., & Weiss, G. (1980). On the number of component failures in systems whose component lives are exchangeable. *Mathematics of Operations Research, 5*, 358–365.

Rychlik, T. (2001). *Projecting statistical functionals. Lecture notes in statistics* (Vol. 160). New York: Springer.

Samaniego, F. (1985). On closure of the IFR class under formation of coherent systems. *IEEE Transactions on Reliability, R-34*, 69–72.
Samaniego, F. (2007). *System signatures and their applications in engineering reliability. International series in operations research & management science* (Vol. 110). New York: Springer.
Schoenberg, I. J. (1959). On variation diminishing approximation methods. In Langer, R. E. (ed.). *On Numerical Approximation. Proceedings of a Symposium, Madison, April 21–23, 1958* (Publication no. 1) (pp. 249–274). Madison: The Mathematics Research Center, U.S. Army, University of Wisconsin, The University of Wisconsin Press.
Wang, B. X. (2012). Statistical inference for reliability of system stress-strength model under exponential distribution (Chinese). *Applied Mathematics-A Journal of Chinese Universities, Series A, 27*, 265–273.
Wang, J. (2015). On reversed hazard ordering of parallel systems with exponential components. *Far East Journal of Theoretical Statistics, 50*, 1–9.
Wang, J., & Zhao, P. (2016). On likelihood ratio ordering of parallel systems with exponential components. *Mathematical Methods of Statistics, 25*, 145–150.
Zhao, P., & Balakrishnan, N. (2009). Characterization of MRL order of fail-safe systems with heterogeneous exponential components. *Journal of Statistical Planning and Inference, 139*, 3027–3037.
Zhao, P., & Balakrishnan, N. (2011). Dispersive ordering of fail-safe systems with heterogeneous exponential components. *Metrika, 74*, 203–210.

Part II
Univariate Distribution Theory

A Note on the Product of Independent Beta Random Variables

Filipe J. Marques, Indranil Ghosh, Johan Ferreira, and Andriëtte Bekker

Abstract In this work, approximations for the distribution of the product of independent Beta random variables, based on mixtures of generalized Gamma distributions, are proposed. These mixtures are finite, and the parameters involved are determined using a two-step moment matching technique. A numerical study is conducted in order to assess the precision of the approximation proposed when compared with other approximations based on mixtures of Gamma distributions or mixtures of Beta distributions. Some observations related with the computational implementation of each type of approximations are discussed, particularly that these approximations may be simple yet efficient alternatives to several other approaches which are more complex in nature.

1 Introduction

The distribution of the product of independent Beta random variables was studied extensively in the last century. Several approaches have been proposed based on different representations, for example, in the form of series expansions (Moschopoulos 1986; Tang and Gupta 1984), Meijer G-function (Meijer 1946; Nagar et al. 1985), or Fox H-function (Carter and Springer 1977; Fox 1961) representations, among others (see Coelho and Alberto (2012) and the references cited therein). However, as

F. J. Marques (✉)
Centro de Matemática e Aplicações (CMA), FCT, UNL and Departamento de Matemática, FCT, UNL, Lisbon, Portugal
e-mail: fjm@fct.unl.pt

I. Ghosh
Department of Mathematics and Statistics, University of North Carolina Wilmington, Wilmington, NC, USA
e-mail: ghoshi@uncw.edu

J. Ferreira · A. Bekker
University of Pretoria, Pretoria, South Africa
e-mail: Johan.Ferreira@up.ac.za; Andriette.Bekker@up.ac.za

I. Ghosh et al. (eds.), *Advances in Statistics - Theory and Applications*, Emerging Topics in Statistics and Biostatistics, https://doi.org/10.1007/978-3-030-62900-7_4

already mentioned by other authors (Coelho and Alberto 2012), despite the existing computational power, these representations are not always easy or straightforward to implement. Recently, new approximations have been proposed, based on the concept of near-exact distributions (Coelho 2004), which have been used with excellent results in terms of precision and that can be implemented in computational terms (Coelho 2004; Coelho and Alberto 2012).

The importance and significance of the distribution of the product of independent Beta random variables can be easily justified, since it is the distribution of Wilks's lambda statistic and the distribution of most of the likelihood ratio statistics used to test the structure of a covariance matrix such as the sphericity, block independence, circularity, and compound symmetry structures of a covariance matrix (see, for example, (Coelho et al. 2010; Marques and Coelho 2008, 2013a,b; Marques et al. 2011) and the references cited therein).

The aim of this paper is to provide an approximation based on mixtures of generalized Gamma distributions to approximate the distribution of the product of independent Beta random variables, which is simple in practice, and at the same time precise. Moreover, we aim to analyze and discuss the performance of other simple approximations. The motivation for this approximation arises from the work of Marques et al. (2019), where it was shown that a generalized Gamma distribution can be represented as a mixture of generalized Gamma distributions with weights given by the probability mass function (p.m.f.) of a negative Binomial distribution and with the shape parameters of the associated generalized Gamma distributions given by a sequence of the type $a + n$ with $n = 0, \ldots$ and $a > 0$. This result has motivated, in the same reference, the use of mixtures of Generalized Gamma distributions to approximate the distributions of the sum of independent Gamma, Weibull, or Rayleigh random variables, which turned out to be a useful strategy.

To establish the notation, if the random variable Y_i has a Beta distribution with parameters a_i and b_i, we write $Y_i \sim Beta(a_i, b_i), i = 1, \ldots, p$, then $W_i = -\log Y_i$ has a Logbeta distribution with parameters a_i and b_i. It is well known that a single Logbeta distribution may be represented as an infinite mixture of Exponential distributions, and since the Exponential distribution is a particular case of the generalized Gamma distribution, we may use the results in Marques et al. (2019) to show that a Logbeta distribution may be represented as an infinite mixture of generalized Gamma distributions. Consequently, the study of the distribution of the product of independent Beta random variables is the same as the study of the sum of independent Logbeta distributions. A similar procedure to the one considered in Marques et al. (2019) may thus be used to address the distribution of the sum of independent Logbeta random variables.

The paper is organized as follows. In Sect. 2, the approximation based on mixtures of generalized Gamma distributions is derived. Additionally, other approximations, one based on a single Beta distribution and/or the mixture of two Beta distributions and the others based on the mixture of Gamma distributions, are also presented. In Sect. 3, numerical studies and simulations are carried out to assess the precision and advantages in using the mixtures presented in Sect. 2. Finally, some concluding remarks are presented in Sect. 4.

2 Approximations Based on Mixtures

In this section, we present the approximations considered for the probability density function (p.d.f.) and cumulative distribution function (c.d.f.) of the product of independent Beta random variables. If $Y_1, \ldots, Y_p$ are independent random variables with $Y_i \sim Beta(a_i, b_i)$ $i = 1, \ldots, p$, with p.d.f. given by

$$f_{Y_i}(y) = \frac{1}{B(a_i, b_i)}(1-y)^{b_i-1}\, y^{a_i-1}\,, \quad 0 < y < 1\,, \quad a_i > 0\,, \quad b_i > 0\,,$$

we are interested in the distribution of $Y = \prod_{i=1}^{p} Y_i$. However, in most of the cases, it is easier to consider

$$W = -\log\left(\prod_{i=1}^{p} Y_i\right) = -\sum_{i=1}^{p} \log Y_i = \sum_{i=1}^{p} W_i\,,$$

where $W_i = -\log Y_i$. We say that the random variable $W_i = -\log Y_i$ has a Logbeta distribution with parameters $a_i > 0$ and $b_i > 0$, and we denote this fact by $W_i \sim$ Logbeta(a_i, b_i), if its p.d.f. is given by

$$f_{W_i}(w) = \frac{1}{B(a_i, b_i)} \exp\{-a_i w\}(1 - \exp\{-w\})^{b_i-1}\,, \quad w > 0\,. \tag{1}$$

Once the approximating p.d.f. and c.d.f. are obtained for W, by simple transformation, we may obtain the corresponding p.d.f. and c.d.f. for Y.

The approximations proposed are based on mixtures of distributions, or on a single Beta distribution, and on a moment matching technique. With regard to the h-th moment of $Y = \prod_{i=1}^{p} Y_i$, where Y_i are independent, the moments Y can be easily obtained as

$$E(Y^h) = \prod_{i=1}^{p} E(Y_i^h) = \prod_{i=1}^{p} \frac{\Gamma(a_i + b_i)}{\Gamma(a_i)} \frac{\Gamma(a_i + h)}{\Gamma(a_i + b_i + h)}\,.$$

Since the random variable W has moments of any order, its moments may be obtained through the derivatives of the corresponding characteristic function, that is,

$$E(W^h) = \mathrm{i}^{-h} \left.\frac{\partial^h \Phi_W(t)}{\partial t^h}\right|_{t=0}, \tag{2}$$

where

$$\Phi_W(t) = \prod_{i=1}^{p} \frac{\Gamma(a_i + b_i)}{\Gamma(a_i)} \frac{\Gamma(a_i - \mathrm{i}t)}{\Gamma(a_i + b_i - \mathrm{i}t)} . \tag{3}$$

Since the approximating distributions for the distribution of Y and W are based on mixtures of distributions with moments of any order, the expression of the h-th moment can be easily derived. More details are given in the next subsections.

2.1 Mixtures of Generalized Gamma Distributions

In Marques et al. (2019), it was shown that a single generalized Gamma distribution can be represented as a mixture of generalized Gamma distributions. More precisely, if a random variable X has a generalized Gamma distribution with p.d.f. given by

$$f(x) = \frac{\gamma e^{-\left(\frac{x-\mu}{\beta}\right)^{\gamma}} \left(\frac{x-\mu}{\beta}\right)^{\alpha\gamma-1}}{\beta\Gamma(\alpha)} ,$$

$\alpha > 0$, $\beta > 0$, $\gamma > 0$, and $\mu \in \mathbb{R}$, which we denote by $X \sim G\Gamma(\alpha, \beta, \gamma, \mu)$, then the p.d.f. $f(x)$, for $\lambda > 0$ such that $\lambda < \beta$, may be represented in the following form:

$$f_X(x) = \sum_{n=0}^{\infty} f_{\mathrm{NB}\left(\alpha, \left(\frac{\beta}{\lambda}\right)^{-\gamma}\right)}(n) f_{G\Gamma(n+\alpha,\lambda,\gamma,\mu)}(x) , \ x > 0 , \tag{4}$$

where $f_{\mathrm{NB}\left(\alpha, \left(\frac{\beta}{\lambda}\right)^{-\gamma}\right)}(.)$ is the p.m.f. of a negative Binomial distribution with parameters α and $\left(\frac{\beta}{\lambda}\right)^{-\gamma}$, and for a given n, $f_{G\Gamma(n+\alpha,\lambda,\gamma,\mu)}(.)$ is the p.d.f. of a generalized Gamma distribution with parameters $(n + \alpha)$, λ, γ, μ. Note that a random variable Y has a negative binomial distribution, denoted by $Y \sim \mathrm{NB}(r, p)$ with $r > 0$ and success probability p, if its p.m.f. is given by

$$f_Y(n) = (1 - p)^n p^r \binom{n + r - 1}{r - 1} , n \geq 0 .$$

The expression in (4) is the p.d.f. of a mixture of generalized Gamma distributions with parameters $(n + \alpha)$, λ, γ, and μ and with weights given by the p.m.f. of a negative Binomial distribution. This representation motivated the use of mixtures of generalized Gamma distributions for the sum of independent Gamma, Weibull, and Rayleigh random variables in Marques et al. (2019), which are all particular cases of the generalized Gamma distribution. Interestingly, we may also represent a Logbeta distribution as a mixture of generalized Gamma distributions: if the random variables Y_i have a Beta distribution with parameters a_i and b_i, $Y_i \sim Beta(a_i, b_i)$, then $W_i = -\log Y_i \sim \text{Logbeta}(a_i, b_i)$, and if we expand the factor $(1 - \exp\{-w\})^{b_i - 1}$ in the p.d.f. of W_i in (1), we obtain

$$f_{W_i}(w) = \sum_{j=0}^{\infty} \frac{(-1)^j \binom{b_i - 1}{j}}{B(a_i, b_i)(a_i + j)} (a_i + j) \exp\{-(a_i + j)w\}, \; w > 0,$$

which corresponds to an infinite mixture of Exponential distributions with parameters $1/(a_i + j)$. Note that if b_i is an integer, then the mixture is finite with the upper limit of the sum equal to $b_i - 1$. The Exponential distribution is a particular case of the Gamma distribution and clearly also a particular case of the generalized Gamma distribution; thus, it follows from the results in Marques et al. (2019), for some $\lambda > 0$, that

$$f_{W_i}(w) = \sum_{j=0}^{\infty} \frac{(-1)^j \binom{b_i - 1}{j}}{B(a_i, b_i)(a_i + j)} \sum_{n=0}^{\infty} f_{\text{NB}(1, \lambda(a_i + j))}(n) f_{G\Gamma(1+n, \lambda, 1, 0)}(w) \tag{5}$$

$$= \sum_{j=0}^{\infty} \sum_{n=0}^{\infty} \frac{(-1)^j \lambda \binom{b_i - 1}{j} (1 - \lambda(a_i + j))^n}{B(a_i, b_i)} f_{G\Gamma(1+n, \lambda, 1, 0)}(w), \; w > 0, \tag{6}$$

where in expression (5), $f_{\text{NB}(1, \lambda(a_i + j))}(.)$ is the p.m.f. of a negative binomial distribution with parameters 1 and $\lambda(a_i + j)$, and for a given n, $f_{G\Gamma(1+n, \lambda, 1, 0)}(.)$ is the p.d.f. of a generalized gamma distribution with parameters $1 + n$, λ, 1, and 0. From expression (6), we may conclude that a Logbeta distribution may be represented as a mixture of generalized Gamma distributions with weights given by

$$\frac{(-1)^j \lambda \binom{b_i - 1}{j} (1 - \lambda(a_i + j))^n}{B(a_i, b_i)}$$

and with the component distributions being generalized Gamma distributions with parameters $1 + n$, λ, 1, and 0, which correspond to Gamma distributions with parameters $1 + n$ and λ.

Motivated by the previous results, and following the methodology proposed in Marques et al. (2019), we will consider mixtures of generalized Gamma distributions as approximating distributions for the distribution of the sum of independent Logbeta random variables. The p.d.f. and c.d.f. of W will be approximated, respectively, by

$$f_{\widetilde{W}_1}(w) = \sum_{n=0}^{m} \pi_n f_{G\Gamma(\alpha+n, \beta, \gamma, 0)}(w) \tag{7}$$

and

$$F_{\widetilde{W}_1}(w) = \sum_{n=0}^{m} \pi_n F_{G\Gamma(\alpha+n,\beta,\gamma,0)}(w)\,, \tag{8}$$

where π_n are the weights, and $f_{G\Gamma(\alpha+n,\beta,\gamma,0)}(.)$ and $F_{G\Gamma(\alpha+n,\beta,\gamma,0)}(.)$ are the p.d.f. and c.d.f. of a generalized gamma distribution with parameters $\alpha+n$, β, γ, and 0.

The parameters and weights in (7) and (8) will be determined using the algorithm given below.

Algorithm 1 Mixtures of generalized Gamma distributions

(i) First, we simulate a small sample from the distribution of W, and then we fit a generalized Gamma distribution to the data in order to obtain the initial values for α, β, and γ;

(ii) then, using initial values of α, β, and γ obtained in the previous step, the "true" values for α, β, and γ are determined numerically in such a way that the first three moments of the approximating distribution are the same as the first exact three moments; that is, α, β, and γ are obtained as solutions of the system of equations

$$E(W^h) = E(X^h)$$

$$\mathrm{i}^{-h} \left.\frac{\partial^h \Phi_W(t)}{\partial t^h}\right|_{t=0} = \frac{\beta^h \Gamma\left(\alpha+\frac{h}{\gamma}\right)}{\Gamma(\alpha)} \tag{9}$$

for $h = 1, \ldots, 3$ with $X \sim G\Gamma(\alpha, \beta, \gamma, 0)$ and with $\Phi_W(t)$ in (3);

(iii) for a given integer m and the values of α, β, and γ defined in the previous step, the first m weights in the mixture are determined in such a way that the first m moments of the approximating distribution are equal to the first exact m moments; note that the last weight is equal to $\pi_m = 1 - \sum_{n=0}^{m-1} \pi_n$. Thus, the first m weights in the mixture are determined as solutions of the system of equations

$$\mathrm{i}^{-h} \left.\frac{\partial^h \Phi_W(t)}{\partial t^h}\right|_{t=0} = \sum_{n=0}^{m} \pi_n \frac{\beta^h \Gamma\left(\alpha+n+\frac{h}{\gamma}\right)}{\Gamma(\alpha+n)} \tag{10}$$

for $h = 1, \ldots, m$, with $\pi_m = 1 - \sum_{n=0}^{m-1} \pi_n$ and $\Phi_W(t)$ in (3).

With this procedure, it is possible to control the precision of the approximation by increasing or decreasing the value of m. Once the approximating p.d.f and c.d.f. are obtained for the distribution of W, it is easy by simple transformation, to obtain the corresponding approximations for the distribution $Y = \prod_{i=1}^{p} Y_i$. The precision of such approximations is examined in Sect. 3.

2.2 A Single Beta or a Mixture of Two Beta Distributions

Since the support of $Y = \prod_{i=1}^{p} Y_i$ is the set (0, 1), it is also intuitive to consider a Beta distribution or mixtures of Beta distributions to approximate the distribution of Y. The approximation based on a single Beta distribution is quite easy to implement, and the corresponding approximating p.d.f. and c.d.f. of Y are given by

$$f_{\widetilde{W}_2}(w) = f_{Beta(c,d)}(w) \tag{11}$$

and

$$F_{\widetilde{W}_2}(w) = F_{Beta(c,d)}(w)\,, \tag{12}$$

where $f_{Beta(c,d)}(.)$ and $F_{Beta(c,d)}(.)$ are the p.d.f. and c.d.f. of a Beta distribution with parameters c and d. The parameters c and d are obtained using a moment matching technique, that is, by matching the first two exact moments, and thus as solution of the following system of equations

$$\prod_{i=1}^{p} \frac{\Gamma(a_i+b_i)}{\Gamma(a_i)} \frac{\Gamma(a_i+h)}{\Gamma(a_i+b_i+h)} = \frac{\Gamma(c+d)}{\Gamma(c)} \frac{\Gamma(c+h)}{\Gamma(c+d+h)}\,, \tag{13}$$

for $h = 1, 2$.

However, we face additional problems (illustrated in the next section) if we want to consider mixtures of Beta distributions, since the numerical computation of the parameters is not easy. For the mixture of two Beta distributions, we have to determine the five parameters of the distribution, that is, one weight and four parameters. In this case, the p.d.f. and c.d.f. of Y will be approximated, respectively, by

$$f_{\widetilde{W}_3}(w) = \pi_1 f_{Beta(c,d)}(w) + (1-\pi_1) f_{Beta(e,f)}(w) \tag{14}$$

and

$$F_{\widetilde{W}_3}(w) = \pi_1 F_{Beta(c,d)}(w) + (1-\pi_1) F_{Beta(e,f)}(w)\,, \tag{15}$$

where π_1 and $1-\pi_1$ are the weights. The parameters π_1, c, d, e, and f are determined by matching the first five exact moments and thus as solution of the system of equations

$$\begin{aligned}\prod_{i=1}^{p} \frac{\Gamma(a_i+b_i)}{\Gamma(a_i)} \frac{\Gamma(a_i+h)}{\Gamma(a_i+b_i+h)} &= \pi_1 \frac{\Gamma(c+d)}{\Gamma(c)} \frac{\Gamma(c+h)}{\Gamma(c+d+h)} \\ &\quad + (1-\pi_1) \frac{\Gamma(e+f)}{\Gamma(e)} \frac{\Gamma(e+h)}{\Gamma(e+f+h)}\,,\end{aligned} \tag{16}$$

for $h = 1, \ldots, 5$. In this case, we do not consider mixtures of more than two Beta distributions, since it becomes challenging to obtain a numeric solution for the system of equations in (16). The process may be summarized in the following algorithm.

Algorithm 2 A single Beta or a mixture of two Beta distributions

(i) First, we simulate a small sample from the distribution of Y, and then we fit to the data (A) a single Beta distribution in order to obtain the initial values for c and d or (B) a mixture of two Beta distributions such that we may obtain initial values for c, d, e, f, and π_1;

(ii) then, using as initial values for c, d, e, f, and π_1 obtained in the previous step, the "true" values for c, d, e, f, and π_1 are determined numerically in such a way that (A) the first two moments of single Beta distribution are the same as the first two exact moments, that is, c and d are obtained as solution of the system in (13) and (B) the first five moments of a mixture of two Beta distribution are the same as the first five exact moments, that is, c, d, e, f, and π_1 are determined as solutions of the system of equations in (16).

2.3 *Mixtures of Gamma Distributions: Type I*

Here, we consider mixtures of Gamma distributions as an approximation for the distribution of $W = \sum_{i=1}^{p} W_i$. This approximation is based on the results derived for the ratio of two Gamma functions by Tricomi and Erdélyi (1951), which after some algebraic manipulation (see Coelho et al. (2010) for further details) can be used to show that the distribution of W may be approximated by an infinite mixture of Gamma distributions all with the same rate parameter λ and with shape parameters $r + n$ for $n = 0, 1, \ldots$. In order to overcome the computational limitations involved when working with the referred infinite mixture, we consider a truncated version of this result, being the approximating p.d.f. and c.d.f. given by

$$f_{\widetilde{W}_4}(w) = \sum_{n=0}^{m} \pi_n f_{\Gamma(r+n,\lambda)}(w) \tag{17}$$

and

$$F_{\widetilde{W}_4}(w) = \sum_{n=0}^{m} \pi_n F_{\Gamma(r+n,\lambda)}(w), \tag{18}$$

where π_n are the weights, and $f_{\Gamma(r+n,\lambda)}(w)(.)$ and $F_{\Gamma(r+n,\lambda)}(w)(.)$ are the p.d.f. and c.d.f. of a Gamma distribution with rate parameter λ and shape parameters $r+n$, $n = 0, \ldots, m$, where m is the number of exact moments matched by the approximating distribution. This approximation is implemented as follows.

Algorithm 3 Mixtures of Gamma distributions: Type I

(i) First, the parameters r and λ are defined in the following way (as suggested in Coelho et al. (2010)): (a) the parameter r is chosen to be equal to the sum of the second parameters of the Logbeta distributions of W_i, and thus $r = \sum_{i=1}^{p} b_i$ and (b) the parameter λ is chosen to be equal to the rate parameter of a mixture of two Gamma distributions (with the same rate parameter), which matches the first four exact moments; thus, it is determined together with the weight θ and the shape parameters r_1 and r_2, such that

$$\mathrm{i}^{-h} \left.\frac{\partial^h \Phi_W(t)}{\partial t^h}\right|_{t=0} = \theta\,\lambda^h \frac{\Gamma(r_1+h)}{\Gamma(r_1)} + (1-\theta)\lambda^h \frac{\Gamma(r_2+h)}{\Gamma(r_2)}\,, \tag{19}$$

for $h = 1, \ldots, 4$ and $\Phi_W(t)$ in (3). It is easy to solve the system of equations in (19), but in some cases, we may need to perform some prior simulation to have starting values for θ, r_1, r_2, and λ;

(ii) after defining the values of r and λ, the weights π_n $(n = 0, \ldots, m-1)$ are determined as solutions of the following system of equations:

$$\mathrm{i}^{-h} \left.\frac{\partial^h \Phi_W(t)}{\partial t^h}\right|_{t=0} = \sum_{n=0}^{m} \pi_n \lambda^h \frac{\Gamma(r+n+h)}{\Gamma(r+n)}\,, \qquad h = 1, \ldots, m\,, \tag{20}$$

with $\pi_m = 1 - \sum_{n=0}^{m-1} \pi_n$ and $\Phi_W(t)$ in (3). This ensures that the first m moments of the approximating distribution are equal to the corresponding exact moments.

In the next section, the precision of asymptotic approximation in (17) and (18) will be analyzed, and it will be shown that in some cases, it is not the best option to approximate the sum of independent Logbeta random variables.

2.4 *Mixtures of Gamma Distributions: Type II*

Finally, we also consider mixtures of Gamma distributions; however, in this case, the shape parameter r is not equal to the sum of the second parameters of the Logbeta distributions of W_i, as it happened in the previous section, but it will be obtained, together with λ, as solution of the system of equations in (21). More precisely, we consider as approximating p.d.f. and c.d.f. for the distribution of W, respectively, the expressions in (17) and (18) but now, the parameters r and λ are both determined as the parameters of a Gamma distribution which match the first two exact moments; thus, this approximation is implemented by replacing the first step in Algorithm 3 as follows.

Note that, in step (i), we have analytical expressions, so the values of r and λ are obtained in a straightforward manner.

Algorithm 4 Mixtures of Gamma distributions: Type II

(i) First, the parameters r and λ are defined as the solution of the system of equations

$$\mathrm{i}^{-h} \left.\frac{\partial^h \Phi_W(t)}{\partial t^h}\right|_{t=0} = \lambda^h \frac{\Gamma(r+h)}{\Gamma(r)}, \tag{21}$$

for $h = 1, 2$ and $\Phi_W(t)$ in (3). The solution of this system of equations is equal to

$$r = -\frac{m_1^2}{m_1^2 - m_2} \quad \text{and} \quad \lambda = \frac{-m_1^2 + m_2}{m_1},$$

where

$$m_1 = \mathrm{i}^{-1} \left.\frac{\partial \Phi_W(t)}{\partial t}\right|_{t=0} \quad \text{and} \quad m_2 = -\left.\frac{\partial^2 \Phi_W(t)}{\partial t^2}\right|_{t=0}.$$

(ii) After defining the values of r and λ, the weights π_n $(n = 0, \ldots, m-1)$ are determined as solutions of the system of equations in (20) with $\pi_m = 1 - \sum_{n=0}^{m-1} \pi_n$.

3 Simulation Study

In order to analyze the precision of the approximations proposed in Sect. 2, we computed the empirical quantiles of Y and W by simulation. We simulated samples of sizes 2,000,000, and we computed the empirical quantiles of Y and W, denoted by q_ℓ, for $\ell = 0.05, 0.1, 0.5, 0.9, 0.95$. Next, we determined the value of the approximating c.d.f.'s computed for the empirical quantiles. Since the approximation proposed in Sect. 2.2 is for the c.d.f. of Y, in this case, we consider the quantiles of Y, and in the remaining cases, the empirical quantiles of W were considered. All the computations, simulations, and plots were obtained using the software Mathematica, Version 10.0 with an Intel(R) Core(TM) i7-7500U CPU@2.70GHz. In Tables 1, 2, 3, and 4 and in Figs. 1, 2, 3, and 4, we considered the following scenarios:

1. Scenario I: $a_i = \{1/2, 1/5\}$ and $b_i = \{1/3, 1/6\}$;
2. Scenario II: $a_i = \{1/2, 1/5\}$ and $b_i = \{14/3, 6/5\}$;
3. Scenario III: $a_i = \{1, 1/2, 1/3\}$ and $b_i = \{1, 2, 3\}$;
4. Scenario IV: $a_i = \{1/2, 5, 7/3, 4/5\}$ and $b_i = \{1, 1/6, 11/2, 3\}$;

Table 1 Scenario I—computed values of the approximating c.d.f.'s for the empirical quantiles q_ℓ with $\ell = 0.05, 0.1, 0.5, 0.90, 0.95$

m	$MG\Gamma_2$	$MG\Gamma_4$	$MG\Gamma_6$	MB_2	MB_5	$M\Gamma_2$	$M\Gamma_4$	$M\Gamma_6$	$M\Gamma_2^*$	$M\Gamma_4^*$	$M\Gamma_6^*$
$q_{0.05}$	0.044	0.044	0.044	0.038	0.050	0.051	0.050	0.050	0.032	0.033	0.034
$q_{0.10}$	0.092	0.092	0.092	0.085	0.100	0.102	0.100	0.100	0.075	0.077	0.080
$q_{0.50}$	0.501	0.502	0.503	0.501	0.500	0.503	0.501	0.500	0.496	0.503	0.506
$q_{0.90}$	0.900	0.900	0.899	0.898	0.900	0.899	0.900	0.900	0.903	0.900	0.898
$q_{0.95}$	0.950	0.950	0.950	0.948	0.950	0.950	0.950	0.950	0.951	0.948	0.948

Table 2 Scenario II—computed values of the approximating c.d.f.'s for the empirical quantiles q_ℓ with $\ell = 0.05, 0.1, 0.5, 0.90, 0.95$

m	$MG\Gamma_2$	$MG\Gamma_4$	$MG\Gamma_6$	MB_2	MB_5	$M\Gamma_2$	$M\Gamma_4$	$M\Gamma_6$	$M\Gamma_2^*$	$M\Gamma_4^*$	$M\Gamma_6^*$
$q_{0.05}$	0.056	0.053	0.050	0.150	0.179	0.006	0.014	0.024	0.081	0.064	0.054
$q_{0.10}$	0.105	0.102	0.100	0.222	0.256	0.017	0.040	0.063	0.130	0.109	0.100
$q_{0.50}$	0.495	0.497	0.500	0.575	0.604	0.366	0.551	0.581	0.485	0.485	0.497
$q_{0.90}$	0.901	0.901	0.900	0.896	0.901	1.061	0.839	0.848	0.896	0.907	0.900
$q_{0.95}$	0.951	0.950	0.950	0.946	0.948	1.022	0.870	0.977	0.952	0.953	0.948

Table 3 Scenario III—computed values of the approximating c.d.f.'s for the empirical quantiles q_ℓ with $\ell = 0.05, 0.1, 0.5, 0.90, 0.95$

m	$MG\Gamma_2$	$MG\Gamma_4$	$MG\Gamma_6$	MB_2	MB_5	$M\Gamma_2$	$M\Gamma_4$	$M\Gamma_6$	$M\Gamma_2^*$	$M\Gamma_4^*$	$M\Gamma_6^*$
$q_{0.05}$	0.051	0.050	0.050	0.235	0.070	0.035	0.045	0.049	0.065	0.054	0.050
$q_{0.10}$	0.101	0.100	0.100	0.307	0.116	0.077	0.095	0.100	0.115	0.102	0.099
$q_{0.50}$	0.499	0.500	0.500	0.611	0.444	0.506	0.509	0.500	0.489	0.494	0.500
$q_{0.90}$	0.900	0.900	0.900	0.892	0.888	0.910	0.895	0.901	0.898	0.903	0.900
$q_{0.95}$	0.951	0.950	0.950	0.943	0.956	0.947	0.949	0.951	0.951	0.951	0.949

Table 4 Scenario IV—computed values of the approximating c.d.f.'s for the empirical quantiles q_ℓ with $\ell = 0.05, 0.1, 0.5, 0.90, 0.95$

m	$MG\Gamma_2$	$MG\Gamma_4$	$MG\Gamma_6$	MB_2	MB_5	$M\Gamma_2$	$M\Gamma_4$	$M\Gamma_6$	$M\Gamma_2^*$	$M\Gamma_4^*$	$M\Gamma_6^*$
$q_{0.05}$	0.052	0.050	0.050	0.111	0.139	0.009	0.022	0.035	0.073	0.055	0.051
$q_{0.10}$	0.102	0.101	0.100	0.173	0.206	0.025	0.058	0.085	0.122	0.102	0.101
$q_{0.50}$	0.497	0.499	0.500	0.528	0.560	0.420	0.573	0.542	0.483	0.492	0.500
$q_{0.90}$	0.901	0.900	0.900	0.893	0.899	1.037	0.825	0.896	0.897	0.904	0.899
$q_{0.95}$	0.951	0.950	0.950	0.947	0.949	0.995	0.894	0.987	0.953	0.951	0.949

and we denote by $MG\Gamma_m$, MB_m, $M\Gamma_m$, and $M\Gamma_m^*$ the approximations developed, respectively, in Sects. 2.1, 2.2, 2.3, and 2.4, where m stands for the number of exact moments matched by each of the approximating distributions.

From Tables 1, 2, 3, and 4, we may conclude that the approximations $M\Gamma_m$ do not perform well in Scenarios 2 and 4, and the justification for this pattern is discussed in the final section and is also illustrated in Figs. 2 and 4. The approximations based on a single Beta or on mixtures of Beta distributions, in most of the cases, only represent good precision for the quantiles 0.90 and 0.95. In all scenarios, the approximations $MG\Gamma_m$ and $M\Gamma_m^*$ have similar behaviors displaying precise results in most of the cases considered. However, it seems that the approximations $MG\Gamma_m$ need to match less exact moments in order to obtain precise results. The results obtained for the different scenarios are illustrated in Figs. 1, 2, 3, and 4, where the approximating p.d.f.'s are plotted together with the histograms obtained from the simulated values of Y or W.

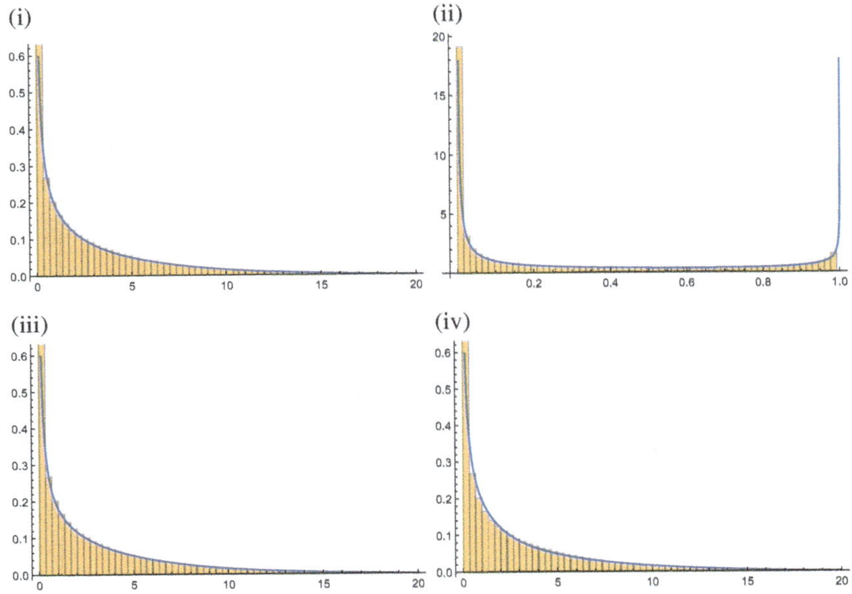

Fig. 1 Scenario 1—Plots for the approximating p.d.f.'s of $MG\Gamma_6$ (i), MB_5 (ii), $M\Gamma_6$ (iii), and $M\Gamma_6^*$ (iv) and for the histograms obtained from the simulated values of W (i), (iii), and (iv) and from the simulated values of Y (ii)

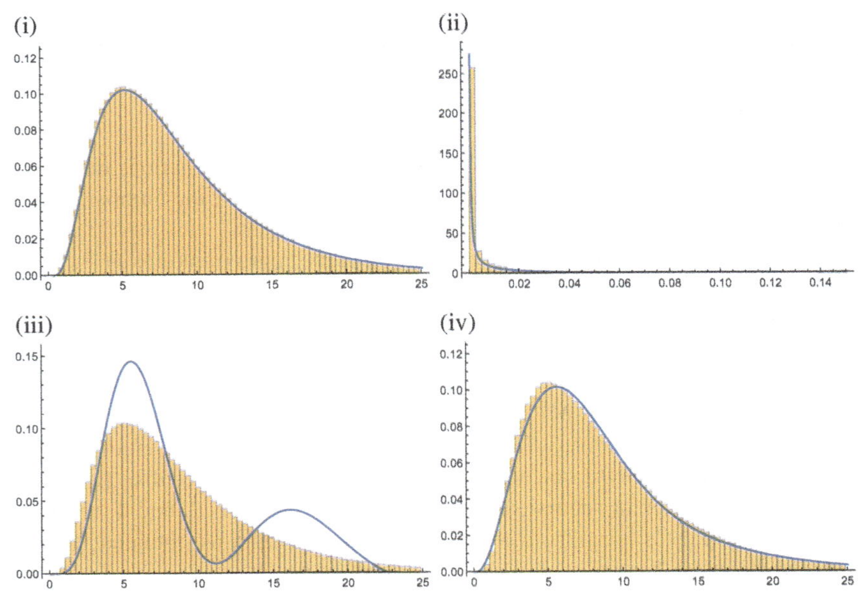

Fig. 2 Scenario 2—Plots for the approximating p.d.f.'s of $MG\Gamma_6$ (i), MB_5 (ii), $M\Gamma_6$ (iii), and $M\Gamma_6^*$ (iv) and for the histograms obtained from the simulated values of W (i), (iii), and (iv) and from the simulated values of Y (ii)

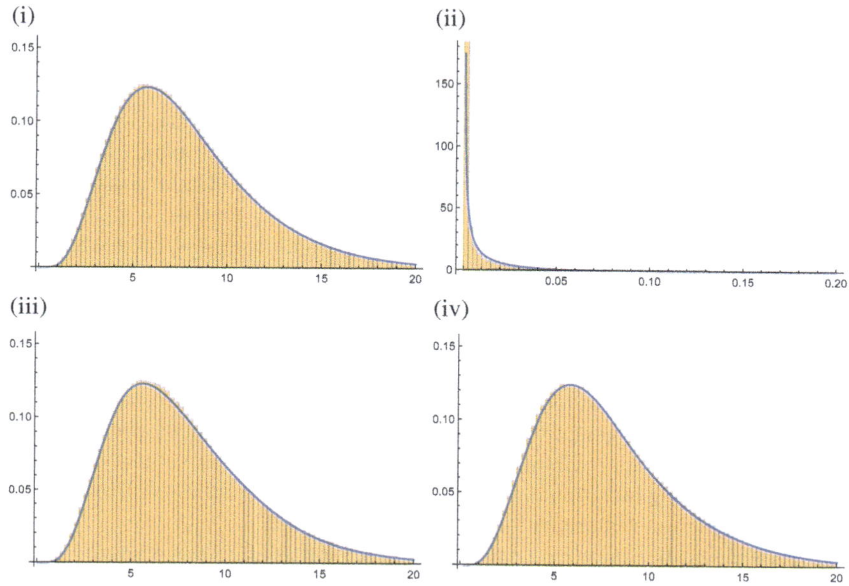

Fig. 3 Scenario 3—Plots for the approximating p.d.f.'s of $MG\Gamma_6$ (i), MB_5 (ii), $M\Gamma_6$ (iii), and $M\Gamma_6^*$ (iv) and for the histograms obtained from the simulated values of W (i), (iii), and (iv) and from the simulated values of Y (ii)

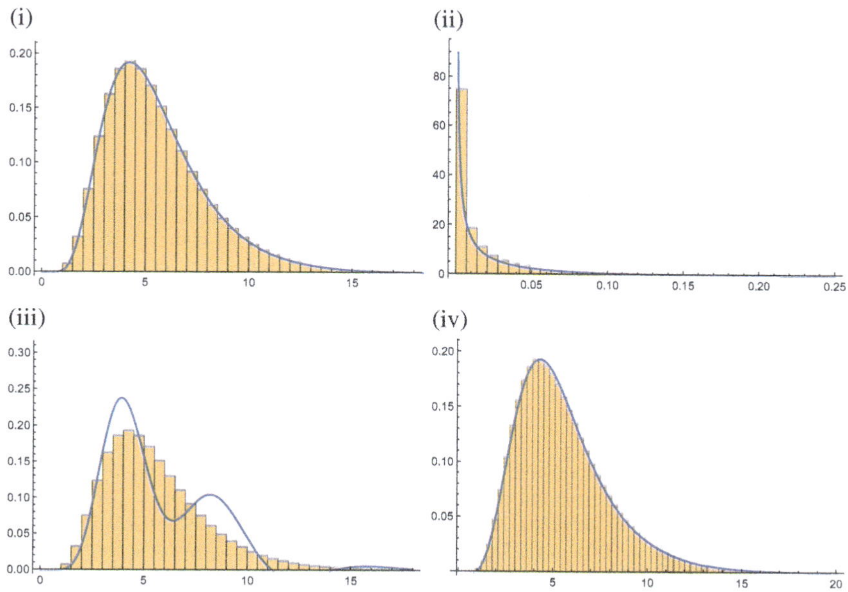

Fig. 4 Scenario 4—Plots for the approximating p.d.f.'s of $MG\Gamma_6$ (i), MB_5 (ii), $M\Gamma_6$ (iii), and $M\Gamma_6^*$ (iv) and for the histograms obtained from the simulated values of W (i), (iii), and (iv) and from the simulated values of Y (ii)

4 Concluding Remarks

Based on our simulation study, some comments are in order. In some of the scenarios, the approximations, designated by $M\Gamma_m$, do not perform well. It seems that the approximations denoted by $MG\Gamma_m$ and $M\Gamma_m^*$ are stable and precise. However, the approximation based on mixtures of generalized Gamma distributions, $MG\Gamma_m$, reaches better results with lower values of m, that is, with less exact moments matched. On the other hand, the approximations based on a single Beta or on mixtures of two Beta distributions, denoted by MB_m, in most of the cases, only provide reasonable results for the 0.90 and 0.95 quantiles. When mixtures of Beta distributions are considered, the solutions of the system in (16) are not easy to obtain with a reasonable precision.

Although we only considered $m = 2, 4$, and 6 for the approximations based on mixtures of Gamma or generalized Gamma distributions, the methodology used to derive these type of approximations allows to consider higher values of m. Since m is the number of exact moments matched by the approximating distributions, we expect to obtain even better results for higher values of m.

To achieve further improvements in the precision of the approximations based on mixtures of Gamma or generalized Gamma distributions, we may also consider a similar procedure to the one used in Marques et al. (2019), where a tuning parameter was introduced in the shape parameters with positive results in the precision of the approximations.

Finally, we should note that it is quite simple to use the approximations discussed in this work, since these approximations are represented as finite mixtures of well-known distributions. With the approximations $MG\Gamma_m$ and $M\Gamma_m^*$, it is possible and simple to obtain results with 3 or 4 exact decimal places. If more precision is required, whenever desired, the near-exact approximations should be considered.

Acknowledgments This work was partially supported by the Fundação para a Ciência e a Tecnologia (Portuguese Foundation for Science and Technology) through the project UIDB/00297/2020 (Centro de Matemática e Aplicações) and also based upon research supported by the National Research Foundation, South Africa (SRUG190308422768 nr. 120839) and the Research Development Programme at University of Pretoria 296/2019.

References

Coelho, C. A. (2004). The generalized near-integer gamma distribution: A basis for 'near-exact' approximations to the distribution of statistics which are the product of an odd number of independent beta random variables. *Journal of Multivariate Analysis, 89*, 191–218.

Carter, B. D., & Springer, M. D. (1977). The distribution of products, quotients and powers of independent H-function variates. *SIAM Journal of Applied Mathematics, 33*, 542–558.

Coelho, C. A., Arnold, B. C., & Marques, F. J. (2010). Near-exact distributions for certain likelihood ratio test statistics. *Journal of Statistical Theory and Practice, 4*, 711–725.

Coelho, C. A., & Alberto, R. P. (2012). On the distribution of the product of independent beta random variables applications. Technical Report, CMA, FCTNOVA (vol. 12).

Fox, C. (1961). The G and H functions as symmetrical kernels. *Transactions of the American Mathematical Society, 98*, 395–429.

Marques, F. J., & Coelho, C. A. (2008). Near-exact distributions for the sphericity likelihood ratio test statistic. *Journal of Statistical Planning and Inference, 138*, 726–741.

Marques, F. J., & Coelho, C. A. (2013a). Obtaining the exact and near-exact distributions of the likelihood ratio statistic to test circular symmetry through the use of characteristic functions. *Computational Statistics, 28*, 2091–2115.

Marques, F. J., & Coelho, C. A. (2013b). The multisample block-diagonal equicorrelation and equivariance test. *AIP Conference Proceedings, 1558*, 793–796.

Marques, F. J., Coelho, C. A. & Arnold, B. C. (2011). A general near-exact distribution theory for the most common likelihood ratio test statistics used in multivariate analysis. *Test, 20*, 180–203.

Marques, F. J., Loots, M. T., & Bekker, A. (2019). Series representations for densities functions of a family of distributions–Application to sums of independent random variables. *Mathematical Methods in the Applied Sciences*, 1–18.

Meijer, C. S. (1946). On the G-function I–VIII. *Proc. Koninklijk Nederlandse Akademie van Weteenschappen, 49*, 227–237, 344–356, 457–469, 632–641, 765–772, 936–943, 1063–1072, 1165–1175.

Moschopoulos, P. G. (1986). New representations for the distribution function of a class of likelihood ratio criteria. *Journal of Statistical Research, 20*, 13–20.

Nagar, D. K., Jain, S. K., & Gupta A. K. (1985). Distribution of LRC for testing sphericity of a complex multivariate Gaussian model. *International Journal of Mathematics & Mathematical Science, 8*, 555–562.

Tang, J., & Gupta, A. K. (1984). On the distribution of the product of independent beta random variables. *Statistics & Probability Letters, 2*, 165–168.

Tricomi, F. G., & Erdélyi, A. (1951). The asymptotic expansion of a ratio of Gamma functions. *Pacific Journal of Mathematics, 1*, 133–142.

On the Distribution of the Product of Independent Beta Random Variables — Applications

Carlos A. Coelho and Rui P. Alberto

Abstract A first approach, based on recently obtained asymptotic expansions of ratios of gamma functions, enables the obtention of the distribution of the product of independent and identically distributed random variables in a much manageable form. However, for the general case, this approach leads to a form which although being very manageable and in line with some previous results, suffers from serious problems of precision and convergence, which have been completely overlooked by other authors and which in most cases prevent its practical use. Nevertheless, it is based on these first results that the authors, using the concept of near-exact distribution, are able to obtain highly manageable but extremely accurate approximations for all cases of the distribution of the product of independent Beta random variables. These near-exact approximations, given their high manageability, accuracy, and proximity to the exact distribution, may in practice be used instead of the exact distribution.

1 Introduction

The distribution of the product of independent Beta random variables (r.v.'s) is a distribution which plays a key role in Statistics. There are many likelihood ratio test (l.r.t.) statistics, namely in Multivariate Analysis, whose distribution has been

Electronic Supplementary Material The online version of this article (https://doi.org/10.1007/978-3-030-62900-7_5) contains supplementary material, which is available to authorized users.

C. A. Coelho (✉)
Departamento de Matemática and Centro de Matemática e Aplicações, FCT NOVA, NOVA University of Lisbon, Lisbon, Portugal
e-mail: cmac@fct.unl.pt

R. P. Alberto
Centro de Matemática e Aplicações, FCT NOVA, NOVA University of Lisbon, Lisbon, Portugal
e-mail: rui.pesado@sapo.pt

I. Ghosh et al. (eds.), *Advances in Statistics - Theory and Applications*, Emerging Topics in Statistics and Biostatistics, https://doi.org/10.1007/978-3-030-62900-7_5

shown to be that of the product of a number of independent Beta r.v.'s, as for example the l.r.t. statistics to test, under multivariate normality, or rather, under multivariate elliptically contoured or left orthogonal-invariant distributions, the independence of several sets of variables, the equality of several mean vectors, the equality of several variance–covariance matrices or sphericity of the covariance matrix (Anderson 2003; Kshirsagar 1972; Marques et al. 2011; Muirhead 2005), the l.r.t. statistics to test similar hypotheses under the complex multivariate normal setting (Coelho et al. 2015; Gupta 1971; Khatri 1965a; Pillai and Jouris 1971), the l.r.t. statistics to test multi-sample sphericity or block-scalar or block-matrix sphericity (Coelho and Marques 2011a; Marques and Coelho 2011a,b), the l.r.t. statistic to test reality of a covariance matrix in a complex Normal distribution (Khatri 1965b) or the l.r.t. statistics to test circularity of the covariance matrix and stationarity (Olkin and Press 1961), or even the l.r.t. statistic to test the equality of several exponential distributions, in the case of equal sample sizes (Coelho and Marques 2011b).

Although along the years many authors have worked on obtaining the distribution of the product of independent Beta r.v.'s in a manageable form or otherwise obtaining manageable approximations for its distribution (Bharbava and Khatri 1981; Carter and Springer 1977; Mathai 1984; Nagar et al. 1985; Nagarsenker and Das 1975; Nagarsenker and Suniaga 1983; Nandi 1980; Pederzoli 1985; Springer 1979; Springer and Thompson 1966, 1970; Tang and Gupta 1984, 1986; Tretter and Walster 1975; Tukey and Wilks 1946; Walster and Tretter 1980), obtaining an explicit, accurate, and highly manageable expression for both the probability density function (p.d.f.) and the cumulative distribution function (c.d.f.) of this distribution has been a hard task and we are absolutely sure that there is still much room left for improvement.

Our aim is exactly to obtain explicit highly manageable expressions for both the p.d.f. and c.d.f. of extremely well-fitting approximations for this distribution, based on highly accurate and manageable mixture expansions.

One popular form to represent the exact p.d.f. and c.d.f. of the distribution of the product of independent Beta r.v.'s has been the use of either the Meijer G or Fox's H functions (Carter and Springer 1977; Springer 1979). However, although this is a very handy way to represent these distributions, these representations are not very adequate in practical terms since both Fox's H function and Meijer G function implementations have their drawbacks not only in terms of precision, but mainly in terms of computation time in all the commonly available software.

Other authors like Bharbava and Khatri (1981) and Pederzoli (1985) used multiple series representations where each summation corresponds to a different Beta r.v. in the product, yielding a too much complicated structure for the distribution, mainly when the number of Beta r.v.'s involved is rather large.

Yet other authors like Nagarsenker and Das (1975), Nandi (1980), Nagarsenker and Suniaga (1983), and Tang and Gupta (1984) express the distribution of the product of independent Beta r.v.'s as infinite mixtures of Beta distributions. However these representations have the drawback of needing, in the general case, a large number of terms to attain the desired accuracy and not allowing for the development of further better performing approximations, while are also not able to take advantage from those cases where some of the Beta r.v.'s have the same distribution. Furthermore, the distribution in Nandi (1980) and Tang and Gupta (1984) depends on the particular ordering of the Beta r.v.'s considered, while the series in Nagarsenker and Das (1975) and Nagarsenker and Suniaga (1983) have highly complicated coefficients.

The papers by Tang and Gupta (1986), Mathai (1984), and Nagar et al. (1985) present results which match the results of what is our first approach to the problem; however, without any reference to accuracy and convergence issues which indeed occur with the series obtained. Moreover, opposite to the results obtained in the present paper, in Nagar et al. (1985) the weights in the infinite mixture have a very complicated formulation, while in Tang and Gupta (1986) there is a parameter left with a not well-defined value.

Yet, our approach enables the use of more adequate expansions for the cases where some of the Beta r.v.'s involved in the product have the same distribution. In a further step we will determine the weights in our mixture distributions by matching some of the first exact moments, what will enable us to obtain distributions which will converge on the whole support of the r.v., overcoming the problems mentioned in Lemma 3.1 and Remark 3.1 in Tang and Gupta (1986). We may note that this moment matching approach is supported by the well known fact that the product of independent Beta r.v.'s, having a bounded support, has its distribution determined by its moments.

In this paper the authors show how, based on asymptotic expansions of the ratio of two gamma functions, presented by Burić and Elezović (2011) but for which much simpler proofs are shown in Appendix A, it is possible to obtain a single mixture of exponentiated gamma distributions as an asymptotic approximation for the exact distribution of the product of any number of independent Beta r.v.'s, with easily computable coefficients. However, in practical terms this approach leads to almost impossible to handle difficulties, arising from the fact that the resulting series distributions are either very slowly convergent or even divergent.

To overcome these difficulties the authors, recover the concept of near-exact distribution (see Sect. 4), and based on this approach they develop near-exact approximations which lie very close to the exact distribution of the product of independent Beta r.v.'s, although remaining highly manageable, while displaying much better performances than previous approaches proposed by different authors.

As already mentioned, many likelihood ratio test statistics have the same distribution as that of a product of independent Beta r.v.'s. In these cases, the first parameter in the distribution of these Beta r.v.'s is directly related with the sample sizes, while the second parameter is commonly directly related with the number of variables. The near-exact distributions developed by the authors, when applied to these settings, show very good performances even for situations in which the sample sizes are very small, that is, barely exceeding the number of variables, even when the number of variables involved is large.

The setup: let

$$X_j \sim Beta(a_j, b_j) \quad \text{and} \quad Y_j = -\log X_j\,, \qquad j = 1, \ldots, p\,, \tag{1}$$

be a set of p independent random variables and let

$$Z=\prod_{j=1}^{p} X_j\,, \qquad W=-\log\,Z=-\sum_{j=1}^{p}\log\,X_j=\sum_{j=1}^{p} Y_j\,. \tag{2}$$

We will say that the random variable $Y=-\log\,X$ has a $Logbeta(a,b)$ distribution and we are interested in the distribution of Z, or, somehow equivalently, in the distribution of W.

At first sight we may think that a good idea to work around the difficulties of the representation of the distribution of Z might be to try to express the distribution of each X_j or Y_j as a mixture.

In order to obtain an asymptotic expansion for the distribution of a Logbeta r.v., we might think about using expression following expression (18) together with expression (19) in Tricomi and Erdélyi (1951) or expression (1) in Fields (1966) which may be written, for $|arg(z+\alpha)|<\pi$, as $z\to\infty$, as

$$\frac{\Gamma(z+\alpha)}{\Gamma(z+\beta)}\approx\sum_{k=0}^{\infty}\frac{1}{k!}\,\frac{\Gamma(1+\alpha-\beta)}{\Gamma(1+\alpha-\beta-k)}\,B_k^{(1+\alpha-\beta)}(\alpha)\,z^{\alpha-\beta-k}\,, \tag{3}$$

where $B_j^{(n)}(\,\cdot\,)$ is the generalized Bernoulli polynomial of degree j and order n.

In fact, an application of expression (3), with $z=a-\mathrm{i}t$, $\alpha=0$ and $\beta=b$, yields

$$\frac{\Gamma(a-\mathrm{i}t)}{\Gamma(a+b-\mathrm{i}t)}\approx\sum_{k=0}^{\infty}p_k(b)\,(a-\mathrm{i}t)^{-b-k}\quad(\text{as } a\to\infty) \tag{4}$$

where

$$p_k(b)=\frac{1}{k!}\,\frac{\Gamma(1-b)}{\Gamma(1-b-k)}\,B_k^{(1-b)}(0)$$

with $B_k^{(1-b)}(0)$ being the generalized Bernoulli number of degree k and order $1-b$.

The result in (4) enables us to represent asymptotically any $Logbeta(a,b)$ distribution as an infinite mixture of $\Gamma(b+k,a)$ distributions ($k=0,1,\ldots$)—see Appendix B in Coelho and Alberto (2020) for the notation used for the gamma distribution. Indeed, from (4) we may then write the characteristic function (c.f.) of Y_j as

$$\begin{aligned}\Phi_{Y_j}(t)&=E\left(e^{\mathrm{i}tY_j}\right)=E\left(X_j^{-\mathrm{i}t}\right)=\frac{\Gamma(a_j+b_j)}{\Gamma(a_j)}\,\frac{\Gamma(a_j-\mathrm{i}t)}{\Gamma(a_j+b_j-\mathrm{i}t)}\\&\approx\sum_{k=0}^{\infty}\underbrace{\frac{\Gamma(a_j+b_j)}{\Gamma(a_j)}\,\frac{p_k(b_j)}{a_j^{b_j+k}}}_{p_k^*(a_j,b_j)}\,a_j^{b_j+k}\,(a_j-\mathrm{i}t)^{-(b_j+k)}\,,\quad(\text{as } a_j\to\infty)\end{aligned}$$

which is the c.f. of an infinite mixture of $\Gamma(b_j + k, a_j)$ distributions, with weights $p_k^*(a_j, b_j)$ $(k = 0, 1, \dots)$.

Then in order to obtain an asymptotic representation for the distribution of W we might think about convoluting p independent Logbeta distributions in the form of mixtures of Gamma distributions, to obtain then, by exponentiation, the distribution of the corresponding product of independent Beta r.v.'s.

However, the problem is that in this case the asymptotic distribution of W would be an infinite mixture of sums of independent gamma random variables, with possibly different rate parameters a_j. Then, the distribution of each of these sums would have itself to be expressed in the form of a mixture, rendering the final expression for the whole distribution not manageable at all.

To overcome these difficulties, our aim is to approximate asymptotically the distribution of W by a single infinite mixture of gamma distributions. This will be achieved with the approach followed in the next section.

2 Some Results Concerning Ratios of Gamma Functions

Let, for the a_j in (1),

$$a = \min(a_1, a_2, \dots, a_p)\,, \tag{5}$$

and then, for

$$\alpha_j = a_j - a \quad \text{and} \quad \beta_j = a_j + b_j - a = \alpha_j + b_j\,, \qquad (j = 1, \dots, p)\,, \tag{6}$$

using (3) with $z = a - \mathrm{i}t$, write (as $a \to \infty$)

$$\begin{aligned}
\frac{\Gamma(a_j - \mathrm{i}t)}{\Gamma(a_j + b_j - \mathrm{i}t)} &= \frac{\Gamma(a - \mathrm{i}t + \alpha_j)}{\Gamma(a - \mathrm{i}t + \beta_j)} \\
&\approx \sum_{k=0}^{\infty} \frac{1}{k!} \frac{\Gamma(1 - b_j)}{\Gamma(1 - b_j - k)} B_k^{(1-b_j)}(\alpha_j)\,(a - \mathrm{i}t)^{-b_j - k} \\
&= \Gamma(1-b_j)\,(a-\mathrm{i}t)^{-b_j} \sum_{k=0}^{\infty} \frac{1}{k!\,\Gamma(1-b_j-k)} B_k^{(1-b_j)}(\alpha_j)\,(a-\mathrm{i}t)^{-k}\,.
\end{aligned}$$

Then, for W in (2), we may write, as $a \to \infty$,

$$\Phi_W(t) = \prod_{j=1}^{p} \frac{\Gamma(a_j + b_j)}{\Gamma(a_j)} \frac{\Gamma(a_j - \mathrm{i}t)}{\Gamma(a_j + b_j - \mathrm{i}t)} \tag{7}$$

$$\approx C\,(a-\mathrm{i}t)^{-b}\prod_{j=1}^{p}\sum_{k=0}^{\infty}\underbrace{\frac{1}{k!\,\Gamma(1-b_j-k)}\,B_k^{(1-b_j)}(\alpha_j)}_{q_{jk}}\,(a-\mathrm{i}t)^{-k}\,, \quad (8)$$

where

$$C=\prod_{j=1}^{p}\frac{\Gamma(1-b_j)\,\Gamma(a_j+b_j)}{\Gamma(a_j)} \quad \text{and} \quad b=\sum_{j=1}^{p}b_j\,. \quad (9)$$

In (8) we have

$$\prod_{j=1}^{p}\sum_{k=0}^{\infty}q_{jk}\,(a-\mathrm{i}t)^{-k}=\sum_{k=0}^{\infty}w_k\,(a-\mathrm{i}t)^{-k}\,,$$

where

$$w_k=\sum_{r_1+r_2+\cdots+r_p=k}q_{1r_1}q_{2r_2}\cdots q_{pr_p}\,,$$

with each sequence $\{r_1,r_2,\ldots,r_p\}$ being a weak composition of the integer k into p parts, and being the sum extended to the complete set of the above compositions, which cardinality is $\binom{k+p-1}{p-1}=\binom{k+p-1}{k}$ (see for example Heuback and Mansour (2009)).

We may thus write

$$\Phi_W(t)\approx C\sum_{k=0}^{\infty}\frac{w_k}{a^{b+k}}\,a^{b+k}\,(a-\mathrm{i}t)^{-(b+k)} \quad (\text{as } a\to\infty) \quad (10)$$

which shows that for large enough a and for b in (9) the c.f. of W in (2) should be well approximated by the c.f. of an infinite mixture of $\Gamma(b+k,a)$ $(k=0,1,\ldots)$ distributions, with weights Cw_k/a^{b+k}.

However, in the more general case we may have each pair (a_j,b_j) in (7) repeated say m_j times. Although in this case we could still use the same approach as above, it happens that for each set of random variables with the same set of parameters (a_j,b_j) the computation of the weights in the mixture will be much more efficient if carried out through a slightly different way. In this case, instead of (3) we should use the more general expression

$$\left(\frac{\Gamma(z+\alpha)}{\Gamma(z+\beta)}\right)^{m}\approx\sum_{k=0}^{\infty}\nu_{k,m}(\alpha,\beta)\,z^{m(\alpha-\beta)-k}\,, \quad (\text{as } z\to\infty,\ |arg(z+\alpha)|<\pi)\,, \quad (11)$$

with

$$\nu_{k,m}(\alpha,\beta)=\frac{1}{k}\sum_{j=1}^{k} j\,\delta_{j,m}(\alpha,\beta)\,\nu_{k-j,m}(\alpha,\beta)\,,\quad (k=1,2,\dots),\quad \nu_{0,m}(\alpha,\beta)=1\,,\tag{12}$$

where

$$\delta_{j,m}(\alpha,\beta)=(-1)^j m\,\frac{B_{j+1}(\beta)-B_{j+1}(\alpha)}{j(j+1)}\,,\tag{13}$$

and where $B_j(a)$ represents the value of the Bernoulli polynomial of degree j in a.

Expression (11) is expression (2.1) in Burić and Elezović (2011) and it may be quite easily obtained from Barnes expression (37). See Appendix A for a simpler and straightforward demonstration. The use of (11) is shown in the next section.

3 Main Results Concerning the Exact Distribution of the Product of Independent Beta Random Variables

3.1 The General Case

In this "general case" we will allow some of the Beta r.v.'s to be identically distributed. Let then

$$X_\ell \sim Beta(a_\ell, b_\ell) \qquad \ell=1,\dots,p$$

be a set of p independent random variables. Let then q be the number of distinct pairs of parameters (a_ℓ, b_ℓ) among the p random variables X_ℓ and let (a_j, b_j) $(j=1,\dots,q)$ represent the set of distinct pairs (a_ℓ, b_ℓ) $(\ell=1,\dots,p)$. Let further m_j be the number of times the pair of parameters (a_j, b_j) appears among the p random variables X_ℓ, thus with

$$p=\sum_{j=1}^{q} m_j\,,$$

and of course with $q=p$ if all $m_j=1$.

Since from (11), taking a as defined in (5), $z=a-\mathrm{i}t$, and α_j and β_j as in (6), we may write

$$\left(\frac{\Gamma(a_j-\mathrm{i}t)}{\Gamma(a_j+b_j-\mathrm{i}t)}\right)^{m_j}=\left(\frac{\Gamma(a-\mathrm{i}t+\alpha_j)}{\Gamma(a-\mathrm{i}t+\beta_j)}\right)^{m_j}\approx\sum_{k=0}^{\infty}\nu_{k,m_j}(\alpha_j,\beta_j)\,(a-\mathrm{i}t)^{-m_jb_j-k}\,,\tag{14}$$

we may thus write, for W in (2),

$$\Phi_W(t) = \prod_{j=1}^{q} \left(\frac{\Gamma(a_j+b_j)}{\Gamma(a_j)}\right)^{m_j} \left(\frac{\Gamma(a_j-\mathrm{i}t)}{\Gamma(a_j+b_j-\mathrm{i}t)}\right)^{m_j} \tag{15}$$

$$\approx C\,(a-\mathrm{i}t)^{-b} \prod_{j=1}^{q}\sum_{k=0}^{\infty} \nu_{k,m_j}(\alpha_j,\beta_j)\,(a-\mathrm{i}t)^{-k} \quad (\text{as } a\to\infty) \tag{16}$$

where $\nu_{k,m_j}(\alpha_j,\beta_j)$ $(k=0,1,\ldots;\ j=1,\ldots,q)$ are given by (12)–(13) and

$$C = \prod_{j=1}^{q}\left(\frac{\Gamma(a_j+b_j)}{\Gamma(a_j)}\right)^{m_j} \quad \text{and} \quad b = \sum_{j=1}^{q} m_j b_j\,. \tag{17}$$

In (16), we may set

$$\prod_{j=1}^{q}\sum_{k=0}^{\infty} \nu_{k,m_j}(\alpha_j,\beta_j)\,(a-\mathrm{i}t)^{-k} = \sum_{k=0}^{\infty}\omega_k\,(a-\mathrm{i}t)^{-k}$$

with

$$\omega_k = \sum_{r_1+r_2+\cdots+r_q=k} \nu_{r_1,m_1}(\alpha_1,\beta_1)\,\nu_{r_2,m_2}(\alpha_2,\beta_2)\,\ldots\,\nu_{r_q,m_q}(\alpha_q,\beta_q)\,, \tag{18}$$

where, as in the previous section, each sequence $\{r_1, r_2, \ldots, r_q\}$ is a weak composition of the integer k into q parts, and the sum is extended to the complete set of these compositions, whose cardinality is $\binom{k+q-1}{q-1} = \binom{k+q-1}{k}$.

From (16) and (18) we may write

$$\Phi_W(t) \approx C\sum_{k=0}^{\infty}\frac{\omega_k}{a^{b+k}}\,a^{b+k}\,(a-\mathrm{i}t)^{-(b+k)} \quad (\text{as } a\to\infty) \tag{19}$$

for a as in (5), C and b given by (17), and ω_k given by (18).

Expression (19) shows that for sufficiently large a the exact distribution of W is well approximated by an infinite mixture of $\Gamma(b+k,a)$ distributions, with weights $C\omega_k/a^{b+k}$ $(k=0,1,\ldots)$, and as such, the exact distribution of $Z=e^{-W}$ will be also well approximated by the corresponding mixture, that is, with the same weights, of exponentiated $\Gamma(b+k,a)$ distributions.

From (19) we may thus write

$$f_W(w) \approx C\sum_{k=0}^{\infty}\frac{\omega_k}{\Gamma(b+k)}\,e^{-aw}\,w^{b+k-1}\,, \quad (w>0)\,,$$

and

$$F_W(w) \approx C \sum_{k=0}^{\infty} \omega_k \, \frac{\Gamma^*(b+k, aw)}{\Gamma(b+k)}\,, \qquad (w > 0)\,,$$

where

$$\Gamma^*(b+k, aw) = \int_0^{aw} e^{-aw} \, w^{b+k-1} \, dw$$

is a version of the incomplete gamma function, and therefore also

$$f_Z(z) \approx C \sum_{k=0}^{\infty} \frac{\omega_k}{\Gamma(b+k)} \, z^{a-1} \, (-\log z)^{b+k-1}\,, \qquad (0 < z < 1)\,,$$

and

$$F_Z(z) \approx 1 - C \sum_{k=0}^{\infty} \omega_k \, \frac{\Gamma^*(b+k, -a \log z)}{\Gamma(b+k)}\,, \qquad (0 < z < 1)\,.$$

However, as we will see in Sect. 6, with the help of some numerical studies, the practical implementation of these representations faces some problems which are not easy to solve and which are related with the facts that

(i) while for sets of Beta r.v.'s with values of a_j which show a moderately large variability we may need an unsoundly large number of terms in the series to get a good approximation,
(ii) on the other hand, the use of a larger number of terms may start to give worse approximations, namely for sets of Beta r.v.'s with values of a_j which show a small variability, while the use of a moderately large number of terms may still not give the desired precision.

We should remark that these problems are not brought to our attention by other authors who, although using different approaches, obtain similar results, as it is the case of Tang and Gupta (1986), Mathai (1984), and Nagar et al. (1985).

We should also note here that the approach followed, in case all m_j in (14) and (16) are equal to 1, yields the approach of Moschopoulos (1986). Although the use of the m_j with values different from 1 may seem a minor detail, that is indeed not so, since this approach, where general m_j are used, may allow for much better approximations than the ones that would be obtained if such approach is not taken. This is true even when we will be interested in developing near-exact distributions, rather than just common asymptotic distributions, as it is shown later in Sect. 7.1, where the use of such expressions enables the obtention of even better near-exact distributions than the ones previously obtained.

If some restrictions are met by the parameters of the Beta distributed r.v.'s in (1) and (2), the distribution of Z and also that of W in (2) may then have a finite closed form representation, and a number of l.r.t. statistics fall in this case. For details on this topic we refer the reader to Coelho and Arnold (2019).

3.2 *The Particular Case of All Different Sets of Pairs of Parameters*

In case each Beta r.v. has a different set of parameters, then all the m_j defined in the previous subsection will be equal to 1 and we will have $q = p$. In this case W will have an approximate c.f. still given by (16) and (19) in the previous subsection, for all $m_j = 1$, or, if we prefer, given by (8) or (10) in Sect. 2.

3.3 *The Particular Case of All Equal Sets of Pairs of Parameters*

In case all p random variables X_j have the same distribution, although remaining independent, then we may either take $q = p$, with all $m_j = 1$ and then apply the results in Sect. 3.1, or take $q = 1$, with $m_1 = p$ and then apply the results in Sect. 3.1. From the derivations in Sect. 2 we are able to see that the second choice is far more efficient in terms of the computation of the weights ω_k.

However, using expression (45) in Appendix A, we may obtain a much faster converging series or mixture distribution. This expression is expression (7.1) in Burić and Elezović (2011), for which we provide a much simpler and straightforward demonstration path in Appendix A.

In this case, if we take $a_j = a$ and $b_j = b$ $(j = 1, \ldots, p)$, and if we also take in (45), $z = a - \mathrm{i}t$, $\alpha = 0$ and $\beta = b$, we may write

$$
\begin{aligned}
\Phi_W(t) &= \left(\frac{\Gamma(a+b)}{\Gamma(a)}\,\frac{\Gamma(a-\mathrm{i}t)}{\Gamma(a+b-\mathrm{i}t)}\right)^p \\
&\approx C\sum_{k=0}^{\infty} \nu_{2k,p}(-k, b-k)\left(a-\mathrm{i}t+\frac{b-1}{2}\right)^{-pb-2k} \\
&= C\sum_{k=0}^{\infty} \frac{\nu_{2k,p}(-k, b-k)}{\left(a+\frac{b-1}{2}\right)^{pb+2k}}\left(a+\frac{b-1}{2}\right)^{pb+2k}\left(a+\frac{b-1}{2}-\mathrm{i}t\right)^{-(pb+2k)}
\end{aligned}
$$

with $\nu_{2k,p}(-k, b-k)$ given by (12)–(13) and

$$C = \left(\frac{\Gamma(a+b)}{\Gamma(a)}\right)^p ,$$

which shows that in this case the distribution of W is asymptotically approximated, for increasing $a+\frac{b-1}{2}$, by an infinite mixture of $\Gamma\left(pb+2k, a+\frac{b-1}{2}\right)$ distributions with weights $C\nu_{2k,p}(-k, b-k)\Big/\left(a+\frac{b-1}{2}\right)^{pb+2k}$ $(k = 0, 1, \ldots)$.

3.4 *The Distribution of the Product of Powers of Independent Beta Random Variables*

So far we have only dealt with the distribution of the product of independent Beta r.v.'s as expressed in (2), that is, with the Beta r.v.'s raised to the power 1. Of course, the results obtained are easily extended to the case where all the Beta r.v.'s are raised to some common positive power. In this case one only has to consider the distribution of the product of the random variable $W = -\log Z$ considered so far, multiplied by that power or the distribution of the exponential of this random variable, if the distribution of Z is desired, being both very simple to obtain by simple transformation.

However, there may be cases where we are interested in the distribution of the random variable

$$Z = \prod_{j=1}^{p} X_j^{c_j}$$

where X_j are as in (2) and the c_j are positive reals. In this case the problem becomes much harder to tackle.

As in Sect. 3.1, let us suppose that among the p random variables X_ℓ $(\ell = 1, \ldots, p)$ there are $q \le p$ of them with different first and second parameter or raised to a different power, that is, let us suppose that there are $q \le p$ different triplets (a_j, b_j, c_j) $(j = 1, \ldots, q)$.

Let us further suppose that the triplet (a_j, b_j, c_j) appears m_j times $(j = 1, \ldots, q)$, once again with $p = \sum_{j=1}^{q} m_j$. Then, for $a = \min(a_1, \ldots, a_q)$ and for α_j and β_j given by (6), we may write the c.f. of $W = -\log Z$ as

$$\begin{aligned}
\Phi_W(t) &= \prod_{j=1}^{q} \left(\frac{\Gamma(a_j+b_j)}{\Gamma(a_j)}\right)^{m_j} \left(\frac{\Gamma(a_j - c_j\mathrm{i}t)}{\Gamma(a_j+b_j-c_j\mathrm{i}t)}\right)^{m_j} \\
&\approx C \prod_{j=1}^{q} \sum_{k=0}^{\infty} \nu_{k,m_j}(\alpha_j, \beta_j)\,(a - c_j\mathrm{i}t)^{-(m_j b_j + k)} \\
&= C \prod_{j=1}^{q} \sum_{k=0}^{\infty} \nu_{k,m_j}(\alpha_j, \beta_j) \left(\frac{a}{c_j} - \mathrm{i}t\right)^{-(m_j b_j + k)} (c_j)^{-(m_j b_j + k)} .
\end{aligned}$$

The problem now is hard to tackle because the rate parameters a/c_j are now function of j, that is, their value varies now with j, and there is no simple way to work around this fact.

Of course we may take each set of Beta r.v.'s with parameters (a_j, b_j, c_j) individually and take the approach first outlined in Sect. 2, but this, as stated in Sect. 2, would lead us to an almost intractable infinite mixture of infinite mixtures, with the further concomitant even arduous problems related with the convergence of truncations of these distributions, if we try to use them in applications.

Although in this case the Fox H function gives a nice way to express both the exact p.d.f. and c.d.f. of Z, there seems to be no really satisfactory formulation for the distribution of Z for practical uses, in this case. However, as we will see in Sects. 5 and 7, the near-exact approach is able to handle this case with no big problems and extremely satisfactory results. See Sect. 5.2 for the theoretical developments and Sect. 7.3 for an application and some numerical results.

4 The Practical Implementation of the Exact Distribution in Sect. 3 — Another Look at the Exact Distribution on the Way to Near-Exact Distributions

Since in any of the cases addressed in Sect. 3 the exact distribution always takes the form of an infinite mixture, in practice when using these distributions we will have to truncate them.

For a truncation corresponding to a c.f. of the form

$$C \sum_{k=0}^{m} \frac{\omega_k}{a^{b+k}}\, a^{b+k}\, (a - \mathrm{i}t)^{-(b+k)} \tag{20}$$

an upper-bound for the truncation error is

$$1 - C \sum_{k=0}^{m} \frac{\omega_k}{a^{b+k}} .$$

But, as we may see from the results in Sect. 6, we may do much better by using a truncation with completion of the weights in such a way that they add up to 1, that is, by using in (20) ω_k given by (18) and (12)–(13) for $k = 0, \ldots, m-1$, and

$$\omega_m = \frac{a^{b+m}}{C} - \sum_{k=0}^{m-1} \omega_k\, a^{m-k}\,. \tag{21}$$

Although for quite small values of k the computation of the weights ω_k does not pose any serious problem, that is not anymore the case for large values of k, where the weights ω_k, given the summation in (18), become quite heavy to compute.

Since we have indeed the exact c.f. of W at hand in the form in (15), we may think about determining the weights ω_k in (20), for $k = 0, \ldots, m-1$, in such a manner that the first m derivatives of the c.f. in (20), at $t = 0$, match the corresponding derivatives of $\Phi_W(t)$ in (15), setting then ω_m to the value given by (21).

This approach will indeed give much better results than the computation of the weights ω_k through their original expression. See the results in Sect. 6.

Yet, in order to better analyze the behavior of these approximations we will consider in Sect. 6 truncations where the first ω_k are computed from (18) and (12)–(13) and the remaining are computed by matching some of the exact moments, that is, we will use a c.f.

$$C \sum_{k=0}^{m^*} \frac{\omega_k}{a^{b+k}}\, a^{b+k}\, (a - \mathrm{i}t)^{-(b+k)} + \sum_{k=m^*+1}^{m^{**}} \pi_{k-m^*}\, a^{b+k}\, (a - \mathrm{i}t)^{-(b+k)}, \tag{22}$$

where ω_k $(k = 0, \ldots, m^*)$ are computed from (18) and (12)–(13) and π_{k-m^*} $(k = m^* + 1, \ldots, m^{**})$ are computed by matching the first $m^{**} - m^*$ derivatives at $t = 0$ of the c.f. in (22) and $\Phi_W(t)$.

One other thing we may notice is that, either computing the weights through their original expression or by matching derivatives, that is, by matching exact moments, for a given number of terms used in (20), the approximations are always much better when the b_j's fall between zero and one. The ascertainment of this fact may lead us to a different approach in which we would "extract" the integer part of the b_j's and somehow set it apart, whenever any of the b_j's exceeds the value of one. This is indeed the approach pursued in the next section.

We should remark that although the notation used in this section is the one used in Sect. 3.1, in order to encompass the case treated in Sect. 3.3 one only has to consider $\omega_k = \nu_{2k,p}(-k, b-k)$.

5 Near-Exact Distributions for the Product of Independent Beta Random Variables

5.1 Near-Exact Distributions for Z in (2)

In trying to "extract" the integer part of the b_j's and set it apart, whenever any of the b_j's exceeds the value of one, this will indeed lead us to the use of what has been called 'near-exact distributions'.

In simple terms, near-exact distributions are distributions which keep intact a good part of the exact distribution and which approximate asymptotically the remaining part.

In order to try to keep intact a good part of the exact c.f. when at least one of the b_j's is greater than 1, we may work through the exact c.f. of W as it is done below, using the fact that for any real or complex a and positive integer n we may write

$$\frac{\Gamma(a+n)}{\Gamma(a)} = \prod_{\ell=0}^{n-1}(a+\ell)\,. \tag{23}$$

In fact, using (23), taking $b_j^* = \lfloor b_j \rfloor$ and $b_j^{**} = b_j - b_j^*$, we may write, for the general case of the distribution of W in Sect. 3.1,

$$\begin{aligned}
\Phi_W(t) &= \prod_{j=1}^{q}\left(\frac{\Gamma(a_j+b_j)}{\Gamma(a_j)}\right)^{m_j}\left(\frac{\Gamma(a_j-\mathrm{i}t)}{\Gamma(a_j+b_j-\mathrm{i}t)}\right)^{m_j}\\
&= \prod_{j=1}^{q}\left(\frac{\Gamma(a_j+b_j)}{\Gamma(a_j+b_j^*)}\,\frac{\Gamma(a_j+b_j^*)}{\Gamma(a_j)}\right)^{m_j}\left(\frac{\Gamma(a_j-\mathrm{i}t)}{\Gamma(a_j+b_j^*-\mathrm{i}t)}\,\frac{\Gamma(a_j+b_j^*-\mathrm{i}t)}{\Gamma(a_j+b_j-\mathrm{i}t)}\right)^{m_j}\\
&= \prod_{j=1}^{q}\left(\frac{\Gamma(a_j+b_j)}{\Gamma(a_j+b_j^*)}\,\frac{\Gamma(a_j+b_j^*-\mathrm{i}t)}{\Gamma(a_j+b_j-\mathrm{i}t)}\right)^{m_j}\prod_{\ell=0}^{b_j^*-1}(a_j+\ell)^{m_j}(a_j+\ell-\mathrm{i}t)^{-m_j}\\
&= \underbrace{\left\{\prod_{j=1}^{q}\prod_{\ell=0}^{b_j^*-1}(a_j+\ell)^{m_j}(a_j+\ell-\mathrm{i}t)^{-m_j}\right\}}_{\Phi_{1,W}(t)}\\
&\qquad\times\underbrace{\left\{\prod_{j=1}^{q}\left(\frac{\Gamma(a_j+b_j)}{\Gamma(a_j+b_j^*)}\,\frac{\Gamma(a_j+b_j^*-\mathrm{i}t)}{\Gamma(a_j+b_j-\mathrm{i}t)}\right)^{m_j}\right\}}_{\Phi_{2,W}(t)}
\end{aligned} \tag{24}$$

where $\Phi_{1,W}(t)$ is the c.f. of a sum of $\sum_{j=1}^{q} b_j^*$ independent Gamma random variables, with integer shape parameters m_j and rate parameters $a_j + \ell$ ($\ell = 0, \dots, b_j^* - 1$; $j = 1, \dots, q$), which is a GIG distribution (Coelho 1998) of depth $\sum_{j=1}^{q} b_j^*$, with rate parameters $a_j + \ell$ and shape parameters m_j ($j = 1, \dots, q$; $\ell = 0, \dots, b_j^* - 1$) and $\Phi_{2,W}(t)$ is the c.f. of a sum of $p = \sum_{j=1}^{q} m_j$ independent Logbeta r.v.'s, m_j of which have the set of parameters $(a_j + b_j^*, b_j^{**})$ ($j = 1, \dots, q$).

We may note that if in (24) some b_j is smaller than 1, then the corresponding b_j^* equals zero and the corresponding term in $\Phi_{1,W}(t)$ simply vanishes, i.e., equals 1.

Since, opposite to $\Phi_{2,W}(t)$, $\Phi_{1,W}(t)$ corresponds to a very manageable distribution, in building the near-exact distribution for W we will leave $\Phi_{1,W}(t)$ unchanged and we will approximate $\Phi_{2,W}(t)$ in a similar manner to the one used in Sect. 3 to approximate $\Phi_W(t)$.

We will take

$$a = \min(a_1 + b_1^*, \dots, a_q + b_q^*)\,, \quad \alpha_j = a_j + b_j - a\,, \quad \text{and} \quad \beta_j = b_j^{**} = b_j - b_j^*\,, \tag{25}$$

and we will write

$$\Phi_{2,W}(t) \approx C \sum_{k=0}^{\infty} \frac{\omega_k}{a^{b+k}}\, a^{b+k}\, (a - \mathrm{i}t)^{-(b+k)}\,,$$

where

$$C = \prod_{j=1}^{q} \left(\frac{\Gamma(a_j + b_j)}{\Gamma(a_j + b_j^*)} \right)^{m_j} \quad \text{and} \quad b = \sum_{j=1}^{q} m_j (b_j - b_j^*)\,, \tag{26}$$

and where ω_k is computed using (18), now with α_j and β_j given by (25). We will then use as near-exact c.f. for W the c.f.

$$\Phi_W^*(t) = \Phi_{1,W}(t)\, C \sum_{k=0}^{m} \pi_k\, a^{b+k}\, (a - \mathrm{i}t)^{-(b+k)}, \tag{27}$$

where the weights π_k will be determined in such a way that

$$\frac{d^h}{dt^h} C \sum_{k=0}^{m} \pi_k\, a^{b+k}\, (a - \mathrm{i}t)^{-(b+k)} \bigg|_{t=0} = \frac{d^h}{dt^h} \Phi_{2,W}(t) \bigg|_{t=0}\,, \qquad h = 1, \dots, m$$

or, equivalently, in such a way that

$$\frac{d^h}{dt^h}\Phi_W^*(t)\bigg|_{t=0} = \frac{d^h}{dt^h}\Phi_W(t)\bigg|_{t=0}, \qquad h = 1, \ldots, m\,.$$

The reason to compute the weights π_k in this way is twofold: computed this way, instead of using expressions (18) and (12)–(13), the weights π_k (i) will yield better approximations and (ii) will be easier to compute for moderately large values of k.

The distribution corresponding to the c.f. $\Phi_W^*(t)$ in (27) is a finite mixture of GNIG (Generalized Near-Integer Gamma) distributions (see Coelho (2004) for the definition of this distribution and Appendix B of Coelho and Alberto (2020) for a definition of its p.d.f. and c.d.f.) which in case all $a_j + \ell$ $(j=1, \ldots, q;\ \ell=0, \ldots, b_j^*-1)$ are different will have depth $1 + \sum_{j=1}^{q} b_j^*$ with shape parameters

$$\underbrace{m_1, \ldots, m_1}_{b_1^*\text{ times}}, \ldots, \underbrace{m_j, \ldots, m_j}_{b_j^*\text{ times}}, \ldots, \underbrace{m_q, \ldots, m_q}_{b_q^*\text{ times}}, b+k$$

and rate parameters $\{a_j + 0, \ldots, a_j + b_j^* - 1 (j = 1, \ldots, q), a\}$.

For the general case, where some of the $a_j + \ell$ may have the same value, let

$$\left\{a_\nu^*;\ \nu = 1, \ldots, q^* \leq \textstyle\sum_{j=1}^{q} b_j^*\right\} = \{\{a_j + \ell;\ \ell = 0, \ldots, b_j^* - 1;\ j = 1, \ldots, q\}\}$$

represent the set of all different rate parameters $a_j + \ell$, that is, the set of all different values of $a_j + \ell$ $(\ell = 0, \ldots, b_j^* - 1;\ j = 1, \ldots, q)$ and let

$$\left\{m_\nu^*;\ \nu=1, \ldots, q^* \leq \textstyle\sum_{j=1}^{q} b_j^*\right\} = \{\{m_{j\ell}=m_j;\ \ell=0, \ldots, b_j^* - 1;\ j=1, \ldots, q\}\}_{\{a_j+\ell\}}$$

be the set of the corresponding shape parameters, where the shape parameter m_ν^* is the shape parameter corresponding to a_ν^*, that is, it is the sum of all $m_{j\ell} = m_j$ corresponding to the ν-th distinct value $a_j + \ell$. Then the p.d.f. and c.d.f. corresponding to the c.f. in (27), using the notation in Appendix B of Coelho and Alberto (2020) for the GNIG distribution would be respectively

$$f_W^*(w) = \sum_{k=0}^{m} \pi_k f^{GNIG}\left(w \mid \{a_\nu^*\}_{\nu=1:q^*}, b+k;\ \{a_\nu^*\}_{\nu=1:q^*}, a;\ q^* + 1\right)$$

and

$$F_W^*(w) = \sum_{k=0}^{m} \pi_k F^{GNIG}\left(w \mid \{a_\nu^*\}_{\nu=1:q^*}, b+k;\ \{a_\nu^*\}_{\nu=1:q^*}, a;\ q^* + 1\right)$$

and the corresponding p.d.f. and c.d.f. for $Z = e^{-W}$ would be

$$f_Z^*(z) = \sum_{k=0}^{m} \pi_k f^{GNIG}\left(-\log z \,|\, \{a_\nu^*\}_{\nu=1:q^*}, b+k;\, \{a_\nu^*\}_{\nu=1:q^*}, a;\, q^*+1\right) \frac{1}{z}$$

and

$$F_Z^*(z) = 1 - \sum_{k=0}^{m} \pi_k F^{GNIG}\left(-\log z \,|\, \{a_\nu^*\}_{\nu=1:q^*}, b+k;\, \{a_\nu^*\}_{\nu=1:q^*}, a;\, q^*+1\right).$$

We may note that in case b in (26) is an integer the GNIG distributions will indeed be GIG (Generalized Integer Gamma) distributions.

Built in this way, the near-exact distribution which c.f. is in (27) will provide extremely good approximations to the exact distribution, while remaining quite manageable. Some of the several vast advantages of these near-exact distributions are that:

(i) they provide the exact distribution in cases where all b_j are integer (in the form of a GIG distribution for $W = -\log Z$ or an EGIG distribution (Arnold et al. 2013) for Z),
(ii) the approximations provided will be even better for cases where the b_j are larger,
(iii) they have a much stable performance for a wide range of values of the parameters a_j, b_j, and m_j,
(iv) they will perform even slightly better in the situations where the other approximations show severe difficulties.

Actually, since the weights π_k in (27) are not going to be computed from (18) and (12)–(13), we may also think about a couple of alternative ways to compute the parameter a in (27). These may be to take a in (27) as one of the following choices:

$$\begin{gathered}
\text{i) } a = \min_{j=1,\dots,q}(a_j + b_j^*) \quad \text{ii) } a = \frac{1}{q}\sum_{j=1}^{q}(a_j+b_j^*) \quad \text{iii) } a = \frac{\sum_{j=1}^{q}(b_j-b_j^*)(a_j+b_j^*)}{\sum_{j=1}^{q}(b_j-b_j^*)}\\
\text{iv) } a = \frac{\sum_{j=1}^{q} m_j(a_j+b_j^*)}{\sum_{j=1}^{q} m_j} \qquad \text{v) } a = \frac{\sum_{j=1}^{q} m_j(b_j-b_j^*)(a_j+b_j^*)}{\sum_{j=1}^{q} m_j(b_j-b_j^*)}\\
\text{vi) the rate parameter } a \text{ in } \Phi^{**}(t) = a^s(a-\mathrm{i}t)^{-s}, \text{ where}\\
\left.\frac{\partial^h}{\partial t^h}\Phi^{**}(t)\right|_{t=0} = \left.\frac{\partial^h}{\partial t^h}\Phi_{2,W}(t)\right|_{t=0}, \quad h=1,2\\
\text{vii) the rate parameter } a \text{ in } \Phi^{***}(t) = \pi a^{s_1}(a-\mathrm{i}t)^{-s_1} + (1-\pi)a^{s_2}(a-\mathrm{i}t)^{-s_2}, \text{ where}\\
\left.\frac{\partial^h}{\partial t^h}\Phi^{***}(t)\right|_{t=0} = \left.\frac{\partial^h}{\partial t^h}\Phi_{2,W}(t)\right|_{t=0}, \quad h=1,\dots,4.
\end{gathered} \tag{28}$$

Details on the performance of such near-exact approximations may be analyzed in the next section and also in Sect. 7.

Mathematica modules to compute these as well as all the other approximations developed in this manuscript are available, on demand, from the authors.

These different strategies for the choice of a will be used only for approximations which correspond to the situations studied in Sects. 3.1 and 3.2, since for the situation addressed in Sect. 3.3 there is no doubt in the choice of a, having only to consider that in this case the parameter a in (27) has to be taken as $a + \frac{b-1}{2}$, where b is the common value of the second parameter for all the Beta r.v.'s involved.

In cases where all the b_j are smaller than 1, the near-exact distribution will then provide an asymptotic distribution of the same kind of the ones in Sect. 3. Anyway, for these cases the distributions in Sect. 3, which are indeed asymptotic distributions, work very well, as we may see from the results in Sect. 6. Furthermore, these are not the most common cases that occur, mainly when these distributions refer to likelihood ratio test statistics, and, as we may also see from the results in Sect. 6, by determining some of the weights through equating some of the first exact moments we may obtain approximations which lie very close to the exact distribution.

Actually, in these latter cases where all b_j are smaller than 1, as it may be seen from the results analyzed in Sect. 6 and reported in Appendix C of Coelho and Alberto (2020), a good balance between a number of weights determined through (18) and (12)–(13) and a number of weights determined by equating some of the first exact moments leads usually to the best results and although this approach might also be applied to the general near-exact distributions, for reasons of simplicity and extent of the manuscript we decided to use in the near-exact distributions only weights determined by equating exact moments. The adaptation of the approach followed to this other one of determining some of the weights through their formulation in (18) and (12)–(13) is quite easy and straightforward, although the computation of the weights through (18) and (12)–(13), namely for higher orders, may require more computation than their determination by equating exact moments.

5.2 *Near-Exact Distributions for the Product of Independent Beta Random Variables Raised to Different Powers*

However, it is interesting to note that this case of different powers c_j poses indeed no big problems when we adopt the near-exact approach. It indeed poses no problem at all in what concerns the handling of the part of the c.f. $\Phi_W(t)$ which will be left unchanged, that is, $\Phi_{1,W}(t)$, anyway posing a similar problem to the one described above for $\Phi_{2,W}(t)$, the part of the c.f. $\Phi_W(t)$ to be asymptotically approximated, since in the present case, following the same lines as in (24) we have

$$
\begin{aligned}
\Phi_W(t) &= \left\{\prod_{j=1}^{q}\prod_{\ell=0}^{b_j^*-1}(a_j+\ell)^{m_j}\,(a_j+\ell-c_j\mathrm{i}t)^{-m_j}\right\}\\
&\qquad\times\left\{\prod_{j=1}^{q}\left(\frac{\Gamma(a_j+b_j)}{\Gamma(a_j+b_j^*)}\,\frac{\Gamma(a_j+b_j^*-c_j\mathrm{i}t)}{\Gamma(a_j+b_j-c_j\mathrm{i}t)}\right)^{m_j}\right\}\\
&= \underbrace{\left\{\prod_{j=1}^{q}\prod_{\ell=0}^{b_j^*-1}\left(\frac{a_j+\ell}{c_j}\right)^{m_j}\left(\frac{a_j+\ell}{c_j}-\mathrm{i}t\right)^{-m_j}\right\}}_{\Phi_{1,W}(t)}\\
&\qquad\times\underbrace{\left\{\prod_{j=1}^{q}\left(\frac{\Gamma(a_j+b_j)}{\Gamma(a_j+b_j^*)}\,\frac{\Gamma(a_j+b_j^*-c_j\mathrm{i}t)}{\Gamma(a_j+b_j-c_j\mathrm{i}t)}\right)^{m_j}\right\}}_{\Phi_{2,W}(t)}
\end{aligned}
$$

where now $\Phi_{1,W}(t)$ is the c.f. of a sum of $\sum\limits_{j=1}^{q} b_j^*$ independent Gamma random variables, with integer shape parameters m_j and rate parameters $(a_j+\ell)/c_j$ ($\ell = 0,\dots,b_j^*-1$; $j=1,\dots,q$), which is a GIG distribution of depth $\sum\limits_{j=1}^{q} b_j^*$, with rate parameters $(a_j+\ell)/c_j$ and shape parameters m_j ($j=1,\dots,q$; $\ell=0,\dots,b_j^*-1$) and $\Phi_{2,W}(t)$ is the c.f. of a sum of $p=\sum_{j=1}^{q} m_j$ independent Logbeta r.v.'s, m_j of which have parameters $(a_j+b_j^*, b_j^{**})$ and are multiplied by c_j ($j=1,\dots,q$).

Then, based on a heuristic approach, in building the near-exact distribution for W we will leave $\Phi_{1,W}(t)$ unchanged and we will now approximate $\Phi_{2,W}(t)$ in exactly the same way we did in the previous subsection, now taking a in (27) as one of the choices in (28), with $a_j+b_j^*$ replaced by $(a_j+b_j^*)/c_j$.

As it happened in the previous subsection, these different strategies for the choice of a will be used only for approximations which correspond to the situations studied in Sects. 3.1 and 3.2, since for the situation addressed in Sect. 3.3, once again there is no doubt in the choice of a, having now to consider that in this case not only the first and second parameters of all the Beta r.v.'s have to be equal but also all the powers to which they are raised have also to be the same. Then we may either take the parameter a in (27) as $\left(a+\frac{b-1}{2}\right)/c$, where a and b are respectively the common values of the first and second parameters for all the Beta r.v.'s involved and c the common power, or just take the transformation procedure outlined in Sect. 3.4.

From the results in the next section as well as in Sect. 7.3, we may see that this approach really works well in practice.

6 Some Evidence Better Analyzed from Numerical Studies

While we clearly expect the "completed" truncation to perform much better than the simple truncation, and the version with the weights computed from the moments to perform even much better, we also expect the near-exact distributions to display an even much better performance than any of these. The results coming out of a few numerical studies may indeed help us in better figuring out the fine behavior of each of these approximations and also to better see that the near-exact approximations are indeed the only ones with a remarkable outstanding performance in all situations, that is, for any combination of values of the parameters involved. These results may be analyzed in detail in Coelho and Alberto (2020).

In order to assess the proximity between the exact distributions of W and Z and the approximations suggested in this manuscript we use the measure

$$\Delta = \frac{1}{2\pi}\int_{-\infty}^{+\infty}\left|\frac{\Phi_W(t)-\Phi^*(t)}{t}\right| dt \tag{29}$$

with

$$\max_{w\in S_W}\left|F_W(w)-F_W^*(w)\right| = \max_{z\in S_Z}\left|F_Z(z)-F_Z^*(z)\right| \leq \Delta\,,$$

where $\Phi_W(t)$ represents the exact c.f. of W given by (7) or (16) and $\Phi^*(t)$ the approximate c.f. corresponding to the approximation being used, and where $F_W(w)$ and $F_W^*(w)$ represent the c.d.f.'s corresponding to $\Phi_W(t)$ and $\Phi^*(t)$, and $F_Z(z)$ and $F_Z^*(z)$ the corresponding c.d.f.'s of Z. Therefore smaller values of Δ correspond to better approximations.

The measure in (29) may be seen as related with the Berry–Esseen bound (Berry 1941; Esseen 1945; Hsu 1945; Hwang 1998) and has been used in several studies as a measure of proximity between distributions (Coelho et al. 2010, 2015; Marques and Coelho 2011a; Marques et al. 2011).

From the results in Tables 1-23 in Appendix C in Coelho and Alberto (2020), we may see how the approximations based on the c.f. in (20) only give somewhat satisfactory results for the scenarios with b_j's smaller than 1, with completely nonsense results for the scenarios with larger spans of the a_j, with values of Δ larger than 1, indicating that indeed the supposedly approximating c.f.'s are not indeed true c.f.'s, that is, they do not even correspond to true distributions. Anyway the behavior of the approximation based on (20) that uses the completion of weights is in all cases much better than the one that does not use the weight completion, and the approximation based on (20) with the weights computed by matching exact moments has always a much better performance than the approximations that compute the weights through (18) and (12)–(13), with quite satisfactory results for all scenarios. However, all these approaches suffer from the problem of starting to yield worse approximations when the number of terms m goes above some threshold for which it is not easy to obtain an "a priori" guess. This problem is more pronounced for the approximation based on (20) with weights given by (18) and (12)–(13) without weight completion and much less pronounced for the approximation that uses weights obtained by equating moments, and it also starts at much larger values of m for this latter approximation.

The results show that in general there is no advantage of having some of the first weights computed through their exact expressions, that is, they show that it is indeed more advantageous to have all weights computed by matching exact moments.

However for the scenarios with b_j's smaller than 1 some combinations of moderate values of m^* with somehow larger values of $m^{**} - m^*$ in (22) may give somewhat better results than those obtained when all the weights are obtained by equating the first exact moments.

This shows that this approach might be useful to be implemented for the near-exact approximations, where the remaining part of the c.f. left to be asymptotically approximated corresponds indeed to a product of independent Beta r.v.'s, all with b_j parameters smaller than 1. However, for reasons related with the already large length of this manuscript, such approaches were not explored, although they may be easily implemented from the approaches developed.

For the same number of exact moments matched, and for the same number of terms in the mixtures, the near-exact distributions yield approximations which exhibit values of Δ which are several millions of times smaller than those for the corresponding approximations based on simple truncations of the c.f., that is the ones based on the c.f.'s in (20) and (22). Moreover, the near-exact distributions show a much stable behavior across all scenarios, actually tending to show slightly better performances in those scenarios where the other approaches tend to behave worse, which are the scenarios where the a_j show larger spans, or scenarios where the b_j have larger values, or yet scenarios where there are more Beta r.v.'s involved, showing this way their great ability and adequacy to handle more complicated situations.

Although for situations where we consider the distribution of the product of different powers of independent Beta r.v.'s, the near-exact approximations exhibit rather larger values of the measure Δ than what they do for situations where no powers are considered, they still have very good performances, with the near-exact approximations with a in (27) given by the minimum of the $(a_j - b_j^*)/c_j$ being the one with a less good performance and the near-exact approximations with a in (27) given by vi) or vii) in (28) being the ones with the best performance. This also shows that there are good reasons to consider the different choices for a in (28), although introduced then in a somewhat heuristic way. As we will also see in Sect. 7.3, these near-exact approximations also perform very well when applied to the distribution of likelihood ratio test statistics.

7 Applications

In this section we have chosen the likelihood ratio test statistics to test (i) the independence of several sets of variables, (ii) sphericity, and (iii) equality of several covariance matrices, under multivariate normal or elliptically contoured distributions to illustrate the performance of the near-exact distributions suggested in Sect. 5 and the different cases addressed in Sects. 3 and 5. In this section we will indeed only use near-exact distributions, given the evidence that these distributions give much better approximations, while remaining highly manageable.

For each type of near-exact distribution studied, 4, 6, 10, or 15 exact moments are matched, in order to make it easier to compare the results obtained with the ones published elsewhere for other near-exact distributions which equated exactly the same numbers of exact moments. As it may be seen from the numerical results, some of the near-exact distributions suggested in this paper, for the general case of the product of independent Beta r.v.'s, yield even slightly better results than the best performing near-exact distributions earlier expressly developed for each of the statistics used as examples.

7.1 The Distribution of the Likelihood Ratio Test Statistic to Test Independence of Sets of Variables

According to Marques et al. (2011), the distribution of Λ_1, the likelihood ratio test statistic to test the independence of m groups of variables, the k-th of them having p_k variables, based on a sample of size n from a multivariate normal or elliptically contoured distribution is the same as the distribution of

$$\prod_{k=1}^{m-1}\prod_{j=1}^{p_k}\left(Y_{jk}\right)^{n/2} \qquad \text{where} \qquad Y_{jk}\sim Beta\left(\frac{n-q_k-j}{2},\frac{q_k}{2}\right) \tag{30}$$

or the distribution of

$$\left\{\prod_{j=3}^{p}e^{-Z_j}\right\}\left\{\prod_{j=1}^{k^*}\left(Y_j^*\right)^{n/2}\right\} \quad \text{where} \quad Z_j\sim\Gamma\left(r_j,\frac{n-j}{n}\right) \quad \text{and} \quad Y_j^*\sim Beta\left(\frac{n-2}{2},\frac{1}{2}\right) \tag{31}$$

with

$$p=\sum_{k=1}^{m}p_k\,,\quad q_k=p_{k+1}+\cdots+p_m \quad \text{and} \quad k^*=\left\lfloor\frac{\ell}{2}\right\rfloor$$

where ℓ is the number of sets of variables with an odd number of variables and where r_j $(j=3,\ldots,p)$ are given by (A.2)-(A.3) in Marques et al. (2011).

We may note that the non-integer part of the second parameters of the Beta r.v.'s in (30) is always either zero or $1/2$, thus rendering the near-exact approach for the distribution in (31) quite simple and much adequate, while in case $k^* = 0$, that is, when at most one of the sets has an odd number of variables, it is clear from (31) above, that we have in this case the exact distribution of Λ_1 as an EGIG distribution.

The way the distribution of Λ_1 is presented in (31), although requiring more elaborate work on the c.f. of $-\log \Lambda_1$, it will allow for much more precise approximations than the ones obtained so far. The c.f. corresponding to $\prod_{j=3}^{p} e^{Z_j}$ in (31) plays the role of $\Phi_{1,W}^*(t)$ in (24), while the c.f. corresponding to $\prod_{j=1}^{k^*} \left(Y_j^*\right)^{n/2}$ in (31) plays the role of $\Phi_{2,W}(t)$ in (24). In this case, in order to approximate $\Phi_{2,W}(t)$ we will use the approach outlined in Sect. 5, corresponding to the case studied in Sect. 3.3.

In Table 28 in Appendix D of Coelho and Alberto (2020) we have values of the measure Δ in (29) for near-exact distributions for Λ_1 for different numbers of sets of variables, different numbers of variables in each set, and different sample sizes. In this table, NE-1, NE-2, NE-6, and NE-7 refer to the near-exact distributions based on the expression of the distribution of Λ_1 in the form in (30) and corresponding different choices for a in (28), while NE-II refers to the near-exact distribution obtained using the form of the distribution in (31) and the approach described in Sect. 3.3, which uses a mixture of gamma distributions, all with rate parameters equal to $\frac{n-2}{2} - \frac{1}{4}$ and shape parameters $\frac{k^*}{2} + 2k$, for $k = 0, \ldots, m$. We should note that given the fact that for the representation of the distribution of Λ_1 in (30) all $b_j^* = \lfloor b_j \rfloor$ are equal to either zero or 1/2 and all m_j are equal to 1, then the near-exact distributions NE-2 through NE-5, corresponding to the choices for a in ii) through v) in (28) yield exactly the same near-exact distributions.

We may note that the form of the distribution in (31) allows for much better approximations. Actually, the results obtained for this form of the distribution by using the approach described in Sects. 5 and 3.3 allow for much better approximations than any of the ones obtained before for this statistic. However, it is interesting to note that the bus approach of building near-exact approximations based directly on the form of the distribution in (30) gives very sharp near-exact approximations which are only barely worse than the ones previously obtained for this statistic when using a dedicated approach (see Coelho et al. (2010) and Marques et al. (2011)).

Some more detailed comments on the performance of the several near-exact distributions are:

- as expected, all the near-exact distributions show a clear asymptotic behavior both for increasing values of m, the number of exact moments matched, and n, the sample size,
- NE-II is by far the best performing near-exact distribution, with a performance even much better than the near-exact distributions in Coelho et al. (2010) and Marques et al. (2011).

- NE-1 through NE-7, which use what we may call a "bus" approach, do not give much worse results than the near-exact distributions in Coelho et al. (2010) and Marques et al. (2011), specifically developed for Λ_1,
- for increasing values of $p = \sum_{k=1}^{\nu} p_k$, keeping $n - p$ fixed, even for very small values of $n-p$ and reduced values of m (the number of exact moments matched), the performance of the near-exact approximations NE-1 through NE-7 does not worsen while the performance of NE-II even improves, what may be seen as a much desirable feature,
- NE-1 is the worse performing near-exact approximation, what amply justifies the choices for the rate parameter a in ii)–vii) of (28) in Sect. 5, which then seemed to be a somewhat heuristic approach,
- the near-exact approximation NE-6, with the rate parameter a based on only two moments, performs always better than NE-7, with a rate parameter a based on four moments, and this latter one better than NE-2.

7.2 The Distribution of the Likelihood Ratio Test Statistic to Test Sphericity

Once again according to Marques et al. (2011), the distribution of Λ_2, the likelihood ratio test statistic to test sphericity in a p-multivariate normal or elliptically contoured distribution, based on a sample of size n has the same distribution as

$$\prod_{j=2}^{p} (Y_j)^{n/2} \qquad \text{where} \qquad Y_j \sim Beta\left(\frac{n-j}{2}, \frac{j-1}{p} + \frac{j-1}{2}\right) \tag{32}$$

or

$$\left\{\prod_{j=2}^{p} e^{-Z_j}\right\}\left\{\prod_{j=2}^{p-k^*} \left(Y_j^*\right)^{n/2}\right\}\left\{\prod_{j=p-k^*+1}^{p} \left(Y_j^{**}\right)^{n/2}\right\}, \tag{33}$$

where $k^* = \lfloor p/2 \rfloor$, and

$$Z_j \sim \Gamma\left(r_j, \frac{n-j}{n}\right), \quad Y_j^* \sim Beta\left(\frac{n-1}{2}, \frac{j-1}{p}\right) \quad \text{and} \quad Y_j^{**} \sim Beta\left(\frac{n}{2}, \frac{j-1}{p} - \frac{1}{2}\right)$$

with

$$r_j = \left\lfloor \frac{p-j+2}{2} \right\rfloor, \qquad j = 2, \ldots, p\,.$$

Since all Beta r.v.'s in either (32) or (33) are all different, with different first and second parameters, in this case all the m_j will be equal to 1 and the near-exact distributions corresponding to the choices of a in ii) and iv) of (28), on one side, and the ones corresponding to iii) and v) in (28) will yield the same result.

As such, in Tables 29-31, in Subsect. D.2 of Appendix D in Coelho and Alberto (2020), we refer to the near-exact distributions for the distribution of Λ_2 as depicted in (32) by NE-1 through NE-7, not using NE-4 neither NE-5, and by NE2-1 through NE2-7 for the representation of the distribution in (33), not using NE2-4 neither NE2-5. For this statistic,

- as it also happens with the statistic Λ_1 in the previous subsection, and as it was expected, all near-exact approximations show a marked asymptotic behavior for increasing values of n, the sample size, and m, the number of exact moments matched,
- an important characteristic of all the near-exact approximations for Λ_2 is that they are also asymptotic in p, that is, for all values of m, even the smaller ones, they perform even better for larger values of p, when keeping $n-p$ constant, even for very small values of $n-p$,
- for the first approach, the NE-2 near-exact distribution presents the worse performance, while NE-1 is comparable to NE-3, with NE-6 and NE-7, which are comparable, exhibiting the best performance,
- for the second approach, NE2-6 and NE2-7 are comparable, showing a better performance than NE2-2 and NE2-3, which are comparable,
- also for the second approach, and for the larger values of m, NE2-1 generally performs better than NE2-6 and NE2-7 for smaller values of n, and the other way around for larger values of n,
- generally, the near-exact distributions based on the second approach show a better performance than the ones based on the first approach, although the gain may be rather slim and tends to reduce for larger values of m.

As the near-exact distributions based on the first approach, based on (32), need less work on the exact c.f. and the gains with the second approach, based on (33), tend to be rather slim, the "bus" near-exact distributions based on the first approach may represent a good choice.

7.3 The Distribution of the Likelihood Ratio Test Statistic to Test Equality of Covariance Matrices

Once again according to Marques et al. (2011), the distribution of Λ_3, the likelihood ratio test statistic to test the equality of q covariance matrices, based on q independent samples, all with size n, from as many p-multivariate normal or elliptically contoured distributions, has the same distribution as

$$\prod_{\substack{j=1 \\ \text{except } j=k=1}}^{p} \prod_{k=1}^{q} \left(Y_{jk}\right)^{n/2} \quad \text{where} \quad Y_{jk} \sim Beta\left(\frac{n-j}{2}, \frac{j(q-1)+2k-1-q}{2q}\right), \tag{34}$$

or

$$\left\{\prod_{j=2}^{p} e^{-Z_j}\right\}\left\{\prod_{j=1}^{\lfloor p/2 \rfloor}\prod_{k=1}^{q}\left(Y_{jk}^{*}\right)^{n}\right\}\left\{\prod_{k=1}^{q}\left(Y_{k}^{*}\right)^{n/2}\right\}^{p \perp\!\!\!\perp 2} \tag{35}$$

where $p \perp\!\!\!\perp 2$ is the remainder of the integer division of p by 2, or equivalently, the indicator function of p being odd,

$$Z_j \sim \Gamma\left(r_j, \frac{n-j}{n}\right), \quad Y_{jk}^{*} \sim Beta\left(a_j + b_{jk}^{*}, b_{jk} - b_{jk}^{*}\right)$$
$$\text{and} \quad Y_j^{**} \sim Beta\left(a_p + b_{pk}^{*}, b_{pk} - b_{pk}^{*}\right)$$

with

$$a_j = n - 2j, \quad b_{jk} = 2j - 1 + \frac{k-2j}{q}, \quad b_{jk}^{*} = \lfloor b_{jk} \rfloor,$$

$$a_p = \frac{n-p}{2}, \quad b_{pk} = \frac{pq - q - p + 2k - 1}{2q}, \quad b_{pk}^{*} = \lfloor b_{pk} \rfloor,$$

and r_j given by (A.12)-(A.16) in Marques et al. (2011).

Also in the distribution of Λ_3 all Beta r.v.'s in either (34) or (35) are all different. As such, in Tables 32-34 in Appendix D of Coelho and Alberto (2020), similar to what was done for Λ_2, we do not use the near-exact distributions NE-4 neither NE-5, NE2-4, NE2-5. In these Tables NE-1 through NE-7 refer to the form of the distribution of Λ_3 in (34) and NE2-1 through NE2-7 refer to the form of the distribution of Λ_3 in (35).

We should also note that for odd p, when using the representation of the distribution of Λ_3 in (35), we will have two products of Beta r.v.'s where in each product the Beta r.v.'s involved are raised to a different power. As such, when using this representation of the distribution for odd p, we will have to use the approach outlined in Sect. 5.2. As overall comments we may see that

- once again, and as expected, all near-exact approximations show a marked asymptotic behavior for increasing values of n, the sample size, and m, the number of exact moments matched,
- NE-6, NE-7, NE2-6, and NE2-7, which are the best performing approximations, even seem to improve quite a bit with the increase in q, what is a token in favor of these near-exact approximations, or, if we want, in favor of the choice of the

computation of the parameter a as in vi) and vii) of (28), and, as in Sect. 7.1, it shows that what might have seemed then as mostly heuristic choices for the computation of the parameter a, are indeed well justified, moreover since this behavior even seems to be more accentuated for larger values of m and n,
- generally the second approach, based on (35) yields somewhat better results, although the difference to the first approach is rather slim mainly for NE-6 and NE-7, what shows that these two near-exact approximations, based on a simpler and more crude approach may indeed constitute good alternatives to NE2-6 and NE2-7,
- very good approximations are obtained, namely when using NE2-6 and NE2-7, but also NE-6 and NE-7, even for small values of $n - p$, which is a much desirable feature.

8 Conclusions

Although the asymptotic distributions which are finite mixtures of beta or exponentiated gamma distributions, are simpler and as such easier to compute, in most situations they do not provide the necessary precision, yielding in many situations completely inadequate approximations. However, opposite to these, the near-exact approximations provide high quality approximations for all situations, even though remaining much manageable. Mainly in situations where the parameters b_j have large values, the a_j present large spans and/or the number of Beta r.v's involved in the product is moderately large or large, the near-exact distributions, which are finite mixtures of GNIG or GIG distributions, provide the sensible approach and the adequate answer to the problem of approximating the distribution of the product of independent Beta r.v.'s with high quality but manageable approximations. These approximations also show very stable performances for all kinds of situations. That is, they show values of the measure Δ which seem to be not much affected by changes in the number of Beta r.v.'s in the product, or the span of the values of the a_j, actually giving even better approximations for situations where the number of Beta r.v.'s involved in the product increase or the values of the parameters b_j increase, and this in clear contrast with all other asymptotic approximations.

In what concerns the l.r.t. statistics used in Multivariate Analysis addressed in Sect. 7, all near-exact distributions show very good performances even for very small sample sizes, and an asymptotic behavior not only for increasing sample sizes but also for increasing number of variables involved. Among all near-exact distributions, the ones with the parameter a defined by vi) or vii) in (28) are usually the best performing ones. The fact that NE-II was by far the best performing near-exact approximation for Λ_1 and that the near-exact distributions corresponding to the "second approaches" for both Λ_2 and Λ_3 yield in general the best approaches, indicates that specific further work on the exact c.f.'s in order to develop near-exact distributions which may lead to the ability of keeping as much as possible of the original c.f. under its exact form, usually pays off. However, for both Λ_1 and Λ_2

this gain is rather slim, while for Λ_3 this gain is extremely slim for smaller values of p (the number of variables involved) and larger for larger values of p, indicating that the application of the near-exact approach and near-exact distributions to a more crude process obtained by working directly on the original product of independent Beta r.v.'s also leads to very accurate approximations, with c.d.f.'s which may easily lie apart from the original by much less than a hundredth of a millionth part, which would never be possible to attain with any other approach.

In fact, the results in this chapter have an even much wider scope than the one analyzed so far. Actually, the distribution of W in (15) is not only the distribution of the negative logarithm of a large number of l.r.t. statistics but it is also the distribution of a linear combination of independent gamma random variables.

Indeed, although in the setting that expression (15) is taken in Sect. 3, all m_j were there taken as positive integers, m in (11) does not have to be an integer. In fact, if in (15) we take $b_j = 1$ and m_j as positive reals ($j = 1, \ldots, q$), the c.f. of W may be written as

$$\Phi_W(t) = \prod_{j=1}^{q} (a_j)^{m_j} (a_j - \mathrm{i}t)^{-m_j} \tag{36}$$

which is the c.f. of a sum of independent $\Gamma(m_j, a_j)$ random variables, which is also the c.f. of a linear combination of independent gamma distributed random variables.

If in (36) we take $m_j = k_j/2$ for some positive integers m_j ($j = 1, \ldots, q$), we may write

$$\Phi_W(t) = \prod_{j=1}^{q} (a_j)^{k_j/2} (a_j - \mathrm{i}t)^{-k_j/2} = \prod_{j=1}^{q} \left(\frac{1}{2}\right)^{k_j/2} \left(\frac{1}{2} - \frac{1}{2a_j}\mathrm{i}t\right)^{-k_j/2},$$

which is the c.f. of a linear combination of independent $\chi^2_{k_j}$ random variables with coefficients $\frac{1}{2a_j}$ ($j = 1, \ldots, q$). This distribution is of key importance since it is intimately related with the distribution of quadratic forms, more precisely, quadratic forms in normal variables (Baksalary et al. 1994; Imhof 1961; Kotz et al. 1967a,b; Shah 1963) which arise in many estimation and testing problems related with Gaussian processes and normal models, or which arise as limiting distributions in non-normal processes (Jensen and Solomon 1972; Khatri 1980).

Acknowledgments This work was partially supported by Fundação para a Ciência e a Tecnologia (Portuguese Foundation for Science and Technology) through projects UID/MAT/ 00297/2013 and UIDB/00297/2020 (Centro de Matemática e Aplicações, CMA-FCT/UNL).

Appendix A: Simple Proofs for Expressions (11) and (45)

The asymptotic expansions in (39) and (45) were first proved by Burić and Elezović (2011). We propose here simpler and straightforward demonstrations.

Barnes (1899) established an asymptotic expansion for the logarithm of the gamma function in the form

$$\log \Gamma(x+h) \approx \log \sqrt{2\pi} + \left(x+h-\tfrac{1}{2}\right)\log x - x - \sum_{r=1}^{\infty} (-1)^r \tfrac{B_{r+1}(h)}{r(r+1)x^r}, \quad (x \to \infty) \tag{37}$$

for any $x, h \in \mathbb{C}$ and where $B_r(\cdot)$ is the Bernoulli polynomial of degree r.

Assuming $z, \alpha, \beta \in \mathbb{C}$ and $m \in \mathbb{R}$, the application of (37) leads to

$$\log \left[\frac{\Gamma(z+\alpha)}{\Gamma(z+\beta)}\right]^m \approx m\,(\alpha-\beta)\log z + \sum_{r=1}^{\infty} \delta_{r,m}(\alpha,\beta)\, z^{-r}, \qquad (z \to \infty)$$

where

$$\delta_{r,m}(\alpha,\beta) = (-1)^r m\, \frac{B_{r+1}(\beta) - B_{r+1}(\alpha)}{r(r+1)}. \tag{38}$$

Therefore, we may write

$$\left[\frac{\Gamma(z+\alpha)}{\Gamma(z+\beta)}\right]^m \approx z^{m\,(\alpha-\beta)}\, e^{\sum_{r=1}^{\infty} \delta_{r,m}(\alpha,\beta)\, z^{-r}}, \qquad (z \to \infty),$$

from which, expanding the exponential function according to expressions (2.7) and (2.8) in Moschopoulos (1985) we obtain the asymptotic expansion

$$\left[\frac{\Gamma(z+\alpha)}{\Gamma(z+\beta)}\right]^m \approx \sum_{k=0}^{\infty} \nu_{k,m}(\alpha,\beta)\, z^{m\,(\alpha-\beta)-k}, \qquad (z \to \infty), \tag{39}$$

for the power of a ratio of two gamma functions, with $\nu_{k,m}(\alpha,\beta)$ given by (12).

However, it is indeed possible to improve the series expansion in (39), achieving a faster convergence series after a convenient parameter manipulation, in case we are willing to use a power basis which is also function of α and β.

From the property of the Bernoulli polynomials stated in expression 23.1.8 in Abramowitz and Stegun (1972), we note that, when n is even,

$$B_n(1-x) = B_n(x). \tag{40}$$

Consider now $c \in \mathbb{C}$ and let $z^* = z + c$, $\alpha^* = \alpha - c$, and $\beta^* = \beta - c$. Then, from (39) we may write

$$\left[\frac{\Gamma(z^* + \alpha^*)}{\Gamma(z^* + \beta^*)}\right]^m \approx \sum_{k=0}^{\infty} \nu_{k,m}(\alpha^*, \beta^*)\,(z^*)^{m\,(\alpha-\beta)-k}, \qquad (z \to \infty)\,. \tag{41}$$

Now, the proper choice of c will allow us to reduce the number of terms in the above series. For this purpose we will force $\nu_{1,m}(\alpha^*, \beta^*) = 0$. Since $\nu_{1,m}(\alpha^*, \beta^*) = \delta_{1,m}(\alpha^*, \beta^*)$, it is enough to determine c such that

$$B_2(\beta - c) = B_2(\alpha - c)\,. \tag{42}$$

But then, according to (40), we have

$$B_2(\beta - c) = B_2(1 - (\beta - c))\,,$$

which, together with (42), entails

$$c = (\alpha + \beta - 1)/2\,. \tag{43}$$

Moreover, this choice of c implies that, for every odd j

$$\delta_{j,m}(\alpha - k, \beta - k) = 0\,. \tag{44}$$

Thus, from (43) and (44), we may prove that, for every odd k

$$\nu_{k,m}(\alpha - c, \beta - c) = 0\,,$$

and that therefore all the odd terms of the series represented in (41) vanish.

The proof is done by induction. As induction basis, the statement $\nu_{1,m}(\alpha - c, \beta - c) = 0$ holds, according to the choice of c in (43). Assuming as induction hypothesis that, for any given odd k, the statement

$$\begin{aligned}\nu_{1,m}(\alpha - c, \beta - c) = \nu_{3,m}(\alpha - c, \beta - c) = \ldots = \nu_{k-2,m}(\alpha - c, \beta - c)\\ = \nu_{k,m}(\alpha - c, \beta - c) = 0\end{aligned}$$

is true, we have, by (38),

$$\nu_{k+2,m}(\alpha - c, \beta - c) = \frac{1}{k+2} \sum_{j=1}^{k+2} j\, \delta_{j,m}(\alpha - c, \beta - c)\, \nu_{k+2-j,m}(\alpha - c, \beta - c)\,.$$

Now all the terms in the summation are zero since, when j is odd the factor $\delta_{j,m}(\alpha - c, \beta - c)$ is zero, according to (44). Otherwise, when j is even, the index $k + 2 - j$

is odd and, by the induction hypothesis, the correspondent coefficient $\nu_{k+2-j,m}(\alpha - c, \beta - c)$ is also zero.

Finally, expression (41) may be written as

$$\left[\frac{\Gamma(z+\alpha)}{\Gamma(z+\beta)}\right]^m \approx \sum_{k=0}^{\infty} \nu_{2k,m}(\alpha - c, \beta - c)\,(z + \tfrac{\alpha+\beta-1}{2})^{m(\alpha-\beta)-2k}, \quad (z \to \infty)\,, \tag{45}$$

where each coefficient $\nu_{2k,m}(\alpha - c, \beta - c)$ is given by (12), with $c = (\alpha + \beta - 1)/2$.

Setting $m = 1$ in (39) we obtain a power expansion which is equivalent to the asymptotic series expansion for the ratio of two gamma functions proposed by Tricomi and Erdélyi (1951), here in the form given by Fields (1966), while by setting $m = 1$ in (45) we obtain the equivalent to the asymptotic series expansion for the ratio of two gamma functions proposed by Fields (1966).

References

Abramowitz, M., & Stegun, I. (eds.) (1972). *Handbook of mathematical functions: with formulas, graphs, and mathematical tables*. New York: Dover.

Anderson, T. W. (2003). *An introduction to multivariate statistical analysis* (3rd edn.). New York: J. Wiley & Sons.

Arnold, B. C., Coelho, C. A., & Marques, F. J. (2013). The distribution of the product of powers of independent uniform random variables – a simple but useful tool to address and better understand the structure of some distributions. *Journal of Multivariate Analysis, 113*, 19–36.

Baksalary, J. K., Hauke, J., & Styan, G. P. H. (1994). On some distributional properties of quadratic forms in normal variables and on some associated matrix partial orderings. In *Multivariate analysis and its applications, IMS Lecture Notes Monogr. Ser.* (Vol. 24, pp. 111–121). Hayward, CA: Inst. Math. Statist.

Barnes, E. W. (1899). The theory of the gamma function. *Messenger of Mathematics, 29*, 64–128.

Berry, A. C. (1941). The accuracy of the Gaussian approximation to the sum of independent variates. *Transactions of the American Mathematical Society, 49*, 122–136.

Bhargava, R. P., & Khatri, C. G. (1981). The distribution of product of independent Beta r.v.'s with applications to multivariate analysis. *Annals of the Institute of Statistical Mathematics, Series A, 33*, 287–296.

Burić, T., & Elezović, N. (2011). Bernoulli polynomials and asymptotic expansions of the quotient of gamma functions. *Journal of Computational and Applied Mathematics, 235*, 3315–3331.

Carter, B. D., & Springer, M. D. (1977). The distribution of products, quotients and powers of independent H-function variates. *SIAM Journal on Applied Mathematics, 33*, 542–558.

Coelho, C. A. (1998). The generalized integer gamma distribution – a basis for distributions in multivariate statistics. *Journal of Multivariate Analysis, 64*, 86–102.

Coelho, C. A. (2004). The generalized near-integer gamma distribution: a basis for 'near-exact' approximations to the distribution of statistics which are the product of an odd number of independent Beta r.v.'s. *Journal of Multivariate Analysis, 89*, 191–218.

Coelho, C. A., & Alberto, R. P. (2020). Supplementary material for 'On the distribution of the Product of Independent Beta Random Variables — Applications' at https://sites.google.com/site/productofbetas.

Coelho, C. A., & Arnold, B. C. (2019). *Finite form representations for Meijer G and Fox H functions: Applied to multivariate likelihood ratio tests using Mathematica®*, MAXIMA and R. Springer International Publishing.
Coelho, C. A., & Marques, F. J. (2011a). The multi-sample block-scalar sphericity test: exact and near-exact distributions for its likelihood ratio test statistic. *Communications in Statistics: Theory and Methods, 42*, 1153–1175.
Coelho, C. A., & Marques, F. J. (2011b). On the exact, asymptotic and near-exact distributions for the likelihood ratio statistics to test equality of several exponential distributions. *AIP Conference Proceedings, 1389*, 1471–1474.
Coelho, C. A., Marques, F. J., & Arnold, B. C. (2010). Near-exact distributions for certain likelihood ratio test statistics. *Journal of Statistical Theory and Practice, 4*, 711–725.
Coelho, C. A., Marques, F. J., & Arnold, B. C. (2015). The exact and near-exact distributions of the main likelihood ratio test statistics used in the complex multivariate normal setting. *Test, 24*, 386–416.
Esseen, C.-G. (1945). Fourier analysis of distribution functions - a mathematical study of the Laplace-Gaussian law. *Acta Mathematica, 77*, 1–125.
Fields, J. L. (1966). A note on the asymptotic expansion of a ratio of gamma functions. *Proceedings of the Edinburgh Mathematical Society, 15*, 43–45.
Gupta, A. K. (1971). Distribution of Wilks' likelihood-ratio criterion in the complex case. *Annals of the Institute of Statistical Mathematics, 23*, 77–87.
Heuback, S., & Mansour, T. (2009). *Combinatorics of compositions and words*. Boca Raton: Chapman and Hall/CRC Press.
Hsu, P. L. (1945). The approximate distributions of the mean and variance of a sample of independent variables. *Annals of Mathematical Statistics, 15*, 1–29.
Hwang, H.-K. (1998). On convergence rates in the central limit theorems for combinatorial structures. *European Journal of Combinatorial, 19*, 329–343.
Imhof, J. P. (1961). Computing the distribution of quadratic forms in normal variables. *Biometrika, 48*, 419–426.
Jensen, D. R., & Solomon, H. (1972). A Gaussian approximation to the distribution of a definite quadratic form. *Journal of the American Statistical Association, 67*, 898–902.
Khatri, C. G. (1965a). Classical statistical analysis based on a certain multivariate complex Gaussian distribution. *Annals of Mathematical Statistics, 36*, 98–114.
Khatri, C. G. (1965b). A test for reality of a covariance matrix in a certain complex Gaussian distribution. *Annals of Mathematical Statistics, 36*, 115–119.
Khatri, C. G. (1980). Quadratic forms in normal variables. In P. R. Krishnaiah (Ed.), *Handbook of statistics, Volume 1: Analysis of variance* (pp. 443–469). Amsterdam: North-Holland.
Kotz, S., Johnson, N. L., & Boyd, D. W. (1967a). Series representations of distributions of quadratic forms in Normal variables I - central case. *Annals of Mathematical Statistics, 38*, 823–837.
Kotz, S., Johnson, N. L., & Boyd, D. W. (1967b). Series representations of distributions of quadratic forms in Normal variables II - non-central case. *Annals of Mathematical Statistics, 38*, 838–848.
Kshirsagar, A. M. (1972). *Multivariate analysis*. New York: Marcel Dekker.
Marques, F. J., & Coelho, C. A. (2011a). The block sphericity test – exact and near-exact distributions for the likelihood ratio statistic. *Mathematical Methods in the Applied Sciences, 35*, 373–383.
Marques, F. J., & Coelho, C. A. (2011b). The multi-sample block-matrix sphericity test. *AIP Conference Proceedings, 1389*, 1479–1482.
Marques, F. J., Coelho, C. A., & Arnold, B. C. (2011). A general near-exact distribution theory for the most common likelihood ratio test statistics used in multivariate analysis. *TEST, 20*, 180–203.
Mathai, A. M. (1984). Extensions of Wilks' integral equations and distributions of test statistics. *Annals of the Institute of Statistical Mathematics, 36*(Part A), 271–288.
Moschopoulos, P. G. (1985). The distribution of the sum of independent gamma random variables. *Annals of the Institute of Statistical Mathematics, 37*(Part A), 541–544.

Moschopoulos, P. G. (1986). New representations for the distribution function of a class of likelihood ratio criteria. *Journal of Statistical Research, 20*, 13–20.
Muirhead, R. J. (2005). *Aspects of multivariate statistical theory* (2nd edn.). New York: J. Wiley & Sons.
Nagar, D. K., Jain, S. K., & Gupta, A. K. (1985). Distribution of LRC for testing sphericity of a complex multivariate Gaussian model. *International Journal of Mathematics and Mathematical Sciences, 8*, 555–562.
Nagarsenker, B. N., & Das, M. M. (1975). Exact distribution of sphericity criterion in the complex case and its percentage points. *Communications in Statistics, 4*, 363–374.
Nagarsenker, B. N., & Suniaga, J. (1983). Distributions of a class of statistics useful in multivariate analysis. *Journal of the American Statistical Association, 78*, 472–475.
Nandi, S. B. (1980). The exact distributions of certain likelihood ratio criteria. *Sankhya, Series B, 42*, 187–196.
Olkin, I., & Press, S. J. (1961). Testing and estimation for a circular stationary model. *Annals of Mathematical Statistics, 40*, 1358–1373.
Pederzoli, G. (1985). Some properties of beta functions and the distribution for the product of independent beta random variables. *Trabajos de Estadistica y de Investigacion Operativa, 36*, 122–128.
Pillai, K. C. S., & Jouris, G. M. (1971). Distribution of Wilks' likelihood-ratio criterion in the complex case. *Annals of Mathematical Statistics, 42*, 517–525.
Shah, B. K. (1963). Distribution of definite and indefinite quadratic forms from a non-central normal distribution. *Annals of Mathematical Statistics, 34*, 186–190.
Springer, M. D. (1979). *The algebra of random variables*. New York: J. Wiley & Sons.
Springer, M. D., & Thompson, W. E. (1966). The distribution of products of independent random variables. *SIAM Journal of Applied Mathematics, 14*, 511–526.
Springer, M. D., & Thompson, W. E. (1970). The distribution of products of beta, gamma and Gaussian random variables. *SIAM Journal of Applied Mathematics, 18*, 721–737.
Tang, J., & Gupta, A. K. (1984). On the distribution of the product of independent Beta random variables. *Statistics & Probability Letters, 2*, 165–168.
Tang, J., & Gupta, A. K. (1986). Exact distribution of certain general test statistics in multivariate analysis. *Australian Journal of Statistics, 28*, 107–114.
Tretter, M. J., & Walster, G. W. (1975). Central and noncentral distribution of Wilks' statistics in MANOVA as mixtures of incomplete beta functions. *Annals of Statistics, 3*, 467–472.
Tricomi, F. G., & Erdélyi, A. (1951). The asymptotic expansion of a ratio of gamma functions. *Pacific Journal of Mathematics, 1*, 133–142.
Tukey, J. W., & Wilks, S. S. (1946). Approximation of the distribution of the product of beta variables by a single beta variable. *Annals of Mathematical Statistics, 17*, 318–324.
Walster, G. W., & Tretter, M. J. (1980). Exact noncentral distributions of Wilks Lambda and Wilks-Lawley U criteria as mixtures of incomplete Beta functions: for three tests. *Annals of Statistics, 8*, 1388–1390.

On the Exact Statistical Distribution of Econometric Estimators and Test Statistics

Yong Bao, Xiaotian Liu, and Aman Ullah

Abstract Barry Arnold has made many fundamental and innovative contributions in different areas of statistics and econometrics, including estimation and inference, distribution theory, Bayesian inference, order statistics, income inequality measures, and characterization problems. His extensive work in the area of distribution theory includes studies on income distributions and Lorenz curves, the exact sampling distribution theory of test statistics, and the characterization of distributions. In our paper, we consider the problem of developing exact sampling distributions of various econometric and statistical estimators and test statistics. The motivation stems from the fact that inference procedures based on the asymptotic distributions may provide misleading results if the sample size is small or moderately large. In view of this, we develop a unified procedure by first observing that a large number of econometric and statistical estimators can be written as ratios of quadratic forms. Their distributions can then be straightforwardly analyzed by using Imhof's (Biometrika 48:419–426, 1961) method. We show the applications of this procedure to develop the distribution of some commonly used statistics in applied work. The exact results developed will be helpful for practitioners to conduct appropriate inference for any given size of the sample data.

1 Introduction

In the early twentieth century, Sir R. A. Fisher and others set in motion what is known today as the classical parametric approach to statistical estimation of a finite number of population parameters using sample data. Thus began the practice

Y. Bao · X. Liu
Department of Economics, Krannert School of Management, Purdue University, West Lafayette, IN, USA
e-mail: ybao@purdue.edu; liu2004@purdue.edu

A. Ullah (✉)
Department of Economics, University of California, Riverside, CA, USA
e-mail: aman.ullah@ucr.edu

I. Ghosh et al. (eds.), *Advances in Statistics - Theory and Applications*, Emerging Topics in Statistics and Biostatistics, https://doi.org/10.1007/978-3-030-62900-7_6

of statistical inference within the framework of estimation and hypothesis testing of univariate and multivariate probability distributions. The extensive study of conditional probability distributions followed, and hence, the estimation and testing in the conditional mean (regression) and conditional variance (volatility) models became a norm in econometrics and statistics. The estimation of parameters of regression and other models gave rise to the development of statistical properties of econometric estimators of such models like their bias, mean squared error (MSE), and distributions. Within this and in related contexts, Barry Arnold has made many fundamental and innovative contributions in different areas of statistics and econometrics, including estimation and testing, distribution theory and characterization of distributions, income distribution theory and Lorenz curves, among others. See, for example, Arnold (1983, 1987, 2012, 2015), Arnold et al. (1987), Arnold and Sarabia (2018), Coelho and Arnold (2014), Marques et al. (2011), and Villaseñor and Arnold (1984, 1989). All of these have made significant impact on the profession and have been instrumental in advancing statistics and econometrics.

The large sample limiting distribution theory was well developed, but there were challenges to develop needed analytical finite sample distributional results. In general, the large sample properties did not necessarily imply the small sample properties, and if they were used in small or moderately large sample cases, they may give misleading policy implications. This problem was posed since most of econometric estimators were nonlinear functions of multivariate random variables and it was not easy to develop their exact distributional properties. Nagar (1959) developed finite sample approximate bias and MSE of the two-stage least squares (2SLS) estimator of the parameters in a structural model. This was followed by an extensive work of many other econometrians and statisticians on the exact bias and MSE, and some on the exact distribution, of the 2SLS estimator. This literature is summarized in Ullah (2004), also see Anderson and Sawa (1973), Phillips (1980, 1986), and Bao et al. (2017). However, the exact distribution of many other econometric and statistical estimators is not yet developed.

In view of this in this paper, we develop a unified procedure to analyze the exact distribution by observing that many econometric and statistical estimators can be written as ratios of quadratic forms. Their distributions can then be straightforwardly developed by using Imhof's (1961) result on the distribution of an indefinite quadratic form. We show the applications of this procedure to develop the distribution of some statistics used in applied work. These include squared coefficient of variation for measuring income inequality, squared Sharpe ratio commonly used in financial management, Durbin–Watson test statistic for serial correlation routinely used in practice, Moran's test statistic for spatial correlation, and goodness of fit in regression models. The exact results developed here will be helpful for practitioners to conduct appropriate inference for any given size of the sample data.

This paper is organized as follows. In Sect. 2, we present the exact distributional results. Then in Sect. 3, we provide a numerical analysis of the exact distribution of a goodness of fit measure. Finally, the conclusion is given in Sect. 4. Throughout, $\boldsymbol{I} = \boldsymbol{I}_n$ is the $n \times n$ identity matrix, $\boldsymbol{\iota} = \boldsymbol{\iota}_n$ is an $n \times 1$ vector of ones, and $\boldsymbol{M}_0 = \boldsymbol{I} - n^{-1}\boldsymbol{\iota}\boldsymbol{\iota}'$.

2 The Exact Distribution

Let us consider the ratio of quadratic forms as

$$q = \frac{\boldsymbol{y}'\boldsymbol{N}_1\boldsymbol{y}}{\boldsymbol{y}'\boldsymbol{N}_2\boldsymbol{y}}, \tag{1}$$

where $\boldsymbol{y}$ is an $n \times 1$ normal random vector with $\mathrm{E}(\boldsymbol{y}) = \boldsymbol{\mu}$ and $\mathrm{Var}(\boldsymbol{y}) = \boldsymbol{\Sigma}$ being positive definite, $\boldsymbol{N}_1$ and $\boldsymbol{N}_2$ are $n \times n$ nonstochastic symmetric matrices, and $\boldsymbol{N}_2$ is a positive semi-definite.[1] The cumulative distribution function (CDF) of this ratio is

$$F(q_0) = \Pr(q \le q_0) = \Pr(\boldsymbol{y}'\boldsymbol{N}\boldsymbol{y} \le 0),$$

where $\boldsymbol{N}{=}\boldsymbol{N}_1{-}q_0\boldsymbol{N}_2$. Note that $\boldsymbol{y}'\boldsymbol{N}\boldsymbol{y}{=}\boldsymbol{y}'\boldsymbol{\Sigma}^{-1/2}\boldsymbol{Q}\boldsymbol{Q}'\boldsymbol{\Sigma}^{1/2}\boldsymbol{N}\boldsymbol{\Sigma}^{1/2}\boldsymbol{Q}\boldsymbol{Q}'\boldsymbol{\Sigma}^{-1/2}\boldsymbol{y} \equiv \boldsymbol{z}'\boldsymbol{\Lambda}\boldsymbol{z}$, where $\boldsymbol{z} = \boldsymbol{Q}'\boldsymbol{\Sigma}^{-1/2}\boldsymbol{y} \sim \mathrm{N}(\boldsymbol{\mu}_z, \boldsymbol{I})$, $\boldsymbol{\mu}_z = \boldsymbol{Q}'\boldsymbol{\Sigma}^{-1/2}\boldsymbol{\mu}$, $\boldsymbol{\Lambda}$ is a diagonal matrix of eigenvalues of $\boldsymbol{\Sigma}^{1/2}\boldsymbol{N}\boldsymbol{\Sigma}^{1/2}$, and $\boldsymbol{Q}$ is an orthogonal matrix of eigenvectors of $\boldsymbol{\Sigma}^{1/2}\boldsymbol{N}\boldsymbol{\Sigma}^{1/2}$ such that $\boldsymbol{Q}'\boldsymbol{\Sigma}^{1/2}\boldsymbol{N}\boldsymbol{\Sigma}^{1/2}\boldsymbol{Q} = \boldsymbol{\Lambda}$. So the distribution of the ratio of quadratic forms translates to that of a linear combination of independent non-central chi-squared random variables. Without loss of generality, let λ_j, $j = 1, \ldots, r \le n$, denote non-zero distinct elements of $\boldsymbol{\Lambda}$, n_j be the corresponding mutiplicities, $\delta_j = \sum_{i \to j} \mu_{z_i}^2$, where $\sum_{i\to j}$ denotes summing over i such that the ith element of $\boldsymbol{\Lambda}$ equals λ_j. Then, $\boldsymbol{z}'\boldsymbol{\Lambda}\boldsymbol{z} = \sum_{j=1}^{r} \lambda_j \zeta_j^2$, where $\zeta_j^2 \sim \chi^2_{n_j}(\delta_j)$, and they are independent of each other. For a linear combination (with weights λ_j) of independent non-central chi-squared variables ζ_j^2 (with non-centrality parameter δ_j and degrees of freedom n_j), Imhof (1961) showed that

$$\Pr\left(\sum_{j=1}^{r} \lambda_j \zeta_j^2 \le q_0^*\right) = \frac{1}{2} - \frac{1}{\pi}\int_0^\infty \frac{\sin\theta(v)}{v\rho(v)} \mathrm{d}v, \tag{2}$$

where

[1] If they are not symmetric, we can simply replace $\boldsymbol{N}_1$ and $\boldsymbol{N}_2$ by $(\boldsymbol{N}_1 + \boldsymbol{N}_1')/2$ and $(\boldsymbol{N}_2 + \boldsymbol{N}_2')/2$, respectively.

$$\theta(v) = -\frac{q_0^* v}{2} + \sum_{j=1}^{r}\left[\frac{n_j}{2}\tan^{-1}(\lambda_j v) + \frac{\lambda_j \delta_j v}{2(1+\lambda_j^2 v^2)}\right],$$

$$\rho(v) = \prod_{j=1}^{r}(1+\lambda_j^2 v^2)^{n_j/4}\exp\left[\frac{\lambda_j^2 v^2 \delta_j}{2(1+\lambda_j^2 v^2)}\right].$$

Setting $q_0^* = 0$, we have $F(q_0) = \Pr(\boldsymbol{y}'\boldsymbol{N}\boldsymbol{y} \leq 0) = \Pr(\boldsymbol{y}'\boldsymbol{N}_1\boldsymbol{y}/\boldsymbol{y}'\boldsymbol{N}_2\boldsymbol{y} \leq q_0)$.

2.1 Goodness of Fit Statistic R^2

For the linear regression model $\boldsymbol{y} = \boldsymbol{X}\boldsymbol{\beta} + \boldsymbol{u}$, where $\boldsymbol{y} = (y_1, \ldots, y_n)'$ is an $n \times 1$ vector of observations on the dependent variable, $\boldsymbol{X} = (\boldsymbol{x}_1, \ldots, \boldsymbol{x}_n)'$ is an $n \times k$ nonstochastic matrix of covariates (including a constant term) with coefficient vector $\boldsymbol{\beta}$, and $\boldsymbol{u} = (u_1, \ldots, u_n)'$ collects normally distributed error terms, a goodness of fit statistic is

$$R^2 = \frac{\sum_{i=1}^n (y_i - \bar{y})(\hat{y}_i - \bar{y})}{\sum_{i=1}^n (y_i - \bar{y})^2} = \frac{\boldsymbol{y}'\boldsymbol{M}_0\boldsymbol{P}\boldsymbol{y}}{\boldsymbol{y}'\boldsymbol{M}_0\boldsymbol{y}}, \tag{3}$$

where $\bar{y} = n^{-1}\sum_{i=1}^n y_i$, $\hat{y}_i = \boldsymbol{x}_i'\hat{\boldsymbol{\beta}}$, and $\boldsymbol{P} = \boldsymbol{X}(\boldsymbol{X}'\boldsymbol{X})^{-1}\boldsymbol{X}'$. We can thus evaluate the distribution of R^2 with $\boldsymbol{N}_1 = \boldsymbol{M}_0\boldsymbol{P}$ and $\boldsymbol{N}_2 = \boldsymbol{M}_0$ by applying (2).

Denote $\boldsymbol{M} = \boldsymbol{I} - \boldsymbol{P}$ and $\boldsymbol{P}_0 = n^{-1}\boldsymbol{\iota}\boldsymbol{\iota}'$. Then, we can put $\boldsymbol{N} = \boldsymbol{M}_0\boldsymbol{P} - a\boldsymbol{M}_0 = \boldsymbol{M}_0((1-a)\boldsymbol{P} - a\boldsymbol{M}) = \boldsymbol{P} + (a-1)\boldsymbol{P}_0 - a\boldsymbol{I}$. Note that $\boldsymbol{P}$ is idempotent with eigenvalues 1 (of multiplicity k) and 0 (of multiplicity $n-k$), and $\boldsymbol{P}_0$ is also idempotent with eigenvalues 1 (of multiplicity 1) and 0 (of multiplicity $n-1$). Since $\boldsymbol{P}_0\boldsymbol{v} = (\boldsymbol{P}_0\boldsymbol{P})\boldsymbol{v} = \boldsymbol{P}_0(\boldsymbol{P}\boldsymbol{v})$ for any conformable vector $\boldsymbol{v}$, we see that if $\boldsymbol{v}$ is an eigenvector of $\boldsymbol{P}$ associated with eigenvalue 0, then it must also be an eigenvector of $\boldsymbol{P}_0$ corresponding to its eigenvalue 0. There are $n-k$ linearly independent such vectors. Denote them by $\boldsymbol{v}_i$, $i = 1, \ldots, n-k$. Further, $\boldsymbol{N}\boldsymbol{v}_i = [\boldsymbol{P} + (a-1)\boldsymbol{P}_0 - a\boldsymbol{I}]\boldsymbol{v}_i = [0 + (a-1)\cdot 0 - a \cdot 1]\boldsymbol{v}_i = -a \cdot \boldsymbol{v}_i$, implying that $\boldsymbol{N}$ has eigenvalue $-a$ with the corresponding eigenvectors $\boldsymbol{v}_i$. Similarly, if $\boldsymbol{w}$ is an eigenvector of $\boldsymbol{P}_0$ associated with eigenvalue 1, so it is an eigenvector of $\boldsymbol{P}$ corresponding to its eigenvalue 1, and $\boldsymbol{N}\boldsymbol{w} = [\boldsymbol{P} + (a-1)\boldsymbol{P}_0 - a\boldsymbol{I}]\boldsymbol{w} = [1 + (a-1)\cdot 1 - a \cdot 1]\boldsymbol{w} = 0 \cdot \boldsymbol{w}$, implying that $\boldsymbol{N}$ has eigenvalue 0 with a corresponding eigenvector $\boldsymbol{w}$. Further, $\boldsymbol{v}_i$ and $\boldsymbol{w}$ are linearly independent. Since $\boldsymbol{N}$, $\boldsymbol{P}$, and $\boldsymbol{P}_0$ are all symmetric matrices, their eigenvectors span $\mathbb{R}^n$ (see page 179, Exercise 7.48 of Abadir and Magnus 2005). Thus, there must exist $k-1$ linearly independent vectors $\boldsymbol{z}_j \in \mathbb{R}^n$, $j = 1, \ldots, k-1$ (also linearly independent of $\boldsymbol{v}_i$ and $\boldsymbol{w}$) to be eigenvectors of $\boldsymbol{N}$, $\boldsymbol{P}$, and $\boldsymbol{P}_0$. Eigenvectors $\boldsymbol{z}_j$ correspond to eigenvalue 1 of $\boldsymbol{P}$ since $\boldsymbol{z}_j$ and $\boldsymbol{v}_i$ are linearly independent. Eigenvectors $\boldsymbol{z}_j$ also correspond to eigenvalue 0 of $\boldsymbol{P}_0$ since $\boldsymbol{z}_j$ and $\boldsymbol{w}$ are linearly independent. As such,

$\boldsymbol{N}\boldsymbol{z}_j = [\boldsymbol{P} + (a-1)\boldsymbol{P}_0 - a\boldsymbol{I}]\boldsymbol{z}_j = [1 + (a-1)\cdot 0 - a\cdot 1]\boldsymbol{z}_j = (1-a)\cdot \boldsymbol{z}_j$, implying that $\boldsymbol{N}$ has eigenvalue $1-a$ with the corresponding eigenvectors $\boldsymbol{z}_j$.

Given that $\boldsymbol{N} = \boldsymbol{M}_0((1-a)\boldsymbol{P} - a\boldsymbol{M})$ has two non-zero eigenvalues, $1-a$ and $-a$, with the corresponding mutiplicities $k-1$ and $n-k$, respectively, it is convenient for us to rewrite

$$R^2 = \frac{\boldsymbol{y}'\boldsymbol{M}_0\boldsymbol{P}\boldsymbol{y}}{\boldsymbol{y}'\boldsymbol{M}_0\boldsymbol{P}\boldsymbol{y} + \boldsymbol{y}'\boldsymbol{M}\boldsymbol{y}}. \tag{4}$$

If the error terms are independent and identically distributed (i.i.d) with variance σ_u^2, then $\boldsymbol{y}'\boldsymbol{M}_0\boldsymbol{P}\boldsymbol{y}/\sigma_u^2 \sim \chi_{k-1}^2(\boldsymbol{\beta}'\boldsymbol{X}'\boldsymbol{M}_0\boldsymbol{X}\boldsymbol{\beta})$, $\boldsymbol{y}'\boldsymbol{M}\boldsymbol{y}/\sigma_u^2 \sim \chi_{n-k}^2(0)$, and they are independent of each other. As such, R^2 follows a singly non-central beta distribution (see Koerts and Abrahamse 1969), and its distribution takes on the following form:

$$\Pr(R^2 \le r_0) = \sum_{j=0}^{\infty} \frac{1}{j!}\left(\frac{\boldsymbol{\beta}'\boldsymbol{X}'\boldsymbol{M}_0\boldsymbol{X}\boldsymbol{\beta}}{2\sigma_u^2}\right)^j \exp\left(-\frac{\boldsymbol{\beta}'\boldsymbol{X}'\boldsymbol{M}_0\boldsymbol{X}\boldsymbol{\beta}}{2\sigma_u^2}\right)$$
$$I\left(r_0 | \frac{k-1}{2} + j, \frac{n-k}{2}\right), \tag{5}$$

where $I(x|a,b) = \int_0^x z^{a-1}(1-z)^{b-1}\mathrm{d}z$ is the incomplete beta function with parameters a and b. Alternatively, the distribution function can be calculated by (2) with $\lambda_1 = 1-a$, $\lambda_2 = -a$, $n_1 = k-1$, $n_2 = n-k$, $\delta_1 = \boldsymbol{\beta}'\boldsymbol{X}'\boldsymbol{M}_0\boldsymbol{X}\boldsymbol{\beta}/\sigma_u^2$, and $\delta_2 = 0$.[2]

2.2 *Squared Sharpe Ratio*

In financial portfolio management, a routine task is to assess a portfolio's performance. The most widely used metric may be the Sharpe ratio, introduced by Sharpe (1966). Recently, Barillas and Shanken (2017) discussed how to compare asset pricing models under the classic Sharpe metric and showed that the quadratic form in the investment alphas is equivalent to the improvement in the squared Sharpe ratio when investment in other assets is permitted in addition to the given model's factors.

The squared Sharpe ratio of an asset is defined as $s = \mu^2/\sigma^2$, where μ is the is mean of the asset's excess return and σ^2 is its variance. Given a sample $\boldsymbol{y} = (y_1, \ldots, y_n)'$ of excess returns, the sample squared Sharpe ratio is

[2]The linkage between Imhof's formula and the non-central F (see the next subsections) and beta distribution functions was discussed in Ennis and Johnson (1993).

$$\hat{s} = \left(\frac{\hat{\mu}}{\hat{\sigma}}\right)^2 = \frac{\boldsymbol{y}'\boldsymbol{\iota}\boldsymbol{\iota}'\boldsymbol{y}/n^2}{\boldsymbol{y}'\boldsymbol{M}_0\boldsymbol{y}/(n-1)} = \frac{\boldsymbol{y}'\left(\frac{\boldsymbol{\iota}\boldsymbol{\iota}'}{n^2}\right)\boldsymbol{y}}{\boldsymbol{y}'\left(\frac{\boldsymbol{M}_0}{n-1}\right)\boldsymbol{y}}, \tag{6}$$

and (2) can be sued to evaluate its exact finite sample distribution with $\boldsymbol{N}_1 = \boldsymbol{\iota}\boldsymbol{\iota}'/n^2$ and $\boldsymbol{N}_2 = \boldsymbol{M}_0/(n-1)$.

When the excess return series is i.i.d. normal, the sample Sharpe ratio $\hat{\xi} = \hat{\mu}/\hat{\sigma}$, when scaled by $\sqrt{n}$, is equivalent to a non-central t random variable with degrees of freedom $n-1$ and non-centrality parameter $\sqrt{n}\xi$.[3] As such, the sample squared Sharpe ratio (scaled by n) follows a singly non-central F-distribution, $F_{1,n-1}(ns, 0)$.[4] So we have

$$\Pr(\hat{s} \le s_0) = \sum_{j=0}^{\infty}\left(\frac{(\frac{ns}{2})^j}{j!}\exp\left(-\frac{ns}{2}\right)\right) I\left(\frac{ns_0}{n-1+ns_0}\,\middle|\,\frac{1}{2}+j, \frac{n-1}{2}\right). \tag{7}$$

2.3 *Squared Coefficient of Variation*

The coefficient of variation (CV) has long been used in the literature as one of the income inequality indexes across regions or over time. It is defined as the ratio of the standard deviation of the variable of interest (e.g., household income) to its mean value, namely, σ/μ. A closely related measure is the squared CV, usually called the coefficient of variation squared (CV2), denoted by $\alpha = \sigma^2/\mu^2$. When the mean value of the variable of interest is positive, CV and CV2 are monotonic transformation of each other. As neither the population mean nor the standard deviation is known, in practice, we usually use their sample analogues to calculate CV and CV2.

Specifically, the sample CV2 is defined as

$$\hat{\alpha} = \frac{\hat{\sigma}^2}{\hat{\mu}^2} = \frac{\boldsymbol{y}'\boldsymbol{M}_0\boldsymbol{y}/(n-1)}{\boldsymbol{y}'\boldsymbol{\iota}\boldsymbol{\iota}'\boldsymbol{y}/n^2} = \frac{\boldsymbol{y}'\left(\frac{\boldsymbol{M}_0}{n-1}\right)\boldsymbol{y}}{\boldsymbol{y}'\left(\frac{\boldsymbol{\iota}\boldsymbol{\iota}'}{n^2}\right)\boldsymbol{y}}. \tag{8}$$

Obviously, we can set $\boldsymbol{N}_1 = \boldsymbol{M}_0/(n-1)$ and $\boldsymbol{N}_2 = \boldsymbol{\iota}\boldsymbol{\iota}'/n^2$ in (2) to evaluate the exact distribution $\Pr(\hat{\alpha} \le a)$.

If we further assume that the data is i.i.d., then from the discussion in the previous subsection, it is obvious that the distribution of $\hat{\alpha}$ (scaled by n^{-1}) is $F_{n-1,1}(0, ns)$,

[3]The connection of the Sharpe ratio to the t-distribution seems to originate in Miller and Gehr's (1978) note on the bias of the Sharpe ratio.

[4]This notation is from the double non-central F-distribution with non-centrality parameters δ_1 and δ_2 and the corresponding degrees of freedom d_1 and d_2, denoted by $F_{d_1,d_2}(\delta_1, \delta_2)$.

where $s = 1/\alpha$. This is a special case of double non-central F-distribution, and since it is the reciprocal of $F_{1,n-1}(ns, 0)$, we have

$$\begin{aligned}\Pr(\hat{\alpha} \le \alpha_0) &= 1 - \Pr(\hat{\alpha} \ge \alpha_0)\\ &= 1 - \Pr\left(\frac{1}{\hat{\alpha}} \le \frac{1}{\alpha_0}\right)\\ &= 1 - \sum_{j=0}^{\infty}\left(\frac{(\frac{n}{2\alpha})^j}{j!}\exp\left(-\frac{n}{2\alpha}\right)\right) I\left(\frac{\frac{n}{\alpha_0}}{n-1+\frac{n}{\alpha_0}}\middle| \frac{1}{2}+j, \frac{n-1}{2}\right).\end{aligned} \tag{9}$$

2.4 The Durbin–Watson Statistic and Moran's I

For testing the first-order autocorrelation in the error term in the classical linear regression model, the Durbin–Watson statistic for testing $H_0 : \rho = 0$ against $H_1 : \rho \neq 0$ in $u_i = \rho u_{i-1} + e_i$, where e_i is an i.i.d. innovation term, is calculated as

$$d = \frac{\sum_{i=2}^{n}(\hat{u}_i - \hat{u}_{i-1})^2}{\sum_{i=1}^{n}\hat{u}_i^2} = \frac{\hat{\boldsymbol{u}}'\boldsymbol{A}\hat{\boldsymbol{u}}}{\hat{\boldsymbol{u}}'\hat{\boldsymbol{u}}} = \frac{\boldsymbol{y}'\boldsymbol{MAMy}}{\boldsymbol{y}'\boldsymbol{My}}, \tag{10}$$

where $\hat{\boldsymbol{u}} = (\hat{u}_1, \ldots, \hat{u}_n)'$, $\hat{u}_i = y_i - \hat{y}_i$, is the residual vector, and $\boldsymbol{A}$ is a tri-diagonal matrix with -1 on the super- and sub-diagonal positions, $a_{11} = a_{nn} = 1$, and $a_{ii} = 2, i = 2, \ldots, n$. So setting $\boldsymbol{N}_1 = \boldsymbol{MAM}$ and $\boldsymbol{N}_2 = \boldsymbol{M}$ in (2), we can evaluate the exact distribution of the Durbin–Watson statistic. Srivastava (1987) derived the asymptotic distribution of Durbin–Watson statistic under the null hypothesis $u_i \sim \mathrm{N}(0, \sigma_u^2\boldsymbol{I})$ as $[(n-k)d - \mathrm{tr}(\boldsymbol{AM})]/\sqrt{2\mathrm{tr}(\boldsymbol{AM})^2} \to \mathrm{N}(0, 1)$.

For spatial data, Moran's I statistic is to test for possible correlation across space. It is calculated as

$$I = \frac{n}{\boldsymbol{1}'\boldsymbol{W}\boldsymbol{1}}\frac{\boldsymbol{y}'\boldsymbol{M}_0\boldsymbol{W}\boldsymbol{M}_0\boldsymbol{y}}{\boldsymbol{y}'\boldsymbol{M}_0\boldsymbol{y}}, \tag{11}$$

where $\boldsymbol{W}$ is the so-called spatial weights matrix with zeros on the diagonal.[5] Again, its exact distribution can be straightforwardly evaluated by (2).

---

[5]If we are interested instead in testing whether the spatial correlation arises from the unobservable error term in a linear regression model, Moran's I can be calculated with $\boldsymbol{M}$ replacing $\boldsymbol{M}_0$ in (11).

3 Illustration

In this section, we illustrate the performance of the exact result via (2) in comparison with the asymptotic distributional results. We focus on the statistic R^2. As discussed in Xu (2014), in the statistical and public health communities, reliable inference on R^2 has attracted a lot of attention. The literature on statistical inference of R^2 has been scarce; however, Xu (2014) developed the asymptotic distribution of R^2 in linear regression models with possibly nonnormal errors and discussed the F-distribution approximation with degrees of freedom adjustment. In Xu's (2014) setup, the data is demeaned such that $\bar{y} = 0$. Here, we relax this restriction. We begin with the general case when the error distribution may be nonnormal. In what follows, let γ_1 and γ_2 denote the skewness and excess kurtosis coefficients of the error distribution. Obviously, when the error is normal, $\gamma_1 = \gamma_2 = 0$.

Recall that we have written $R^2 = \boldsymbol{y}'\boldsymbol{M}_0\boldsymbol{P}\boldsymbol{y}/(\boldsymbol{y}'\boldsymbol{M}_0\boldsymbol{P}\boldsymbol{y} + \boldsymbol{y}'\boldsymbol{M}\boldsymbol{y})$. Below we present the asymptotic distributions of R^2 and two monotonic transformations of it.

Theorem 1 *For the linear regression model,* $\boldsymbol{y} = \boldsymbol{X\beta}+\boldsymbol{u}$, *where* $\boldsymbol{X}$ *is nonstochastic and* $\boldsymbol{u}$ *consists of i.i.d. errors,* R^2, $R^2/(1-R^2)$, *and* $\log(R^2/(1-R^2))$ *have the following asymptotic distributions:*

$$\sqrt{n}\left(R^2 - \frac{\beta'\boldsymbol{X}'\boldsymbol{M}_0\boldsymbol{X}\beta}{\beta'\boldsymbol{X}'\boldsymbol{M}_0\boldsymbol{X}\beta + n\sigma_u^2}\right) \xrightarrow{d} \mathrm{N}\left(0, \frac{\frac{4\beta'\Sigma\beta}{\sigma_u^2} + (2+\gamma_2)\left(\frac{\beta'\Sigma\beta}{\sigma_u^2}\right)^2}{\left(\frac{\beta'\Sigma\beta}{/\sigma_u^2}+1\right)^4}\right), \tag{12}$$

$$\sqrt{n}\left(\frac{R^2}{1-R^2} - \frac{\boldsymbol{\beta}'\boldsymbol{X}'\boldsymbol{M}_0\boldsymbol{X}\boldsymbol{\beta}}{n\sigma_u^2}\right) \xrightarrow{d} \mathrm{N}\left(0, \frac{4\boldsymbol{\beta}'\boldsymbol{\Sigma}\boldsymbol{\beta}}{\sigma_u^2} + \frac{(2+\gamma_2)(\boldsymbol{\beta}'\boldsymbol{\Sigma}\boldsymbol{\beta})^2}{\sigma_u^4}\right), \tag{13}$$

$$\sqrt{n}\left(\log\left(\frac{R^2}{1-R^2}\right) - \log\left(\frac{\boldsymbol{\beta}'\boldsymbol{X}'\boldsymbol{M}_0\boldsymbol{X}\boldsymbol{\beta}}{n\sigma_u^2}\right)\right) \xrightarrow{d} \mathrm{N}\left(0, \frac{4\sigma_u^2}{\boldsymbol{\beta}'\boldsymbol{\Sigma}\boldsymbol{\beta}} + 2 + \gamma_2\right). \tag{14}$$

Proof By substitution, $\boldsymbol{y}'\boldsymbol{M}_0\boldsymbol{P}\boldsymbol{y} = (\boldsymbol{X\beta}+\boldsymbol{u})'\boldsymbol{M}_0\boldsymbol{P}(\boldsymbol{X\beta}+\boldsymbol{u}) = \boldsymbol{\beta}'\boldsymbol{X}'\boldsymbol{M}_0\boldsymbol{X\beta} + \boldsymbol{u}'\boldsymbol{M}_0\boldsymbol{P}\boldsymbol{u} + 2\boldsymbol{u}'\boldsymbol{M}_0\boldsymbol{X\beta}$. Using results on the moments of quadratic forms in nonnormal random vectors (see, for example, Bao and Ullah 2010), we have $\mathrm{E}(\boldsymbol{u}'\boldsymbol{M}_0\boldsymbol{P}\boldsymbol{u}) = \sigma_u^2\mathrm{tr}(\boldsymbol{M}_0\boldsymbol{P}) = k\sigma_u^2 - n^{-1}\boldsymbol{1}'\boldsymbol{P}\boldsymbol{1}$ and $\mathrm{Var}(\boldsymbol{u}'\boldsymbol{M}_0\boldsymbol{P}\boldsymbol{u}) = \sigma_u^4[\gamma_2\mathrm{tr}(\boldsymbol{M}_0\boldsymbol{P}\odot\boldsymbol{M}_0\boldsymbol{P})+2\mathrm{tr}(\boldsymbol{M}_0\boldsymbol{P}\boldsymbol{M}_0\boldsymbol{P})]$, where $\odot$ denotes the Hadamard product operator. Since the idempotent matrix $\boldsymbol{P}$ has elements of order $O(n^{-1})$ and $\boldsymbol{M}_0$ is uniformly bounded in row and column sums, we can write $\mathrm{Var}(\boldsymbol{u}'\boldsymbol{M}_0\boldsymbol{P}\boldsymbol{u}) = 2\sigma_u^4\mathrm{tr}(\boldsymbol{M}_0\boldsymbol{P}\boldsymbol{M}_0\boldsymbol{P}) + o(1) = 2\sigma_u^4[\mathrm{tr}(\boldsymbol{P}) - 2n^{-1}\boldsymbol{1}'\boldsymbol{P}\boldsymbol{P}\boldsymbol{1} + n^{-2}(\boldsymbol{1}'\boldsymbol{P}\boldsymbol{1})^2] + o(1) = O(1)$. Thus we can claim $n^{-1/2}\boldsymbol{u}'\boldsymbol{M}_0\boldsymbol{P}\boldsymbol{u} = o_P(1)$. Using the central limit theorem on linear and quadratic forms in random vectors (see Kelejian and Prucha 2001), we have $n^{-1/2}\boldsymbol{u}'\boldsymbol{M}_0\boldsymbol{X\beta} \xrightarrow{d} \mathrm{N}(0, \sigma_u^2\boldsymbol{\beta}'\boldsymbol{\Sigma}\boldsymbol{\beta})$, where $\boldsymbol{\Sigma} = \lim_{n\to\infty} n^{-1}\boldsymbol{X}'\boldsymbol{M}_0\boldsymbol{X}$. So $n^{-1/2}(\boldsymbol{y}'\boldsymbol{M}_0\boldsymbol{P}\boldsymbol{y} - \boldsymbol{\beta}'\boldsymbol{X}'\boldsymbol{M}_0\boldsymbol{X\beta}) = 2n^{-1/2}\boldsymbol{u}'\boldsymbol{M}_0\boldsymbol{X\beta} + o_P(1) \xrightarrow{d} \mathrm{N}(0, 4\sigma_u^2\boldsymbol{\beta}'\boldsymbol{\Sigma}\boldsymbol{\beta})$. Similarly, $n^{-1/2}\boldsymbol{u}'\boldsymbol{M}\boldsymbol{u} = n^{-1/2}\boldsymbol{u}'\boldsymbol{u} + o_P(1) \xrightarrow{d} \mathrm{N}(\sigma_u^2, \sigma_u^4(2+\gamma_2))$. Further, $\mathrm{Cov}(\boldsymbol{u}'\boldsymbol{M}_0\boldsymbol{X\beta}, \boldsymbol{u}'\boldsymbol{u}) = \mathrm{E}(\boldsymbol{\beta}'\boldsymbol{X}'\boldsymbol{M}_0\boldsymbol{u}\boldsymbol{u}'\boldsymbol{u}) = \gamma_1\boldsymbol{\beta}'\boldsymbol{X}'\boldsymbol{M}_0\boldsymbol{\iota} = 0$. Following

Kelejian and Prucha (2001) again, we can show that any linear combination of $n^{-1/2}\boldsymbol{u}'\boldsymbol{M}_0\boldsymbol{X}\boldsymbol{\beta}$ and $n^{-1/2}\boldsymbol{u}'\boldsymbol{u} - \sigma_u^2$ (say, $l_1 n^{-1/2}\boldsymbol{u}'\boldsymbol{M}_0\boldsymbol{X}\boldsymbol{\beta} + l_2(n^{-1/2}\boldsymbol{u}'\boldsymbol{u} - \sigma_u^2)$, where l_1 and l_2 are non-zero constants) is asymptotically normal ($\mathrm{N}(0, l_1^2\sigma_u^2\boldsymbol{\beta}'\boldsymbol{\Sigma}\boldsymbol{\beta} + l_2^2\sigma_u^4(2+\gamma_2))$). Therefore,

$$\sqrt{n}\begin{pmatrix} n^{-1}\boldsymbol{y}'\boldsymbol{M}_0\boldsymbol{P}\boldsymbol{y} - n^{-1}\boldsymbol{\beta}'\boldsymbol{X}'\boldsymbol{M}_0\boldsymbol{X}\boldsymbol{\beta} \\ n^{-1}\boldsymbol{u}'\boldsymbol{M}\boldsymbol{u} - \sigma_u^2 \end{pmatrix} \xrightarrow{d} \mathrm{N}\left(\begin{pmatrix} 0 \\ 0 \end{pmatrix}, \begin{pmatrix} 4\sigma_u^2\boldsymbol{\beta}'\boldsymbol{\Sigma}\boldsymbol{\beta} & 0 \\ 0 & \sigma_u^4(2+\gamma_2) \end{pmatrix}\right).$$

The asymptotic distributions of $R^2 = \boldsymbol{y}'\boldsymbol{M}_0\boldsymbol{P}\boldsymbol{y}/(\boldsymbol{y}'\boldsymbol{M}_0\boldsymbol{P}\boldsymbol{y} + \boldsymbol{u}'\boldsymbol{M}\boldsymbol{u})$, $R^2/(1 - R^2) = \boldsymbol{y}'\boldsymbol{M}_0\boldsymbol{P}\boldsymbol{y}/\boldsymbol{u}'\boldsymbol{M}\boldsymbol{u}$, and $\log(R^2/(1-R^2)) = \log(\boldsymbol{y}'\boldsymbol{M}_0\boldsymbol{P}\boldsymbol{y}/\boldsymbol{u}'\boldsymbol{M}\boldsymbol{u})$ then follow immediately from the delta method. □

Note that R^2, $R^2/(1 - R^2)$, and $\log(R^2/(1 - R^2))$ are monotonic transformations of each other. Thus,

$$\Pr(R^2 \le r_0) = \Pr\left(\frac{R^2}{1-R^2} \le \frac{r_0}{1-r_0}\right) = \Pr\left[\log\left(\frac{R^2}{1-R^2}\right) \le \log\left(\frac{r_0}{1-r_0}\right)\right]. \tag{15}$$

When the error is normally distributed, by using (2) and setting $\boldsymbol{N}_1 = \boldsymbol{M}_0\boldsymbol{P}$ and $\boldsymbol{N}_2 = \boldsymbol{M}_0$, we can calculate the exact distribution of R^2 and, equivalently, that of $R^2/(1-R^2)$ or $\log(R^2/(1-R^2))$, in light of the above relationship. The asymptotic distribution, however, crucially depends on which statistic we are using. From (13)–(14), we see that when the signal to noise ratio, measured by $\boldsymbol{\beta}'\boldsymbol{\Sigma}\boldsymbol{\beta}/\sigma_u^2$, increases, the asymptotic distribution of $R^2/(1 - R^2)$ becomes more dispersed, whereas the asymptotic distribution of $\log(R^2/(1 - R^2))$ becomes more concentrated. Its effect on the asymptotic distribution of R^2 is ambiguous, and it depends on the strength of the signal to noise ratio.[6] An interesting case is the extreme case when $\boldsymbol{\beta} = \boldsymbol{0}$. In this case, while R^2 and $R^2/(1 - R^2)$ have well-defined asymptotic distributions, $\log(R^2/(1 - R^2))$ does not have a properly defined asymptotic distribution.[7] The exact distribution is free of this kind of pitfall and can be calculated regardless of the strength of the signal to noise ratio.

Figures 1, 2, 3, and 4 plot the cumulative distribution functions of the three statistics by comparing the true, exact, and asymptotic distributions for samples sizes 10, 20, 50, and 100, based on averages across 100,000 simulations.[8] The data generating process is $y = \beta_0 + \beta_1 x_1 + \beta_2 x_2 + u$, where x_1 and x_2 are generated from two independent i.i.d. N(0, 4) random variables, and the error term is simulated as

---

[6]More specifically, when $\boldsymbol{\beta}'\boldsymbol{\Sigma}\boldsymbol{\beta}/\sigma_u^2 < 1$, as $\boldsymbol{\beta}'\boldsymbol{\Sigma}\boldsymbol{\beta}/\sigma_u^2$ goes up, the asymptotic distribution of R^2 gets more dispersed. But when $\boldsymbol{\beta}'\boldsymbol{\Sigma}\boldsymbol{\beta}/\sigma_u^2 > 1$, as $\boldsymbol{\beta}'\boldsymbol{\Sigma}\boldsymbol{\beta}/\sigma_u^2$ goes up, the asymptotic distribution of R^2 gets more concentrated.

[7]Recall that the null distribution of the F statistic for testing the overall significance of a linear regression, which is proportional to $R^2/(1 - R^2)$, has a well-defined distribution.

[8]We never know the true distribution. But we believe that averaging 100,000 simulations should give results very close to the truth. In calculating the exact distributions via (2), we used Matlab's `integral` function.

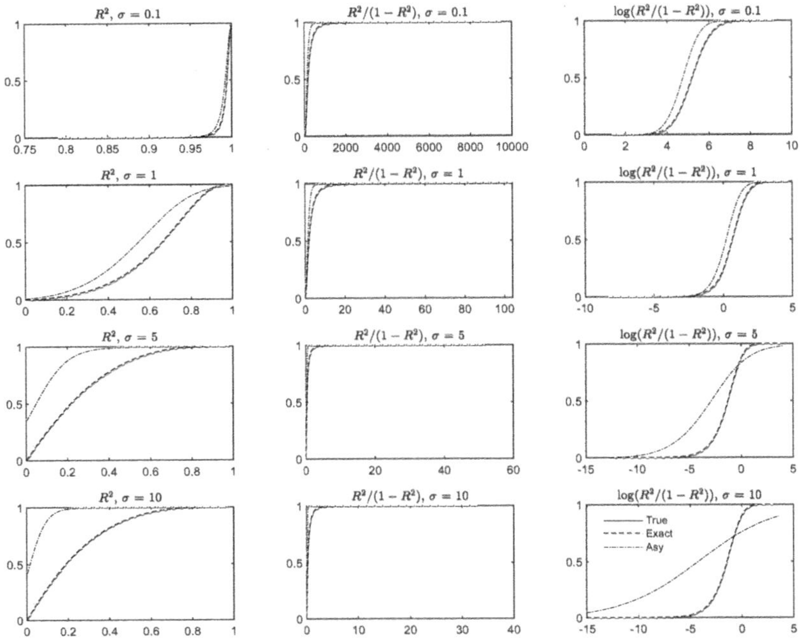

Fig. 1 CDF plots of R^2, $R^2/(1-R^2)$, and $\log(R^2/(1-R^2))$, $n = 10$

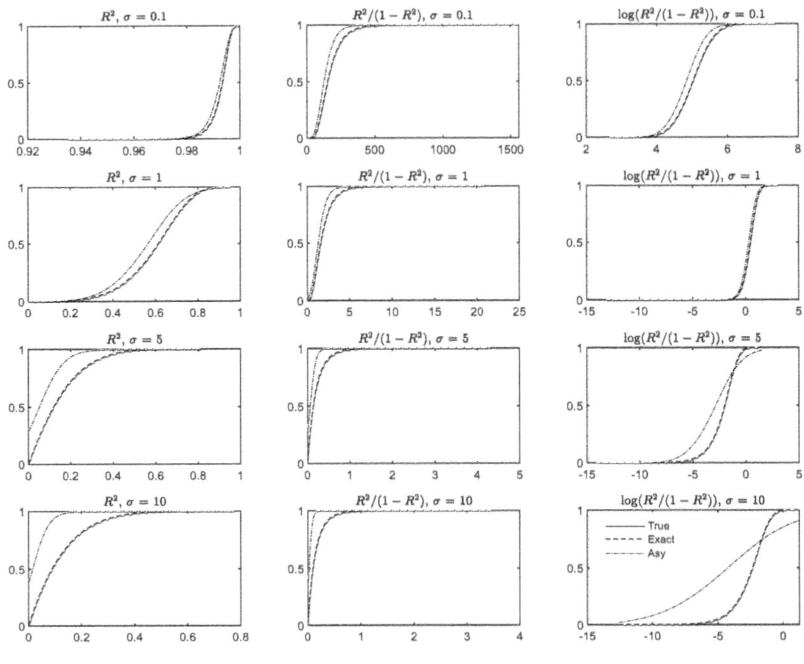

Fig. 2 CDF plots of R^2, $R^2/(1-R^2)$, and $\log(R^2/(1-R^2))$, $n = 20$

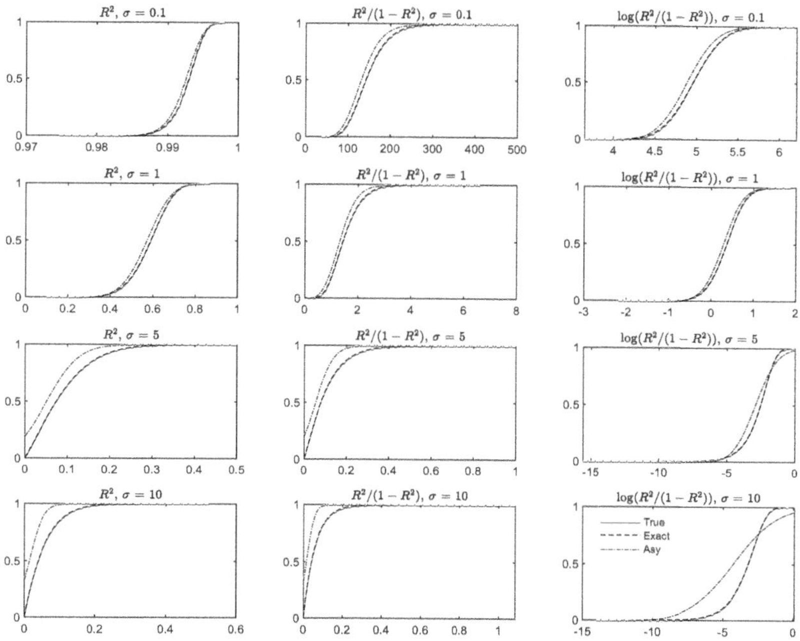

Fig. 3 CDF plots of R^2, $R^2/(1 - R^2)$, and $\log(R^2/(1 - R^2))$, $n = 50$

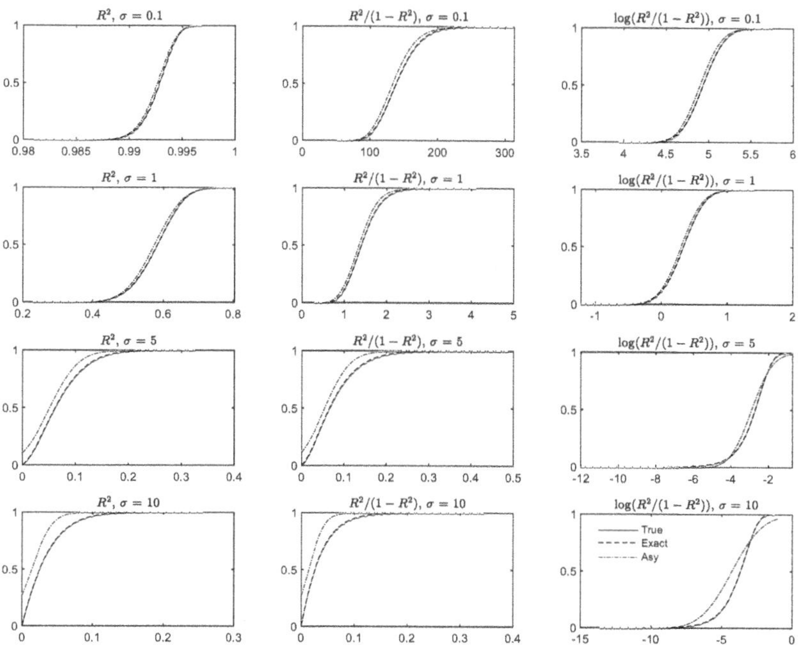

Fig. 4 CDF plots of R^2, $R^2/(1 - R^2)$, and $\log(R^2/(1 - R^2))$, $n = 100$

i.i.d. N(0, σ_u^2). We fix $\boldsymbol{\beta} = (\beta_0, \beta_1, \beta_2)' = (1, 0.3, 0.5)'$ and set $\sigma_u = 0.1, 1, 5, 10$, corresponding to scenarios from high to low signal to noise ratios. We observe that regardless of the sample size and the signal to noise ratio, the exact distribution matches precisely the true distribution. The asymptotic distributions fare reasonably well in small samples with $n = 10$ when $\sigma = 0.1$, corresponding to the situation of high signal to noise ratio. When $\sigma = 10$, the asymptotic distributions can be quite off the exact distribution in small samples. Xu (2014) recommended using $\log(R^2/(1 - R^2))$ by arguing that its asymptotic distribution is more stable. We see here clearly that this is not necessarily the case, as it depends on the signal to noise ratio.

4 Concluding Remarks

In this paper, we have presented a unified development of the exact distributions of many econometric statistics. These results can be straightforwardly implemented by numerical integration. In the context of the exact distribution of a goodness of fit measure, we numerically demonstrate that the asymptotic distribution may not carry forward in the small sample case. The exact distributional results developed in the paper could be easily extended to a class of some other econometric and statistical estimators used in practice that can be written as ratios of quadratic forms.

Acknowledgments We are grateful to an anonymous referee for very helpful comments.

References

Abadir, K. M., & Magnus, J. R. (2005). *Matrix algebra*. New York: Cambridge University Press.

Anderson, T. W., & Sawa, T. (1973). Distributions of estimates of coefficients of a single equation in a simultaneous system and their asymptotic expansions. *Econometrica, 41*, 683–714.

Arnold, B. C. (1983). *Pareto distributions*. Fairland: International Cooperative Publishing House.

Arnold, B. C. (1987). *Majorization and the Lorenz curve*. New York: Springer.

Arnold, B. C. (2012). On the Amato inequality index. *Statistics and Probability Letters, 82*, 1504–1506.

Arnold, B. C. (2015). *Pareto distributions* (2nd ed.). Boca Raton: CRC Press.

Arnold, B. C., & Sarabia, J. M. (2018). Analytic expressions for multivariate Lorenz surfaces. *Sankhya A, 80*, 84–111.

Arnold, B. C., Robertson, C. A., Brockett, P. L., & Shu, B.-Y. (1987). Generating ordered families of Lorenz curves by strongly unimodal distributions. *Journal of Business & Economic Statistics, 5*, 305–308

Bao, Y., & Ullah, A. (2010). Expectation of quadratic forms in normal and nonnormal variables with applications. *Journal of Statistical Planning and Inference, 140*, 193–1205.

Bao, Y., Ullah, A., & Wang, Y. (2017). Distribution of the mean reversion estimator in the Ornstein–Uhlenbeck process. *Econometric Reviews, 36*, 1039–1056.

Barillas, F., & Shanken, J. (2017). Which alpha? *Review of Financial Studies, 30*, 1316–1338

Coelho, C. A., & Arnold, B. C. (2014). On the exact and near-exact distributions of the product of generalized Gamma random variables and the generalized variance. *Communications in Statistics Theory and Methods, 43*, 2007–2033.

Ennis, D. M., & Johnson, N. L. (1993). Noncentral and central chi-square, F and beta distribution functions as special cases of the distribution function of an indefinite quadratic form. *Communications in Statistics Theory and Methods, 22*, 897–905.

Imhof, J. P. (1961). Computing the distribution of quadratic forms in normal variables. *Biometrika, 48*, 419–426.

Kelejian, H. H., & Prucha, I. R. (2001). On the asymptotic distribution of the Moran I test statistic with applications. *Journal of Econometrics, 104*, 219–257.

Koerts, J., & Abrahamse, A. P. J. (1969). *On the theory and application of the general linear model.* Rotterdam: Universitaire Pers Rotterdam

Marques, F. J., Coelho, C. A., & Arnold, B. C. (2011). A general near-exact distribution theory for the most common likelihood ratio test statistics used in multivariate analysis. *TEST, 20*, 180–203.

Miller, R. E., & Gehr, A. K. (1978). Sample size bias and Sharpe's performance measure: A note. *The Journal of Financial and Quantitative Analysis, 13*, 943–946.

Nagar, A. L. (1959). The bias and moment matrix of the general k-class estimators of the parameters in simultaneous equations. *Econometrica, 27*, 575–595.

Phillips, P. C. B. (1980). Finite sample theory and the distributions of alternative estimators of the marginal propensity to consume. *Review of Economic Studies, 47*, 183–224.

Phillips, P. C. B. (1986). The exact distribution of the Wald statistic. *Econometrica, 54*, 881–895.

Sharpe, W. F. (1966). Mutual fund performance. *The Journal of Business, 39*, 119–138.

Srivastava, M. S. (1987). Asymptotic distribution of Durbin-Watson statistic. *Economics Letters, 24*, 157–160.

Ullah, A. (2004). *Finite sample econometrics*. New York: Oxford University Press.

Villaseñor, J. A., & Arnold, B. C. (1984). *Some examples of fitted general quadratic Lorenz curves.* Technical report no. 130, Riverside, CA: Statistics Department, University of California.

Villaseñor, J. A., & Arnold, B. C. (1989). Elliptical Lorenz curves. *Journal of Econometrics, 40*, 327–338.

Xu, L. (2014). *R-squared Inference under Non-normal Error.* Dissertation, Department of Statistics, University of Washington.

Hidden Truncation in Non-Normal Models: A Brief Survey

Indranil Ghosh and Hon Keung Tony Ng

Following Arnold and Beaver (2000, *Sankhyā A*, **62**, 23–35), we revisit the hidden truncation paradigm for non-normal models with a feature that the resulting hidden truncated distribution arises from two different families of distributions with the same support set as well as from the same family. In the bivariate case, we illustrate the situations where the normalizing constant is in a closed form and situations where the normalizing constant is not in a closed form. Distributional properties of such models are investigated. Discussions on some conjectures related to hidden truncation paradigm for non-normal models are also provided.

1 Introduction

The theory and applications of hidden truncation models have a long history in the statistics literature. Some of the earliest works include Galton (1898) and Pearson and Lee (1908), who introduced the basic concepts of left and right truncated distributions. Thereafter, several different types of truncated distributions, both in the discrete domain and in the continuous domain, have been developed. For discrete distributions, one may refer to the papers by David and Johnson (1952) and Moore (1954), who implemented a truncated Poisson distribution to examine the number of accidents per worker. Finney (1947) and Sampford (1955) discussed the doubly

I. Ghosh (✉)
Department of Mathematics and Statistics, University of North Carolina Wilmington, Wilmington, NC, USA
e-mail: ghoshi@uncw.edu

H. K. T. Ng
Department of Statistical Sciences, Southern Methodist University, Dallas, TX, USA
e-mail: ngh@mail.smu.edu

I. Ghosh et al. (eds.), *Advances in Statistics - Theory and Applications*, Emerging Topics in Statistics and Biostatistics, https://doi.org/10.1007/978-3-030-62900-7_7

truncated binomial and negative-binomial distributions with applications in biology with respect to the number of abnormal sibships of specified size. Hidden truncation paradigm in non-normal models has received a great attention since the inception of it in the modern era. Truncated gamma, Pareto, exponential, Cauchy, t, F, normal, Weibull, and beta distributions have also been studied by many researchers. Chapman (1956) discussed a truncated gamma distribution with right truncation to analyze an animal migration pattern. A truncated Pareto distribution was considered to find the appropriate distribution due to the lack of the Pareto distribution, in which the whole range of income and tax is not rarely fitted over, in income statistics by Bhattacharya (1963). Cosentino et al. (1977) investigated the frequency magnitude relationship to solve a problem concerning the statistical analysis of earthquakes with a truncated exponential distribution. A truncated Cauchy distribution was introduced to overcome the weakness of the Cauchy distribution by Nadarajah and Kotz (2006). Nadarajah and Kotz (2008) introduced the truncated t and F distributions to inspect the moments and estimation procedures by the method of moments and the method of maximum likelihood. A truncated Weibull distribution was studied to solve the problem of nonexistence of the maximum likelihood estimators by Mittal and Dahiya (1989). Jamalizadeh et al. (2009) examined the cumulative distribution function (c.d.f.) and the moment generating function (m.g.f.) of a truncated skew normal distribution. Zaninetti (2013) found that a left truncated beta distribution provides a better fit to the initial mass function for stars compared to the lognormal distribution, which has been commonly used in astrophysics. The details of formation of distributions through truncation have also been discussed in Kotz et al. (2000, Chapter 44). Arnold (2009) developed and studied several univariate, bivariate, and multivariate parametric families of flexible models based on hidden truncation. Arnold and Ghosh (2011, 2013) discussed and studied hidden truncation in bivariate and multivariate Pareto data and applied to income modeling, especially in data sets where a hidden truncation has occurred. In particular, for a hidden truncation of a bivariate Pareto (type II), see Ghosh and Nadarajah (2015), and for a hidden truncation of a bivariate Pareto (type IV), see Ghosh and Balakrishnan (2017). Although a general framework to construct non-normal hidden truncation models was described by Arnold and Beaver (2000), much of the attention was given to the Gaussian family of distributions. Arnold and Beaver (2002) came up with a new characterization of a skew normal distribution via a hidden truncation mechanism. The hidden truncation models are also known as frontier models in the economics literature (see, for example, Kumbhakar and Knox Lovell 2000).

In this article, we motivate the study from Arnold and Beaver (2000) that many hidden truncation models with non-normal component densities undoubtedly deserve further attention. In many cases, as we will observe in this article, the normalizing constant may not be obtained in a closed form. During this course, we will also discuss some useful structural properties of those hidden truncation models. The rest of this paper is organized as follows. In Sect. 2, we provide the basic two-component models of hidden truncated distributions for non-normal component models. Section 3 discusses some illustrative examples from non-normal component densities in which the normalizing constant is either comprised of special mathematical functions and/or analytically intractable expressions. In Sect. 4, we discuss some useful structural properties of the hidden truncated models developed in Sect. 3. In Sect. 5, we discuss some inferential issues related to non-normal hidden truncated densities and briefly explore some conjectures related to hidden truncated models obtained via non-normal components. Finally, some concluding remarks are presented in Sect. 6.

2 Hidden Truncation in Non-Normal Models

Consider a hidden truncation model in which the observed data is truncated with respect to an unobserved co-variable. We examine two hidden truncation mechanisms that are slightly different from each other. The first type of hidden truncation, denoted as HD(Type I), starts with two independent random variables, while the second type of hidden truncation, denoted as HD(Type II), starts with two concomitant random variables. HD(Type II) is a more general mechanism in nature as it describes the hidden truncation from below, hidden truncation from above, and hidden truncation from both sides. Note that the outset that hidden truncation from below will not augment the original model since the resulting density will be again a member in the same family of distributions with only a reparametrization of the parent model. Consequently, we focus primarily on hidden truncation from both sides in the more general framework as hidden truncation from below and/or from above will be simply a particular case of the hidden truncation from both sides.

For the first type of hidden truncation, HD(Type I), we start with the basic definition as described in Arnold and Beaver (2000). Let U_1 and U_2 be two independent random variables with c.d.f. (probability density function (p.d.f.)) $\Psi_1(\cdot)(\psi_1(\cdot))$ and $\Psi_2(\cdot)(\psi_2(\cdot))$, respectively. Then, the conditional p.d.f. of U_1 given $\lambda_0 + \lambda_1 U_1 > U_2$, for any $\lambda_0 \in \mathbb{R}$ and $\lambda_1 \neq 0$, can be written as

$$f_{U_1|U_2<\lambda_0+\lambda_1 U_1}(u_1|U_2 < \lambda_0 + \lambda_1 U_1) = \frac{\Psi_1(u_1)\Psi_2(\lambda_0 + \lambda_1 u_1)}{\Pr(\lambda_0 + \lambda_1 U_1 > U_2)}. \tag{1}$$

In Eq. (1), if we consider the conditional density as $\lambda_0 \to \infty$, then the limit will be $\psi_1(\cdot)$, which is the non-truncated (alias unconditional) version of the density of U_1. If we consider $\lambda_1 = 0$, then we have the conditional density of U_1 given $U_2 < \lambda_0$, which is the same as the unconditional density of U_1, (i.e., $\psi_1(\cdot)$) because of U_1 and U_2 are independent. Noticeably, if we include the location (μ) and the scale parameter (σ) for U_1, a four-parameter model corresponding to Eq. (1) will be

$$f_{U_1|U_2<\lambda_0+\lambda_1 U_1}(u_1|U_2 < \lambda_0 + \lambda_1 U_1) = \frac{\Psi_1(\frac{u_1-\mu}{\sigma})\Psi_2\left(\lambda_0 + \lambda_1\left(\frac{u_1-\mu}{\sigma}\right)\right)}{\Pr\left(\lambda_0 + \lambda_1\left(\frac{U_1-\mu}{\sigma}\right) > U_2\right)}.$$

If both U_1 and U_2 belong to the same family of distributions, then the resulting hidden truncation model is again a member of the same family (possibly with a reparametrization). Therefore, it does not augment the parent distribution in such a case. On the contrary, under the same set of conditions, if we consider the conditional density of U_1 given that $\lambda_0 + \lambda_1 U_1 \leq U_2$, then the resulting hidden truncation model will be a distribution different from their parent distributions. We will consider truncation from both sides as well. We will illustrate this phenomenon with several examples in Sect. 3.

For the second type of hidden truncation, denoted as HD(Type II), we start with a bivariate model in which X and Y are concomitant variables with three different forms of hidden truncation. Suppose (X, Y) is a two-dimensional absolutely continuous random vector, we consider the conditional distribution of X given $Y \in M$, where M is a Borel set in $\mathbb{R}$. We can write the conditional p.d.f. of X given $Y \in M$ as

$$f_{X|Y\in M}(x) = f_X(x)\frac{\Pr(Y \in M|X = x)}{\Pr(Y \in M)}. \tag{2}$$

The following three forms of hidden truncation model are considered:

(i) truncation from below (also known as lower truncation): $M = (a, \infty)$, where a is the lower truncation point;
(ii) truncation from above (also known as upper truncation): $M = (-\infty, b)$, where b is the upper truncation point;
(iii) two-sided truncation: $M = (a, b]$, where a and b are the lower and upper truncation points, respectively.

For a two-sided hidden truncation, the observations are only available for X's whose concomitant variable Y is between $(a, b]$, $a < b$,, and Eq. (2) reduces to

$$f_{(a,b]}(x) = f(x|a < Y \leq b) = f_X(x)\frac{\Pr(a < Y \leq b|X = x)}{\Pr(a < Y \leq b)}. \tag{3}$$

This kind of hidden truncation model is characterized by

- the underlying distribution of X, which can be specified by the p.d.f. $f_X(x)$;
- the conditional distribution of Y given $X = x$, which can be specified by the conditional p.d.f. $f_{Y|X}(y|x)$;
- the specified values of the truncation points a and b;
- some other model parameters in addition to a and b.

For the conditional p.d.f. in Eq. (3), if we consider $a \to -\infty$ and $b \to +\infty$, the p.d.f. reduces to the unconditional density of X. The shape of the conditional p.d.f. will be more sensitive for smaller values of the lower truncation point a as compared to small or large values of the upper truncation point b.

3 Model Descriptions

In this section, we focus on several specific hidden truncation models with non-normal distributions. We will utilize either of the two hidden truncation paradigms, HD(Type I) and HD(Type II), as described in Sect. 2.

3.1 *Bivariate Cauchy distribution*

Consider the bivariate standard Cauchy distribution with joint p.d.f.

$$f(x, y) = \frac{1}{2\pi}\left(1 + x^2 + y^2\right)^{-3/2} I(-\infty < x < \infty; -\infty < y < \infty),$$

where $I(A)$ is the indication function with $I(A) = 1$ when event A is true and $I(A) = 0$ when event A is false. In this case, both the marginals of X and Y are univariate standard Cauchy distributed. For more details on the bivariate Cauchy distribution, one may refer to Nadarajah and Kotz (2007). Several properties of the bivariate Cauchy distributions can also be found in Balakrishnan and Lai (2009, Chapter 9).

Under the bivariate Cauchy distribution, the second type of hidden truncation, HD(Type II), described in Sect. 2 is considered. The conditional p.d.f. of Y given $X = x$ is

$$f(y|X = x) = \frac{1}{2}\left(1 + \frac{y^2}{1+x^2}\right)^{-3/2}\left(1 + x^2\right)^{-1/2} I(-\infty < y < \infty).$$

For the hidden truncation model, we assume that the random variable X is observed if and only if $d_1 < Y \leq d_2$, for any $(d_1, d_2) \in S(Y)$, where $S(Y)$ is the set of support of Y. The associated hidden truncated p.d.f. of X given $d_1 < Y \leq d_2$ in Eq. (2) can be expressed as

$$f(x|d_1 < Y \leq d_2) = \frac{f(x)\Pr(d_1 < Y \leq d_2|X = x)}{\Pr(d_1 < Y \leq d_2)} I(-\infty < x < \infty), \tag{4}$$

where

$$\Pr(d_1 < Y \leq d_2) = \int_{d_1}^{d_2} \frac{1}{\pi}\left(1 + y^2\right) dy = \frac{1}{\pi}\left[\tan^{-1}(d_2) - \tan^{-1}(d_1)\right], \tag{5}$$

and

$$\begin{aligned}
&\Pr\left(d_1 < Y \le d_2 | X = x\right) \\
&= \frac{1}{\pi}\int_{d_1}^{d_2} \frac{1}{2}\left(1+\frac{y^2}{1+x^2}\right)^{-3/2}\left(1+x^2\right)^{-1/2} dy \\
&= \frac{1}{2\pi}\left\{d_2\left[1+x^2+d_2^2\right]^{-1/2} - d_1\left[1+x^2+d_1^2\right]^{-1/2}\right\}. \qquad (6)
\end{aligned}$$

Therefore, with Eqs. (5) and (6), the hidden truncated p.d.f. of X given $d_1 < Y \le d_2$ in Eq. (4) can be expressed as

$$\begin{aligned}
&f\left(x|d_1 < Y \le d_2\right) \\
&= \frac{\left\{d_2\left[1+x^2+d_2^2\right]^{-1/2} - d_1\left[1+x^2+d_1^2\right]^{-1/2}\right\}}{2\pi\left(1+x^2\right)\left[\tan^{-1}(d_2) - \tan^{-1}(d_1)\right]} I(-\infty < x < \infty). \quad (7)
\end{aligned}$$

Figure 1 presents the hidden truncated p.d.f.s of X given $d_1 < Y \le d_2$ for different values of d_1 and d_2 based on the bivariate Cauchy distribution along with the non-truncated Cauchy distribution.

From Fig. 1, we can observe that when the left truncation point (i.e., d_1) assumes larger negative values (i.e, far away from 0), regardless of the right truncation point (i.e., d_2), the spread remains almost the same. For positive value of d_1, the spread of the distribution increases as the value of the right truncation point d_2 increases.

3.2 Bivariate Generalized Pareto Distribution

Consider the generalized bivariate Pareto distribution with joint p.d.f.

$$f(x, y) = \frac{K(xy)^{p-1}}{(\alpha + \beta x + \gamma y + \delta xy)^{p+q}} I(0 < x < \infty, 0 < y < \infty), \qquad (8)$$

where $p \in \mathbb{Z}$, $q \in \mathbb{Z}$, $\alpha > 0$, $\beta > 0$, $\gamma > 0$, and $\delta > 0$ are the model parameters, and K is the normalizing constant that can be evaluated as

$$K = \left[\int_0^{\infty}\int_0^{\infty} \frac{(xy)^{p-1}}{(\alpha + \beta x + \gamma y + \delta xy)^{p+q}} dx\, dy\right]^{-1}.$$

The bivariate distribution considered in Eq. (8) is the class of bivariate distributions with second kind beta conditionals (or bivariate distributions with Pearson type VI conditionals). Some aspects of this class of distributions have been studied in Castillo and Sarabia (1990) (see also, Arnold et al. 1999, Section 5.3). Moreover,

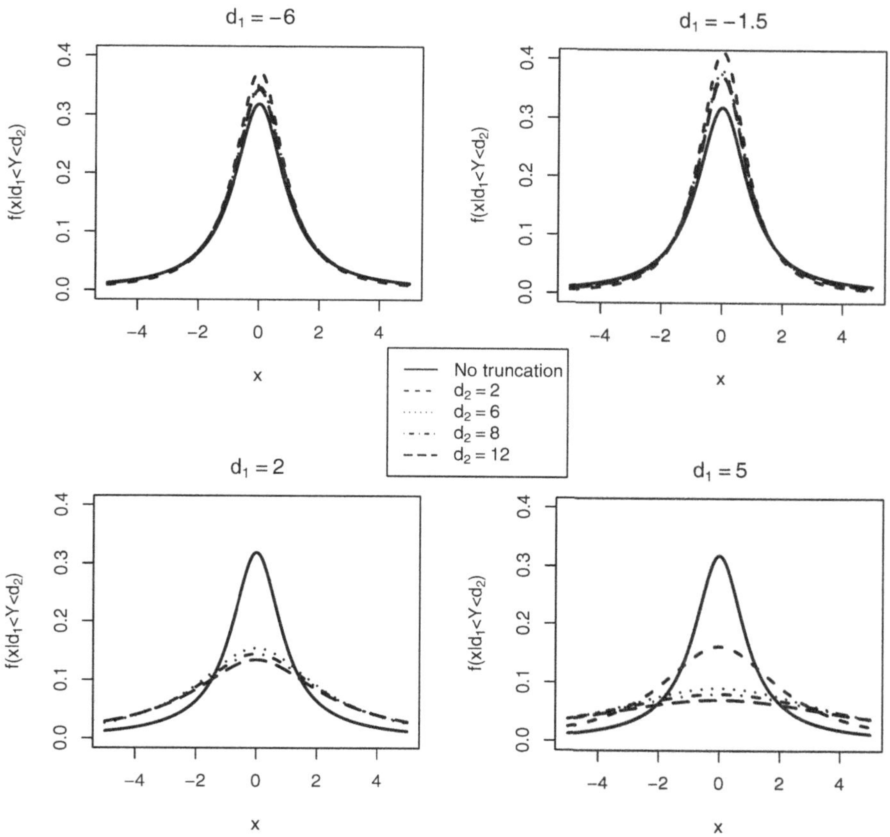

Fig. 1 Hidden truncated p.d.f.s of X given $d_1 < Y \leq d_2$ for different values of d_1 and d_2 based on bivariate Cauchy distribution along with the non-truncated Cauchy distribution

Eq. (8) is an extension of the class of bivariate distributions with Pareto conditionals considered by Arnold (1987).

For more details on the bivariate generalized Pareto distribution, see Ali and Nadarajah (2007) and Ghosh and Banks (2020). To construct a hidden truncation model based on HD(Type II) in Sect. 2, we need the following result.

Result 1 For $0 < \alpha < p$,

$$\int_0^\infty \frac{x^{\alpha-1}}{(x+z)^p} dx = z^{\alpha-p} B(p, p-\alpha),$$

where $B(a, b) = \int_0^1 w^{a-1}(1-w)^{b-1} dw$ with $a > 0$ and $b > 0$ is the beta function. □

From Ghosh and Banks (2020), if (X, Y) follows the bivariate generalized Pareto distribution in Eq. (8), then using Result 1, the marginal p.d.f. of X is

$$f_X(x) = Kx^{p-1}(\alpha + \beta x)^{-q}(\gamma + \delta x)^{-p} B(p, q) I(0 < x < \infty). \tag{9}$$

Similarly, the marginal p.d.f. of Y is

$$f_Y(y) = Ky^{p-1}(\alpha + \gamma y)^{-q}(\beta + \delta y)^{-p} B(p, q) I(0 < y < \infty).$$

Therefore, the normalizing constant can be evaluated using a one-dimensional integral instead of a two-dimensional integral as

$$\begin{aligned} K &= \left[B(p, q)\int_0^\infty x^{p-1}(\alpha + \beta x)^{-q}(\gamma + \delta x)^{-p}\,dx\right]^{-1} \\ &= \left[B(p, q)\int_0^\infty y^{p-1}(\alpha + \gamma y)^{-q}(\beta + \delta y)^{-p}\,dy\right]^{-1}. \end{aligned}$$

The conditional p.d.f. of Y given $X = x$ can be expressed as

$$f(y|X = x) = \frac{y^{p-1}}{B(p, q)}\left[1 + y\left(\frac{\gamma + \delta x}{\alpha + \beta x}\right)\right]^{-p-q}\left(\frac{\gamma + \delta x}{\alpha + \beta x}\right)^p \mathrm{I}(0 < y < \infty).$$

Note that the random variable

$$Y\left(\frac{\gamma + \delta X}{\alpha + \beta X}\right)\Bigg| X = x$$

follows the beta prime distribution (also known as the beta distribution of second kind or inverted beta distribution) with parameters p and q. Similarly, we can show that the random variable

$$X\left(\frac{\beta + \delta Y}{\alpha + \gamma Y}\right)\Bigg| Y = y$$

also follows the beta prime distribution with parameters p and q. Based on the marginal p.d.f. of Y, we can compute

$$\begin{aligned} \Pr(d_1 < Y \le d_2) &= KB(p, q)\int_{d_1}^{d_2} y^{p-1}(\alpha + \gamma y)^{-q}(\beta + \delta y)^{-p}\,dy \\ &= p^{-1}KB(p, q) \\ &\times\left[d_1^p\left(\frac{\delta d_1}{\beta} + 1\right)^p(\beta + \delta d_1)^{-p}(\alpha + \gamma d_1)^{-q}\left(\frac{\gamma d_1}{\alpha} + 1\right)^q\right. \end{aligned}$$

$$\times F_1\left(p; q, p; p+1; -\frac{d_1\gamma}{\alpha}, -\frac{d_1\delta}{\beta}\right)$$
$$+d_2^p(\beta+\delta d_2)^{-p}\left(\frac{\delta d_2}{\beta}+1\right)^p(\alpha+\gamma d_2)^{-q}\left(\frac{\gamma d_2}{\alpha}+1\right)^q$$
$$\times F_1\left(p; q; p; p+1; -\frac{d_2\gamma}{\alpha}, -\frac{d_2\delta}{\beta}\right)\Bigg], \tag{10}$$

$$\Pr(d_1 < Y \le d_2)$$
$$= p^{-1}KB(p,q)$$
$$\times\left[d_1^p\left(\frac{\delta d_1}{\beta}+1\right)^p(\beta+\delta d_1)^{-p}(\alpha+\gamma d_1)^{-q}\left(\frac{\gamma d_1}{\alpha}+1\right)^q\right.$$
$$\times F_1\left(p; q, p; p+1; -\frac{d_1\gamma}{\alpha}, -\frac{d_1\delta}{\beta}\right)$$
$$+d_2^p(\beta+\delta d_2)^{-p}\left(\frac{\delta d_2}{\beta}+1\right)^p(\alpha+\gamma d_2)^{-q}\left(\frac{\gamma d_2}{\alpha}+1\right)^q$$
$$\left.\times F_1\left(p; q; p; p+1; -\frac{d_2\gamma}{\alpha}, -\frac{d_2\delta}{\beta}\right)\right], \tag{11}$$

where $F_1\,(a; b; c; d, u, v)$ is the Appell hypergeometric function defined as

$$F_1(a; b; c; d, u, v)$$
$$= \frac{\Gamma(d)}{\Gamma(a)\Gamma(d-a)}\int_0^1 w^{a-1}(1-w)^{d-a-1}(1-wu)^{-b}(1-wv)^{-c}dw$$

and $\Gamma(a) = \int_0^\infty w^{a-1}e^{-w}dw$ denotes the gamma function.

Then, we obtain the conditional probability

$$\Pr(d_1 < Y \le d_2 | X = x)$$
$$= \left(\frac{\gamma+\delta x}{\alpha+\beta x}\right)^p \frac{1}{B(p,q)}\int_{d_1}^{d_2} y^{p-1}\left[1+y\left(\frac{\gamma+\delta x}{\alpha+\beta x}\right)\right]^{-p-q} dy$$
$$= \left(\frac{\alpha+x\beta}{(\gamma+\delta x)\,B(p,q)}\right)$$
$$\times\left[d_2^p\Gamma(p)\,{}_2\tilde{F}_1\left(p, p+q; p+1; -\frac{d_2(\gamma+x\delta)}{\alpha+x\beta}\right)\right.$$
$$\left.-d_1^p\Gamma(p)\,{}_2\tilde{F}_1\left(p, p+q; p+1; -\frac{d_1(\gamma+x\delta)}{\alpha+x\beta}\right)\right], \tag{12}$$

where ${}_2\tilde{F}_1(a, b; c; z) = {}_2F_1(a, b; c; z)/\Gamma(c)$ is the regularized hypergeometric function. As a result, the hidden truncated p.d.f. of X given $d_1 < Y \leq d_2$ in Eq. (4) can be obtained by using Eqs. (9), (11), and (12) as

$$
\begin{aligned}
f(x|d_1 < Y \leq d_2) = & \frac{px^{p-1}}{B(p,q)}(\alpha+\beta x)^{-q+1}(\gamma+\delta x)^{-p-1} \\
& \times\left[d_2^p\Gamma(p)\,{}_2\tilde{F}_1\left(p, p+q; p+1; -\frac{d_2(\gamma+x\delta)}{\alpha+x\beta}\right)\right. \\
& \left.-d_1^p\Gamma(p)\,{}_2\tilde{F}_1\left(p, p+q; p+1; -\frac{d_1(\gamma+x\delta)}{\alpha+x\beta}\right)\right] \\
& \times\left[d_1^p\left(\frac{\delta d_1}{\beta}+1\right)^p(\beta+\delta d_1)^{-p}(\alpha+\gamma d_1)^{-q}\left(\frac{\gamma d_1}{\alpha}+1\right)^q\right. \\
& \times F_1\left(p; q, p; p+1; -\frac{d_1\gamma}{\alpha}, -\frac{d_1\delta}{\beta}\right) \\
& +d_2^p(\beta+\delta d_2)^{-p}\left(\frac{\delta d_2}{\beta}+1\right)^p(\alpha+\gamma d_2)^{-q}\left(\frac{\gamma d_2}{\alpha}+1\right)^q \\
& \left.\times F_1\left(p; q, p; p+1; -\frac{d_2\gamma}{\alpha}, -\frac{d_2\delta}{\beta}\right)\right]^{-1}.
\end{aligned}
$$

Figure 2 presents the hidden truncated p.d.f.s of X given $d_1 < Y \leq d_2$ for different values of d_1 and d_2 based on the bivariate generalized Pareto distribution along with the non-truncated Pareto distribution. From Fig. 2, we can observe that the non-truncated and hidden truncated p.d.f.s (regardless of the choices of the lower and upper truncation points, d_1 and d_2, respectively) are always positively skewed. For fixed values of α, β, γ, δ, p, and d_1, when d_2 and q increase, the skewness of the hidden truncated p.d.f. increases. For fixed values of α, β, γ, δ, p, q, and d_2, when d_1 increases, the hidden truncated p.d.f. behaves similarly to a non-truncated version in terms of the overall shape.

3.3 Arnold and Strauss Bivariate Exponential Distribution

The joint p.d.f. of the Arnold and Strauss (1988) bivariate exponential distribution is

$$
f(x, y) = K\exp[-(ax+by+cxy)], \tag{13}
$$

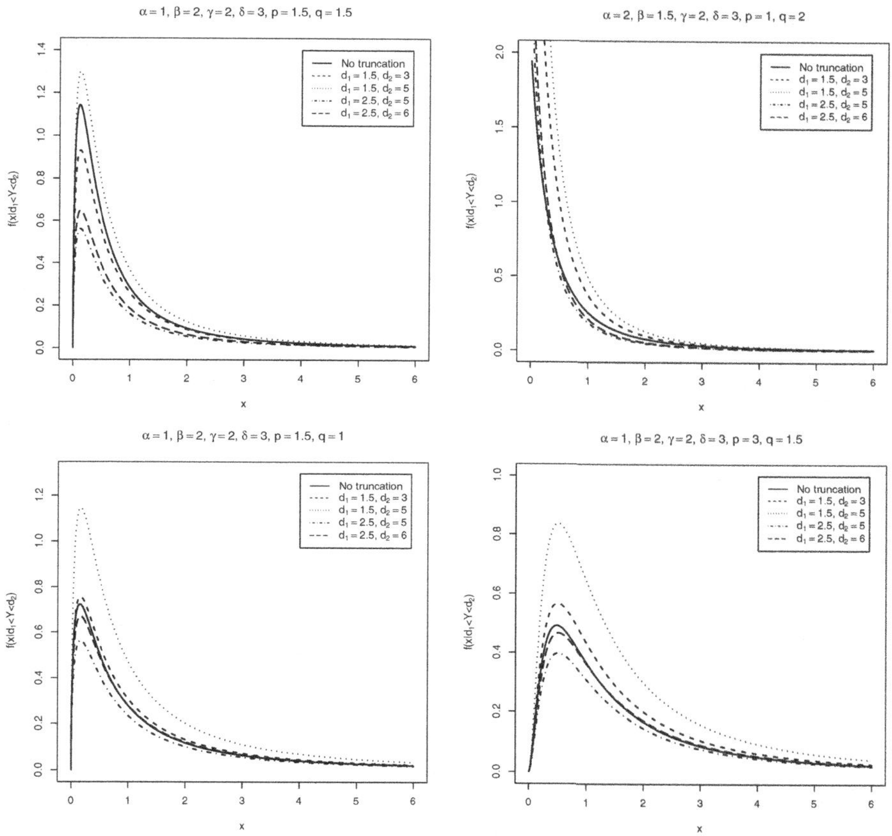

Fig. 2 Hidden truncated p.d.f.s of X given $d_1 < Y \leq d_2$ for different values of d_1 and d_2 based on the bivariate generalized Pareto distribution along with the non-truncated Pareto distribution

where $x > 0$, $y > 0$, $a > 0$, $b > 0$, $c > 0$, and K is the normalizing constant, which is defined as

$$K^{-1} = -c \exp\left(\frac{ab}{c}\right) Ei\left(-\frac{ab}{c}\right),$$

with $Ei(x)$ be the exponential integral function defined by $Ei(x) = \int_{-\infty}^{x} t^{-1} \exp(t) dt$.

For Arnold and Strauss (1988) bivariate exponential distribution, we can obtain the following:

- The marginal density of X is given by

$$f_X(x) = \frac{K \exp(-ax)}{b + cx}, \quad x > 0. \tag{14}$$

- Similarly, the marginal density of Y is given by

$$f_Y(y) = \frac{K \exp(-by)}{a + cy}, \quad y > 0.$$

- Conditional p.d.f. of Y given $X = x$ is

$$f_{Y|x}(y|X = x) = (b + cx)\exp(-(b + cx)y),\ y > 0.$$

Let us consider the two-sided hidden truncation for Y, say $d_1 < Y \leq d_2$, where $(d_1, d_2) \in S(Y)$, i.e., a HD(Type II) model from Sect. 2. Observe that

$$\Pr(d_1 < Y \leq d_2 | X{=}x) = \int_{d_1}^{d_2} (b{+}cx)\exp[-(b{+}cx)y]\, dy = A_1(d_1, d_2, b, c, x),$$

where $A_1(d_1, d_2, b, c, x) = \exp[-d_1(b + cx)] - \exp[-d_2(b + cx)]$. Then, we have

$$\begin{aligned}
\Pr(d_1 < Y \leq d_2) &= \int_{d_1}^{d_2} \frac{K \exp(-by)}{a + cy} dy \\
&= \int_0^{d_2} \frac{K \exp(-by)}{a + cy} dy - \int_0^{d_1} \frac{K \exp(-by)}{a + cy} dy \\
&= K\left\{ - \frac{e^{\frac{ab}{c}}\left[Ei\left(-\frac{b(a+cd_1)}{c}\right) - Ei\left(-\frac{b(a+cd_2)}{c}\right)\right]}{c}\right\} = M_1 \quad \text{say.}
\end{aligned}$$

Therefore, the conditional p.d.f. of X given $d_1 < Y \leq d_2$, based on the HD(Type II) mechanism, can be expressed as

$$f(x | d_1 < Y \leq d_2) = \frac{\exp(-ax)(b + cx)^{-1} A_1(d_1, d_2, b, c, x)}{\frac{b}{c}\exp\left(-\frac{ab}{c}\right) M_1}, \quad x > 0. \tag{15}$$

Here, numerical integration is needed to compute $A_1(d_1, d_2, b, c, x)$. Figure 3 presents the hidden truncated p.d.f.s of X given $d_1 < Y \leq d_2$ for different values of d_1 and d_2 based on the Arnold and Strauss bivariate exponential distribution along with the non-truncated exponential distribution.

From Fig. 3, we can observe that regardless of the choices of model parameters a, b, c and with non-zero values of d_1 and d_2,, the hidden truncated p.d.f.s are always positively skewed with varying intensity. The results in this subsection can be extended to the case of gamma conditionals (see Section 4.6 in Arnold et al. (1999) and Castillo et al. (1990)).

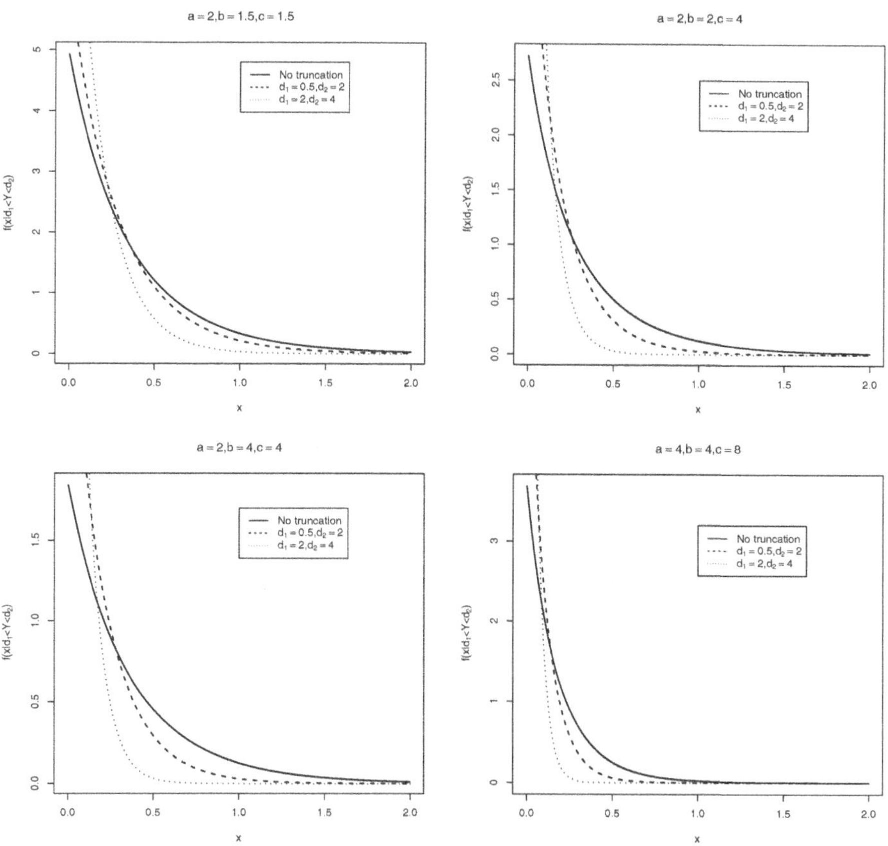

Fig. 3 Hidden truncated p.d.f.s of X given $d_1 < Y \leq d_2$ for different values of d_1 and d_2 based on the Arnold and Strauss bivariate exponential distribution along with the non-truncated exponential distribution

3.4 Pareto (Type II) and Pareto (Type IV) Model

For this model, the first type of hidden truncation, HD(Type I), described in Sect. 2 is considered. Suppose $U_1 \sim Pareto(type\ II)(\mu = 0, \alpha, \delta)$ and $U_2 \sim Pareto(type\ IV)(\mu = 0, \alpha, \delta, \gamma)$ with p.d.f.s

$$f_1(u_1) = \frac{\alpha}{\delta}\left(1 + \frac{u_1}{\delta}\right)^{-(\alpha+1)}, \quad u_1 \geq 0$$

$$\text{and } f_2(u_2) = \frac{\alpha}{\delta\gamma}\left(\frac{u_2}{\delta}\right)^{1/\gamma-1}\left[1 + \left(\frac{u_2}{\delta}\right)^{1/\gamma}\right]^{-(\alpha+1)}, \quad u_2 \geq 0,$$

respectively. Therefore, the denominator in Eq. (1) can be expressed as

$$\Pr(\lambda_0 + \lambda_1 U_1 > U_2) = \Pr(W < U_1), \quad \text{where} \quad W = \frac{U_2 - \lambda_0}{\lambda_1}.$$

The p.d.f. of W is

$$f_W(w) = \frac{\alpha}{\gamma\delta}\left(\frac{\lambda_0 + \lambda_1 w}{\delta}\right)^{1/\gamma - 1}\left[1 + \left(\frac{\lambda_0 + \lambda_1 w}{\delta}\right)^{1/\gamma}\right]^{-(\alpha+1)} I\left(-\frac{\lambda_0}{\lambda_1} < w < \infty\right).$$

The associated c.d.f. of W can be obtained as

$$\begin{aligned} F_W(w) &= \int_{-\frac{\lambda_0}{\lambda_1}}^{w}\left(\frac{\alpha}{\gamma\delta}\right)\left(\frac{\lambda_0 + \lambda_1 t}{\delta}\right)^{1/\gamma - 1}\left[1 + \left(\frac{\lambda_0 + \lambda_1 t}{\delta}\right)^{1/\gamma}\right]^{-(\alpha+1)} dt \\ &= 1 - \left[1 + \left(\frac{\lambda_0 + \lambda_1 w}{\delta}\right)^{\frac{1}{\gamma}}\right]^{-\alpha}. \end{aligned}$$

Therefore, the denominator of Eq. (1) can be written as

$$\begin{aligned} &\Pr(W < U_1) \\ &= \int_0^{\infty} F_W(u_1) f_1(u_1) du_1 \\ &= \frac{\alpha}{\delta}\int_0^{\infty}\left\{1 - \left[1 + \left(\frac{\lambda_0 + \lambda_1 u_1}{\delta}\right)^{\frac{1}{\gamma}}\right]^{-\alpha}\right\}\left(1 + \frac{u_1}{\delta}\right)^{-(\alpha+1)} du_1 = C_1, \quad \text{say}. \end{aligned}$$

Hence, the hidden truncated density from Eq. (1) is

$$\begin{aligned} &f(u_1 | U_2 < \lambda_0 + \lambda_1 U_1) \\ &= C_1^{-1}\frac{\alpha}{\delta}\left(1 + \frac{u_1}{\delta}\right)^{-(\alpha+1)}\left\{1 - \left[1 + \left(\frac{\lambda_0 + \lambda_1 u_1}{\delta}\right)^{\frac{1}{\gamma}}\right]^{-\alpha}\right\} I(0 < u_1 < \infty). \end{aligned} \tag{16}$$

Figure 4 presents the hidden truncated p.d.f.s of U_1 given $U_2 < \lambda_0 + \lambda_1 U_1$ for different values of λ_1 and λ_2 based on the Pareto(type II) and Pareto(type IV) models along with the Pareto(type II) distribution.

From Fig. 4, it appears that for any choices of the model parameters, α, δ, and γ, and for any finite choices of λ_0 and λ_1 (i.e., $|\lambda_0| < \infty$ and $|\lambda_1| < \infty$), the associated p.d.f.s are positively skewed.

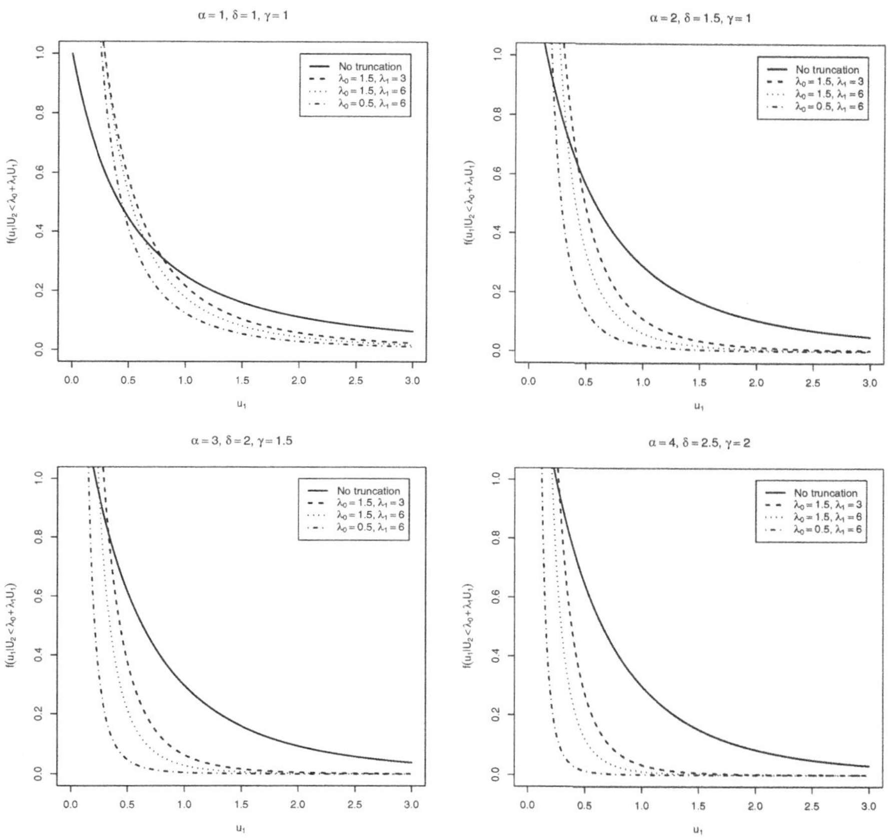

Fig. 4 Hidden truncated p.d.f.s of U_1 given $U_2 < \lambda_0 + \lambda_1 U_1$ for different values of λ_0 and λ_1 based on the Pareto(type II) and Pareto(type IV) models along with the Pareto(type II) distribution

3.5 *Cauchy–Cauchy Hidden Truncated Model*

In this subsection, we revisit the hidden truncation model discussed in Arnold and Gomez (2008) based on the two independent standard Cauchy distributions. Specifically, the standard Cauchy random variables U_1 and U_2 have c.d.f.

$$\Psi_1(x) = \Psi_2(x) = \frac{1}{2} + \pi^{-1} \tan^{-1} x,$$

and p.d.f.

$$\psi_1(x) = \psi_2(x) = \frac{1}{\pi\left(1 + x^2\right)} I(-\infty < x < \infty).$$

Observe that $U_i \sim Cauchy\,(0,1)$, $i = 1, 2$, and we have $U_2 - \lambda_1 U_1 \sim Cauchy\,(0, 1 + |\lambda_1|)$. Consequently,

$$\Pr\left(U_2 < \lambda_0 + \lambda_1 U_1\right) = \Psi\left(\frac{\lambda_0}{1 + |\lambda_1|}\right).$$

The associated hidden truncated model via the HD(type I) mechanism is

$$f\left(u_1 | U_2 < \lambda_0 + \lambda_1 U_1\right) = \frac{1}{\pi\left(1 + u_1^2\right)} \times \left[\frac{\frac{1}{2} + \pi^{-1}\tan^{-1}\left(\lambda_0 + \lambda_1 u_1\right)}{\frac{1}{2} + \pi^{-1}\tan^{-1}\left(\frac{\lambda_0}{1+|\lambda_1|}\right)}\right] I(-\infty < x < \infty). \tag{17}$$

Figure 5 presents the hidden truncated p.d.f.s of U_1 given $U_2 < \lambda_0 + \lambda_1 U_1$ for different values of λ_0 and λ_2 based on the Cauchy–Cauchy hidden truncated model

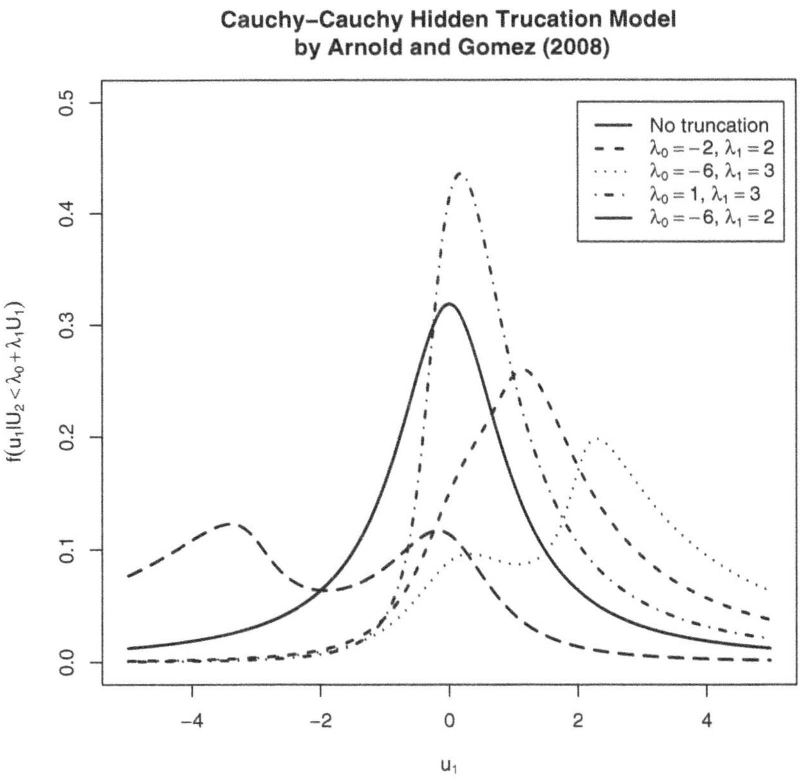

Fig. 5 Hidden truncated p.d.f.s of U_1 given $U_2 < \lambda_0 + \lambda_1 U_1$ for different values of λ_0 and λ_2 based on the Cauchy–Cauchy hidden truncated model in Arnold and Gomez (2008) along with the non-truncated Cauchy distribution

in Arnold and Gomez (2008) along with the non-truncated Cauchy distribution. From Fig. 5, we can observe that depending on the choices of λ_0 and λ_1, the hidden truncated density given in Eq. (17) can assume to be approximately left-skewed and can have more than one peak in the distribution.

4 Distributional Properties of Non-normal Hidden Truncation Models

In this section, we discuss some useful structural properties of the hidden truncated densities developed in Sect. 3. We begin our discussion with the both-sided hidden truncated Cauchy model. Here, we will primarily focus on identifying the shape of the density functions, the shape of the hazard functions, the raw moments of order $r(r \geq 2)$, and several different types of stochastic orderings. All the mathematical calculations are obtained using the *Mathematica* software. Note that in the situations where a closed form or an analytically tractable form of the normalizing constant is not found, one will have to consider the strategy involving the use of numerical integration.

4.1 *Structural Properties for Hidden Truncated Cauchy Model*

In this subsection, we discuss the structural properties of the hidden truncated Cauchy model presented in Sect. 3.1.

4.1.1 Moments

For the hidden truncated Cauchy model with p.d.f. in Eq. (7), the moments of order $r(r \geq 1)$ can be obtained as

$$
\begin{aligned}
&E\left(X^r | d_1 < Y \leq d_2\right)\\
&= \left(4\sqrt{\pi} d_1 d_2\right)^{-1} \Bigg\{ -\left[(-1)^r + 1\right] \exp\left(-\frac{1}{2} i \pi r\right) \sin\left(\frac{\pi r}{2}\right) \left[\cot\left(\frac{\pi r}{2}\right) + i\right] \\
&\times \Bigg[d_1 d_2 \Gamma\left(-\frac{r}{2}\right) \Gamma\left(\frac{r+1}{2}\right) \Bigg[d_1 \left(d_1^2 + 1\right)^{r/2} {}_2F_1\left(1, \frac{r+1}{2}; \frac{r+2}{2}; d_1^2 + 1\right) \\
&- d_2 \left(d_2^2 + 1\right)^{r/2} {}_2F_1\left(1, \frac{r+1}{2}; \frac{r+2}{2}; d_2^2 + 1\right) \Bigg] \\
&+ \pi^{3/2} \left(d_1 \sqrt{-d_2^2} - d_2 \sqrt{-d_1^2}\right) \csc\left(\frac{\pi r}{2}\right) \Bigg] \Bigg\},
\end{aligned}
$$

where $i = \sqrt{-1}$. The variance and other moment-based measures such as skewness and kurtosis of the hidden truncated random variable $X|d_1 < Y \leq d_2$ can be obtained from the above expression.

4.1.2 Stochastic Ordering

Ordering probability distributions, particularly among lifetime distributions, play an important role in the statistical literature and distribution theory, see, for example, Johnson et al. (1995) and the references therein. Here, we consider four different stochastic orders including the conventional order, the hazard rate order, the mean residual life order, and the likelihood ratio order for the hidden truncated distributions constructed in Sect. 3. There are numerous statistical applications of these stochastic orders. For instance, if a family of distributions has a likelihood ratio ordering, then it has the monotone likelihood ratio property. This implies that there exists a uniformly most powerful test for any one-sided hypothesis when the other parameters are known. If X_1 and X_2 are independent random variables with c.d.f.s F_{X_1} and F_{X_2}, respectively, then X_1 is said to be smaller than X_2 in the

- stochastic order ($X_1 \geq_{st} X_2$), if $F_{X_1}(x) \leq F_{X_2}(x)$ for all x;
- hazard rate order ($X_1 \geq_{hr} X_2$), if $h_{X_1}(x) \leq h_{X_2}(x)$ for all x;
- mean residual life order ($X_1 \geq_{mrl} X_2$), if $m_{X_1}(x) \leq m_{X_2}(x)$ for all x;
- likelihood ratio order ($X_1 \geq_{lr} X_2$), if $\frac{f_{X_1}(x)}{f_{X_2}(x)}$ decreases in x.

The following well-known results for establishing stochastic orders of distributions are due to Shaked and Shanthikumar (1995):

$$\begin{array}{c} X_1 \leq_{lr} X_2 \Rightarrow X_1 \leq_{hr} X_2 \Rightarrow X_1 \leq_{mrl} X_2 \\ \Downarrow \\ X_1 \leq_{st} X_2. \end{array}$$

We begin with the p.d.f. in Eq. (7), and for notational simplicity, we denote the hidden truncated Cauchy distribution with truncation points d_1 and d_2 as $TC\,(d_1, d_2)$. The $TC\,(d_1, d_2)$ distribution is ordered with respect to the strongest "likelihood ratio" ordering as shown in the following Theorem 1. It shows the flexibility of a two-parameter $TC\,(d_1, d_2)$ distribution.

Theorem 1 *Let* $X_1 \sim TC\,(a, b)$ *and* $X_2 \sim TC\,(c, d)$. *If* $a < \min\{b, d\}$ *and* $d < b < c$, *then* $X_1 \geq_{lr} x_2$, $X_1 \geq_{hr} X_2$, $X_1 \geq_{mrl} X_2$, *and* $X_1 \leq_{st} X_2$.

Proof Taking the derivative of the natural logarithm of the ratio of the p.d.f.s of X_1 and X_2, where $X_1 \sim TC\,(a, b)$ and $X_2 \sim TC\,(c, d)$, we have

$$\frac{d}{dx}\log\frac{f_{X_1}(x|a<Y\le b)}{f_{X_2}(x|c<Y\le d)}$$

$$=\frac{\left(\frac{d}{\sqrt{d^2+x^2+1}}-\frac{c}{\sqrt{c^2+x^2+1}}\right)}{\left(\frac{b}{\sqrt{b^2+x^2+1}}-\frac{a}{\sqrt{a^2+x^2+1}}\right)\left(\frac{c}{\sqrt{c^2+x^2+1}}-\frac{d}{\sqrt{d^2+x^2+1}}\right)^2}$$

$$\times\left\{\frac{ax\left[\frac{c(a^2-c^2)}{(c^2+x^2+1)^{3/2}}+\frac{d^3-a^2d}{(d^2+x^2+1)^{3/2}}\right]}{\left(a^2+x^2+1\right)^{3/2}}+\frac{bx\left[\frac{c(c^2-b^2)}{(c^2+x^2+1)^{3/2}}+\frac{d(b^2-d^2)}{(d^2+x^2+1)^{3/2}}\right]}{\left(b^2+x^2+1\right)^{3/2}}\right\}.$$

If $a<\min\{b,d\}$ and $d<b<c$, then $\frac{d}{dx}\log\frac{f_{X_1}(x)}{f_{X_2}(x)}\ge 0$, which implies that $X_1\ge_{lr}X_2$ and, hence, $X_1\ge_{lr}X_2$, $X_1\ge_{hr}X_2$, $X_1\ge_{mrl}X_2$, and $X_1\ge_{st}X_2$. □

4.1.3 Shape of the Probability Density Function

For the p.d.f. presented in Eq. (7), we have the first derivative of the logarithm of p.d.f. as

$$\frac{\partial\log f(x|d_1<Y\le d_2)}{\partial x}=\frac{\frac{d_1x(2d_1^2+3x^2+3)}{(d_1^2+x^2+1)^{3/2}}-\frac{d_2x(2d_2^2+3x^2+3)}{(d_2^2+x^2+1)^{3/2}}}{\left(x^2+1\right)\left(\frac{d_2}{\sqrt{d_2^2+x^2+1}}-\frac{d_1}{\sqrt{d_1^2+x^2+1}}\right)}. \quad (18)$$

From Eq. (18), it can be shown that the p.d.f. is log-concave. The proof is available from the authors upon request.

4.1.4 Shape of the Hazard Function

For the hidden truncated Cauchy model with p.d.f. in Eq. (7), the associated hazard function is decreasing provided that $d_1<d_2$. The details are presented in Appendix.

4.2 *Structural Properties of the Hidden Truncated in Arnold and Strauss Bivariate Exponential Distribution*

In this subsection, we discuss the structural properties of the hidden truncated model based on the Arnold and Strauss bivariate exponential distribution presented in Sect. 3.3.

4.2.1 Moments

For the hidden truncated model based on the Arnold and Strauss bivariate exponential distribution with p.d.f. in Eq. (15), the moments of order $r(r \geq 1)$ can be obtained as

$$E\left(X^r|d_1 < Y \leq d_2\right) = \left[b\exp\left(-\frac{ab}{c}\right)M_1\right]^{-1}\left(\frac{c}{b}\right)^{-r}\Gamma(r+1)\exp\left(\frac{ab}{c}\right) \times\left[\exp(-bd_1)\Gamma\left(-r,\frac{b(a+cd_1)}{c}\right)-\exp(-bd_2)\Gamma\left(-r,\frac{b(a+cd_2)}{c}\right)\right]. \quad (19)$$

4.2.2 Stochastic Ordering

We denote the hidden truncated model based on the Arnold and Strauss bivariate exponential distribution with parameters a, b, and c, and truncation points d_1 and d_2 as $HTExp\,(a, b, c, d_1, d_2)$. The $HTExp\,(a, b, c, d_1, d_2)$ distribution is ordered with respect to the strongest "likelihood ratio" ordering as shown in the following Theorem 2.

Theorem 2 *Let* $X_1 \sim HTExp\,(a, b, c, d_1, d_2)$ *and* $X_2 \sim HTExp\,(a, b, c, \ell_1, \ell_2)$. *If* $d_1 < d_2$ *and* $\ell_1 < \ell_2$, $\ell_1 < \min\{d_1, d_2\}$, *then* $X_1 \geq_{lr} X_2$, $X_1 \geq_{hr} X_2$, $X_1 \geq_{mrl} X_2$, *and* $X_1 \leq_{st} X_2$.

Proof Taking the derivative of the natural logarithm of the ratio of two p.d.f.s of X_1 and X_2, where $X_1 \sim HTExp\,(a, b, c, d_1, d_2)$ and $X_2 \sim HTExp\,(a, b, c, \ell_1, \ell_2)$, we have

$$\frac{d}{dx}\log\frac{f_{X_1}(x)}{f_{X_2}(x)} = \left\{c\left[d_2\left(e^{(d_1+\ell_2)(b+cx)}-e^{(d_1+\ell_1)(b+cx)}\right) +d_1\left(e^{(d_2+\ell_1)(b+cx)}-e^{(d_2+\ell_2)(b+cx)}\right) +\left(e^{d_1(b+cx)}-e^{d_2(b+cx)}\right)\left(\ell_2 e^{\ell_1(b+cx)}-\ell_1 e^{\ell_2(b+cx)}\right)\right]\right\} \times\left[\left(e^{d_1(b+cx)}-e^{d_2(b+cx)}\right)\left(e^{\ell_1(b+cx)}-e^{\ell_2(b+cx)}\right)\right]^{-1}.$$

Observe that if $d_1 < d_2$ and $\ell_1 < \ell_2$, with $\ell_1 < \min\{d_1, d_2\}$, $\frac{d}{dx} \log \frac{f_{X_1}(x)}{f_{X_2}(x)} \geq 0$, which implies that $X_1 \geq_{lr} X_2$, $X_1 \geq_{hr} X_2$, $X_1 \geq_{mrl} X_2$, and $X_1 \leq_{st} X_2$. □

4.2.3 Shape of the Probability Density Function

For the hidden truncated model based on the Arnold and Strauss bivariate exponential distribution with p.d.f. presented in Eq. (15), we have the first derivative of the logarithm of p.d.f. as

$$\begin{aligned}
&\frac{\partial \log f(x|d_1 < Y \leq d_2)}{\partial x} \\
&\quad = (b+cx)^{-2} \\
&\quad\times\Big\{e^{-x(a+c(d_1+d_2))-b(d_1+d_2)}\Big[a(b+cx)\left(e^{d_1(b+cx)} - e^{d_2(b+cx)}\right) \\
&\quad -c(bd_1+cd_1x+1)e^{d_2(b+cx)} + ce^{d_1(b+cx)}(bd_2+cd_2x+1)\Big]\Big\}.
\end{aligned}$$

We can also obtain the second derivative of the logarithm of p.d.f. as

$$\begin{aligned}
&\frac{\partial^2 \log f(x|d_1 < Y \leq d_2)}{\partial x^2} \\
&= (b+cx)^{-3} \\
&\times\Big\{e^{-x(a+c(d_1+d_2))-b(d_1+d_2)}\Big[-a^2(b+cx)^2\left(e^{d_1(b+cx)} - e^{d_2(b+cx)}\right) \\
&-2ac(b+cx)\left[e^{d_1(b+cx)}(bd_2+cd_2x+1) - (bd_1+cd_1x+1)e^{d_2(b+cx)}\right] \\
&+c^2\Big[-\Big(e^{d_1(b+cx)}\left(b^2d_2^2+2bd_2(cd_2x+1)+c^2d_2^2x^2+2cd_2x+2\right) \\
&-\left(b^2d_1^2+2bd_1(cd_1x+1)+c^2d_1^2x^2+2cd_1x+2\right)e^{d_2(b+cx)}\Big)\Big]\Big\}. \qquad (20)
\end{aligned}$$

From Eq. (20), we can observe that for all choices of the parameters a, b, c, d_1, d_2, $\frac{\partial^2 \log f(x)}{\partial x^2} \leq 0$. This implies that the hidden truncated p.d.f. based on the Arnold and Strauss bivariate exponential distribution is log-concave and unimodal. □

4.2.4 Shape of the Hazard Function

For the hidden truncated model based on the Arnold and Strauss bivariate exponential distribution with p.d.f. presented in Eq. (15), we show that the associated hazard function is increasing in the following theorem.

Theorem 3 *The hazard rate function is increasing for any $\mu \in \mathscr{R}$, $\delta \in \mathscr{R}^+$.*

Proof For the hidden truncated model based on the Arnold and Strauss bivariate exponential distribution, we have

$$\eta(x) = -\Big\{ - a(b+cx)\left(e^{d_1(b+cx)} - e^{d_2(b+cx)}\right) + c\,(bd_1 + cd_1x + 1)\,e^{d_2(b+cx)} \\ -ce^{d_1(b+cx)}\,(bd_2 + cd_2x + 1)\Big\} \\ \times\Big\{(b+cx)\left(e^{d_1(b+cx)} - e^{d_2(b+cx)}\right)\Big\}^{-1}.$$

Then, we have

$$\frac{\partial\eta(x)}{\partial x} = \frac{c^2}{(b+cx)^2\,(\exp[d_1(b+cx)] - \exp[d_2(b+cx)])^2} \\ \times\Big\{\exp[(d_1+d_2)(b+cx)] \\ \times\left[b^2(d_1-d_2)^2 + 2bcx(d_1-d_2)^2 + c^2x^2(d_1-d_2)^2 + 2\right] \\ - \exp[2d_1(b+cx)] - \exp[2d_2(b+cx)]\Big\}. \tag{21}$$

Note that from Eq. (21), we can show that $\frac{\partial\eta(x)}{\partial x} > 0$, for any $\mu \in \mathscr{R}, \delta \in \mathscr{R}^+$, and therefore, from Glaser (1980), the hazard function is increasing. □

4.3 *Structural Properties for Hidden Truncated Pareto Mixture Model*

In this subsection, we discuss the structural properties of the hidden truncated model based on the Pareto(type II) and Pareto(type IV) models presented in Sect. 3.4.

4.3.1 Moments

For the hidden truncated model based on the Pareto(type II) and Pareto(type IV) models with p.d.f. presented in Eq. (17), the moments of order $r(r \geq 1)$ can be obtained as

$$
\begin{aligned}
&E\left(U_1^r | U_2 < \lambda_0 + \lambda_1 U_1\right)\\
&= \sum_{j_1=0}^{\infty}\sum_{j_2=0}^{\infty}(-1)^{j_1}\binom{-\alpha}{j_1}\binom{j_1}{j_2}C_1^{-1}\\
&\times\left\{\left[\delta\lambda_1\Gamma(\alpha+1)\Gamma\left(-\frac{j_2}{\gamma}\right)\right]^{-1}\right\}\alpha\left(\frac{\lambda_1}{\lambda_0}\right)^{-r}\\
&\times\left(\frac{\lambda_0}{\delta}\right)^{j_2/\gamma}\left\{\delta\lambda_1\Gamma\left(-\frac{j_2}{\gamma}\right)\Gamma\left(\frac{j_2}{\gamma}+r+1\right)\Gamma\left(-\frac{j_2}{\gamma}-r+\alpha\right)\left(\frac{\delta\lambda_1}{\lambda_0}\right)^{\frac{j_2}{\gamma}+r}\right.\\
&\times{}_2F_1\left(-\frac{j_2}{\gamma}-r+\alpha,-\frac{j_2}{\gamma};-\frac{j_2+r\gamma}{\gamma};\frac{\lambda_0}{\delta\lambda_1}\right)\\
&+\lambda_0\Gamma(\alpha+1)\Gamma(r+1)\Gamma\left(-\frac{j_2+r\gamma+\gamma}{\gamma}\right){}_2F_1\\
&\left.\times\left(r+1,\alpha+1;\frac{j_2}{\gamma}+r+2;\frac{\lambda_0}{\delta\lambda_1}\right)\right\}.
\end{aligned}
$$

Note If j_1 is an integer, the second sum will be up to j_1.

4.3.2 Shape of the Probability Density Function

For the hidden truncated model based on the Pareto(type II) and Pareto(type IV) models with p.d.f. presented in Eq. (17), we have the first derivative of the logarithm of p.d.f. as

$$
\frac{\partial \log f(u|U_2<\lambda_0+\lambda_1 U_1)}{\partial u} = C_1^{-1}\left\{\frac{\alpha\lambda_1\left(\frac{\lambda_0+\lambda_1 u}{\delta}\right)^{\frac{1}{\gamma}-1}}{\gamma\delta\left[\left(\frac{\lambda_0+\lambda_1 u}{\delta}\right)^{\frac{1}{\gamma}}+1\right]\left[\left[\left(\frac{\lambda_0+\lambda_1 u}{\delta}\right)^{\frac{1}{\gamma}}+1\right]^{\alpha}-1\right]}-\frac{\alpha+1}{\delta+u}\right\}.
$$

From this first derivative of p.d.f., it can be shown that the p.d.f. is log-concave. The proof is available from the authors upon request.

4.3.3 Shape of the Hazard Function

For the hidden truncated model based on the Pareto(type II) and Pareto(type IV) models with p.d.f. presented in Eq. (17), the associated hazard function is decreasing if $\delta > \max\{\lambda_0, \lambda_1\}$ and $1 \leq \gamma \leq \delta$. The proof is available from the authors upon request.

5 Inferential Issues and Conjectures

5.1 *Inferential Issues*

In this subsection, we discuss the relative merits and/or demerits of the classical and Bayesian inferential aspects related to the hidden truncated models for non-normal densities exist in the literature. A full scale simulation study along with some useful applications of the hidden truncation models developed in Sect. 3 will be the subject matter of a separate report. Except for the hidden truncation model based on the Arnold and Strauss bivariate exponential distribution presented in Sect. 3.3, the hidden truncation models discussed in this article do not constitute exponential family of densities. As a consequence, essentially no reduction in the complexity of the model can be obtained by introducing the sufficiency arguments. In general, the method of maximum likelihood can be used for parameter estimation; however, the likelihood functions associated with these models often do not have easily identified modes. For hidden truncated Pareto models, there has been a reasonable amount of successes when it comes to classical parameter estimation. For instance, Arnold and Ghosh (2011) studied the hidden truncated bivariate Pareto(type II) model and discussed the parameter estimation via the method of maximum likelihood, fractional method of moments, and the quartile estimation method with appreciable amount of errors in the maximum likelihood method for small sample sizes. Arnold and Ghosh (2011) provided a foundation to the theory and applications of hidden truncated Pareto-type models. Consequently, several research papers in the literature focused on particular members of the Pareto family of distributions and addressed the issue of statistical inference primarily under the classical setup. Ghosh and Nadarajah (2015) and Ghosh and Balakrishnan (2017) studied the hidden truncation models (both-sided truncation) starting from a bivariate Pareto(type II) and a bivariate Pareto(type IV) distribution, respectively. In the Bayesian paradigm, Ghosh (2014) discussed the Bayesian estimation for a hidden truncated Pareto(type II) model. Recently, Ghosh (2020) discussed the Bayesian estimation for a hidden truncated Pareto(type IV) model. In Arnold and Ghosh (2013), hidden truncation in a multivariate Pareto setting is discussed. For a comprehensive review on skewed and/or hidden truncation models, one may refer to Arnold (2015) and the references therein.

Besides the Pareto-type hidden truncated models, there is not much work done for the other non-normal models, especially for the models with a ubiquitous normalizing constant. In case that the normalizing constant involves some special functions/series (e.g., the Gauss hypergeometric function), certain software packages such as *Mathematica* can handle this issue as these software packages have built-in functions to compute these special functions that are readily available. However, there are cases that the normalizing constant cannot be written in a closed form. In such scenarios, one can consider the Bayesian paradigm in which the likelihood is updated with judicious prior choices of the model parameters, and the posterior distribution can be approximated without knowing the normalizing constant. On the other hand, frequentist approach with profile likelihood method or expectation maximization (EM) algorithm can be used. The usual strategy (specially for multi-parameter models) is to pick initial values using the method of moments estimates and then use in a variation of the Newton–Raphson approach to finding the maximum of the surface.

5.2 Conjectures

In this subsection, we postulate some conjectures related to hidden truncation. General proofs are left to readers as open research problems.

Conjecture 1 Let X be a random variable defined over $\mathscr{R}$ or in any subset of $\mathscr{R}$ with a finite mean (μ) and variance (σ^2). Let X_T denote the truncated version of the original random variable X. Then, regardless of the hidden truncation mechanism (i.e., HD(type I) or HD(type II)), and the type of truncation (left, right, or both-sided), the variance of X_T, say, σ_T^2 will be smaller than or equal to σ^2. □

As an illustration, we sketch the approach to access the result described in Conjecture 1 for the hidden truncated model constructed based on the Arnold and Strauss bivariate exponential distribution discussed in Sect. 3.3. Let X be a random variable with marginal density in Eq. (14) based on the Arnold and Strauss bivariate exponential distribution and $X_T \sim HTPExp(a, b, c, d_1, d_2)$, and let $Var(X)$ and $Var(X_T)$ be the variances of X and X_T, respectively. To show that $Var(X_T) \leq Var(X)$, we obtain

$$
\begin{aligned}
Var(X) = c^{-4} \Bigg\{ c \Bigg[a^2 \log(b) \left(-e^{\frac{ab}{c}}\right) + a^2 e^{\frac{ab}{c}} \log\left(\frac{c}{a}\right) \\
+ a^2 e^{\frac{ab}{c}} \left(\log\left(\frac{ab}{c}\right) + \Gamma\left(\frac{ab}{c}\right) \right) - \frac{ac}{b} + \frac{c^2}{b^2} \Bigg] \\
- \frac{\left[c - abe^{\frac{ab}{c}} \left(\log\left(\frac{ab}{c}\right) + \Gamma\left(\frac{ab}{c}\right) + \log\left(\frac{c}{a}\right) - \log(b) \right) \right]^2}{b^2} \Bigg\},
\end{aligned}
$$

and

$$Var(X_T) = \left\{2M_1^{-1}c^{-2}\exp\left(\frac{2ab}{c}\right)\right.$$
$$\left.\times\left[\Gamma\left(-2, \frac{b(a+cd_1)}{c}\right) - \Gamma\left(-2, \frac{b(a+cd_2)}{c}\right)\right]\right\}$$
$$-\left\{\exp\left(\frac{2ab}{c}\right)M_1^{-1}\left[\Gamma\left(-1, \frac{b(a+cd_1)}{c}\right) - \Gamma\left(-1, \frac{b(a+cd_2)}{c}\right)\right]\right\}^2.$$

With some tedious algebraic simplification, it can be shown that $Var(X) - Var(X_T) \geq 0$. □

Conjecture 2 If the original density for random variable X is log-concave, then the hidden truncated p.d.f. of X_T is also log-concave and hence unimodal.

Conjecture 3 If the hazard function for random variable X is increasing, decreasing, and/or bathtub shape, then the hazard function of the corresponding hidden truncated random variable X_T exhibits similar behavior.

Conjecture 4 The hidden truncated version from any density retains the properties corresponding to several variants of stochastic ordering that holds for the non-truncated version.

6 Concluding Remarks

In this paper, we have explored two different types of hidden truncation mechanism. Noticeably, the hidden truncation models resulting from the two different approaches, HD(Type I) and HD(Type II), will lead to different distributions if we begin with non-normal components. Data sets involving hidden truncation, or in the case of model-misspecification leading to a hidden truncation, require a careful investigation as well as its appropriate applications to real life scenarios. With our naked eye, at times, we may not be able to differentiate/identify whether or not we are actually using a truncated version of an underlying probability model. For example, any statistical analysis involving linear normal models (e.g., analysis of variance, regression, principal components, etc.) can be considered to be potentially a setting in which hidden truncation might have occurred and some effort to investigate the possibility can be clearly justified. Mitra and Das (1989) used the truncated Cauchy distribution in the field of crystallographic statistics. Mitra and Das (1989) stated that "the Cauchy or Lorentzian distribution, having no finite moment apart from above and the first is looked upon with suspicion. But one never works with a distribution function ranging between $\pm\infty$; the function is cut off on the surface of the sphere of reflection." Thus, we are actually dealing with a truncated Cauchy distribution function for which second and higher moments exist. The findings in this article have the potential to impact a wide range of other engineering and science applications such as those found in statistical tolerance analysis, more specifically, tolerance stack analysis methods. We also hope that the results investigated/studied here will ignite much deserved motivation and attention to develop the associated theoretical and methodological works (including but not limited to a thorough comparative study among several different methods of skewing paradigm, such as hidden truncation, additive components, and Jones method of skewing non-normal densities in two and higher dimensions) before it can be applied to real world data involving some forms of hidden truncation.

References

Ali, M. M., & Nadarajah, S. (2007). A truncated bivariate generalized Pareto distribution. *Computer Communications, 30*(8), 1926–1930.

Arnold, B. C. (1987). Bivariate distributions with Pareto conditionals. *Statistics and Probability Letters, 5*, 263–266.

Arnold, B. C. (2009). Flexible univariate and multivariate models based on hidden truncation. *Journal of Statistical Planning and Inference, 139*(11), 3741–3749.

Arnold, B. C. (2015). *Pareto Distributions* (2nd edn.). New York: CRC Press.

Arnold, B. C., Beaver, R.J. (2000). Hidden truncation models. *Sankhyā: The Indian Journal of Statistics, Series A, 62*, 23–35.

Arnold, B. C., & Beaver, R. J. (2002). Skewed multivariate models related to hidden truncation and/or selective reporting (with discussion). *Test, 11*, 7–54.

Arnold, B. C., & Ghosh, I. (2011). Inference for Pareto data subject to hidden truncation. *Journal of the Indian Society for Probability and Statistics, 13*, 1–16.

Arnold, B. C., & Ghosh, I. (2013). Hidden truncation in multivariate Pareto data. In A. Adhikai, M. R. Adhikari & Y. P. Chaubey (Eds.), *Contemporary Topics in Mathematics and Statistics with Applications*, vol. I. New Delhi: Asian Books Pvt. Ltd., 211–226.

Arnold, B. C., & Gomez, H. (2008). Hidden truncation and additive components: Two alternative skewing paradigms. *Calcutta Statistical Association Bulletin, 60* (March & June 2008), 239–240.

Arnold, B. C., & Strauss, D. (1988). Bivariate distributions with exponential conditionals. *Journal of the American Statistical Association, 83*(402), 522–527.

Arnold, B. C., Castillo, E., and Sarabia, J.M. (1999). Conditional Specification of Statistical Models. Springer, New York.

Balakrishnan, N., & Lai, C. D. (2009). *Continuous bivariate distributions* (2nd ed.) New York: Springer.

Bhattacharya, N. (1963). A property of the Pareto distribution. *Sankhyā: The Indian Journal of Statistics, Series B, 25*, 195–196.

Castillo, E., & Sarabia, J.M. (1990). Bivariate distributions with second kind beta conditionals. *Communications in Statistics, Theory and Methods, 19*, 3433–3445.

Castillo, E., Galambos, J., & Sarabia, J.M. (1990). Caracterizacin de modelos bivariantes con distribuciones condicionadas tipo gamma (in Spanish). *Estadistica Espaola, 31*, 439–450.

Chapman, D.G. (1956). Estimating the parameters of a truncated gamma distribution. *The Annals of Mathematical Statistics*, 498–506.

Cosentino, P., Ficarra, V., & Luzio, D. (1977). Truncated exponential frequency-magnitude relationship in earthquake statistics. *Bulletin of the Seismological Society of America, 67*(6), 1615–1623.

David, F. N., & Johnson, N. L. (1952). The truncated Poisson. *Biometrics, 8*(4), 275–285.

Finney, D. J. (1947). The truncated binomial distribution. *Annals of Eugenics, 14*(1), 319–328.
Galton, F. (1898). An examination into the registered speeds of American trotting horses, with remarks on their value as hereditary data. *Proceedings of the Royal Society of London, 62*(379–387), 310–315.
Ghosh, I. (2014). Bayesian inference for hidden truncation Pareto (II) models. *Journal of Applied Statistical Science, 3*. https://doi.org/10.4172/2155-6180.S1.021.
Ghosh, I. (2020). Bayesian inference for hidden truncation Pareto (IV) models. *Journal of Statistical Computation and Simulation, 90*, 2136–2155.
Ghosh, I., & Balakrishnan, N. (2017). On the hidden truncated bivariate Pareto (IV) model and associated inferential issues. *Journal of Statistical Computation and Simulation, 87*, 1467–1487.
Ghosh, I., & Banks, O. (2020). A study of bivariate generalized Pareto distribution and its dependence structure among model parameters. *Sankhyā: The Indian Journal of Statistics, Series B*, 1–30.
Ghosh, I., & Nadarajah, S. (2015). Inference for a hidden truncated (both-sided) bivariate Pareto (II) distribution. *Communications in Statistics–Theory and Methods, 44*, 2136–2150.
Glaser, R. E. (1980). Bathtub and related failure rate characterizations. *Journal of the American Statistical Association, 75*(371), 667–672.
Jamalizadeh, A., Pourmousa, R., & Balakrishnan, N. (2009). Truncated and limited skew-normal and skew distributions: properties and an illustration. *Communications in Statistics–Theory and Methods, 38*(16–17), 2653–2668.
Johnson, N. L., Kotz, S., & Balakrishnan, N. (1995). Continuous Univariate Distributions. Wiley: New York.
Kotz, S., Balakrishnan, N., & Johnson, N. L. (2000). Continuous multivariate distributions. In *Models and Applications*, vol. 1 (2nd ed.). Wiley: New York.
Kumbhakar, S. C., & Knox Lovell, C. A. (2000). *Stochastic frontier analysis*. Cambridge University: Cambridge.
Mitra, G. B., & Das, S. (1989). Cauchy distribution, intensity statistics and phases of reflections from crystal planes. *Acta Crystallographica, A 45*, 314–319.
Mittal, M. M., & Dahiya, R. C. (1989). Estimating the parameters of a truncated Weibull distribution. *Communications in Statistics–Theory and Methods, 18*(6), 2027–2042.
Moore, P. G. (1954). A note on truncated Poisson distributions. *Biometrics, 10*(3), 402–406.
Nadarajah, S., & Kotz, S. (2006): A truncated Cauchy distribution. *International Journal of Mathematical Education in Science and Technology, 37*(5), 605–608.
Nadarajah, S., & Kotz, S. (2007). A truncated bivariate Cauchy distribution. *Bulletin of the Malaysian Mathematical Sciences Society, 30*(2), 185–193.
Nadarajah, S., & Kotz, S. (2008). Moments of truncated t and F distributions. *Portuguese Economic Journal, 7*(1), 63–73.
Pearson, K., & Lee, A. (1908). On the generalised probable error in multiple normal correlation. *Biometrika, 6*(1), 59–68.
Sampford, M. R. (1955). The truncated negative binomial distribution. *Biometrika, 42*(1/2), 58–69.
Shaked, M., & Shanthikumar, J. G. (1995). Hazard rate ordering of k-out-of-n systems. *Statistics and Probability Letters, 23*, 1–8.
Zaninetti, L. (2013). The initial mass function modeled by a left truncated beta distribution. *The Astrophysical Journal, 765*(2), 128.

Part III
Multivariate Distribution Theory

Our Joint Work with Barry Arnold: Conditional Specification and Other Topics

Enrique Castillo and José María Sarabia

Abstract We review some of the joint contributions made with Barry C. Arnold to the Probability and Statistics field during more than 30 years. First, we concentrate on those related to conditional specification, characterization of distributions and Bayesian methodologies with priors based on conditional specification. Also, we review other topics studied jointly with Barry C. Arnold such as multivariate distributions defined in terms of contours, new classes of multivariate distributions based on the Rosenblatt construction and multivariate order statistics and other applications.

1 Introduction

Professor Barry Charles Arnold has made relevant contributions to many different areas of probability and statistics including distribution theory, multivariate analysis, majorization and stochastic ordering, order statistics and record values, classical and Bayesian inference, bounds and orderings, and characterization problems.

When Barry turned 65, we had the opportunity to organize (jointly with Professor N. Balakrishnan) an International Conference on Distribution Theory, Order Statistics, and Inference in his honor in Santander, Spain in June 2004. That conference was a success and some selected papers that were presented at that conference were included in a volume (*Advances in Distribution Theory, Order Statistics, and Inference*, N. Balakrishnan, E. Castillo, J.M. Sarabia Editors, Birkhäuser, Boston, 2006), see Balakrishnan et al. (2006).

E. Castillo
University of Cantabria, Santander, Spain
e-mail: castie@unican.es

J. M. Sarabia (✉)
Department of Economics, University of Cantabria, Santander, Spain
e-mail: sarabiaj@unican.es

I. Ghosh et al. (eds.), *Advances in Statistics - Theory and Applications*, Emerging Topics in Statistics and Biostatistics, https://doi.org/10.1007/978-3-030-62900-7_8

At this time we celebrate Barry's 80th birthday, and our participation consists of this article, as a tribute to his academic and research career, and to all the works we made together with him.

The contents of this chapter are the following. In this first section we continue by describing the first contacts with Professor Barry C. Arnold, in the early eighties of the last century. In Sect. 2, we present our contributions to conditional specification, with reference to some new advances in the topic. In Sect. 3 we discuss other research topics made jointly with Barry. Finally, some conclusions are included in Sect. 4.

1.1 First Contacts with Barry Arnold

The first time Enrique Castillo met Barry Arnold was at the Institute of Advanced Studies of NATO on Statistical Extremes and Applications dedicated to the Memory of E. J. Gumbel, held in Vimeiro, Portugal in 1983. The meeting took 2 weeks and was organized by J. Tiago de Oliveira and it was probably one of the most important meetings on this important topic. In fact, well-known scientists shared their knowledge and contributed to the development of this crucial field, not only in probability and statistics but also in physics and engineering.

Enrique also met Janos Galambos for the first time there, and informed Janos about his desire of a sabbatical year at Temple University to write a book on Extremes and Engineering Applications. This stay started after the Summer in 1985. During this stay, Janos and Enrique wrote some common papers. The first one was born after a Janos invitation to Enrique to participate at a Conference on Weighted distributions at Pen State University. One Friday morning, Janos offered Enrique this opportunity and mentioned that we could travel together by car from Philadelphia. On Monday morning, we discussed a draft of our first joint paper and developed our paper with title "Bivariate distributions with normal conditionals" in which the most general bivariate model with normal conditionals was obtained. It is important to indicate that functional equations played a very important role in that paper and in almost all of the sequence of papers that followed. So, we cannot avoid to mention the books of Janos Aczél, but specially Aczél (1966), who motivated the books Castillo and Ruíz-Cobo (1992) and Castillo et al. (2005).

The paper was presented at the meeting. By chance, Barry Arnold was there and liked the idea. Very soon Barry wrote to Janos, asking for permission to publish a paper with exponential conditionals, based on the methodology proposed by us. I have to point out that Barry did not need our permission, but he was extremely polite and kind to follow this process. In fact, we were really honored by this letter because of the implied recognition to our work. He published the paper in 1988 with David Strauss in *Journal of the American Statistical Association* (see Arnold and Strauss 1988) and in 1991, another paper about bivariate distributions with conditionals in prescribed exponential families (see Arnold and Strauss 1991). In 1989, he

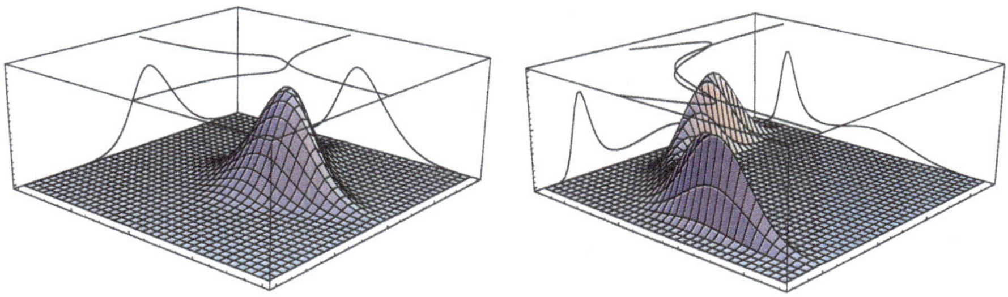

Fig. 1 Bivariate densities with normal conditionals and non-linear regressions with one mode (left) and two modes (right)

published one important paper about compatibility in conditional distribution with Jim Press (see Arnold and Press 1989).

1.2 Parallel Works on Conditional Specification

In the meantime, Enrique and Janos published the normal conditionals paper (see Castillo and Galambos 1989). Two examples of these families are shown in Fig. 1, where the left hand side shows a normal conditionals model with non-linear regressions and the right hand side model is a normal conditionals model with two modes. In Arnold et al. (2000) a normal conditionals model with three modes was presented.

Later, we published one paper in which some conditional considerations allowed to solve a functional equation that generated a fatigue model for the S-N curves, Castillo and Galambos (1987). The idea is as follows. Suppose that several specimens are tested at different stress ranges, $\Delta\sigma^*$, and that their fatigue lives are determined N^*, that is, their S-N curves, shown in red in Fig. 2. If we consider a generic point $(\Delta\sigma^*, N^*)$, and the vertical and horizontal segments of the figure, it is obvious that any S-N curve crossing the horizontal segment, necessarily has to cross the vertical segment, which implies that the shaded areas of the densities of N^* conditioned by $\Delta\sigma^*$ and $\Delta\sigma^*$ conditional by N^*, have to be identical. But those areas correspond to the corresponding conditional distribution functions, so it must be:

$$p = h^*(N^*|\Delta\sigma^*) = g^*(\Delta\sigma^*|N),$$

where h^* and g^* are the conditional distributions. This is a compatibility condition.

If we assume now that the functions h^* and g^* belong to the same family of distributions and that, this is a location and scale family of distributions, which is a very weak hypothesis, since they have to be stable with respect to changes of scale

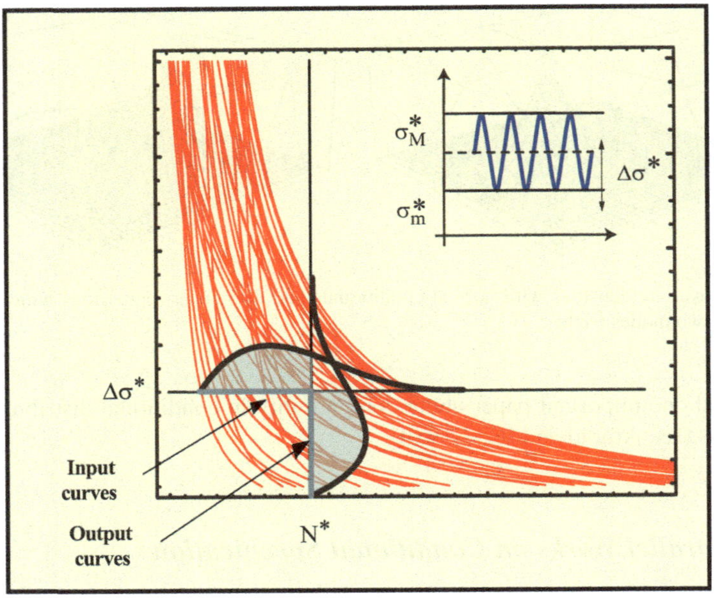

Fig. 2 Compatibility condition of two conditionals leading to the S-N fatigue model

(of units) and of origin, the compatibility condition can be written in the form:

$$\frac{N^* - \mu_1^*(\Delta\sigma^*)}{\sigma_1^*(\Delta\sigma^*)} = \frac{\Delta\sigma^* - \mu_2^*(N^*)}{\sigma_2^*(N^*)}, \tag{1}$$

which is a functional equation with four unknown functions, whose solution, as shown in Castillo and Galambos (1987), leads to the following models:

$$\text{Model 1}: \; p = h^* \left(\frac{(N^* - B^*)(\Delta\sigma^* - C^*) - \lambda^*}{\delta} \right), \tag{2}$$

$$\text{Model 2}: \; p = h^* \left(A^* N^* + B^* \Delta\sigma^* + C^* \right), \tag{3}$$

where λ^* and δ^* are location and scale parameters, respectively, and A^*, B^*, and C^* are other parameters, and this is independent on the selected function h^*.

Later, they also studied the conditional families specified by Weibull conditionals in Castillo and Galambos (1990), and later by gamma conditionals in Castillo et al. (1990), this work joint with José María Sarabia.

2 Contributions to Conditional Specification

In this section we present our main contributions with Barry in the field of conditional specification of statistical models.

2.1 *The Lecture Notes in Statistics Monograph*

A short period of time working in similar papers having the conditional specification as the main topic motivated an invitation from Enrique and José María to Barry in order to work on a joint book. The invitation was immediately accepted by Barry and the book project started. After several stays of Barry at the University of Cantabria in Santander, we produced a Monograph that was presented to Springer for its publication in the Lecture Notes Series on Probability and Statistics and published as Monograph N. 73, in 1992 (see Arnold et al. 1992).

Some common works on conditional specification of families of distributions include: (a) second kind beta conditionals in Castillo and Sarabia (1990) and classical beta conditionals and its generalizations in Arnold et al. (2004b), (b) the generalized Pareto conditionals model, in Arnold et al. (1993b), (c) distributions with conditionals in truncated weighted families, in Arnold et al. (2005), (d) the conditional characterization of the Mardia multivariate Pareto in Arnold et al. (1994b), (e) the conditionally specified multivariate skewed distributions, in Arnold et al. (2002a), and (f) conditionally specified multivariate generalized skewed distributions in Arnold et al. (2007a).

In a few years, the edition was sold out and, then, we decided to write a second book on the conditional specification of distributions, to include the new advances produced from and after the previous monograph. After some hard work, we produced a new book, that was published by Springer in 1999, in its prestigious Springer Series in Statistics (Arnold et al. 1999).

Immediately after publication of this book, we published an invited paper (Arnold et al. 2001b) in the journal *Statistical Science* with a summary of the material included in the book and some new results and applications.

2.2 *Some Work on Characterizations of the Normal Family*

First of all we want to emphasize the importance of characterizing families of distributions. If we characterize a family of distributions in different ways, we have alternative definitions of these families. This implied a better and deeper knowledge of these classes of distributions. It also means that we were able to derive conclusions about these families from different points of view or starting points. Logically, some definitions will make easier to derive certain conclusions, and other definitions will do the same for other conclusions. Thus, having at hand different characterizations allow us to analyze and solve more problems and in different ways, because we can start proofs from different alternative definitions

The next theorem provides a relevant characterization of the bivariate normal distribution (see Castillo and Galambos 1989).

Theorem 1 (Characterization of the Bivariate Normal Distribution) *The density $f(x, y)$ is a classical bivariate normal density if and only if all conditional distributions, both of X given Y and of Y given X, are normal and any one of the following properties holds:*

- $\sigma_2^2(x) = Var(Y|X = x)$ *or* $\sigma_1^2(y) = Var(X|Y = y)$ *is constant.*
- $\lim_{y\to\infty} y^2\sigma_1^2(y) = \infty$ *or* $\lim_{x\to\infty} x^2\sigma_1^2(x) = \infty$.
- $\lim_{y\to\infty}\sigma_1(y) \neq 0$ *or* $\lim_{\to\infty} \sigma_2(x) \neq 0$.
- $E(Y|X = x)$ *or* $E(X|Y = y)$ *is linear and non-constant.*

These results for the bidimensional case were extended to the conditional characterization of the multivariate normal family in terms of classical conditional distributions of (X_i, X_j) given $\underline{X}_{(i,j)}$, where $\underline{X} = (X_1, X_2, \ldots, X_n)$ and $\underline{X}_{(i,j)}$ refers to $\underline{X}$ with X_i and X_j deleted, which appear in Arnold et al. (1994a).

Later, these results were extended to the case of classical conditional distributions of $X_i|\underline{X}_{(i)} = \underline{x}_{(i)}$ and $X_i|\underline{X}_{(i,j)} = \underline{x}_{(i,j)}$ (see Arnold et al. 1994c).

Finally, an extension to $(k - 1)$-dimensional marginal densities was provided in Arnold et al. (2007b).

2.3 *Compatibility and Near Compatibility*

In Arnold et al. (2001c), the authors move further from the problem of conditional specification of distributions dealing with the problem of determining whether or not a given set of constraints, including marginal and conditional probabilities and expectations of given functions are compatible. They deal with the finite discrete case and convert it into a problem of linear equations in restricted domains. When compatibility was not possible, they introduced the concept of near compatibility and ϵ-compatibility of conditional distributions. A general solution was provided in Arnold et al. (2002b).

In Arnold et al. (2004a), the authors dealt with the problem of whether or not a set of conditional probabilities are compatible, and obtaining all the possible solutions. The authors propose the "rank one extension" technique as the most convenient for identifying all possible compatible distributions associated with complete and partial conditional specifications including the case with zero probabilities. The case of a sequential assessment of compatible conditional probabilities and the possible extensions to higher dimensions are also discussed. The proposed methods are illustrated with several examples. The rank-based compatibility method allows us to conclude whether or not two conditional probability arrays are compatible and, if the answer is positive, to obtain the set of all compatible joint distributions. The method works for all cases, even if the conditional probability matrices are not strictly positive. The method is valid for cases including the partial specification and can be used to help human experts to make the assessments sequentially by giving adequate compatibility intervals for each desired parameter being assessed.

2.4 Conditionally Specified Bivariate Gumbel Models

Assume that for every y, the conditional distribution of X given $Y = y$ is Gumbel $(\mu_1(y), \sigma_1(y))$ and that for every x, the conditional distribution of Y given $X = x$ is Gumbel $(\mu_2(x), \sigma_2(x))$. The family of densities satisfying this condition is the family of distributions with conditional Gumbel densities that was identified in Arnold et al. (1998b).

It is interesting to point out that the classical bivariate Gumbel models are limited in the sense that they include only non-negative correlation, while the conditional models exhibit non-positive correlation. Three examples are given in Fig. 3, where the positive and negative correlations become apparent.

2.5 Bivariate Distributions Characterized by One Family of Conditionals and Conditional Percentile or Mode Functions

As illustrated above, the knowledge of all conditional distributions will typically serve to completely characterize a bivariate distribution if they are compatible. In addition, a partial knowledge can also be sufficient, as it is the case of the conditional distribution of X given Y and the conditional mean of Y given X.

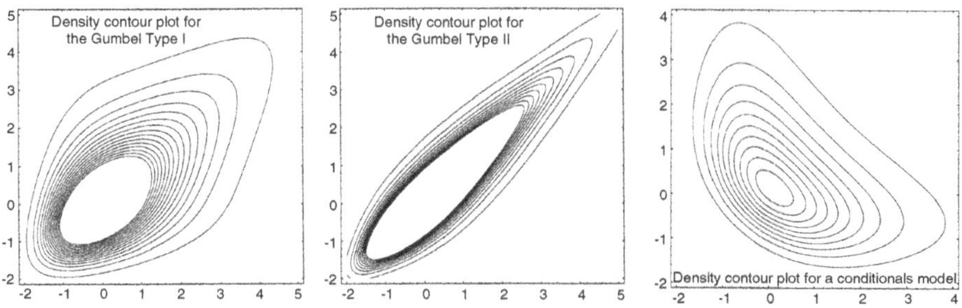

Fig. 3 Contour plots corresponding to classical bivariate Gumbel models (left and center) and bivariate densities with conditional Gumbel distributions (right)

Thus, it is natural to ask whether or not a conditional percentile or mode function (of Y given X) together with knowledge of the conditional distribution of X given Y characterize the joint distribution.

In Arnold et al. (2008a), the authors investigate the required conditions for the characterization problem in the following two cases: (a) given $\Pr(X \leq x|Y \leq y)$ and a conditional percentile function of Y given $\{X \leq x\}$, and (b) given $f_{X|Y}(x|y)$ and the conditional mode function of Y given $\{X = x\}$. As a corollary, they obtain the following normal characterization theorem,

Theorem 2 *The classical bivariate normal distribution is characterized as the unique absolutely continuous bivariate distribution with normal conditionals of X given Y with linear regression and a constant conditional variance function together with a linear conditional mode function of Y given X.*

2.6 Distributions with Generalized Skewed Conditionals and Mixtures of Such Distributions

The class of skew-normal distributions introduced by Azzalini has received a lot of attention in the recent statistical literature. The paper Arnold et al. (2002a) identifies first the classes of bivariate distributions with skewed normal, linearly skewed normal, rotation and quadratic skewed normal conditionals, and also some multivariate extensions. In the bivariate case, this class of distributions (without including location and scale parameters) is given by

$$f_{X,Y}(x, y; \lambda) = 2\phi(x)\phi(y)\Phi(\lambda xy), \quad (x, y) \in \mathbb{R}^2, \tag{4}$$

and $\lambda \in \mathbb{R}$. One of the relevant property of (4) is its bimodality. If $|\lambda| > \sqrt{\pi/2}$, the density (4) presents two modes. This property is also presented in more general multivariate skew-normal distributions. They also deal with non-normal variants and polynomially skewed normal models.

A probability density function (pdf) is said to have a generalized skewed distribution if

$$f(x) = 2f_0(x)G\{w(x)\}; \quad -\infty < x < \infty, \tag{5}$$

where f_0 is a one-dimensional probability density function, symmetric about 0, and G is a one-dimensional distribution function such that G' exists and is symmetric about 0. The paper Arnold et al. (2007a) considers the choice $w(x) = w(x; \theta)$, where θ is a vector of parameters, obtaining new classes of multivariate distributions with conditionals of the type (5), when $w(x; \theta)$ are scale functions or high-order odd polynomials. Some examples of these densities are shown in Fig. 4. A class of skewed distributions with applications in environmental data has been provided by Ghosh and Ng (2019).

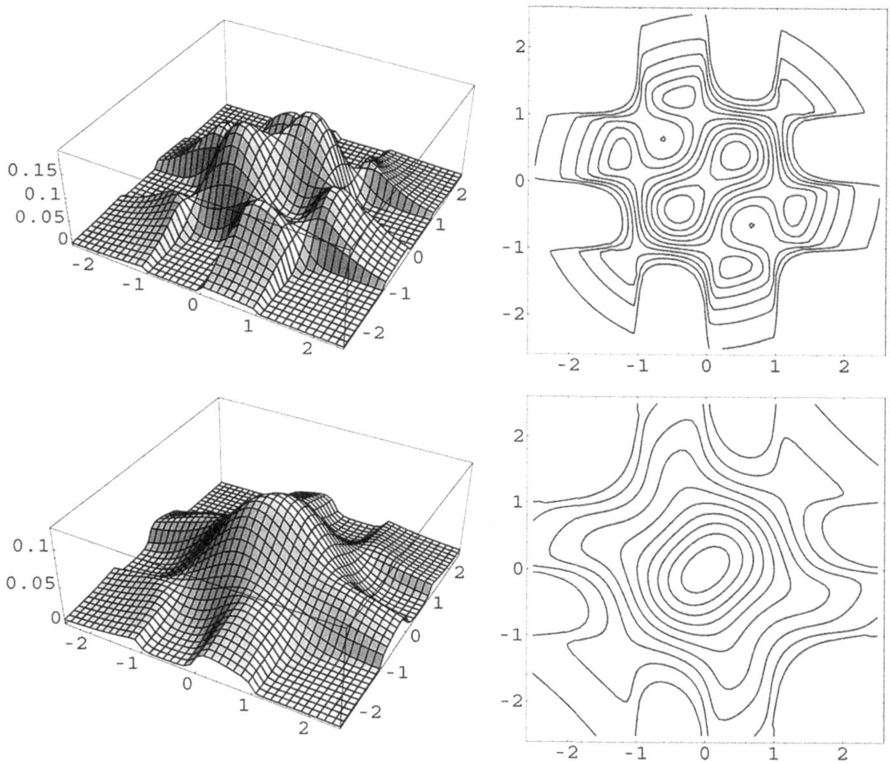

Fig. 4 Some examples of densities with generalized skew conditionals with $w(x;\theta)$ a scale function

2.7 Some Bayesian Applications

We have collaborated in some Bayesian models in which we had explored the power of functional equations to obtain the most general models with priors and likelihoods in exponential families, in Arnold et al. (1993a), and later the most general models with priors and posteriors, not necessarily in the same but, in well-known posterior families, in Arnold et al. (1996b).

More specifically, this methodology has been used for the Bayesian estimation of the parameters of classical distributions, including normal and classical Pareto distributions and simple linear regression (see Arnold et al. 1993a, Arnold et al. 1998a and Sarabia et al. 2005) and in the Bayesian estimation of ratios of gamma scale parameters (see Arnold et al. 1998c and Moschopoulos and Sha 2005). In Sarabia et al. (2008) we have proposed the use of this methodology for the Bayesian analysis of hurdle count data models and the estimation with incomplete count data. A more recent application of these methodologies can be found in Sarabia and Shahtahmassebi (2017).

2.8 Other Topics in Conditional Specification

In this section we discuss briefly other research topics related to conditional specification were studied.

Motivated by our research in conditional specification and by the paper by Gelman and Speed (see Gelman and Speed 1993), we studied the problem of specification of distributions by combinations of marginal and conditional distributions. A k-dimensional probability density function can be determined by certain combinations of marginal and conditional densities. The paper Arnold et al. (1996c) identifies all possible such specifications. As well, appropriate compatibility conditions are described as sufficient conditions for uniqueness of the resulting density which must, in general, be checked for integrability.

A particular and very interesting case of conditional specification is the case of Bayesian networks, which are defined by an acyclic graph of the set of nodes (variables) and a set of conditional distributions of each variable given its parents. The interesting thing is that the graph defines the dependence structure of the multivariate model, and the set of conditional distributions quantifies it. More important this definition is always compatible provided that the conditional distributions are well defined and that the graph is acyclic. The reader can see all these properties in Castillo et al. (1997), together with some interesting applications.

A multivariate version of Stein's identity with applications to moment calculations and estimation of conditionally specified distributions is included in Arnold et al. (2001a). The resulting identity is useful for generating recurrence formulae for mixed moments and for deriving consistent moment based estimates of parameters. The technique is illustrated in a spectrum of one-dimensional multiparameter cases and in a variety of bivariate conditionally specified distribution settings, including non-exponential families of distributions.

The modeling of the fatigue life of longitudinal elements is studied in Arnold et al. (1996a). In this paper using functional equations, a simple consensus model for fatigue life of longitudinal elements based on engineering principles is obtained. As well, by the application of proportional hazard techniques and subsequent likelihood analysis, simple parsimonious Weibull models are obtained.

2.9 Some Recent Topics and Applications in Conditional Specification

The field of conditional specification has served as inspiration for the study and development of other topics in probability and statistical applications. In this section we include some recent applications, some of them discussed initially in Arnold (2008) and in Sarabia et al. (2008).

An application in the field of economics is the specification of multivariate income distributions. The catalogue of multivariate income distributions is limited and is usually reduced to the use of to the classical multivariate lognormal distribution. However, this distribution presents some shortcomings. It is well known that the range of the correlation coefficient is more narrowed than the normal case. An alternative model has been proposed in Sarabia et al. (2007), where the class of bivariate distributions with lognormal conditionals has been considered. This model includes the classical lognormal distribution and is more flexible for fitting bivariate income data.

Actuarial statistics and risk analysis are other important fields of application of the conditional specification models. In Sarabia et al. (2005), we have considered a new methodology for obtaining a premium based on a broad class of conjugate priors, assuming lognormal claims. Other models with broad application in risk theory in the classical collective model (see Sarabia et al. 2004 and Sarabia and Guillén 2008) are the mixture conditional distributions. These models correspond to distributions where one of the conditional distributions is of the type discrete and the other one is of the type continuous. More relevant applications in risk analysis have also been provided in Gómez-Déniz and Calderín (2014).

Another recent application of the conditional specification models is in some topics in reliability. The concept of equilibrium distribution plays an important role in reliability, survival analysis, and insurance studies. In Navarro and Sarabia (2010) several alternative definitions of bivariate equilibrium distributions are studied, some of them based on the conditional specification idea. Reliability properties in two classes of bivariate continuous distributions based on specification of conditional hazard functions are considered in Navarro and Sarabia (2013). These classes were constructed by conditioning on two different kinds of events proposed in Arnold and Kim (1996). New classes of bivariate distributions based on conditional specification satisfying the proportional generalized odds rate model were considered in Navarro et al. (2015). More recently, families of bivariate distributions with generalized three-parameter beta conditionals and transmuted conditionals have been studied in Sarabia and Castillo (2006) and Sarabia et al. (2020), respectively.

3 Other Research Topics

In this section we include other topics studied in our joint research work with Barry.

3.1 Multivariate Distributions Involving the Rosenblatt Construction

Other joint research with Barry (see Arnold et al. 2006) was on the construction of families of multivariate distributions involving the Rosenblatt transformation. In this work we proposed a method for generating extensions of multivariate parametric models that provides extra flexibility by means of the beta parameters.

The idea in this paper is as follows: It is well known (see Rosenblatt 1952) that if $\underline{X}$ has distribution function $F_{\underline{X}}(\underline{x};\underline{\theta})$ and if we define

$$\begin{aligned} U_1 &= F_1(X_1;\underline{\theta}) \\ U_2 &= F_2(X_2|X_1;\underline{\theta}) \\ &\ldots\ldots\ldots \\ U_m &= F_m(X_m|X_1,X_2,\ldots,X_{m-1};\underline{\theta}), \end{aligned} \tag{6}$$

then the U_i's are independent Uniform(0, 1) random variables. In the spirit of the quantile function construction in Jones (2004), we can use (6) to generate a random vector with distribution $F_{\underline{X}}(\underline{x};\underline{\theta})$ as follows

$$\begin{aligned} X_1 &= F_1^{-1}(U_1;\underline{\theta}) \\ X_2 &= F_2^{-1}(U_2|X_1;\underline{\theta}) = F_2^{-1}\left(U_2|F_1^{-1}(U_1);\underline{\theta}\right) \\ &\ldots\ldots\ldots \\ X_m &= F_m^{-1}\left(U_m|X_1,\ldots,X_{m-1};\underline{\theta}\right) = F_m^{-1}\left(U_m|F_1^{-1}(U_1;\underline{\theta}),\ldots,\right. \\ &\quad \left. F_{m-1}^{-1}\left(U_{m-1}|F_1^{-1}(U_1;\underline{\theta}),\ldots\right);\underline{\theta}\right), \end{aligned} \tag{7}$$

where the U_i's are independent Uniform(0, 1) random variables.

If we replace the uniformly distributed U's in (7) and independent V's which are assumed to have Beta distribution, we have

$$\begin{aligned} X_1 &= F_1^{-1}(V_1;\underline{\theta}) \\ X_2 &= F_2^{-1}(V_2|X_1;\underline{\theta}) = F_2^{-1}\left(V_2|F_1^{-1}(V_1);\underline{\theta}\right) \\ &\ldots\ldots\ldots \\ X_m &= F_m^{-1}(V_m|X_1,\ldots,X_{m-1};\underline{\theta}) = F_m^{-1}\left(V_m|F_1^{-1}(V_1;\underline{\theta}),\ldots,\right. \\ &\quad \left. F_{m-1}^{-1}\left(V_{m-1}|F_1^{-1}(V_1;\underline{\theta}),\ldots\right);\underline{\theta}\right), \end{aligned} \tag{8}$$

where $V_i \sim \mathcal{B}(\alpha_i,\beta_i);\ i=1,2,\ldots,m.$

The resulting joint density for $\underline{X}$ is then given by

$$f_{\underline{X}}(\underline{x}; \underline{\theta}, \underline{\alpha}, \underline{\beta}) = f(x_1, x_2, \ldots, x_m; \underline{\theta}) \prod_{i=1}^{m} f_{\alpha_i, \beta_i}(F_i(x_i | x_1, \ldots, x_{i-1}; \underline{\theta})) \quad (9)$$

in which f_{α_i, β_i} denotes the density of a Beta(α_i, β_i) random variable, $i = 1, 2, \ldots, m$.

It is evident from (9) that the original joint density $f(x_1, x_2, \ldots, x_m; \underline{\theta})$ is included in (9) as a special case corresponding to the choice $\alpha_i = \beta_i = 1;\ i = 1, 2, \ldots, m$. If the original family of joint densities is

$$\mathcal{F} = \{f(\underline{x}; \underline{\theta}) : \underline{\theta} \in \Theta\}, \quad (10)$$

then we will say that (9) represents the $\mathcal{F}$-Beta family of distributions parameterized now by $\underline{\theta} \in \Theta$ and $\alpha_i, \beta_i \in R^+,\ i = 1, 2, \ldots, m$. Thus, if the original parameter space of $\mathcal{F}$ is of dimension k, then the dimension of the parameter space of the $\mathcal{F}$-Beta family of distributions will be $k + 2m$.

The authors provide several specific models, a very simple estimation method for the parameters of this family of distribution and applications with simulated and real data.

3.2 *Probability Distributions Defined in Terms of Contours*

An interesting alternative to conditional specification presented jointly with Barry Arnold in Arnold et al. (2008b) consists of using contours as the basis for defining probability distributions. To this end, the most general probability densities with given contours are obtained and the particular cases of circular and elliptical contours are discussed. It is demonstrated that the well-known elliptically contoured family of distributions does not include all possible cases to be used in practical applications, which are obtained in this paper.

In particular, the case of contours defined by polar coordinates is analyzed including its simulation and parameter estimation, which become especially simple for this case. Finally, the contours idea is extended to the case of case of cumulative distribution functions, so that the families of distribution functions with given contours are identified and some illustrative examples are presented.

Figure 5 shows two examples of densities with elliptic contours, the left one with parallel axes ellipses and the right one with rotated axes. One original contribution of this paper consists of giving the possibility of extend given families of distributions to improve the fit associated with a given data set and at the same time keeping the initial family of contours.

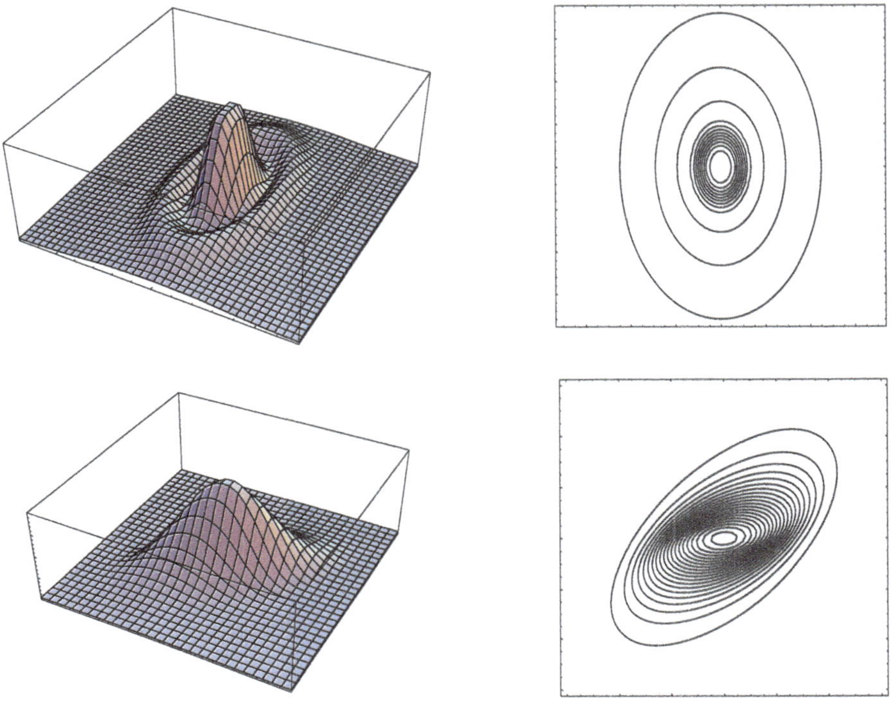

Fig. 5 Bivariate densities with normal conditionals based on contours

3.3 Multivariate Order Statistics

The problem of defining multivariate order statistics is studied in Arnold et al. (2009). In that paper a general class of complete orderings of such random vectors is supplied by viewing them as concomitants of an auxiliary random variable. The resulting definitions of multivariate order statistics subsume and extend orderings that have been previously proposed. As well, analogous concepts of multivariate record values and multivariate generalized order statistics are also proposed.

4 Conclusions

Our joint work with Barry C. Arnold covered several relevant fields of probability and statistics. Many of the most important contributions were made in the topic of conditional specification of distributions, characterization, and estimation of new families of distributions. Other fields of our work include the construction of new families of multivariate distributions, multivariate order statistics, specification of

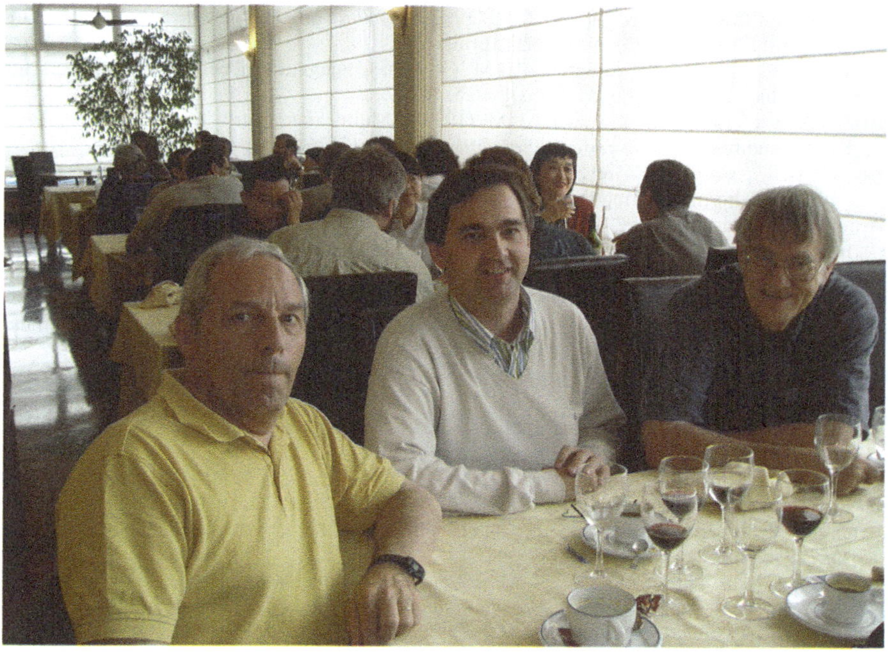

Fig. 6 Barry (right), Enrique (left) and José María in Castro Urdiales (Cantabria, Spain) in June 2004 in the 65th birthday of Barry

fatigue models and Bayesian estimation of parametric families using conditional specification priors. The research in all these topics continues to be an active field of work is current statistical science and should extend to other fields of application including applications in data science and machine learning.

Figure 6 shows a photo taken in the Castro Urdiales (Cantabria, Spain) meeting in June 2004, honoring Barry in his 65th birthday. In this picture he appears with Enrique and José María.

Acknowledgments The authors are grateful for the constructive suggestions provided by the reviewers, which have improved the paper.

References

Aczél, J. (1966). *Lectures on functional equations and their applications. Mathematics in science and engineering* (vol. 19). Cambridge: Academic.

Arnold, B. C. (2008). Enrique Castillo's contributions to conditional specification. In B. C. Arnold, N. Balakrishnan, J. M. Sarabia, R. Mínguez (Eds.), *Advances in mathematical and statistical modeling* (pp. 3–19). Boston: Birkhäuser.

Arnold, B. C., Castillo, E., & Sarabia, J. M. (1992). *Conditionally specified distributions. Lecture notes in statistics* (vol. 73). New York: Springer.
Arnold, B. C., Castillo, E., & Sarabia, J. M. (1993a). Conjugate exponential family priors for exponential family likelihoods. *Statistics, 25*, 71–77.
Arnold, B. C., Castillo, E., & Sarabia, J. M. (1993b). Multivariate distributions with generalized Pareto conditionals. *Statistics and Probability Letters, 17*, 361–368.
Arnold, B. C., Castillo, E., & Sarabia, J. M. (1994a). A conditional characterization of the multivariate normal distribution. *Statistics and Probability Letters, 19*, 313–315.
Arnold, B. C., Castillo, E., & Sarabia, J. M. (1994b). Conditional characterization of the Mardia multivariate pareto distribution. *Pakistan Journal of Statistics, 10*, 143–145.
Arnold, B. C., Castillo, E., & Sarabia, J. M. (1994c). Multivariate normality via conditional specification. *Statistics and Probability Letters, 20*, 353–354.
Arnold, B. C., Castillo, E., & Sarabia, J. M. (1996a). Modelling the fatigue life of longitudinal elements. *Naval Research Logistics, 43*, 885–895.
Arnold, B. C., Castillo, E., & Sarabia, J. M. (1996b). Priors with convenient posteriors. *Statistics, 28*(4), 347–354.
Arnold, B. C., Castillo, E., & Sarabia, J. M. (1996c). Specification of distributions by combinations of marginal and conditional distributions. *Statistics and Probability Letters, 26*, 153–157.
Arnold, B. C., Castillo, E., & Sarabia, J. M. (1998a). Bayesian analysis for classical distributions using conditionally specified priors. *Sankhya, Series B, 60*, 228–245.
Arnold, B. C., Castillo, E., & Sarabia, J. M. (1998b). Some alternative bivariate Gumbel models. *Environmetrics, 9*(6), 599–616.
Arnold, B. C., Castillo, E., & Sarabia, J. M. (1998c). The use of conditionally priors in the study of ratios of gamma scale parameters. *Computational Statistics and Data Analysis, 27*, 125–139.
Arnold, B. C., Castillo, E., & Sarabia, J. M. (1999). *Conditional specification of statistical models. Springer Series in Statistics*. New York: Springer.
Arnold, B. C., Castillo, E., & Sarabia, J. M. (2001a). A multivariate version of Stein's identity con applications to moment calculations and estimation of conditionally specified distributions. *Communications in Statistics, Theory and Methods, 30*, 2517–2542.
Arnold, B. C., Castillo, E., & Sarabia, J. M. (2001b). Conditionally specified distributions: An introduction (with comments and a rejoinder by the authors). *Statistical Science, 16*, 249–274.
Arnold, B. C., Castillo, E., & Sarabia, J. M. (2001c). Quantification of incompatibility of conditional and marginal information. *Communications in Statistics, Theory and Methods, 30*, 381–395.
Arnold, B. C., Castillo, E., & Sarabia, J. M. (2002a). Conditionally specified multivariate skewed distributions. *Sankhya, A, 64*, 206–226.
Arnold, B. C., Castillo, E., & Sarabia, J. M. (2002b). Exact and near compatibility of discrete conditional distributions. *Computational Statistics and Data Analysis, 40*, 231–252.
Arnold, B. C., Castillo, E., & Sarabia, J. M. (2004a). Compatibility of partial or complete conditional probability specifications. *Journal of Statistical Planning and Inference, 123*, 133–159.
Arnold, B. C., Castillo, E., & Sarabia, J. M. (2004b). Distributions with beta conditionals. In A. K. Gupta & S. Nadarajah (Eds.), *Handbook of beta distribution and its applications* (pp. 255–281). New York: Marcell Dekker.
Arnold, B. C., Castillo, E., & Sarabia, J. M. (2005). Distributions with conditionals in truncated weighted families. *Statistics, 39*, 133–147.
Arnold, B. C., Castillo, E., & Sarabia, J. M. (2006). Families of multivariate distributions involving the Rosenblatt construction. *Journal of the American Statistical Association, 101*, 1652–1662.
Arnold, B. C., Castillo, E., & Sarabia, J. M. (2007a). Distributions with generalized skewed conditionals and mixtures of such distributions. *Communications in Statistics, Theory and Methods, 36*(8), 1493–1503.
Arnold, B. C., Castillo, E., & Sarabia, J. M. (2007b). Variations on the classical multivariate normal theme. *Journal of Statistical Planning and Inference, 137*, 3249–3260.

Arnold, B. C., Castillo, E., & Sarabia, J. M. (2008a). Bivariate distributions characterized by one family of conditionals and conditional percentile or mode functions. *Journal of Multivariate Analysis, 99*, 1383–1392.

Arnold, B. C., Castillo, E., & Sarabia, J. M. (2008b). Multivariate distributions defined in terms of contours. *Journal of Statistical Planning and Control, 138*, 4158–4171.

Arnold, B. C., Castillo, E., & Sarabia, J. M. (2009). On multivariate orders statistics with application to ranked set sampling. *Computational Statistics and Data Analysis, 53*, 4555–4569.

Arnold, B. C., Castillo, E., Sarabia, J. M., & González-Vega, L. (2000). Multiple modes in densities with normal conditionals. *Statistics and Probability Letters, 49*, 355–363.

Arnold, B. C., & Kim, Y. H. (1996). Conditional proportional hazard models. In: N. P. Jewell, A. C. Kimber, M. L. T. Lee, & G. A. Whitmore (Eds.), *Lifetime data: Models in reliability and survival analysis* (pp. 21–28). Dordrecht: Kluwer Academic.

Arnold, B. C., & Press, S. J. (1989). Compatible conditional distributions. *Journal of the American Statistical Association, 84*, 152–156.

Arnold, B. C., & Strauss, D. (1988). Bivariate distributions with exponential conditionals. *Journal of the American Statistical Association, 83*, 522–527.

Arnold, B. C., & Strauss, D. J. (1991). Distributions with conditionals in prescribed exponential families. *Journal of the Royal Statistical Society, B, 53*, 365–375.

Balakrishnan, N., Castillo, E., & Sarabia, J. M. (Eds.) (2006). *Advances in distribution theory, order statistics, and inference*. Boston: Birkhäuser.

Castillo, E., & Galambos, J. (1987). Lifetime regression models based on a functional equation of physical nature. *Journal of Applied Probability, 24*, 160–169.

Castillo, E., & Galambos, J. (1989). Conditional distributions and the bivariate normal distribution. *Metrika, 36*, 209–214.

Castillo, E., & Galambos, J. (1990). Bivariate distributions with Weibull conditionals. *Analysis Mathematica, 16*, 3–9.

Castillo, E., Galambos, J., & Sarabia, J. M. (1990). Caracterizaci6n de modelos bivariantes con distribuciones condicionadas tipo gamma. *Estadística Española, 32*, 439–450.

Castillo, E., Gutiérrez, J. M., & Hadi, A. S. (1997). Expert systems and probabilistic networks models. New York: Springer.

Castillo, E., Iglesias, A., & Ruíz-Cobo, R. (2005). *Functional equations in applied sciences. Mathematics in science and engineering* (vol. 199). Amsterdam: Elsevier.

Castillo, E., & Ruíz-Cobo, M. R. (1992). *Functional equations and modelling in science and engineering. Monographs and textbooks in pure and applied mathematics* (vol. 161). New York: Marcel Dekker.

Castillo, E., & Sarabia, J. M. (1990). Bivariate distributions with second kind beta conditionals. *Communications in Statistics, Theory and Methods, 19*, 3433–3445.

Gelman, A., & Speed, T. P. (1993). Characterizing a joint probability distribution by conditionals. *Journal of the Royal Statistical Society, B55*, 185–188.

Ghosh, I., & Ng, H. K. T. (2019). A class of skewed distributions with applications in environmental data. *Communications in Statistics: Case Studies, Data Analysis and Applications, 5*, 346–365.

Gómez-Déniz, E., & Calderín, E. (2014). Unconditional distributions obtained from conditional specifications models with applications in risk theory. *Scandinavian Actuarial Journal, 7*, 602–619.

Jones, M. C. (2004). Families of distributions arising from distributions of order statistics. *Test, 13*, 1–44.

Moschopoulos, P., & Sha, N. (2005). Bayesian inference of scale parameters in exponential family using conditionally specified priors. *Communications in Statistics, Theory and Methods, 34*, 303–318.

Navarro, J., Esna-Ashari, M., Asadi, M., & Sarabia, J. M. (2015). Bivariate distributions with conditionals satisfying the proportional generalized odds rate model. *Metrika, 78*, 691–709.

Navarro, J., & Sarabia, J. M. (2010). Alternative definitions of bivariate equilibrium distributions. *Journal of Statistical Planning and Inference, 140*, 2046–2056.
Navarro, J., & Sarabia, J. M. (2013). Reliability properties of bivariate conditional proportional hazard rate models. *Journal of Multivariate Analysis, 113*, 116–127.
Rosenblatt, M. (1952). Remarks on a multivariate transformation. *The Annals of Mathematical Statistics, 23*, 470–472.
Sarabia, J. M., & Castillo, E. (2006). Bivariate distributions based on the generalized three-parameter beta distribution. In N. Balakrishnan, E. Castillo, & J. M. Sarabia (Eds.), *Advances on distribution theory, order statistics and inference* (pp. 85–110). Boston: Birkhäuser.
Sarabia, J. M., Castillo, E., Gómez-Déniz, E., & Vázquez, F. (2005). A class of conjugate priors for log-normal claims based on conditional specification. *Journal of Risk and Insurance, 72*, 479–495.
Sarabia, J. M., Castillo, E., Pascual, M., & Sarabia, M. (2007). Bivariate income distributions with lognormal conditionals. *Journal of Economic Inequality, 5*, 371–383.
Sarabia, J. M., Gómez-Déniz, E., & Vázquez, F. (2004). On the use of conditional specification models in claim count distributions: An application to bonus-malus systems. *ASTIN Bulletin, 34*, 85–98.
Sarabia, J. M., & Guillén, M. (2008). Joint modelling of the total amount and the number of claims by conditionals. *Insurance: Mathematics and Economics, 43*, 466–473.
Sarabia, J. M., Raja, A. V., & Asha, G. (2020). Bivariate distributions with transmuted conditionals: Models and applications. *Communications in Statistics, Theory and Methods, 49*, 221–242.
Sarabia, J. M., Sarabia, M., & Pascual, M. (2008). Conditionally specified models: New developments and applications. In B. C. Arnold, N. Balakrishnan, J. M. Sarabia, & R. Mínguez (Eds.), *Advances in Mathematical and Statistical Modeling* (pp. 35–43). Boston: Birkhäuser.
Sarabia, J. M., & Shahtahmassebi, G. (2017). Bayesian estimation of incomplete data using conditionally specified priors. *Communications in Statistics, Simulation and Computation, 46*, 3419–3435.

On the Asymptotic Joint Distribution of Multivariate Sample Moments

Reinaldo B. Arellano-Valle, Simone B. Harnik, and Marc G. Genton

Abstract We present the asymptotic joint distribution of the sample central moments and the standardized sample central moments of multivariate random variables. Sample central moments and standardized sample central moments are quantities of interest for statistical inference as the variance and the coefficients of skewness and kurtosis are particular cases. The results described here are known for univariate random variables; now, we extend them to random vectors. After presenting our results, we apply them to multivariate elliptical distributions and the multivariate skew-normal distribution, showing that these expressions can be simplified considerably in specific cases.

1 Introduction

Statistical analyses frequently make use of functions of the sample mean and sample covariance matrix for multivariate inference. In the exponential family, for instance, such statistics are sufficient to estimate the parameters of distributions. In other families, the third and fourth standardized sample moments, respectively, known as the coefficients of skewness and kurtosis, may be of interest. Here, we present the asymptotic joint distribution for multivariate sample moments and apply it to both multivariate elliptical distributions and the multivariate skew-normal family.

R. B. Arellano-Valle
Departamento de Estadística, Facultad de Matemática, Pontificia Universidad Católica de Chile, Santiago, Chile
e-mail: reivalle@mat.puc.cl

S. B. Harnik
Departamento de Estatística, Instituto de Matemática e Estatística, Universidade de São Paulo, São Paulo, Brazil
e-mail: simone.harnik@usp.br

M. G. Genton (✉)
Statistics Program, King Abdullah University of Science and Technology, Thuwal, Saudi Arabia
e-mail: marc.genton@kaust.edu.sa

I. Ghosh et al. (eds.), *Advances in Statistics - Theory and Applications*, Emerging Topics in Statistics and Biostatistics, https://doi.org/10.1007/978-3-030-62900-7_9

Sample moments are used in the method of moments, an estimation technique based on the assumption that unknown parameters can be computed by matching the sample moments with the theoretical ones, and solving a system of p equations and p unknown parameters. The p parameters may be over-identified by the system of equations; so, the Generalized Method of Moments (GMM) was developed to tackle this obstacle. As noted by Harris and Mátyás (1999), the estimation via moments requires fewer assumptions than the maximum likelihood estimation, which needs specification of the whole distribution. Therefore, estimation via moments may be convenient in many situations. The sample moments can also be used for optimization of the likelihood, according to Lehmann and Casella (1998, pp. 456–457).

As the sample moments have numerous applications, these measures and their asymptotic distributions have been vastly explored in the literature. As one of the first in this field, Cramér (1946) dealt with moments, functions of moments, and their asymptotic normality using a technique that later became known as the delta method. Pewsey (2005) derived a general result for the large-sample joint distribution of the mean, the standard deviation, and the coefficients of skewness and kurtosis of a general distribution by employing the Central Limit Theorem (CLT), the Taylor expansion of functions of the moments, and extensive algebraic manipulations. Both these works referred to the univariate context only.

An interesting property of Pewsey's result is that he isolated the asymptotic bias for the coefficients of skewness and kurtosis, so his formulation can be applied in bias corrections of estimators. However, practical simulations from the author with bias correction through subtraction or ratio performed poorly. Bao (2013) derived analytical results for finite sample biases for skewness and kurtosis coefficients in a different way. He achieved a good performance using his asymptotic results for bias correction in an AR(1) process. He also claimed that applying the results to hypothesis tests for normality increased the power of the tests. In the multivariate context, Kollo and von Rosen (2005) presented the asymptotic distribution of the sample mean and the sample covariance matrix, using as a background the law of large numbers and the CLT.

Asymptotic results may be applied to the multivariate skew-normal distribution, a more general class than the normal distribution, as shown by Arnold and Beaver (2002). The authors also exposed different causes yielding skewed distributions, for example, the hidden truncation mechanism. Arnold et al. (1993), motivated by practical problems, such as "selective reporting," i.e., when, intentionally or not, only random vectors related to a truncated variable are recorded, developed these ideas and provided a direct relationship with Azzalini's (1985) skew-normal distribution. As selective reporting is generated by common procedures, this hidden truncation mechanism may be frequent in data analyses and was addressed by a series of papers that Prof. Arnold pioneered.

Here, we apply asymptotic results to multivariate elliptical distributions and the multivariate skew-normal distribution developed by Azzalini and Dalla Valle (1996). In this last scenario, we show that expressions simplify considerably, depending on the parameters. Two key advantages of our results are that we address the higher-order moments, unlike previous works, and we employ intuitive and straightforward notation.

The structure of this paper is as follows. In Sect. 2, we provide the notation and terminology used throughout the paper. In Sect. 3, we present the main results about the asymptotic joint distribution of multivariate sample moments and multivariate standardized sample moments and describe several examples for illustration. In Sect. 4, we apply the results to multivariate elliptical distributions, and in Sect. 5, we evaluate the asymptotic behavior for the skew-normal distribution.

2 Notation and Terminology

To derive the asymptotic joint distribution of central moments from multivariate random variables, we consider a non-degenerate random vector $\boldsymbol{X} = (X_1, \dots, X_d)^\top \sim f(\boldsymbol{x}; \boldsymbol{\theta}), \boldsymbol{x} \in \mathcal{X} \subseteq \mathbb{R}^d, \boldsymbol{\theta} \in \Theta \subset \mathbb{R}^q$, where f is a parametric joint probability density function. We also consider the following theoretical quantities, provided they exist:

- $\mu_{kr} = \mathbb{E}(X_k^r), k = 1, \dots, d,\ r = 1, \dots, p$, is the rth theoretical moment of X_k, and $\mu_{k1} = \mu_k$ is the mean of the kth variable;
- $\kappa_{kr} = \mathbb{E}\{(X_k - \mu_k)^r\}, k = 1, \dots, d,\ r = 1, \dots, p$, is the rth theoretical central moment of X_k about the mean μ_k, where $\kappa_{k1} = 0$ and $\kappa_{k2} = \sigma_k^2$ is the variance;
- $\kappa_{kl,rs} = \mathbb{E}\{(X_k - \mu_k)^r (X_l - \mu_l)^s\}, k, l = 1, \dots, d,\ r, s = 1, \dots, p$, represents the theoretical central cross-moments of orders r and s between the kth and lth variables, $\kappa_{kl,11} = \sigma_{kl}$ is the covariance between the kth and lth variables, and $\kappa_{kk,rs} = \kappa_{k,r+s}$;
- $\rho_{kr} = \frac{\kappa_{kr}}{\kappa_{k2}^{r/2}}, k = 1, \dots, d,\ r = 1, \dots, p$, is the standardized rth theoretical moment of X_k with $\rho_{k1} = 0, \rho_{k2} = 1,\ \rho_{k3} = \gamma_{k1}$ and $\rho_{k4} - 3 = \gamma_{k2}$, where γ_{k1} is the skewness coefficient and γ_{k2} is the excess kurtosis;
- $\rho_{kl,rs} = \frac{\kappa_{kl,rs}}{\kappa_{k2}^{r/2}\kappa_{l2}^{s/2}},\ k, l = 1, \dots, d,\ r, s = 1, \dots, p$, and $\rho_{kk,rs} = \rho_{k,r+s}$, $\rho_{kk,11} = \rho_{k2} = 1$;
- $\bar{\rho}_{kl,rs} = \frac{\kappa_{kl,rs} - \kappa_{kr}\kappa_{ls}}{\kappa_{k2}^{r/2}\kappa_{l2}^{s/2}} = \rho_{kl,rs} - \rho_{kr}\rho_{ls},\ k, l = 1, \dots, d,\ r, s = 1, \dots, p$, and $\bar{\rho}_{kk,rs} = \bar{\rho}_{k,r+s}$, $\bar{\rho}_{kl,1s} = \rho_{kl,1s}$ and $\bar{\rho}_{kl,r1} = \rho_{kl,r1}$.

We also define D_{kr}, S_{kr}, and R_{kr}, which are, respectively, the rth sample central moment about the mean, the rth sample central moment about the sample mean, and the rth standardized sample central moment about the sample mean, for a random sample $\boldsymbol{X}_i = (X_{i1}, \dots, X_{id})^\top, i = 1, \dots, n$, from the random vector $\boldsymbol{X} = (X_1, \dots, X_d)^\top \sim f(\boldsymbol{x}; \boldsymbol{\theta})$ as follows:

$$D_{kr} = \frac{1}{n}\sum_{i=1}^{n}(X_{ik} - \mu_k)^r, k = 1, \dots, d,\ r = 1, \dots, p, \quad (D_{k1} = \bar{X}_k - \mu_k),$$

$$S_{kr} = \frac{1}{n}\sum_{i=1}^{n}(X_{ik} - \bar{X}_k)^r, k = 1, \ldots, d, \ r = 2, \ldots, p, \quad (S_{k1} = 0, \ S_{k2} = S_k^2),$$
$$= \sum_{s=0}^{r}(-1)^{r-s}\binom{r}{s} D_{ks} D_{k1}^{r-s}, \quad (D_{k0} = 1),$$
$$R_{kr} = S_{k2}^{-r/2} S_{kr}, \quad k = 1, \ldots, d, \ r = 3, \ldots, p.$$

The sample central moments (S_{kr}) are strongly consistent estimators of the respective theoretical central moments (κ_{kr}) for each $k = 1, \ldots, d$ and $r = 2, \ldots, p$. Therefore, the standardized sample central moments (R_{kr}) are also strongly consistent estimators of the respective standardized theoretical central moments (ρ_{kr}) for each $k = 1, \ldots, d$ and $r = 2, \ldots, p$, i.e., each univariate marginal. Besides, if the $(2r)$th theoretical moments are finite, then the asymptotic normality of these central statistics is known. In the next section, we deliver the basic elements needed to study the asymptotic distribution in the multivariate context and give some illustrative examples of how to apply the proposed results.

3 Main Results

We let $\boldsymbol{D} = (\boldsymbol{D}_1^\top, \ldots, \boldsymbol{D}_p^\top)^\top$, $\boldsymbol{D}_k = (D_{k1}, \ldots, D_{kp})^\top$, and $\boldsymbol{D}_k = \frac{1}{n}\sum_{i=1}^{n} \boldsymbol{W}_{ik}$, where $\boldsymbol{W}_{ik} = ((X_{ik} - \mu_k)^1, (X_{ik} - \mu_k)^2, \ldots, (X_{ik} - \mu_k)^p)^\top$, $k = 1, \ldots, d$, $i = 1, \ldots, n$. If the mean vector and the variance–covariance matrix of $\boldsymbol{W}_{ik}$ exist, they are, respectively, defined as

$$\mathbb{E}(\boldsymbol{W}_{ik}) = \boldsymbol{\kappa}_k = (\kappa_{k1}, \kappa_{k2}, \ldots, \kappa_{kp})^\top, \text{ and}$$
$$\mathrm{Var}(\boldsymbol{W}_{ik}) = \mathcal{K}_{kk} = \left(\mathrm{Cov}\left\{(X_k - \mu_k)^i, (X_k - \mu_k)^j\right\}\right)_{i,j=1,2,\ldots,p}$$
$$= (\kappa_{kk,ij} - \kappa_{ki}\kappa_{kj})_{i,j=1,2,\ldots,p}, \quad k = 1, \ldots, d.$$

Thus, $\boldsymbol{D} = \frac{1}{n}\sum_{i=1}^{n} \boldsymbol{W}_i$, where $\boldsymbol{W}_i = (\boldsymbol{W}_{i1}^\top, \ldots, \boldsymbol{W}_{id}^\top)^\top$, $i = 1, \ldots, n$, are i.i.d. random vectors, with a mean vector $\boldsymbol{\kappa} = (\boldsymbol{\kappa}_1^\top, \ldots, \boldsymbol{\kappa}_d^\top)^\top$ and a variance–covariance matrix $\mathcal{K} = (\mathcal{K}_{kl})$, $k, l = 1, \ldots, d$, where the block $\mathcal{K}_{kl} = \mathrm{Cov}\{\boldsymbol{W}_k, \boldsymbol{W}_l\}$ is

$$\mathcal{K}_{kl} = \left(\mathrm{Cov}\left\{(X_k - \mu_k)^i, (X_l - \mu_l)^j\right\}\right)_{i,j=1,2,\ldots,p}$$
$$= (\kappa_{kl,ij} - \kappa_{ki}\kappa_{lj})_{i,j=1,2,\ldots,p}, \quad k, l = 1, \ldots, d. \tag{1}$$

With this, we make use of the multivariate Central Limit Theorem (CLT) to obtain the results in Proposition 1:

Proposition 1 *Let* $\boldsymbol{D} = (\boldsymbol{D}_1^\top, \ldots, \boldsymbol{D}_d^\top)^\top$, *and* $\boldsymbol{\kappa} = (\boldsymbol{\kappa}_1^\top, \ldots, \boldsymbol{\kappa}_d^\top)^\top$, *where* $\boldsymbol{D}_k = (D_{k1}, \ldots, D_{kp})^\top$, $D_{k1} = \bar{X}_k - \mu_k$, $\boldsymbol{\kappa}_k = (\kappa_{k1}, \ldots, \kappa_{kp})^\top$, $\kappa_{k1} = 0$, *and* $\kappa_{k2} = \sigma_k^2$, $k = 1, \ldots, d$. *If* $\kappa_{k,2p} < \infty$ *for all* $k = 1, \ldots, d$, *then*

$$\sqrt{n}(\boldsymbol{D} - \boldsymbol{\kappa}) \xrightarrow{d} \mathcal{N}_{dp}(\boldsymbol{0}, \mathcal{K}),$$

where $\mathcal{K}$ *has block elements* $\mathcal{K}_{kl}$ *given by (1). In particular,*

$$\sqrt{n}(\boldsymbol{D}_k - \boldsymbol{\kappa}_k) \xrightarrow{d} \mathcal{N}_p(\boldsymbol{0}, \mathcal{K}_{kk}), \quad k = 1, \ldots, d.$$

Example 1 We illustrate this result with the case in which $p = 4$. Assuming that $\kappa_{k,8} < \infty$, then for all $k = 1, \ldots, d$,

$$\sqrt{n}\begin{pmatrix} D_{k1} - \kappa_{k1} \\ D_{k2} - \kappa_{k2} \\ D_{k3} - \kappa_{k3} \\ D_{k4} - \kappa_{k4} \end{pmatrix} \xrightarrow{d} \mathcal{N}_4\left(\begin{pmatrix} 0 \\ 0 \\ 0 \\ 0 \end{pmatrix}, \begin{pmatrix} \kappa_{k2}-\kappa_{k1}^2 & \kappa_{k3}-\kappa_{k1}\kappa_{k2} & \kappa_{k4}-\kappa_{k1}\kappa_{k3} & \kappa_{k5}-\kappa_{k1}\kappa_{k4} \\ \kappa_{k3}-\kappa_{k2}\kappa_{k1} & \kappa_{k4}-\kappa_{k2}^2 & \kappa_{k5}-\kappa_{k2}\kappa_{k3} & \kappa_{k6}-\kappa_{k2}\kappa_{k4} \\ \kappa_{k4}-\kappa_{k3}\kappa_{k1} & \kappa_{k5}-\kappa_{k3}\kappa_{k2} & \kappa_{k6}-\kappa_{k3}^2 & \kappa_{k7}-\kappa_{k3}\kappa_{k4} \\ \kappa_{k5}-\kappa_{k4}\kappa_{k1} & \kappa_{k6}-\kappa_{k4}\kappa_{k2} & \kappa_{k7}-\kappa_{k4}\kappa_{k3} & \kappa_{k8}-\kappa_{k4}^2 \end{pmatrix}\right).$$

If the distribution of $X_k - \mu_k$ is symmetric around zero, then the result reduces to

$$\sqrt{n}\begin{pmatrix} D_{k1} \\ D_{k2} - \kappa_{k2} \\ D_{k3} \\ D_{k4} - \kappa_{k4} \end{pmatrix} \xrightarrow{d} \mathcal{N}_4\left(\begin{pmatrix} 0 \\ 0 \\ 0 \\ 0 \end{pmatrix}, \begin{pmatrix} \kappa_{k2} & 0 & \kappa_{k4} & 0 \\ 0 & \kappa_{k4}-\kappa_{k2}^2 & 0 & \kappa_{k6}-\kappa_{k2}\kappa_{k4} \\ \kappa_{k4} & 0 & \kappa_{k6} & 0 \\ 0 & \kappa_{k6}-\kappa_{k4}\kappa_{k2} & 0 & \kappa_{k8}-\kappa_{k4}^2 \end{pmatrix}\right),$$

indicating asymptotic independence between the random vectors $\sqrt{n}\,(D_{k1}, D_{k3})^\top$ and $\sqrt{n}\,(D_{k2} - \kappa_{k2}, D_{k4} - \kappa_{k4})^\top$.

Similarly, for sample central moments about the true mean vector, we derive asymptotic distributions for the sample central moments about the sample mean as stated below in Proposition 2. As noted by Afendras et al. (2020), when investigating the limiting behavior of sample central moments in the univariate context, two general assumptions about each of the components of the random vector $\boldsymbol{X} = (X_1, \ldots, X_d)^\top$ are required. First, $\mathbb{E}(|X_k|^{2r}) < \infty$. Second, non-singularity of order r, that is, $\tau_{kr}^2 \neq 0$, for $r = 2, 3, \ldots$. These conditions guarantee the marginal $\sqrt{n}$-convergence of the sample central moments, i.e., each marginal sample central moment $\sqrt{n}\,(S_{kr} - \kappa_{kr})$ converges in distribution to a non-degenerate $\mathcal{N}_1(0, \tau_{kr}^2)$, with $\tau_{kr}^2 > 0$. Under singularity of order r, whenever $\tau_{kr}^2 = 0$, Afendras et al. (2020) verified that $n\,(S_{kr} - \kappa_{kr})$ converges in distribution to a non-normal law of probability.

Proposition 2 *Let* $\boldsymbol{S} = (\boldsymbol{S}_1^\top, \ldots, \boldsymbol{S}_d^\top)^\top$ *and* $\boldsymbol{\kappa} = (\boldsymbol{\kappa}_1^\top, \ldots, \boldsymbol{\kappa}_d^\top)^\top$, *where* $\boldsymbol{S}_k = (D_{k1}, S_{k2}, \ldots, S_{kp})^\top$ *and* $\boldsymbol{\kappa}_k = (\kappa_{k1}, \kappa_{k2}, \ldots, \kappa_{kp})^\top$, $k = 1, \ldots, d$. *If* $\kappa_{k(2p)} < \infty$ *for all* $k = 1, \ldots, d$, *then*

$$\sqrt{n}\,(\boldsymbol{S} - \boldsymbol{\kappa}) \xrightarrow{d} \mathcal{N}_{pd}(\boldsymbol{0}, \boldsymbol{C}\mathcal{K}\boldsymbol{C}^\top),$$

where $\boldsymbol{C} = diag(\boldsymbol{C}_1, \ldots, \boldsymbol{C}_d)$, *and*

$$\boldsymbol{C}_k = \begin{pmatrix} 1 & 0\;0\cdots 0 \\ -2\kappa_{k1} & 1\;0\cdots 0 \\ -3\kappa_{k2} & 0\;1\cdots 0 \\ \vdots & \vdots\;\vdots\;\ddots\;\vdots \\ -p\kappa_{k(p-1)} & 0\;0\cdots 1 \end{pmatrix}, \quad k = 1, \ldots, d,$$

where $\kappa_{k1} = 0$ *and* $\kappa_{k2} = \sigma_k^2$. *In particular,*

$$\sqrt{n}(\boldsymbol{S}_k - \boldsymbol{\kappa}_k) \xrightarrow{d} \mathcal{N}_p(\boldsymbol{0}, \boldsymbol{C}_k\mathcal{K}_{kk}\boldsymbol{C}_k^\top), \quad k = 1, \ldots, d,$$

where the asymptotic variance–covariance matrix $\boldsymbol{C}_k\mathcal{K}_{kk}\boldsymbol{C}_k^\top$ *has entries* $\tau_{k,rs}$, *where* $\tau_{k,rr} = \tau_{k,r}^2$, *and*

$$\begin{aligned}
\tau_{k,11} &= \kappa_{k2} - \kappa_{k1}^2, \\
\tau_{k,1s} &= \tau_{k,s1} = \kappa_{k(s+1)} - s\kappa_{k2}\kappa_{k(s-1)}, \quad s = 2, \ldots, p, \\
\tau_{k,rs} &= \kappa_{k(r+s)} - \kappa_{kr}\kappa_{ks} - r\kappa_{k(r-1)}\kappa_{k(s+1)} \\
&\quad - s\kappa_{k(r+1)}\kappa_{k(s-1)} + rs\kappa_{k2}\kappa_{k(r-1)}\kappa_{k(s-1)}, \quad r, s = 2, \ldots, p.
\end{aligned}$$

Proof of Proposition 2 Since $\bar{X}_k - \mu_k = D_{k1}$ and, for $r = 2, \ldots, p$,

$$\begin{aligned}
S_{kr} &= \sum_{s=0}^{r} (-1)^{r-s}\binom{r}{s} D_{ks} D_{k1}^{r-s} \quad (D_{k0} = \kappa_{k0} = 0,\ D_{k1} = \bar{X}_k - \mu_k) \\
&= (-1)^{r-1}(r-1)D_{k1}^r + \sum_{s=2}^{r-1} (-1)^{r-s}\binom{r}{s}(D_{ks} - \kappa_{ks})D_{k1}^{r-s} \\
&\quad + \sum_{s=2}^{r-1} (-1)^{r-s}\binom{r}{s}\kappa_{ks} D_{k1}^{r-s} + D_{kr}
\end{aligned}$$

$$= -r\kappa_{k,r-1}D_{k1} + D_{kr} + \sum_{s=0}^{r-1}(-1)^{r-s}\binom{r}{s}(D_{ks} - \kappa_{ks})D_{k1}^{r-s}$$

$$+ \sum_{s=0}^{r-2}(-1)^{r-s}\binom{r}{s}\kappa_{ks}D_{k1}^{r-s},$$

we have

$$\begin{aligned}\sqrt{n}\,(S_{kr} - \kappa_{kr}) &= \sqrt{n}\Big(D_{kr} - \kappa_{kr} - r\kappa_{k(r-1)}D_{k1} \\ &\quad + \sum_{s=0}^{r-1}(-1)^{r-s}\binom{r}{s}(D_{ks} - \kappa_{ks})D_{k1}^{r-s} \\ &\quad + \sum_{s=0}^{r-2}(-1)^{r-s}\binom{r}{s}\kappa_{ks}D_{k1}^{r-s}\Big) \\ &= \sqrt{n}\,\big(D_{kr} - \kappa_{kr} - r\kappa_{k(r-1)}D_{k1}\big) \\ &\quad + \sum_{s=0}^{r-1}(-1)^{r-s}\binom{r}{s}\sqrt{n}\,(D_{ks} - \kappa_{ks})D_{k1}^{r-s} \\ &\quad + \sum_{s=0}^{r-2}(-1)^{r-s}\binom{r}{s}\kappa_{ks}\sqrt{n}\,D_{k1}^{r-s}.\end{aligned}$$

By Proposition 1, $\sqrt{n}\,(D_{ks} - \kappa_{ks}) = O_p(1)$ as $n \to \infty$, for all $k = 1, \ldots, d$ and $s = 1, \ldots, p$, implying that:
$D_{k1} = O_p(n^{-1/2}) = o_p(1)$ and $D_{k1}^{r-s} = o_p(1)$, for all $r - s > 0$;
$\sqrt{n}\,(D_{ks} - \kappa_{ks})D_{k1}^{r-s} = O_p(1)o_p(1) = o_p(1)$, for $s = 2, \ldots, r-1$ and $r = 3, \ldots, p$; and
$\sqrt{n}\,D_{k1}^{r-s} = n^{-(r-s-1)/2}(\sqrt{n}\,D_{k1})^{r-s} = o_p(1)O_p(1) = o_p(1)$, for all $r - s \geq 2$.
These facts imply that:

$$\sum_{s=0}^{r-1}(-1)^{r-s}\binom{r}{s}\sqrt{n}\,(D_{ks} - \kappa_{ks})D_{k1}^{r-s} + \sum_{s=0}^{r-2}(-1)^{r-s}\binom{r}{s}\kappa_{ks}\sqrt{n}\,D_{k1}^{r-s} = o_p(1),$$

which holds for all $k = 1, \ldots, d$ and all $r = 2, \ldots, p$.

Hence, we obtain $\sqrt{n}\,(\boldsymbol{S}_k - \boldsymbol{\kappa}_k) = \boldsymbol{C}_k\sqrt{n}(\boldsymbol{D}_k - \boldsymbol{\kappa}_k) + o_p(1)$, for all $k = 1, \ldots, d$, and thus, $\sqrt{n}\,(\boldsymbol{S} - \boldsymbol{\kappa}) = \boldsymbol{C}\sqrt{n}(\boldsymbol{D} - \boldsymbol{\kappa}) + o_p(1)$. The proof is concluded by applying Proposition 1 and Slutsky's theorem. □

Example 2 Similar to Example 1, for $p = 4$, we suppose that $\kappa_{k8} < \infty$. Then, for all $k = 1, \ldots, d$,

$$\sqrt{n}\begin{pmatrix}\bar{X}_k - \mu_k \\ S_{k2} - \kappa_{k2} \\ S_{k3} - \kappa_{k3} \\ S_{k4} - \kappa_{k4}\end{pmatrix}$$

$$= \sqrt{n}\begin{pmatrix} D_{k1} \\ -2\kappa_{k1} D_{k1} + (D_{k2} - \kappa_{k2}) - D_{k1}^2 \\ -3\kappa_{k2} D_{k1} + (D_{k3} - \kappa_{k3}) + 2D_{k1}^2 - 3(D_{k2} - \kappa_{k2}) D_{k1} \\ -4\kappa_{k3} D_{k1} + (D_{k4} - \kappa_{k4}) - 3D_{k1}^2 - 4(D_{k3} - \kappa_{k3}) D_{k1} + 6(D_{k2} - \kappa_{k2}) D_{k1}^2 \end{pmatrix}$$

$$= \begin{pmatrix} 1 & 0 & 0 & 0 \\ -2\kappa_{k1} & 1 & 0 & 0 \\ -3\kappa_{k2} & 0 & 1 & 0 \\ -4\kappa_{k3} & 0 & 0 & 1 \end{pmatrix} \sqrt{n}\begin{pmatrix} D_{k1} \\ D_{k2} - \kappa_{k2} \\ D_{k3} - \kappa_{k3} \\ D_{k4} - \kappa_{k4} \end{pmatrix}$$

$$+ \underbrace{\sqrt{n}\begin{pmatrix} 0 \\ -D_{k1}^2 \\ -3(D_{k2} - \kappa_{k2}) D_{k1} + 2D_{k1}^2 \\ -4(D_{k3} - \kappa_{k3}) D_{k1} + 6(D_{k2} - \kappa_{k2}) D_{k1}^2 - 3D_{k1}^2 \end{pmatrix}}_{o_p(1)}$$

$$\xrightarrow{d} \mathcal{N}_4\left(\begin{pmatrix}0\\0\\0\\0\end{pmatrix}, \begin{pmatrix} \tau_{k,11} & \tau_{k,12} & \tau_{k,13} & \tau_{k,14} \\ \tau_{k,21} & \tau_{k,22} & \tau_{k,23} & \tau_{k,24} \\ \tau_{k,31} & \tau_{k,32} & \tau_{k,33} & \tau_{k,34} \\ \tau_{k,41} & \tau_{k,42} & \tau_{k,43} & \tau_{k,44} \end{pmatrix}\right),$$

where

$$\tau_{k,11} = \tau_{k,1}^2 = \kappa_{k2} - \kappa_{k1}^2,$$

$$\tau_{k,12} = \tau_{k,21} = \kappa_{k3} - 2\kappa_{k2}\kappa_{k1},$$

$$\tau_{k,13} = \tau_{k,31} = \kappa_{k4} - 3\kappa_{k2}^2,$$

$$\tau_{k,14} = \tau_{k,41} = \kappa_{k5} - 4\kappa_{k2}\kappa_{k3},$$

$$\tau_{k,22} = \tau_{k,2}^2 = \kappa_{k4} - \kappa_{k2}^2 - 4\kappa_{k1}\kappa_{k3} + 4\kappa_{k2}\kappa_{k1}^2,$$

$$\tau_{k,23} = \kappa_{k5} - 4\kappa_{k2}\kappa_{k3} - 2\kappa_{k1}\kappa_{k4} + 6\kappa_{k2}^2\kappa_{k1},$$

$$\tau_{k,24} = \kappa_{k6} - \kappa_{k2}\kappa_{k4} - 2\kappa_{k1}\kappa_{k5} - 4\kappa_{k3}^2 + 8\kappa_{k2}\kappa_{k1}\kappa_{k3},$$

$$\tau_{k,33} = \tau_{k,3}^2 = \kappa_{k6} - \kappa_{k3}^2 - 6\kappa_{k2}\kappa_{k4} + 9\kappa_{k,2}^3,$$

$$\tau_{k,34} = \kappa_{k7} - 5\kappa_{k3}\kappa_{k4} - 3\kappa_{k2}\kappa_{k5} + 12\kappa_{k2}^2\kappa_{k3},$$

(continued)

Example 2 (continued)

$$\tau_{k,44} = \tau_{k,4}^2 = \kappa_{k8} - \kappa_{k4}^2 - 8\kappa_{k3}\kappa_{k5} + 16\kappa_{k2}\kappa_{k3}^2,$$

with $\kappa_{k1} = 0$ and $\kappa_{k2} = \sigma_k^2$. In particular, if the marginal distribution of $X_k - \mu_k$ is symmetric around zero, then $\kappa_{kr} = 0$ for odd r, and the asymptotic multivariate normal distribution of $\sqrt{n}\,(\bar{X}_k - \mu_k, S_{k2} - \kappa_{k2}, S_{k3}, S_{k4} - \kappa_{k4})^\top$ reduces to

$$\mathcal{N}_4\left(\begin{pmatrix}0\\0\\0\\0\end{pmatrix}, \begin{pmatrix} \kappa_{k2} & 0 & \kappa_{k4}-3\kappa_{k2}^2 & 0 \\ 0 & \kappa_{k4}-\kappa_{k2}^2 & 0 & \kappa_{k6}-\kappa_{k2}\kappa_{k4} \\ \kappa_{k4}-3\kappa_{k2}^2 & 0 & \kappa_{k6}-6\kappa_{k2}\kappa_{k4}+9\kappa_{k2}^3 & 0 \\ 0 & \kappa_{k6}-\kappa_{k2}\kappa_{k4} & 0 & \kappa_{k8}-\kappa_{k4}^2 \end{pmatrix}\right),$$

which indicates that there is asymptotic independence between the sample central moments of odd and even orders. This is a general result valid for higher-order sample central moments.

The next proposition shows the asymptotic joint distribution of multivariate standardized sample central moments.

Proposition 3 *Let* $\boldsymbol{R} = (\boldsymbol{R}_1^\top, \ldots, \boldsymbol{R}_d^\top)$ *and* $\boldsymbol{\rho} = (\boldsymbol{0}^\top, \boldsymbol{\rho}_1^\top, \ldots, \boldsymbol{\rho}_d^\top)^\top$, *where* $\boldsymbol{R}_k = (D_{k1}, S_{k2}, R_{k3}, \ldots, R_{kp})^\top$ *and* $\boldsymbol{\rho}_k = (0, \kappa_{k2}, \rho_{k3}, \ldots, \rho_{kp})^\top$, $k = 1, \ldots, d$. *If* $\kappa_{k,2p} < \infty$ *for all* $k = 1, \ldots, d$, *then*

$$\sqrt{n}\,(\boldsymbol{R} - \boldsymbol{\rho}) \xrightarrow{d} \mathcal{N}_{dp}(\boldsymbol{0}, \boldsymbol{G}\boldsymbol{C}\mathcal{K}\boldsymbol{C}^\top\boldsymbol{G}^\top),$$

where $\boldsymbol{G}\boldsymbol{C} = diag(\boldsymbol{G}_1\boldsymbol{C}_1, \ldots, \boldsymbol{G}_d\boldsymbol{C}_d)$, *with*

$$\boldsymbol{G}_k\boldsymbol{C}_k = \begin{pmatrix} 1 & 0 & 0 & \cdots & 0 \\ 0 & 1 & \vdots & \ddots & \vdots \\ -\frac{3}{\kappa_{k2}^{1/2}} & -\frac{3}{2}\frac{\rho_{k3}}{\kappa_{k2}} & \frac{1}{\kappa_{k2}^{3/2}} & \cdots & 0 \\ \vdots & \vdots & \vdots & \ddots & \vdots \\ -\frac{p\rho_{k(p-1)}}{\kappa_{k2}^{1/2}} & -\frac{p}{2}\frac{\rho_{kp}}{\kappa_{k2}} & 0 & \cdots & \frac{1}{\kappa_{k2}^{p/2}} \end{pmatrix}.$$

In particular,

$$\sqrt{n}(\boldsymbol{R}_k - \boldsymbol{\rho}_k) \xrightarrow{d} \mathcal{N}_p(\boldsymbol{0}, \boldsymbol{G}_k\boldsymbol{C}_k\mathcal{K}_{kk}\boldsymbol{C}_k^\top\boldsymbol{G}_k^\top), \quad k = 1, \ldots, d.$$

Proof of Proposition 3 We let $\boldsymbol{g}(\boldsymbol{x}) = (\boldsymbol{g}_1(\boldsymbol{x}_1), \ldots, \boldsymbol{g}_d(\boldsymbol{x}_d))^\top$, where $\boldsymbol{x} = (\boldsymbol{x}_1^\top, \ldots, \boldsymbol{x}_d^\top)^\top$, $\boldsymbol{x}_k = (x_{k1}, \ldots, x_{kp})^\top$, $\boldsymbol{g}_k = (g_{k1}, \ldots, g_{kp})^\top$, and

$$g_{kr}(\boldsymbol{x}_k) = \begin{cases} x_{kr}, & r = 1, 2, \\ x_{k2}^{-r/2} x_{kr}, & r = 3, \ldots, p. \end{cases}$$

The Jacobian matrix is $\dot{\boldsymbol{G}}(\boldsymbol{x}) = \operatorname{diag}(\boldsymbol{G}_1(\boldsymbol{x}_1), \ldots, \boldsymbol{G}_k(\boldsymbol{x}_k))$, with $\boldsymbol{G}_k(\boldsymbol{x}_k) = \left(\frac{\partial \boldsymbol{g}_k(\boldsymbol{x}_k)}{\partial \boldsymbol{x}_k}\right)$ given by

$$\boldsymbol{G}_k(\boldsymbol{x}_k) = \begin{pmatrix} 1 & 0 & 0 & \cdots & 0 \\ 0 & 1 & 0 & \cdots & 0 \\ 0 & -\frac{3}{2}\frac{x_{k3}}{x_{k2}^{3/2+1}} & \frac{1}{x_{k2}^{3/2}} & \cdots & 0 \\ \vdots & \vdots & \vdots & \ddots & \vdots \\ 0 & -\frac{p}{2}\frac{x_{kp}}{x_{k2}^{p/2+1}} & 0 & \cdots & \frac{1}{x_{k2}^{p/2}} \end{pmatrix}, \quad k = 1, \ldots, d.$$

Thus, from the delta method, we have $\sqrt{n}\,(\boldsymbol{R} - \boldsymbol{\rho}) = \sqrt{n}\,(\boldsymbol{G}(\boldsymbol{S}) - \boldsymbol{G}(\boldsymbol{\rho})) \xrightarrow{d} \mathcal{N}_{dp}(\boldsymbol{0}, \boldsymbol{G}\boldsymbol{C}\boldsymbol{\mathcal{K}}\boldsymbol{C}^\top\boldsymbol{G}^\top)$, where $\boldsymbol{G} = \boldsymbol{G}(\boldsymbol{\rho}) = \operatorname{diag}(\boldsymbol{G}_1(\boldsymbol{\rho}_1), \ldots, \boldsymbol{G}_d(\boldsymbol{\rho}_d))$ and $\boldsymbol{G}\boldsymbol{C} = \operatorname{diag}(\boldsymbol{G}_1\boldsymbol{C}_1, \ldots, \boldsymbol{G}_d\boldsymbol{C}_d)$, concluding the proof. □

Example 3 For $p = 4$, we have

$$\boldsymbol{G}_k\boldsymbol{C}_k = \begin{pmatrix} 1 & 0 & 0 & 0 \\ 0 & 1 & 0 & 0 \\ -\frac{3}{\kappa_{k2}^{1/2}} & -\frac{3}{2}\frac{\rho_{k3}}{\kappa_{k2}} & \frac{1}{\kappa_{k2}^{3/2}} & 0 \\ -\frac{4\rho_{k3}}{\kappa_{k2}^{1/2}} & -\frac{2\rho_{k4}}{\kappa_{k2}} & 0 & \frac{1}{\kappa_{k2}^{2}} \end{pmatrix}.$$

Hence, as in Example 2, if $\kappa_{k8} < \infty$, then for all $k = 1, \ldots, d$,

$$\sqrt{n}\begin{pmatrix} \bar{X}_k - \mu_k \\ S_{k2} - \kappa_{k2} \\ R_{k3} - \rho_{k3} \\ R_{k4} - \rho_{k4} \end{pmatrix} \xrightarrow{d} \mathcal{N}_4\left(\begin{pmatrix} 0 \\ 0 \\ 0 \\ 0 \end{pmatrix}, \begin{pmatrix} \upsilon_{k,11} & \upsilon_{k,12} & \upsilon_{k,13} & \upsilon_{k,14} \\ \upsilon_{k,21} & \upsilon_{k,22} & \upsilon_{k,23} & \upsilon_{k,24} \\ \upsilon_{k,31} & \upsilon_{k,32} & \upsilon_{k,33} & \upsilon_{k,34} \\ \upsilon_{k,41} & \upsilon_{k,42} & \upsilon_{k,43} & \upsilon_{k,44} \end{pmatrix}\right),$$

where $\upsilon_{k,ij} = \upsilon_{k,ji}$ and $\upsilon_{k,ii} = \upsilon_{k,i}^2$, with

$$\upsilon_{k,11} = \tau_{k,11} = \sigma_k^2,$$

(continued)

Example 3 (continued)

$$\upsilon_{k,12} = \tau_{k,12} = \sigma_k^3 \rho_{k3},$$

$$\upsilon_{k,13} = \sigma_k(-3 - 3\rho_{k3}^2/2 + \rho_{k4}),$$

$$\upsilon_{k,14} = \sigma_k(-4\rho_{k3} - 2\rho_{k3}\rho_{k4} + \rho_{k5}),$$

$$\upsilon_{k,22} = \sigma_k^4(\rho_{k4} - 1),$$

$$\upsilon_{k,23} = -(\sigma_k^2/2)\{\rho_{k3}(5 + 3\rho_{k4}) - 2\rho_{k5}\},$$

$$\upsilon_{k,24} = \sigma_k^2(-4\rho_{k3}^2 + \rho_{k4} - 2\rho_{k4}^2 + \rho_{k6}),$$

$$\upsilon_{k,33} = 9 - 6\rho_{k4} + (\rho_{k3}^2/4)(35 + 9\rho_{k4}) - 3\rho_{k3}\rho_{k5} + \rho_{k6},$$

$$\upsilon_{k,34} = 6\rho_{k3}^3 - (3 + 2\rho_{k4})\rho_{k5} + (3\rho_{k3}/2)(8 + \rho_{k4} + 2\rho_{k4}^2 - \rho_{k6}) + \rho_{k7},$$

$$\upsilon_{k,44} = -\rho_{k4}^2 + 4\rho_{k4}^3 + 16\rho_{k3}^2(1 + \rho_{k4}) - 8\rho_{k3}\rho_{k5} - 4\rho_{k4}\rho_{k6} + \rho_{k8}.$$

In this paper, we developed all the calculations considering S_{k2}, i.e., the second sample central moment (the sample variance). Pewsey (2005), on the other hand, built his results with $S_k = \sqrt{S_{k2}}$, the sample standard deviation, and only for the univariate case. Therefore, Example 3 corresponds to Pewsey's result, if $k = 1$, and we make use of another Jacobian matrix $\boldsymbol{P}_k$:

$$\boldsymbol{P}_k = \begin{pmatrix} 1 & 0 & 0 & 0 \\ 0 & \frac{1}{2\kappa_{k2}^{1/2}} & 0 & 0 \\ 0 & 0 & 1 & 0 \\ 0 & 0 & 0 & 1 \end{pmatrix}.$$

Hence, the variance–covariance matrix for the asymptotic distribution for the kth marginal univariate example, considering Pewsey's approach, is given by the expression $\boldsymbol{P}_k(\boldsymbol{G}_k\boldsymbol{C}_k\mathcal{K}\boldsymbol{C}_k^\top\boldsymbol{G}_k^\top)\boldsymbol{P}_k^\top$.

With Proposition 3, we derive the following corollary:

Corollary 1 *Let* $\boldsymbol{R}_{3\cdot} = (R_{31}, \ldots, R_{3d})^\top$ *and* $\boldsymbol{\rho}_{3\cdot} = (\rho_{31}, \ldots, \rho_{3d})^\top$. *Under the conditions of Proposition 3, we have*

$$\sqrt{n}\,(\boldsymbol{R}_{3\cdot} - \boldsymbol{\rho}_{3\cdot}) \xrightarrow{d} \mathcal{N}_d(\boldsymbol{0}, \boldsymbol{\Upsilon}_3),$$

where

$$\boldsymbol{\Upsilon}_3 = (\boldsymbol{I}_d \otimes \boldsymbol{e}_3^\top)\boldsymbol{G}\boldsymbol{C}\mathcal{K}\boldsymbol{C}^\top\boldsymbol{G}^\top(\boldsymbol{I}_d \otimes \boldsymbol{e}_3),$$

with $\boldsymbol{e}_3 = (0, 0, 1, 0, \ldots, 0)^\top \in \mathbb{R}^p$, *i.e.,* $\boldsymbol{\Upsilon}_3$ *has entries* $\upsilon_{kl}^{\{3\}}$, $k, l = 1, \ldots, d$, *given by*

$$\upsilon_{kl}^{\{3\}} = \boldsymbol{e}_3^\top \boldsymbol{G}_k \boldsymbol{C}_k \mathcal{K}_{kl} \boldsymbol{C}_l^\top \boldsymbol{G}_l^\top \boldsymbol{e}_3 = \left(-\frac{3}{\kappa_{k2}^{1/2}}, -\frac{3\rho_{k3}}{2\kappa_{k2}}, \frac{1}{\kappa_{k2}^{3/2}}, 0, \ldots, 0\right)$$

$$\times \begin{pmatrix} \kappa_{kl,11} - \kappa_{k1}\kappa_{l1} & \kappa_{kl,12} - \kappa_{k1}\kappa_{l2} & \kappa_{kl,13} - \kappa_{k1}\kappa_{l3} & \cdots & \kappa_{kl,1p} - \kappa_{k1}\kappa_{lp} \\ \kappa_{kl,21} - \kappa_{k2}\kappa_{l1} & \kappa_{kl,22} - \kappa_{k2}\kappa_{l2} & \kappa_{kl,23} - \kappa_{k2}\kappa_{l3} & \cdots & \kappa_{kl,2p} - \kappa_{k2}\kappa_{lp} \\ \kappa_{kl,31} - \kappa_{k3}\kappa_{l1} & \kappa_{kl,32} - \kappa_{k3}\kappa_{l2} & \kappa_{kl,33} - \kappa_{k3}\kappa_{l3} & \cdots & \kappa_{kl,3p} - \kappa_{k3}\kappa_{lp} \\ \vdots & \vdots & \vdots & \ddots & \vdots \\ \kappa_{kl,p1} - \kappa_{kp}\kappa_{l1} & \kappa_{kl,p2} - \kappa_{kp}\kappa_{l2} & \kappa_{kl,p3} - \kappa_{kp}\kappa_{l3} & \cdots & \kappa_{kl,pp} - \kappa_{kp}\kappa_{lp} \end{pmatrix} \begin{pmatrix} -\frac{3}{\kappa_{l2}^{1/2}} \\ -\frac{3\rho_{l3}}{2\kappa_{l2}} \\ \frac{1}{\kappa_{l2}^{3/2}} \\ 0 \\ \vdots \\ 0 \end{pmatrix}$$

$$\begin{aligned} &= 9\bar{\rho}_{kl,11} + \frac{9}{2}(\rho_{l3}\bar{\rho}_{kl,12} + \rho_{k3}\bar{\rho}_{kl,21}) + \frac{9}{4}\rho_{k3}\rho_{l3}\bar{\rho}_{kl,22} - 3(\bar{\rho}_{kl,13} + \bar{\rho}_{kl,31}) \\ &\quad - \frac{3}{2}(\rho_{k3}\bar{\rho}_{kl,23} + \rho_{l3}\bar{\rho}_{kl,32}) + \bar{\rho}_{kl,33} \\ &= 9\rho_{kl,11} + \frac{9}{2}(\rho_{l3}\rho_{kl,12} + \rho_{k3}\rho_{kl,21}) \\ &\quad + \frac{9}{4}\rho_{k3}\rho_{l3}(\rho_{kl,22} - \rho_{k2}\rho_{l2}) - 3(\rho_{kl,13} + \rho_{kl,31}) \\ &\quad - \frac{3}{2}\{\rho_{k3}(\rho_{kl,23} - \rho_{k2}\rho_{l3}) + \rho_{l3}(\rho_{kl,32} - \rho_{k3}\rho_{l2})\} + \rho_{kl,33} - \rho_{k3}\rho_{l3}. \end{aligned}$$

In particular,

$$\sqrt{n}\,(R_{k3} - \rho_{k3}) \xrightarrow{d} \mathcal{N}(0, \upsilon_{kk}^{\{3\}}), \quad k = 1, \ldots, d,$$

with

$$\begin{aligned} \upsilon_{kk}^{\{3\}} &= 9\bar{\rho}_{kk,11} + \frac{9}{2}(\rho_{l3}\bar{\rho}_{kk,12} + \rho_{k3}\bar{\rho}_{kk,21}) + \frac{9}{4}\rho_{k3}^2\bar{\rho}_{kk,22} - 3(\bar{\rho}_{kk,13} + \bar{\rho}_{kk,31}) \\ &\quad - \frac{3}{2}\rho_{k3}(\bar{\rho}_{kk,23} + \bar{\rho}_{kk,32}) + \bar{\rho}_{kl,33} \\ &= 9 - 6\rho_{k4} + \frac{1}{4}\rho_{k3}^2(35 + 9\rho_{k4}) - 3\rho_{k3}\rho_{k5} + \rho_{k6}. \end{aligned}$$

Example 4 For symmetric distributions, we have $\rho_{k5} = \rho_{k3} = \rho_{k1} = 0$. Therefore,

$$\sqrt{n}\, R_{k3} \xrightarrow{d} \mathcal{N}(0, 9 - 6\rho_{k4} + \rho_{k6}), \quad k = 1, \ldots, d,$$

where $\rho_{kr} = \frac{\kappa_{kr}}{\kappa_{k2}^{r/2}}$. For the normal model, $9 - 6\rho_{k4} + \rho_{k6} = 9 - 6 \times 3 + 15 = 6$, so

$$\sqrt{n}\, R_{k3} \xrightarrow{d} \mathcal{N}(0, 6), \quad k = 1, \ldots, d.$$

Focusing on the fourth standardized sample central moment, we derive the next corollary:

Corollary 2 *Let* $\boldsymbol{R}_{4\cdot} = (R_{41}, \ldots, R_{4d})^\top$ *and* $\boldsymbol{\rho}_{4\cdot} = (\rho_{41}, \ldots, \rho_{4d})^\top$. *Under the conditions of Proposition 3, we have*

$$\sqrt{n}\,(\boldsymbol{R}_{4\cdot} - \boldsymbol{\rho}_{4\cdot}) \xrightarrow{d} \mathcal{N}_d(\boldsymbol{0}, \boldsymbol{\Upsilon}_4),$$

where

$$\boldsymbol{\Upsilon}_4 = (\boldsymbol{I}_d \otimes \boldsymbol{e}_4^\top)\boldsymbol{G}\boldsymbol{C}\mathcal{K}\boldsymbol{C}^\top\boldsymbol{G}^\top(\boldsymbol{I}_d \otimes \boldsymbol{e}_4),$$

with $\boldsymbol{e}_4 = (0, 0, 1, 0, \ldots, 0)^\top \in \mathbb{R}^p$, *i.e.,* $\boldsymbol{\Upsilon}_4$ *has entries* $\upsilon_{kl}^{\{4\}}$, $k, l = 1, \ldots, d$, *given by*

$$\upsilon_{kl}^{\{4\}} = \boldsymbol{e}_4^\top \boldsymbol{G}_k \boldsymbol{C}_k \mathcal{K}_{kl} \boldsymbol{C}_l^\top \boldsymbol{G}_l^\top \boldsymbol{e}_4 = \left(-\frac{4\rho_{k3}}{\kappa_{k2}^{1/2}},\, -\frac{2\rho_{k4}}{\kappa_{k2}},\, 0,\, \frac{1}{\kappa_{k2}^2},\, 0,\, \ldots,\, 0\right)$$

$$\times \begin{pmatrix} \kappa_{kl,11} - \kappa_{k1}\kappa_{l1} & \kappa_{kl,12} - \kappa_{k1}\kappa_{l2} & \kappa_{kl,13} - \kappa_{k1}\kappa_{l3} & \cdots & \kappa_{kl,1p} - \kappa_{k1}\kappa_{lp} \\ \kappa_{kl,21} - \kappa_{k2}\kappa_{l1} & \kappa_{kl,22} - \kappa_{k2}\kappa_{l2} & \kappa_{kl,23} - \kappa_{k2}\kappa_{l3} & \cdots & \kappa_{kl,2p} - \kappa_{k2}\kappa_{lp} \\ \kappa_{kl,31} - \kappa_{k3}\kappa_{l1} & \kappa_{kl,32} - \kappa_{k3}\kappa_{l2} & \kappa_{kl,33} - \kappa_{k3}\kappa_{l3} & \cdots & \kappa_{kl,3p} - \kappa_{k3}\kappa_{lp} \\ \kappa_{kl,41} - \kappa_{k4}\kappa_{l1} & \kappa_{kl,42} - \kappa_{k4}\kappa_{l2} & \kappa_{kl,43} - \kappa_{k4}\kappa_{l3} & \cdots & \kappa_{kl,4p} - \kappa_{k4}\kappa_{lp} \\ \vdots & \vdots & \vdots & \ldots & \vdots \\ \kappa_{kl,p1} - \kappa_{kp}\kappa_{l1} & \kappa_{kl,p2} - \kappa_{kp}\kappa_{l2} & \kappa_{kl,p3} - \kappa_{kp}\kappa_{l3} & \cdots & \kappa_{kl,pp} - \kappa_{kp}\kappa_{lp} \end{pmatrix} \begin{pmatrix} -\frac{4\rho_{l3}}{\kappa_{l2}^{1/2}} \\ -\frac{2\rho_{l4}}{\kappa_{l2}} \\ 0 \\ \frac{1}{\kappa_{l2}^2} \\ 0 \\ \vdots \\ 0 \end{pmatrix}$$

$$= \bar{\rho}_{kl,44} - 4\bar{\rho}_{kl,41}\rho_{l3} - 2\bar{\rho}_{kl,42}\rho_{l4} - 4\rho_{k3}(\bar{\rho}_{kl,14} - 4\bar{\rho}_{kl,11}\rho_{l3} - 2\bar{\rho}_{kl,12}\rho_{l4})$$
$$+\rho_{k4}(-2\bar{\rho}_{kl,24} + 8\bar{\rho}_{kl,21}\rho_{l3} + 4\bar{\rho}_{kl,22}\rho_{l4}).$$

In particular,

$$\sqrt{n}\,(R_{k4} - \rho_{k4}) \xrightarrow{d} \mathcal{N}(0, \upsilon_{kk}^{\{4\}}), \quad k = 1, \ldots, d,$$

with

$$\begin{aligned}
\upsilon_{kk}^{\{4\}} &= \bar{\rho}_{kk,44} - 4\bar{\rho}_{kk,41}\rho_{k3} - 2\bar{\rho}_{kk,42}\rho_{k4} - 4\rho_{k3}(\bar{\rho}_{kk,14} - 4\bar{\rho}_{kk,11}\rho_{k3} - 2\bar{\rho}_{kk,12}\rho_{k4}) \\
&\quad + \rho_{k4}(-2\bar{\rho}_{kk,24} + 8\bar{\rho}_{kk,21}\rho_{k3} + 4\bar{\rho}_{kk,22}\rho_{k4}) \\
&= \rho_{kk,44} - \rho_{k4}^2 - 4\rho_{k5}\rho_{k3} - 2(\rho_{k6} - \rho_{k4})\rho_{k4} - 4\rho_{k3}(\rho_{k4} - 4\rho_{k3} - 2\rho_{k3}\rho_{k4}) \\
&\quad + \rho_{k4}\{-2(\rho_{k6} - \rho_{k4}) + 8\rho_{k3}^2 + 4(\rho_{k4} - 1)\rho_{k4}\} \\
&= -\rho_{k4}^2 + 4\rho_{k4}^3 + 16\rho_{k3}^2(1 + \rho_{k4}) - 8\rho_{k3}\rho_{k5} - 4\rho_{k4}\rho_{k6} + \rho_{k8}.
\end{aligned}$$

Example 5 When working with symmetric distributions, we have $\rho_{k5} = \rho_{k3} = \rho_{k1} = 0$.
Therefore,

$$\sqrt{n}\,R_{k4} \xrightarrow{d} \mathcal{N}\Big(0, -\rho_{k4}^2 + 4\rho_{k4}^3 - 4\rho_{k4}\rho_{k6} + \rho_{k8}\Big), \quad k = 1, \ldots, d.$$

For the standard normal model, we have $\rho_{k4} = 3$, $\rho_{k6} = 15$, $\rho_{k8} = 108$, and

$$-\rho_{k4}^2 + 4\rho_{k4}^3 - 4\rho_{k4}\rho_{k6} + \rho_{k8} = -9 + 108 - 180 + 105 = 24$$

so $\sqrt{n}\,R_{k4} \xrightarrow{d} \mathcal{N}(0, 24)$, $k = 1, \ldots, d$.

4 Application to Multivariate Elliptical Distributions

In this section, we apply the previous results to a d-dimensional elliptical random vector $\boldsymbol{X} \sim El_d(\boldsymbol{\mu}, \boldsymbol{\Omega}; h)$ with the density function $|\boldsymbol{\Omega}|^{-1/2}h\{(\boldsymbol{x}-\boldsymbol{\mu})^\top\boldsymbol{\Omega}^{-1}(\boldsymbol{x}-\boldsymbol{\mu})\}$, where $\boldsymbol{\mu}$ is a $d \times 1$ location vector, $\boldsymbol{\Omega}$ is a $d \times d$ positive definite scale matrix, and h is the density generator function.

The central moments of $\boldsymbol{X}$ can be obtained from the moments of R and $\boldsymbol{U}$ because $\boldsymbol{X} - \boldsymbol{\mu} = R\,\boldsymbol{\Omega}^{1/2}\boldsymbol{U}$, where R and $\boldsymbol{U}$ are independent random quantities, with $R \stackrel{d}{=} \|\boldsymbol{Z}\|$, a radial variable, and $\boldsymbol{U} \stackrel{d}{=} \frac{\boldsymbol{Z}}{\|\boldsymbol{Z}\|}$, a uniform vector on the unit sphere $\{\boldsymbol{x} \in \mathbb{R}^d : \|\boldsymbol{x}\| = 1\}$, where $\boldsymbol{Z} = \boldsymbol{\Omega}^{-1/2}(\boldsymbol{X} - \boldsymbol{\mu})$ is the spherical version of $\boldsymbol{X}$. The existence of these moments depends on the existence of the associated moments of R. For instance, as we know,

- if $\mathbb{E}(R) < \infty$, then $\mathbb{E}(\boldsymbol{X}) = \boldsymbol{\mu}$, and
- if $\mathbb{E}(R) < \infty$, then $\text{Var}(\boldsymbol{X}) = \sigma_h^2 \boldsymbol{\Omega}$,

where $\sigma_h^2 = \frac{1}{d}\,\mathbb{E}(R^2)$ becomes the marginal variance induced by the density generator function h.

By symmetry, the odd moments of $\boldsymbol{X} - \boldsymbol{\mu}$ are zero, and its even moments can be computed using the results in Berkane and Bentler (1986); see also Lemmas 1 and 2 in Maruyama and Seo (2003). Thus, for $r + s = 2m$ (even), we have

$$\kappa_{kl,rs} = \mathbb{E}\left\{(X_k - \mu_k)^r (X_l - \mu_l)^s\right\} = (\kappa_{(m)} + 1)\nu_{2m}\sigma_{kl}^m, \quad k, l = 1, \dots, d,$$

where $\sigma_{kl} = \text{Cov}(X_k, X_l) = \sigma_h^2 \omega_{kl}$ becomes $\kappa_{kl,11}$, $\nu_{2m} = \frac{(2m)!}{2^m m!}$ is the $(2m)$th moment of $Z \sim \mathcal{N}(0, 1)$, and $\kappa_{(m)} + 1 = \frac{d^m}{d_{(m)}} \frac{\mathbb{E}(R^{2m})}{(\mathbb{E}(R^2))^m}$, with $d_{(m)} = d(d + 2) \cdots (d - 2(m - 1))$ being the mth moment of the chi-square distribution with d degrees of freedom. We note that $\kappa_{(1)} = 0$ and $\kappa_{(2)} = \kappa$ is the kurtosis parameter, which is related to the multivariate kurtosis index of Mardia (1970) of $\boldsymbol{X} \sim El_d(\boldsymbol{\mu}, \boldsymbol{\Omega}; h)$. The $\mathcal{K}_{kl}$ matrix for elliptical distributions can be simplified due to symmetry, which makes the odd central moments equal to zero. As mentioned before, this result implies asymptotic independence between the even and odd sample central moments. The $\mathcal{K}_{kl}$ matrix is given by

$$\mathcal{K}_{kl} = \begin{pmatrix} \kappa_{kl,11} & 0 & \kappa_{kl,13} & 0 & \cdots \\ 0 & \kappa_{kl,22} - \kappa_{k2}\kappa_{l2} & 0 & \kappa_{kl,24} - \kappa_{k2}\kappa_{l4} & \cdots \\ \kappa_{kl,31} & 0 & \kappa_{kl,33} & 0 & \cdots \\ 0 & \kappa_{kl,42} - \kappa_{k4}\kappa_{l2} & 0 & \kappa_{kl,44} - \kappa_{k4}\kappa_{l4} & \cdots \\ \vdots & \vdots & \vdots & \vdots & \cdots \end{pmatrix}.$$

That is, if $r + s = 2m$ (even) and r and s are odd, then the elements of $\mathcal{K}_{kl}$ are $\kappa_{kl,rs}$; if $r+s = 2m$ (even) and r and s are also even, then the elements of $\mathcal{K}_{kl}$ are of the form $\kappa_{kl,rs} - \kappa_{kr}\kappa_{ls}$. When $r + s = 2m - 1$ (odd), then the element in row r and column s of $\mathcal{K}_{kl}$ is zero. If $p = 4$ and we are interested in $\mathcal{K}_{kk}$, then the expression reduces to the following, as $\kappa_{kk,rs} = \kappa_{k,r+s}$:

$$\mathcal{K}_{kk} = \begin{pmatrix} \kappa_{k2} & 0 & \kappa_{k4} & 0 \\ 0 & \kappa_{k4} - \kappa_{k2}^2 & 0 & \kappa_{k6} - \kappa_{k2}\kappa_{k4} \\ \kappa_{k4} & 0 & \kappa_{k6} & 0 \\ 0 & \kappa_{k6} - \kappa_{k4}\kappa_{k2} & 0 & \kappa_{k8} - \kappa_{k4}^2 \end{pmatrix}.$$

Therefore, we see that there is independence between the pairs X_k and S_{k2} and R_{k3} and R_{k4}. Also, by Proposition 3, we have

$$\sqrt{n}(\boldsymbol{R}_k - \boldsymbol{\rho}_k) \xrightarrow{d} \mathcal{N}_p(\boldsymbol{0}, \boldsymbol{G}_k \boldsymbol{C}_k \mathcal{K}_{kk} \boldsymbol{C}_k^\top \boldsymbol{G}_k^\top), \quad k = 1, \dots, d.$$

For elliptical distributions, with $\kappa_{k8} < \infty$, for all $k = 1, \ldots, d$,

$$\boldsymbol{G}_k \boldsymbol{C}_k \mathcal{K}_{kk} \boldsymbol{C}_k^\top \boldsymbol{G}_k^\top = \begin{pmatrix} \upsilon_{k,11} & 0 & \upsilon_{k,13} & 0 \\ 0 & \upsilon_{k,22} & 0 & \upsilon_{k,24} \\ \upsilon_{k,31} & 0 & \upsilon_{k,33} & 0 \\ 0 & \upsilon_{k,42} & 0 & \upsilon_{k,44} \end{pmatrix},$$

where $\upsilon_{ij} = \upsilon_{ji}$, and

$$\begin{aligned}
\upsilon_{k,11} &= \kappa_{k2}, \\
\upsilon_{k,13} &= \frac{-3\kappa_{k2}^2 + \kappa_{k4}}{\kappa_{k2}^{(3/2)}}, \\
\upsilon_{k,22} &= -\kappa_{k2}^2 + \kappa_{k4}, \\
\upsilon_{k,24} &= \frac{\kappa_{k2}^2\kappa_{k4} - 2\kappa_{k4}^2 + \kappa_{k2}\kappa_{k6}}{\kappa_{k2}^3}, \\
\upsilon_{k,33} &= 9 - \frac{6\kappa_{k4}}{\kappa_{k2}^2} + \frac{\kappa_{k6}}{\kappa_{k2}^3}, \\
\upsilon_{k,44} &= \frac{4\kappa_{k4}^3 - 4\kappa_{k2}\kappa_{k4}\kappa_{k6} + \kappa_{k2}^2(-\kappa_{k4}^2 + \kappa_{k8})}{\kappa_{k2}^6}.
\end{aligned}$$

Using the formula for computing $\kappa_{kl,rs}$, we have the following elements:

$$\begin{aligned}
\upsilon_{k,11} &= \sigma_{kk} = \sigma_h^2 \omega_{kk}, \\
\upsilon_{k,13} &= 3\kappa_{(2)}\sigma_h \omega_{kk}^{(1/2)}, \\
\upsilon_{k,22} &= (2 + 3\kappa_{(2)})\sigma_h^4 \omega_{kk}^2, \\
\upsilon_{k,24} &= -3(11\kappa_{(2)} + 6\kappa_{(2)}^2 - 5\kappa_{(3)})\sigma_h^2 \omega_{kk}, \\
\upsilon_{k,33} &= 6 - 18\kappa_{(2)} + 15\kappa_{(3)}, \\
\upsilon_{k,44} &= 3(8 + 105\kappa_{(2)}^2 + 36\kappa_{(2)}^3 + \kappa_{(2)}(42 - 60\kappa_{(3)}) - 60\kappa_{(3)} + 35\kappa_{(4)}).
\end{aligned}$$

For the multivariate normal distribution, according to Maruyama and Seo (2003), $\kappa_{(i)} = 0$, $i = 2, 3, 4$. Considering the standard normal distribution, $\sigma_h^2 = \omega_{kk} = 1$, $\upsilon_{k,11} = 1$, $\upsilon_{k,13} = 0$, $\upsilon_{k,22} = 2$, $\upsilon_{k,24} = 0$, $\upsilon_{k,33} = 6$, and $\upsilon_{k,44} = 24$. For other elliptical distributions, the values for the asymptotic variance–covariance matrix depend on the computation of σ_h^2 and $\kappa_{(i)}$, $i = 2, 3, 4$. For a multivariate Student-t distribution, we have $\sigma_h^2 = \frac{\nu}{\nu-2}$, $\kappa_{(2)} = \frac{2}{\nu-4}$, $\kappa_{(3)} = \frac{6\nu-20}{(\nu-6)(\nu-4)}$ and $\kappa_{(4)} = \frac{12\nu^2-92\nu+184}{(\nu-8)(\nu-6)(\nu-4)}$.

5 Application to Multivariate Skew-Normal Distributions

In this section, we apply the previous results to the multivariate skew-normal distributions of Azzalini and Dalla Valle (1996); see also the books by Genton (2004) and Azzalini and Capitanio (2014). We let $\boldsymbol{X} \sim \mathcal{SN}_d(\boldsymbol{\xi}, \boldsymbol{\Omega}, \boldsymbol{\alpha})$, with the density given by $2\phi_d(\boldsymbol{x} - \boldsymbol{\xi}; \boldsymbol{\Omega})\Phi\{\boldsymbol{\alpha}^\top \boldsymbol{\omega}^{-1}(\boldsymbol{x} - \boldsymbol{\xi})\}, \boldsymbol{x} \in \mathbb{R}^d$, where $\phi_d(\boldsymbol{x}; \boldsymbol{\Omega})$ is the pdf of the $\mathcal{N}_d(\boldsymbol{0}, \boldsymbol{\Omega})$ distribution, and $\Phi(\cdot)$ is the cdf of the univariate standard normal distribution. We know that $\boldsymbol{\mu} = \mathbb{E}(\boldsymbol{X}) = \boldsymbol{\xi} + \boldsymbol{\mu}_0$ and $\boldsymbol{\Sigma} = \mathrm{Var}(\boldsymbol{X}) = \boldsymbol{\Omega} - \boldsymbol{\mu}_0\boldsymbol{\mu}_0^\top$, where $\boldsymbol{\mu}_0 = \mathbb{E}(\boldsymbol{X} - \boldsymbol{\xi}) = \sqrt{2/\pi}\,\boldsymbol{\omega\delta}$, $\boldsymbol{\delta} = \bar{\boldsymbol{\Omega}}\boldsymbol{\alpha}/\sqrt{1 + \boldsymbol{\alpha}^\top \bar{\boldsymbol{\Omega}}\boldsymbol{\alpha}}$, $\bar{\boldsymbol{\Omega}} = \boldsymbol{\omega}^{-1}\boldsymbol{\Omega}\boldsymbol{\omega}^{-1}$, and $\boldsymbol{\omega} = \mathrm{diag}(\boldsymbol{\Omega})^{1/2} = \boldsymbol{\sigma}\{\boldsymbol{I}_d + \mathrm{diag}(\bar{\boldsymbol{\mu}}_0\bar{\boldsymbol{\mu}}_0^\top)\}^{1/2}$, with $\bar{\boldsymbol{\mu}}_0 = \boldsymbol{\sigma}^{-1}\boldsymbol{\mu}_0$ and $\boldsymbol{\sigma} = \mathrm{diag}(\boldsymbol{\Sigma})^{1/2}$.

Here, for any $d \times d$ matrix $\boldsymbol{A} = (a_{ij}) \geq 0$, $\mathrm{diag}(\boldsymbol{A})^{1/2}$ is the diagonal matrix whose diagonal elements are $a_{11}^{1/2}, \ldots, a_{dd}^{1/2}$. We know that

$$\boldsymbol{\alpha} = \frac{\sqrt{\pi/2}\,\boldsymbol{\omega\sigma}^{-1}\bar{\boldsymbol{\Sigma}}^{-1}\bar{\boldsymbol{\mu}}_0}{\sqrt{(1 + \beta_0^2)\left\{1 + (1 - \pi/2)\beta_0^2\right\}}}, \qquad \beta_0^2 = \bar{\boldsymbol{\mu}}_0^\top \bar{\boldsymbol{\Sigma}}^{-1}\bar{\boldsymbol{\mu}}_0,$$

where $\bar{\boldsymbol{\Sigma}} = \boldsymbol{\sigma}^{-1}\boldsymbol{\Sigma}\boldsymbol{\sigma}^{-1}$ and $\boldsymbol{\omega\sigma}^{-1} = \boldsymbol{\sigma}^{-1}\boldsymbol{\omega} = \{\boldsymbol{I}_d + \mathrm{diag}(\bar{\boldsymbol{\mu}}_0\bar{\boldsymbol{\mu}}_0^\top)\}^{1/2}$.

We let $\boldsymbol{Z} = \boldsymbol{\sigma}^{-1}(\boldsymbol{X} - \boldsymbol{\mu}) = \boldsymbol{\sigma}^{-1}(\boldsymbol{X}_0 - \boldsymbol{\mu}_0)$, where $\boldsymbol{X}_0 = \boldsymbol{X} - \boldsymbol{\xi}$. Its density and moment-generating functions are, respectively, given by

$$f_{\boldsymbol{Z}}(\boldsymbol{z}) = 2\phi_d\left(\boldsymbol{z} + \bar{\boldsymbol{\mu}}_0; \bar{\boldsymbol{\Sigma}} + \bar{\boldsymbol{\mu}}_0\bar{\boldsymbol{\mu}}_0^\top\right)\Phi\left\{\boldsymbol{\alpha}^\top\boldsymbol{\omega}^{-1}\boldsymbol{\sigma}(\boldsymbol{z} + \bar{\boldsymbol{\mu}}_0)\right\}, \quad \boldsymbol{z} \in \mathbb{R}^d,$$

and

$$M_{\boldsymbol{Z}}(\boldsymbol{t}) = 2e^{-\boldsymbol{t}^\top\bar{\boldsymbol{\mu}}_0 + \frac{1}{2}\boldsymbol{t}^\top\left(\bar{\boldsymbol{\Sigma}} + \bar{\boldsymbol{\mu}}_0\bar{\boldsymbol{\mu}}_0^\top\right)\boldsymbol{t}}\,\Phi\left(\boldsymbol{t}^\top\boldsymbol{\sigma}^{-1}\boldsymbol{\omega\delta}\right), \quad \boldsymbol{t} \in \mathbb{R}^d,$$

where $\boldsymbol{\omega}^{-1}\boldsymbol{\sigma} = \left\{\boldsymbol{I}_d + \mathrm{diag}(\bar{\boldsymbol{\mu}}_0\boldsymbol{\mu}_0^\top)\right\}^{-1/2} = \mathrm{diag}\left(\bar{\boldsymbol{\Sigma}} + \bar{\boldsymbol{\mu}}_0\bar{\boldsymbol{\mu}}_0^\top\right)^{-1/2}$ and $\boldsymbol{\sigma}^{-1}\boldsymbol{\omega\delta} = \sqrt{\frac{\pi}{2}}\,\bar{\boldsymbol{\mu}}_0$.

Hence, we obtain

$$\boldsymbol{Z} \sim \mathcal{SN}_d\left(-\bar{\boldsymbol{\mu}}_0, \bar{\boldsymbol{\Sigma}} + \bar{\boldsymbol{\mu}}_0\bar{\boldsymbol{\mu}}_0^\top, \boldsymbol{\alpha}\right), \boldsymbol{\alpha} = \frac{\sqrt{\pi/2}\left\{\boldsymbol{I}_d + \mathrm{diag}(\bar{\boldsymbol{\mu}}_0\bar{\boldsymbol{\mu}}_0^\top)\right\}^{1/2}\bar{\boldsymbol{\Sigma}}^{-1}\bar{\boldsymbol{\mu}}_0}{\sqrt{(1 + \beta_0^2)\left\{1 + (1 - \pi/2)\beta_0^2\right\}}},$$

$$\Longrightarrow \boldsymbol{X} = \boldsymbol{\mu} + \boldsymbol{\sigma Z} \sim \mathcal{SN}_d(\boldsymbol{\mu} - \boldsymbol{\mu}_0, \boldsymbol{\Sigma} + \boldsymbol{\mu}_0\boldsymbol{\mu}_0^\top, \boldsymbol{\alpha}).$$

Moreover, $\boldsymbol{Z}$ has univariate and bivariate marginals given by

$$Z_k = \boldsymbol{e}_k^\top \boldsymbol{Z} \sim \mathcal{SN}_1\left(-\bar{\mu}_{0k}, 1+\bar{\mu}_{0k}^2, \frac{\sqrt{\pi/2}\,\bar{\mu}_{0k}}{\sqrt{1+(1-\pi/2)\bar{\mu}_{0k}^2}}\right), \quad k=1,\ldots,d,$$

and

$$\begin{pmatrix} Z_k \\ Z_l \end{pmatrix} \sim \mathcal{SN}_2\left(\begin{pmatrix} -\bar{\mu}_{0k} \\ -\bar{\mu}_{0l} \end{pmatrix}, \begin{pmatrix} 1+\bar{\mu}_{0k}^2 & \bar{\sigma}_{kl}+\bar{\mu}_{0k}\bar{\mu}_{0l} \\ \bar{\sigma}_{kl}+\bar{\mu}_{0k}\bar{\mu}_{0l} & 1+\bar{\mu}_{0l}^2 \end{pmatrix}, \begin{pmatrix} \alpha_k' \\ \alpha_l' \end{pmatrix}\right),$$

where $\bar{\boldsymbol{\Sigma}} = (\bar{\sigma}_{kl})$, with $\bar{\sigma}_{kk} = 1$. To identify the skewness parameters $(\alpha_k', \alpha_l')^\top$, we use the fact that for a $d_B \times d$ matrix $\boldsymbol{B}$ of rank d_B, $\boldsymbol{BZ} \sim \mathcal{SN}_{d_B}(\boldsymbol{B}\bar{\boldsymbol{\mu}}_0, \boldsymbol{B}\bar{\boldsymbol{\Sigma}} + \boldsymbol{B}\bar{\boldsymbol{\mu}}_0\bar{\boldsymbol{\mu}}_0\boldsymbol{B}^\top, \boldsymbol{\alpha_B})$, with

$$\boldsymbol{\alpha_B} = \frac{\sqrt{\pi/2}\,\mathrm{diag}\left(\boldsymbol{B}\bar{\boldsymbol{\Sigma}}\boldsymbol{B}^\top + \boldsymbol{B}\bar{\boldsymbol{\mu}}_0\bar{\boldsymbol{\mu}}_0^\top\boldsymbol{B}^\top\right)^{1/2}\left(\boldsymbol{B}\bar{\boldsymbol{\Sigma}} + \boldsymbol{B}\bar{\boldsymbol{\mu}}_0\bar{\boldsymbol{\mu}}_0^\top\boldsymbol{B}^\top\right)^{-1}\boldsymbol{B}\bar{\boldsymbol{\mu}}_0}{\sqrt{1-(\pi/2)(\boldsymbol{B}\bar{\boldsymbol{\mu}}_0)^\top\left(\boldsymbol{B}\bar{\boldsymbol{\Sigma}} + \boldsymbol{B}\bar{\boldsymbol{\mu}}_0\bar{\boldsymbol{\mu}}_0^\top\boldsymbol{B}^\top\right)^{-1}\boldsymbol{B}\bar{\boldsymbol{\mu}}_0}},$$

and

$$\boldsymbol{\delta_B} = \sqrt{\pi/2}\,\mathrm{diag}\left(\boldsymbol{B}\bar{\boldsymbol{\Sigma}}\boldsymbol{B}^\top + \boldsymbol{B}\bar{\boldsymbol{\mu}}_0\bar{\boldsymbol{\mu}}_0^\top\boldsymbol{B}^\top\right)^{-1/2}\boldsymbol{B}\bar{\boldsymbol{\mu}}_0.$$

We also note that

$$M_{\boldsymbol{BZ}}(\boldsymbol{t}) = M_{\boldsymbol{Z}}(\boldsymbol{B}^\top\boldsymbol{t}) = 2e^{-\boldsymbol{t}^\top\bar{\boldsymbol{\mu}}_0+\frac{1}{2}\boldsymbol{t}^\top\left(\boldsymbol{B}\bar{\boldsymbol{\Sigma}}+\boldsymbol{B}\bar{\boldsymbol{\mu}}_0\bar{\boldsymbol{\mu}}_0^\top\boldsymbol{B}^\top\right)\boldsymbol{t}}\,\Phi\left(\sqrt{\pi/2}\,\boldsymbol{t}^\top\boldsymbol{B}\bar{\boldsymbol{\mu}}_0\right).$$

Thus, for $\boldsymbol{B} = (\boldsymbol{e}_k, \boldsymbol{e}_l)^\top$, we have

$$\boldsymbol{\alpha_B} = \begin{pmatrix} \alpha_k' \\ \alpha_l' \end{pmatrix} = \frac{1}{\sqrt{(1-\rho_{\boldsymbol{B}}^2)\{1-\rho_{\boldsymbol{B}}^2-(\delta_{0k}^2+\delta_{0l}^2-2\rho_{\boldsymbol{B}}\delta_{0k}\delta_{0l})\}}}\begin{pmatrix} \delta_{0k}-\rho_{\boldsymbol{B}}\delta_{0l} \\ \delta_{0l}-\rho_{\boldsymbol{B}}\delta_{0k} \end{pmatrix},$$

and $\boldsymbol{\delta_B} = (\delta_{0k}, \delta_{0l})^\top$, where

$$\delta_{0k} = \frac{\sqrt{\pi/2}\,\bar{\mu}_{0k}}{\sqrt{1+\bar{\mu}_{0k}^2}}, \quad \rho_{\boldsymbol{B}} = \frac{\bar{\sigma}_{kl}+\bar{\mu}_{0k}\bar{\mu}_{0l}}{\sqrt{(1+\bar{\mu}_{0k}^2)(1+\bar{\mu}_{0l}^2)}},$$

and

$$M_{Z_k,Z_l}(t_k,t_l) = 2\exp\left\{-t_k\bar{\mu}_{0k} - t_l\bar{\mu}_{0l} + \frac{1}{2}t_k^2\left(1+\bar{\mu}_{0k}^2\right) + \frac{1}{2}t_l^2\left(1+\bar{\mu}_{0l}^2\right)\right.$$

$$\left. + t_kt_l\left(\bar{\sigma}_{kl}+\bar{\mu}_{0k}\bar{\mu}_{0l}\right)\right\} \times \Phi\left\{\sqrt{\frac{\pi}{2}}\left(t_k\bar{\mu}_{0k}+t_l\bar{\mu}_{0l}\right)\right\}.$$

We compute $\rho_{kr}(Z_k) = \mathbb{E}(Z_k^r)$, $\rho_{kl,rs}(Z_k, Z_l) = \mathbb{E}(Z_k^r Z_l^s)$, and $\bar{\rho}_{kl,rs}(Z_k, Z_l) = \mathbb{E}(Z_k^r Z_l^s) - \mathbb{E}(Z_k^r)\mathbb{E}(Z_l^s) = \rho_{kl,rs}(Z_k, Z_l) - \rho_{kr}(Z_k)\rho_{lr}(Z_k)$.

Now, we let $M(t_k, t_l) = M_{Z_k,Z_l}(t_k, t_l)$, and the cumulant function

$$\begin{aligned} K(t_k, t_l) &= \log M(t_k, t_l) \\ &= -t_k\bar{\mu}_{0k} - t_l\bar{\mu}_{0l} + \frac{1}{2}t_k^2\left(1 + \bar{\mu}_{0k}^2\right) + \frac{1}{2}t_l^2\left(1 + \bar{\mu}_{0l}^2\right) \\ &\quad + t_k t_l\left(\bar{\sigma}_{kl} + \bar{\mu}_{0k}\bar{\mu}_{0l}\right) \\ &\quad + \log\left[2\Phi\left\{\sqrt{\frac{\pi}{2}}\left(t_k\bar{\mu}_{0k} + t_l\bar{\mu}_{0l}\right)\right\}\right]. \end{aligned}$$

We also denote the derivatives as follows:

$$M_k = \frac{\partial M}{\partial t_k}, \quad M_{kk} = \frac{\partial^2 M}{\partial t_k^2}, \quad M_{kl} = \frac{\partial^2 M}{\partial t_k \partial t_l}, \ldots,$$

and

$$K_k = \frac{\partial K}{\partial t_k}, \quad K_{kk} = \frac{\partial^2 K}{\partial t_k^2}, \quad K_{kl} = \frac{\partial^2 K}{\partial t_k \partial t_l}, \ldots.$$

Then, we have

$$\begin{aligned} M_k &= M K_k, \\ M_{kl} &= M_l K_k + M K_{kl}, \\ M_{kll} &= M_{ll} K_k + 2M_l K_{kl} + M K_{kll}, \\ M_{kkl} &= M_{kl} K_k + M_k K_{kl} + M_l K_{kk} + M K_{kkl}, \\ M_{kkkl} &= M_{kkl} K_k + 2M_{kl} K_{kk} + M_{kk} K_{kl} + 2M_k K_{kkl} + M_l K_{kkk} + M K_{kkkl}, \\ M_{kkll} &= M_{kll} K_k + 2M_{kl} K_{kl} + M_k K_{kll} + M_{ll} K_{kk} + 2M_l K_{kkl} + M K_{kkll}, \\ M_{klll} &= M_{lll} K_k + 3M_{ll} K_{kl} + 3M_l K_{kll} + M K_{klll}, \\ M_{kklll} &= M_{klll} K_k + 3M_{kll} K_{kl} + 3M_{kl} K_{kll} + M_k K_{klll} + M_{lll} K_{kk} \\ &\quad + 3M_{ll} K_{kkl} + 3M_l K_{kkll} + M K_{kklll}, \\ M_{kkkll} &= M_{kkll} K_k + 2M_{kll} K_{kk} + 2M_{kkl} K_{kl} + 4M_{kl} K_{kkl} + M_{kk} K_{kll} \\ &\quad + 2M_k K_{kkll} + M_{ll} K_{kkk} + 2M_l K_{kkkl} + M K_{kkkll}, \\ M_{kkklll} &= M_{kklll} K_k + 2M_{klll} K_{kk} + 3M_{kkll} K_{kl} + 6M_{kll} K_{kkl} + 3M_{kkl} K_{kll} \\ &\quad + 6M_{kl} K_{kkll} + M_{lll} K_{kkk} + 3M_{ll} K_{kkkl} + 3M_l K_{kkkll} + M_{kk} K_{klll} \\ &\quad + 2M_k K_{kklll} + M K_{kkklll}, \end{aligned}$$

with

$$
\begin{aligned}
K_k &= -\bar{\mu}_{0k} + t_k(1+\bar{\mu}_{0k}^2) + t_l(\bar{\sigma}_{kl} + \bar{\mu}_{0k}\bar{\mu}_{0l}) \\
&\quad + \zeta_1\{\sqrt{\pi/2}(t_k\bar{\mu}_{0k} + t_l\bar{\mu}_{0l})\}\sqrt{\pi/2}\,\bar{\mu}_{0k}, \\
K_{kl} &= (\bar{\sigma}_{kl} + \bar{\mu}_{0k}\bar{\mu}_{0l}) + \zeta_2\{\sqrt{\pi/2}(t_k\bar{\mu}_{0k} + t_l\bar{\mu}_{0l})\}\{\sqrt{\pi/2}\}^2\bar{\mu}_{0k}\bar{\mu}_{0l}, \\
K_{kll} &= \zeta_3\{\sqrt{\pi/2}(t_k\bar{\mu}_{0k} + t_l\bar{\mu}_{0l})\}\{\sqrt{\pi/2}\}^3\bar{\mu}_{0k}\bar{\mu}_{0l}^2, \\
K_{klll} &= \zeta_4\{\sqrt{\pi/2}(t_k\bar{\mu}_{0k} + t_l\bar{\mu}_{0l})\}\{\sqrt{\pi/2}\}^4\bar{\mu}_{0k}\bar{\mu}_{0l}^3, \\
K_{kkl} &= \zeta_3\{\sqrt{\pi/2}(t_k\bar{\mu}_{0k} + t_l\bar{\mu}_{0l})\}\{\sqrt{\pi/2}\}^3\bar{\mu}_{0k}^2\bar{\mu}_{0l}, \\
K_{kkk} &= \zeta_3\{\sqrt{\pi/2}(t_k\bar{\mu}_{0k} + t_l\bar{\mu}_{0l})\}\{\sqrt{\pi/2}\}^3\bar{\mu}_{0k}^3, \\
K_{kkll} &= \zeta_4\{\sqrt{\pi/2}(t_k\bar{\mu}_{0k} + t_l\bar{\mu}_{0l})\}\{\sqrt{\pi/2}\}^4\bar{\mu}_{0k}^2\bar{\mu}_{0l}^2, \\
K_{kklll} &= \zeta_5\{\sqrt{\pi/2}(t_k\bar{\mu}_{0k} + t_l\bar{\mu}_{0l})\}\{\sqrt{\pi/2}\}^5\bar{\mu}_{0k}^2\bar{\mu}_{0l}^3, \\
K_{kkkll} &= \zeta_5\{\sqrt{\pi/2}(t_k\bar{\mu}_{0k} + t_l\bar{\mu}_{0l})\}\{\sqrt{\pi/2}\}^5\bar{\mu}_{0k}^3\bar{\mu}_{0l}^2, \\
K_{kkklll} &= \zeta_6\{\sqrt{\pi/2}(t_k\bar{\mu}_{0k} + t_l\bar{\mu}_{0l})\}\{\sqrt{\pi/2}\}^6\bar{\mu}_{0k}^3\bar{\mu}_{0l}^3.
\end{aligned}
$$

Here, $\zeta_k(x)$ is the kth derivative of $\zeta_0(x) = \log\{2\Phi(x)\}$, for which

$$
\begin{aligned}
&\zeta_0(0) = 1, \quad \zeta_1(0) = \sqrt{2/\pi} = b, \quad \zeta_2(0) = -b^2, \\
&\zeta_3(0) = b(2b^2-1), \quad \zeta_4(0) = -2b^2(3b^2-2), \\
&\zeta_5(0) = b(24b^4 - 20b^2 + 3), \quad \zeta_6(0) = -4b^2(30b^4 - 30b^2 + 7).
\end{aligned}
$$

Hence,

$$
\begin{aligned}
K_k(0) &= -\bar{\mu}_{0k} + \zeta_1(0)\sqrt{\pi/2}\,\bar{\mu}_{0k} \;=\; 0, \\
K_{kl}(0) &= \bar{\sigma}_{kl} + \bar{\mu}_{0k}\bar{\mu}_{0l} + \zeta_2(0)\{\sqrt{\pi/2}\}^2\bar{\mu}_{0k}\bar{\mu}_{0l} \;=\; \bar{\sigma}_{kl}, \\
K_{kll}(0) &= \zeta_3(0)\{\sqrt{\pi/2}\}^3\bar{\mu}_{0k}\bar{\mu}_{0l}^2 \;=\; (2-\pi/2)\bar{\mu}_{0k}\bar{\mu}_{0l}^2, \\
K_{kkl}(0) &= \zeta_3(0)\{\sqrt{\pi/2}\}^3\bar{\mu}_{0k}^2\bar{\mu}_{0l} \;=\; (2-\pi/2)\bar{\mu}_{0k}^2\bar{\mu}_{0l}, \\
K_{kkk}(0) &= \zeta_3(0)\{\sqrt{\pi/2}\}^3\bar{\mu}_{0k}^3 \;=\; (2-\pi/2)\bar{\mu}_{0k}^3, \\
K_{klll}(0) &= \zeta_4(0)\{\sqrt{\pi/2}\}^4\bar{\mu}_{0k}\bar{\mu}_{0l}^3 \;=\; -2(3-\pi)\bar{\mu}_{0k}\bar{\mu}_{0l}^3, \\
K_{kkkl}(0) &= \zeta_4(0)\{\sqrt{\pi/2}\}^4\bar{\mu}_{0k}^3\bar{\mu}_{0l} \;=\; -2(3-\pi)\bar{\mu}_{0k}^3\bar{\mu}_{0l}, \\
K_{kkll}(0) &= \zeta_4(0)\{\sqrt{\pi/2}\}^4\bar{\mu}_{0k}^2\bar{\mu}_{0l}^2 \;=\; -2(3-\pi)\bar{\mu}_{0k}^2\bar{\mu}_{0l}^2, \\
K_{kklll}(0) &= \zeta_5(0)\{\sqrt{\pi/2}\}^5\bar{\mu}_{0k}^2\bar{\mu}_{0l}^3 \;=\; (3\pi^2/4 - 10\pi + 24)\bar{\mu}_{0k}^2\bar{\mu}_{0l}^3, \\
K_{kkkll}(0) &= \zeta_5(0)\{\sqrt{\pi/2}\}^5\bar{\mu}_{0k}^3\bar{\mu}_{0l}^2 \;=\; (3\pi^2/4 - 10\pi + 24)\bar{\mu}_{0k}^3\bar{\mu}_{0l}^2,
\end{aligned}
$$

$$K_{kkklll}(0) = \zeta_6(0)\{\sqrt{\pi/2}\}^6 \bar{\mu}_{0k}^3 \bar{\mu}_{0l}^3 = (-7\pi^2 + 60\pi - 120)\bar{\mu}_{0k}^3 \bar{\mu}_{0l}^3.$$

Thus, considering that $M(0) = 1$, $\rho_{k1} = M_k(0) = K_k(0) = 0$, and $\rho_{kl,11} = M_{kl}(0) = K_{kl}(0) = \bar{\sigma}_{kl}$, with $\bar{\sigma}_{kk} = \bar{\sigma}_{ll} = 1$, we have

$$\begin{aligned}
\rho_{k1} &= M_k(0) = M(0)K_k(0) = 0,\\
\rho_{k2} &= M_{kk}(0) = M_k(0)K_k(0) + M(0)K_{kk}(0) = 1,\\
\rho_{k3} &= M_{kkk}(0) = M_{kk}(0)K_k(0) + 2M_k(0)K_{kk}(0) + M(0)K_{kkk}(0)\\
&= (2 - \pi/2)\bar{\mu}_{0k}^3,\\
\rho_{k4} &= M_{kkkk}(0) = M_{kkk}(0)K_k(0) + 3M_{kk}(0)K_{kk}(0) + 3M_k(0)K_{kkk}(0)\\
&\quad + M(0)K_{kkkk}(0)\\
&= 3 - 2(3 - \pi/2)\bar{\mu}_{0k}^4,\\
\rho_{k5} &= M_{kkkkk}(0) = M_{kkkk}(0)K_k(0) + 4M_{kkk}(0)K_{kk}(0) + 6M_{kk}(0)K_{kkk}(0)\\
&\quad + 4M_k(0)K_{kkkk}(0) + M(0)K_{kkkkk}(0)\\
&= 10(2 - \pi/2)\bar{\mu}_{0k}^3 + (3\pi^2/4 - 10\pi + 24)\bar{\mu}_{0k}^5,\\
\rho_{k6} &= M_{kkkkkk}(0) = M_{kkkkk}(0)K_k(0) + 5M_{kkkk}(0)K_{kk}(0) + 10M_{kkk}(0)K_{kkk}(0)\\
&\quad + 10M_{kk}(0)K_{kkkk}(0) + 5M_k(0)K_{kkkkk}(0) + M(0)K_{kkkkkk}(0)\\
&= 15 - 30(3 - \pi)\bar{\mu}_{0k}^4 + 10(2 - \pi/2)^2\bar{\mu}_{0k}^6\\
&\quad + (-7\pi^2 + 60\pi - 120)\bar{\mu}_{0k}^6,
\end{aligned}$$

and

$$\begin{aligned}
\rho_{kl,11} &= M_{kl}(0) = M_l(0)K_k(0) + M(0)K_{kl}(0) = \bar{\sigma}_{kl},\\
\rho_{kl,12} &= M_{kll}(0) = M_{ll}(0)K_k(0) + 2M_l(0)K_{kl}(0) + M(0)K_{kll}(0)\\
&= (2 - \pi/2)\bar{\mu}_{0k}\bar{\mu}_{0l}^2,\\
\rho_{kl,21} &= M_{kkl}(0) = M_{kl}(0)K_k(0) + M_k(0)K_{kl}(0) + M_l(0)K_{kk}(0) + M(0)K_{kkl}(0)\\
&= (2 - \pi/2)\bar{\mu}_{0k}^2\bar{\mu}_{0l},\\
\rho_{kl,22} &= M_{kkll}(0) = M_{kll}(0)K_k(0) + 2M_{kl}(0)K_{kl}(0) + M_k(0)K_{kll}(0)\\
&\quad + M_{ll}(0)K_{kk}(0) + 2M_l(0)K_{kkl}(0) + M(0)K_{kkll}(0)\\
&= 2\bar{\sigma}_{kl}^2 + 1 - 2(3 - \pi)\bar{\mu}_{0k}^2\bar{\mu}_{0l}^2,\\
\rho_{kl,13} &= M_{klll}(0) = M_{lll}(0)K_k(0) + 3M_{ll}(0)K_{kl}(0)\\
&\quad + 3M_l(0)K_{kll}(0) + M(0)K_{klll}(0)\\
&= 3\bar{\sigma}_{kl} - 2(3 - \pi)\bar{\mu}_{0k}\bar{\mu}_{0l}^3,
\end{aligned}$$

$$\begin{aligned}
\rho_{kl,31} = M_{kkkl}(0) &= M_{kkl}(0)K_k(0) + 2M_{kl}(0)K_{kk}(0) + M_{kk}(0)K_{kl}(0) \\
&\quad +2M_k(0)K_{kkl}(0) + M_l(0)K_{kkk}(0) + M(0)K_{kkkl}(0) \\
&= 3\bar{\sigma}_{kl} - 2(3-\pi)\bar{\mu}_{0k}^3\bar{\mu}_{0l}, \\
\rho_{kl,23} = M_{kklll}(0) &= M_{klll}(0)K_k(0) + 3M_{kll}(0)K_{kl}(0) + 3M_{kl}(0)K_{kll}(0) \\
&\quad +M_k(0)K_{klll}(0) + M_{lll}(0)K_{kk}(0) + 3M_{ll}(0)K_{kkl}(0) \\
&\quad +3M_l(0)K_{kkll}(0) + M(0)K_{kklll}(0) \\
&= 3(2-\pi/2)\bar{\mu}_{0k}\bar{\mu}_{0l}^2\bar{\sigma}_{kl} + 3(2-\pi/2)\bar{\mu}_{0k}\bar{\mu}_{0l}^2\bar{\sigma}_{kl} \\
&\quad +(2-\pi/2)\bar{\mu}_{0l}^3 \\
&\quad +3(2-\pi/2)\bar{\mu}_{0k}^2\bar{\mu}_{0l} + (3\pi^2/4 - 10\pi + 24)\bar{\mu}_{0k}^2\bar{\mu}_{0l}^3, \\
\rho_{kl,32} = M_{kkkll}(0) &= M_{kkll}(0)K_k(0) + 2M_{kll}(0)K_{kk}(0) + 2M_{kkl}(0)K_{kl}(0) \\
&\quad +4M_{kl}(0)K_{kkl}(0) + M_{kk}(0)K_{kll}(0) + 2M_k(0)K_{kkll}(0) \\
&\quad +M_{ll}(0)K_{kkk}(0) + 2M_l(0)K_{kkkl}(0) + M(0)K_{kkkll}(0) \\
&= 2(2-\pi/2)\bar{\mu}_{0k}\bar{\mu}_{0l}^2 + 2(2-\pi/2)\bar{\mu}_{0k}^2\bar{\mu}_{0l}\bar{\sigma}_{kl} \\
&\quad +4(2-\pi/2)\bar{\mu}_{0k}^2\bar{\mu}_{0l}\bar{\sigma}_{kl} \\
&\quad +(2-\pi/2)\bar{\mu}_{0k}\bar{\mu}_{0l}^2 + (2-\pi/2)\bar{\mu}_{0k}^3 \\
&\quad +(3\pi^2/4 - 10\pi + 24)\bar{\mu}_{0k}^3\bar{\mu}_{0l}^2, \\
\rho_{kl,33} = M_{kkklll}(0) &= M_{kklll}(0)K_k(0) + 2M_{klll}(0)K_{kk}(0) + 3M_{kkll}(0)K_{kl}(0) \\
&\quad +6M_{kll}(0)K_{kkl}(0) + 3M_{kkl}(0)K_{kll}(0) + 6M_{kl}(0)K_{kkll}(0) \\
&\quad +M_{lll}(0)K_{kkk}(0) + 3M_{ll}(0)K_{kkkl}(0) + 3M_l(0)K_{kkkll}(0) \\
&\quad +M_{kk}(0)K_{klll}(0) + 2M_k(0)K_{kklll}(0) + M(0)K_{kkklll}(0) \\
&= 2\{3\bar{\sigma}_{kl} - 2(3-\pi)\bar{\mu}_{0k}\bar{\mu}_{0l}^3\} + 3\{2\bar{\sigma}_{kl}^2 + 1 \\
&\quad -2(3-\pi)\bar{\mu}_{0k}^2\bar{\mu}_{0l}^2\}\bar{\sigma}_{kl} \\
&\quad +10(2-\pi/2)^2\bar{\mu}_{0k}^3\bar{\mu}_{0l}^3 l - 12(3-\pi)\bar{\mu}_{0k}^2\bar{\mu}_{0l}^2\bar{\sigma}_{kl} \\
&\quad -6(3-\pi)\bar{\mu}_{0k}^3\bar{\mu}_{0l} \\
&\quad -2(3-\pi)\bar{\mu}_{0k}\bar{\mu}_{0l}^3 + (-7\pi^2 + 60\pi - 120)\bar{\mu}_{0k}^3\bar{\mu}_{0l}^3.
\end{aligned}$$

Finally, with the purpose of illustrating the application of some of the previous results to the multivariate skew-normal distribution, we present two examples below.

Example 6 From Corollary 1, we have that $\sqrt{n}(\boldsymbol{R}_{3\cdot} - \boldsymbol{\rho}_{3\cdot}) \xrightarrow{d} \mathcal{N}(\boldsymbol{0}, \boldsymbol{\Upsilon}_3)$, $k = 1, \ldots, d$, where $\boldsymbol{\Upsilon}_3$ has elements given by

$$\begin{aligned}
\upsilon_{kl}^{\{3\}} &= 9\rho_{kl,11} + \frac{9}{2}(\rho_{l3}\rho_{kl,12} + \rho_{k3}\rho_{kl,21}) + \frac{9}{4}\rho_{k3}\rho_{l3}(\rho_{kl,22} - \rho_{k2}\rho_{l2}) \\
&\quad -3(\rho_{kl,13} + \rho_{kl,31}) \\
&\quad -\frac{3}{2}\{\rho_{k3}(\rho_{kl,23} - \rho_{k2}\rho_{l3}) + \rho_{l3}(\rho_{kl,32} - \rho_{k3}\rho_{l2})\} + \rho_{kl,33} - \rho_{k3}\rho_{l3} \\
&= 6\bar{\sigma}_{kl}^3 + (9/2)(2 - \pi/2)^2(\bar{\mu}_{0k}\bar{\mu}_{0l}^5 + \bar{\mu}_{0k}^5\bar{\mu}_{0l}) \\
&\quad +\frac{9}{4}(2 - \pi/2)^2\{2\bar{\sigma}_{kl}^2\bar{\mu}_{0k}^3\bar{\mu}_{0l}^3 - 2(3 - \pi)\bar{\mu}_{0k}^5\bar{\mu}_{0l}^5\} \\
&\quad -(9/2)(2 - \pi/2)^2(\bar{\mu}_{0k}^5\bar{\mu}_{0l} + \bar{\mu}_{0k}\bar{\mu}_{0l}^5 + 2\bar{\mu}_{0k}^4\bar{\mu}_{0l}^2\bar{\sigma}_{kl} + 2\bar{\mu}_{0k}^2\bar{\mu}_{0l}^4\bar{\sigma}_{kl}) \\
&\quad -(3/2)(2 - \pi/2)(3\pi^2/4 - 10\pi + 24)(\bar{\mu}_{0k}^5\bar{\mu}_{0l}^3 + \bar{\mu}_{0k}^3\bar{\mu}_{0l}^5)\} \\
&\quad +\{9(2 - \pi/2)^2 - 7\pi^2 + 60\pi - 120\}\bar{\mu}_{0k}^3\bar{\mu}_{0l}^3 - 18(3 - \pi)\bar{\mu}_{0k}^2\bar{\mu}_{0l}^2\bar{\sigma}_{kl}.
\end{aligned}$$

In particular, $\sqrt{n}\,(R_{k3} - \rho_{k3}) \xrightarrow{d} \mathcal{N}(0, \upsilon_{kk}^{\{3\}})$, $k = 1, \ldots, d$, with

$$\begin{aligned}
\upsilon_{kk}^{\{3\}} &= 6 - 18(3-\pi/2)\bar{\mu}_{0k}^4 - \{(9/2)(2-\pi/2)^2 + 7\pi^2 - 60\pi + 120\}\bar{\mu}_{0k}^6 \\
&\quad -3(2-\pi/2)(3\pi^2/4 - 10\pi + 24)\bar{\mu}_{0k}^8 - (9/2)(2-\pi/2)^2(3-\pi/2)\}\bar{\mu}_{0k}^{10}.
\end{aligned}$$

Moreover, for $\bar{\mu}_{0k} = 0$ $(k = 1, \ldots, d)$, we have

$$\upsilon_{kl}^{\{3\}} = 6\bar{\sigma}_{kl}^3,$$

where $\bar{\sigma}_{kl}$ $(k, l = 1, \ldots, d)$ are the entries of the correlation matrix $\bar{\boldsymbol{\Sigma}}$.

In a similar way, from Corollary 2, we can find the asymptotic variance–covariance matrix $\boldsymbol{\Upsilon}_4$ of $\sqrt{n}(\boldsymbol{R}_{4\cdot} - \boldsymbol{\rho}_{4\cdot})$.

The following example provides for each marginal k the joint asymptotic distribution for its sample mean, sample variance, and sample skewness, and from which, we can also find the joint asymptotic distribution of the moment estimators of the respective marginal parameters, namely, $(\xi_k, \omega_k^2, \alpha_k)$, $k = 1, \ldots, d$.

Example 7 From Example 3, we have for all $k = 1, \ldots, d$:

$$\sqrt{n}\begin{pmatrix} \bar{X}_k - \mu_k \\ S_{k2} - \kappa_{k2} \\ R_{k3} - \rho_{k3} \end{pmatrix} \xrightarrow{d} \mathcal{N}_4\left(\begin{pmatrix} 0 \\ 0 \\ 0 \end{pmatrix}, \begin{pmatrix} \upsilon_{k,11} & \upsilon_{k,12} & \upsilon_{k,13} \\ \upsilon_{k,21} & \upsilon_{k,22} & \upsilon_{k,23} \\ \upsilon_{k,31} & \upsilon_{k,32} & \upsilon_{k,33} \end{pmatrix}\right),$$

where

$$\begin{aligned}
\upsilon_{k,11} &= \sigma_k^2, \\
\upsilon_{k,12} &= \sigma_k^3 \rho_{k3}, \\
\upsilon_{k,13} &= \sigma_k(-3 - 3\rho_{k3}^2/2 + \rho_{k4}), \\
\upsilon_{k,22} &= \sigma_k^4(\rho_{k4} - 1), \\
\upsilon_{k,23} &= -(\sigma_k^2/2)(5\rho_{k3} + 3\rho_{k3}\rho_{k4} - 2\rho_{k5}), \\
\upsilon_{k,33} &= 9 - 6\rho_{k4} + (1/4)(35\rho_{k3}^2 + 9\rho_{k3}^2\rho_{k4}) - 3\rho_{k3}\rho_{k5} + \rho_{k6},
\end{aligned}$$

with

$$\begin{aligned}
\rho_{k3} &= (2 - \pi/2)\bar{\mu}_{0k}^3, \\
\rho_{k4} &= 3 - 2(3 - \pi)\bar{\mu}_{0k}^4, \\
\rho_{k5} &= 10(2 - \pi/2)\bar{\mu}_{0k}^3 + (3\pi^2/4 - 10\pi + 24)\bar{\mu}_{0k}^5, \\
\rho_{k6} &= 15 - 30(3 - \pi)\bar{\mu}_{0k}^4 + \{10(2 - \pi/2)^2\bar{\mu}_{0k}^6 - 7\pi^2 + 60\pi - 120\}\bar{\mu}_{0k}^6.
\end{aligned}$$

For $\bar{\mu}_{0k} = 0$, we have

$$\sqrt{n}\begin{pmatrix} \bar{X}_k - \mu_k \\ S_{k2} - \kappa_{k2} \\ R_{k3} - \rho_{k3} \end{pmatrix} \xrightarrow{d} \mathcal{N}_4\left(\begin{pmatrix} 0 \\ 0 \\ 0 \end{pmatrix}, \begin{pmatrix} \sigma_k^2 & 0 & 0 \\ 0 & 2\sigma_k^4 & 0 \\ 0 & 0 & 6 \end{pmatrix}\right), \quad k = 1, \ldots, d.$$

6 Final Remarks

We used standard tools to obtain our results, hence facilitating the comprehension of the derivations. We illustrated the practical capabilities of the developed techniques through several simple examples. Derivations similar to the ones we presented can be carried out for multivariate skew-t and skew-elliptical distributions. Some references on theses distributions include Branco and Dey (2001), Azzalini and Capitanio (2003), Gupta (2003), and Genton and Loperfido (2005).

As a by-product of the derivations, we found that in the context of symmetric distributions, such as the elliptical ones, the known fact of asymptotic independence between the sample mean and the sample variance extends to all the sample central moments of both even and odd orders.

Acknowledgments The authors would like to thank Professor Adelchi Azzalini and a reviewer for their useful suggestions and comments. The second author was financed by the Coordenação de Aperfeiçoamento de Pessoal de Nível Superior—Brasil (CAPES)—Finance Code 001. The work of the last author was supported by the King Abdullah University of Science and Technology (KAUST).

References

Afendras, G., Papadatos, N., & Piperigou, V. E. (2020). On the limiting distribution of sample central moments. *Annals of the Institute of Statistical Mathematics, 72*(2), 399–425.

Arnold, B. C., & Beaver, R. J. (2002). Skewed multivariate models related to hidden truncation and/or selective reporting. *TEST, 11*(1), 7–54.

Arnold, B. C., Beaver, R. J., Groeneveld, R. A., & Meeker, W. Q. (1993). The nontruncated marginal of a truncated bivariate normal distribution. *Psychometrika, 58*(3), 471–488

Azzalini, A. (1985). A class of distributions which includes the normal ones. *Scandinavian Journal of Statistics, 12*(2), 171–178.

Azzalini, A., & Capitanio, A. (2003). Distributions generated by perturbation of symmetry with emphasis on a multivariate skew t-distribution. *Journal of the Royal Statistical Society: Series B (Statistical Methodology), 65*(2), 367–389.

Azzalini, A., & Capitanio, A. (2014). *The skew-normal and related families. IMS monographs.* Cambridge: Cambridge University Press.

Azzalini, A., & Dalla Valle, A. (1996). The multivariate skew-normal distribution. *Biometrika, 83*(4), 715–726.

Bao, Y. (2013). On sample skewness and kurtosis. *Econometric Reviews, 32*(4), 415–448.

Berkane, M., & Bentler, P. (1986). Moments of elliptically distributed random variates. *Statistics & Probability Letters, 4*(6), 333–335.

Branco, M. D., & Dey, D. K. (2001). A general class of multivariate skew-elliptical distributions. *Journal of Multivariate Analysis, 79*(1), 99–113.

Cramér, H. (1946). *Mathematical methods of statistics.* Princeton: Princeton University Press.

Genton, M. G. (Eds.) (2004). *Skew-elliptical distributions and their applications: A journey beyond normality.* Boca Raton: CRC Press.

Genton, M. G., & Loperfido, N. M. (2005). Generalized skew-elliptical distributions and their quadratic forms. *Annals of the Institute of Statistical Mathematics, 57*(2), 389–401.

Gupta, A. K. (2003). Multivariate skew t-distribution. *Statistics: A Journal of Theoretical and Applied Statistics, 37*(4), 359–363.

Harris, D., & Mátyás, L. (1999). Introduction to the generalized method of moments estimation. In L. Mátyás (Ed.), *Generalized method of moments estimation* (pp. 3–30). Cambridge: Cambridge University Press.

Kollo, T., & von Rosen, D. (2005). Distribution expansions. In M. Hazewinkel (Ed.), *Advanced multivariate statistics with matrices* (Vol. 579, Chap. III). Berlin: Springer.

Lehmann, E. L., & Casella, G. (1998). *Theory of point estimation* (2nd ed.). *Springer texts in statistics.* New York: Springer.

Mardia, K. V. (1970). Measures of multivariate skewness and kurtosis with applications. *Biometrika, 57*(3), 519–530.

Maruyama, Y., & Seo, T. (2003). Estimation of moment parameter in elliptical distributions. *Journal of the Japan Statistical Society, 33*(2), 215–229.

Pewsey, A. (2005). The large-sample distribution of the most fundamental of statistical summaries. *Journal of Statistical Planning and Inference, 134*(2), 434–444.

Tail Behavior for Bivariate Distributions Based on Pareto Mixtures

Vincenzo Coia, Harry Joe, and Natalia Nolde

Abstract For conditional tail inferences from multivariate distributions, we desire models with positive dependence for which conditional distributions of one variable given others have extreme value indices that can be functions of the values of conditioning variables. That is, the tails of the conditional distributions behave like Pareto distributions with varying tail parameter. It is shown in Arnold (Stat Probab Lett 5:263–266, 1987) and Arnold et al. (Stat Probab Lett 17:361–368, 1993) in the bivariate case that if all conditional distributions are (generalized) Pareto and the tail parameters are non-constant, then tractable solutions have limited range of dependence. To obtain models with our desired properties, we specify one set of conditional Pareto distributions and one marginal distribution: for example, (a) $F_{Y|X}(\cdot|x)$ is Pareto with tail parameter decreasing in x and/or scale parameter is increasing in x, (b) no specification is made for $F_{X|Y}(\cdot|x)$, and (c) X has a distribution with regularly varying upper tail. Based on this construction, we study the following properties: (1) relation of concordance ordering to the tail parameter function, (2) relations of conditional extreme value indices to marginal extreme value indices, and (3) tail dependence.

1 Introduction

Bivariate and multivariate distributions have been constructed in many ways (Arnold et al. 1999; Balakrishnan and Lai 2009; Joe 2014, and references cited therein). To match with potential applications and different types of inferences, it is important to know about their dependence and tail properties.

Examples of applications that motivated our research include forecasting of conditional extreme quantiles (Coia 2017) and estimation of extreme quantiles as

V. Coia · H. Joe (✉) · N. Nolde
Department of Statistics, University of British Columbia, Vancouver, BC, USA
e-mail: vincen.coia@stat.ubc.ca; Harry.Joe@ubc.ca; natalia@stat.ubc.ca

I. Ghosh et al. (eds.), *Advances in Statistics - Theory and Applications*, Emerging Topics in Statistics and Biostatistics, https://doi.org/10.1007/978-3-030-62900-7_10

a function of covariates in operational risk losses (Chavez-Demoulin et al. 2016) and in heavy internet traffic (Rezaul and Grout 2007).

For applications where conditional tail inferences are important, we would like multivariate and bivariate models to have the flexibility of allowing for conditional distributions with varying extreme value indices. For the bivariate case, this means a bivariate distribution $F_{X,Y}$ for variables X, Y such that $F_{Y|X}(\cdot|x)$ has regular varying (Pareto-like) tails with non-constant extreme value index as x varies. For example, $\overline{F}_{Y|X}(y|x) = 1 - F_{Y|X}(y|x) = O(y^{-\alpha(x)})$ as $y \to \infty$, with $\alpha(x) > 0$ and non-constant. With this notation, the conditional extreme value index function is $\xi_{Y|X}(x) = 1/\alpha(x)$ so that a larger value of ξ implies a heavier tail.

For conditional models based on specifications of functional forms of all possible conditional distributions of one variable given others, one can sometimes get families of bivariate distributions with only negative dependence. This happens in one tractable case with Burr (or generalized Pareto) conditional distributions in Arnold et al. (1993).

For tractable bivariate copula families with a wide range of dependence that have been constructed in different ways, it seems that the conditional extreme value index is constant. One goal is to understand conditions that lead to (1) a non-constant conditional extreme value index function and/or (2) conditional extreme value index values smaller than marginal extreme value index. To achieve these properties, we consider constructions based on one set of conditional distributions (e.g., $\{F_{Y|X}(\cdot|x)\}$) assumed to be Pareto with no specifications made for the other set of conditional distributions (e.g., $\{F_{X|Y}(\cdot|y)\}$). The tail and dependence properties of the resulting joint distribution can be studied with different assumptions on the scale and tail parameters of the conditional distributions and on the mixing distribution over the set of conditional distributions.

The rest of this chapter is organized as follows. Section 2 provides background results for extreme value indices and copulas, because the constructions may be converted to copulas for analysis of tail and dependence properties. Section 3 presents the constructions with different mixtures of conditional Pareto distributions to achieve different tail properties. Section 4 contains theory to show how concordance properties can be verified for the different constructions. Section 5 gives results on comparison of conditional and marginal extreme value indices. Section 6 has results on conditions for upper tail dependence. Section 7 concludes with a discussion.

2 Background for Extreme Value Index and Copula

In this section, we set out the notation for distributions and densities and provide mathematical definitions for concepts such as regular variation, extreme value index, and copula. Some examples are given to show how these are obtained for some copula families.

We use the following notation: F for the cumulative distribution function (cdf), f for the probability density function (pdf), and $\overline{F}$ for the survival function. These have subscripts to indicate the random variable or random vector. Conditional cdfs have the form $F_{Y|X}$ for Y conditional on X.

Definition (Regular Variation and Extreme Value Index of Univariate Distribution with Regularly Varying Upper Tail) Let F be the cdf of a random variable with upper support point of ∞. F is *regularly varying* of order $-\alpha$ at ∞ ($\alpha > 0$), denoted as $F \in \mathrm{RV}_{-\alpha}$, if $\overline{F}(x) = 1 - F(x) \sim x^{-\alpha}\ell(x)$ as $x \to \infty$ for a slowly varying function $\ell(x)$, where a slowly varying function $\ell(x)$ satisfies $\lim_{x\to\infty} \ell(tx)/\ell(x) = 1$ for all $t > 0$. Equivalently, $\lim_{x\to\infty}[1 - F(tx)]/[1 - F(x)] = t^{-\alpha}$ for all $t > 0$. The *extreme value index* for $Z \sim F \in \mathrm{RV}_{-\alpha}$ is $\xi_F = \xi_Z = 1/\alpha > 0$, so that a larger ξ_Z value indicates a heavier upper tail.

Definition (Copula) A copula is a multivariate distribution with $U(0, 1)$ margins.

The copula cdf is denoted with C. Next is Sklar's result (Sklar 1959) for copulas and how it is used.

If F is a d-variate distribution with univariate marginal cdfs $F_1, \ldots, F_d$, then there is a copula C with domain $[0, 1]^d$ such that

$$F(y_1, \ldots, y_d) = C\big(F_1(y_1), \ldots, F_d(y_d)\big), \quad (y_1, \ldots, y_d) \in \Re^d.$$

If F is continuous, the copula is unique and is given by

$$C(u_1, \ldots, u_d) = F\big(F_1^{-1}(u_1), \ldots, F_d^{-1}(u_d)\big), \quad 0 \le u_j \le 1,\ j = 1, \ldots, d,$$

where the F_j^{-1} for $j = 1, \ldots, d$ are the inverse cdfs.

For a given copula family C, one can get a multivariate distribution with univariate margins $F_1^*, \ldots, F_d^*$ from $C(F_1^*, \ldots, F_d^*)$. Similarly, one can get a multivariate survival function with univariate survival functions $\overline{F}_1^*, \ldots, \overline{F}_d^*$ from $C(\overline{F}_1^*, \ldots, \overline{F}_d^*)$.

Definition (Marginal and Conditional Extreme Value Index of Bivariate Distribution) Assume that the marginal and conditional distributions have regularly varying upper tails. Suppose (X, Y) has continuous joint cdf $F_{X,Y}$. The univariate marginal extreme value indices are denoted as ξ_X and ξ_Y. The conditional extreme value index function of $F_{Y|X}(\cdot|x)$ is denoted as $\xi_{Y|X}(x)$, and the conditional extreme value index function of $F_{X|Y}(\cdot|y)$ is denoted as $\xi_{X|Y}(y)$.

Similarly, conditional extreme value index functions can be defined for multivariate distributions, but here we focus on properties for the bivariate case. The conditional extreme value indices are obtained from the conditional distributions of a bivariate or multivariate distribution. They can be calculated with the following steps.

For a bivariate or multivariate distribution, one can convert via probability integral transforms to a copula with $U(0, 1)$ margins and then to Pareto margins with cdf $F_{\text{Pareto}}(x;\alpha) = 1 - x^{-\alpha}$, for $x > 1$ and $\alpha > 0$ with scale parameter 1. This is called type I Pareto in Arnold (2015). The conversion to Pareto margins makes it easier to compute extreme value indices; however, extreme value indices could be defined from the copula and its conditional distributions without Pareto distributions.

One goal is to find or construct models for which the conditional extreme value index function is not constant as the conditioning variables vary. The ideas are clarified after the next example.

Example Consider the bivariate Pareto distribution of Mardia (1962) and Takahasi (1965) with scale parameters of 1. Its survival function and cdf are

$$\overline{F}_{X,Y}(x,y) = \Pr(X > x, Y > y) = (1 + x + y)^{-1/\delta}, \quad x > 0,\ y > 0,\ \delta > 0,$$
$$F_{X,Y}(x,y) = 1 - (1+x)^{-1/\delta} - (1+y)^{-1/\delta} + (1 + x + y)^{-1/\delta},$$

with univariate survival functions $\overline{F}_X(x) = (1+x)^{-1/\delta}$ and $\overline{F}_Y(y) = (1+y)^{-1/\delta}$. Its copula (from probability integral transforms via univariate cdfs) with $u = 1 - \overline{F}_X(x)$ and $v = 1 - \overline{F}_Y(y)$ is

$$C(u,v;\delta) = u + v - 1 + [(1-u)^{-\delta} + (1-v)^{-\delta} - 1]^{-1/\delta},$$
$$0 < u < 1, 0 < v < 1, \delta > 0, \quad (1)$$

and its survival or reflected copula (from probability integral transforms via univariate survival functions) with $u = \overline{F}_X(x)$ and $v = \overline{F}_Y(y)$ is

$$\widehat{C}(u,v;\delta) = [u^{-\delta} + v^{-\delta} - 1]^{-1/\delta}, \quad 0 < u < 1, 0 < v < 1, \delta > 0. \quad (2)$$

For each of these copulas, we convert to bivariate Pareto distributions $F_{X,Y}(x,y) = C(F_X(x), F_Y(y))$ with marginal cdfs $F_X(x) = 1 - x^{-\alpha}$, $F_Y(y) = 1 - y^{-\alpha}$ with $x > 1, y > 1$, and $\alpha > 0$. Then, we will derive the extreme value indices of the conditional cdf $F_{Y|X}(\cdot|x)$ for $x > 1$, making use of the univariate density $f_X(x) = \alpha x^{-\alpha-1}$ for $x > 1$. Because these distributions are permutation symmetric, the behavior is similar for the conditional cdfs $F_{X|Y}(\cdot|y)$ for $y > 1$.

(a) The copula family in (1) leads to

$$F_{X,Y}(x,y) = 1 - x^{-\alpha} - y^{-\alpha} + [x^{\alpha\delta} + y^{\alpha\delta} - 1]^{-1/\delta},$$
$$\frac{\partial F_{X,Y}(x,y)}{\partial x} = \alpha x^{-\alpha-1} - \alpha x^{\alpha\delta-1}[x^{\alpha\delta} + y^{\alpha\delta} - 1]^{-1/\delta-1},$$
$$F_{Y|X}(y|x) = \frac{\partial F_{X,Y}(x,y)}{\partial x} / f_X(x) = 1 - [1 + x^{-\alpha\delta}(y^{\alpha\delta} - 1)]^{-1/\delta-1},$$
$$F_{Y|X}(y|x) \sim 1 - x^{\alpha(1+\delta)} y^{-\alpha(1+\delta)}, \quad y \to \infty.$$

Hence, $F_{Y|X}(y|x) \in \mathrm{RV}_{-\alpha(1+\delta)}$ for all $x > 1$ and $\xi_{Y|X}(x) = \alpha^{-1}(1+\delta)^{-1} < \alpha^{-1} = \xi_Y$ for all $x > 1$.

(b) The copula family in (2) leads to

$$
\begin{aligned}
F_{X,Y}(x,y) &= [(1-x^{-\alpha})^{-\delta} + (1-y^{-\alpha})^{-\delta} - 1]^{-1/\delta},\\
\frac{\partial F_{X,Y}(x,y)}{\partial x} &= \alpha x^{-\alpha-1}(1-x^{-\alpha})^{-\delta-1}[(1-x^{-\alpha})^{-\delta}\\
&\quad +(1-y^{-\alpha})^{-\delta} - 1]^{-1/\delta-1},\\
F_{Y|X}(y|x) &= \frac{\partial F_{X,Y}(x,y)}{\partial x} / f_X(x)\\
&= [1 + (1-x^{-\alpha})^{\delta}\{(1-y^{-\alpha})^{-\delta} - 1\}]^{-1/\delta-1},\\
F_{Y|X}(y|x) &\sim 1 - (\delta+1)(1-x^{-\alpha})^{\delta} y^{-\alpha}, \quad y \to \infty.
\end{aligned}
$$

Hence, $F_{Y|X}(y|x) \in \mathrm{RV}_{-\alpha}$ for all $x > 1$ and $\xi_{Y|X}(x) = \alpha^{-1} = \xi_Y$ for all $x > 1$.

The above example raises some questions on how dependence properties of a copula are related to the conditional and marginal extreme value indices.

1. What is a condition for $\xi_{Y|X}(x) = \xi_Y$ for all x?
2. What is a condition for $\sup_x \xi_{Y|X}(x) < \xi_Y$?
3. Is it possible for $\xi_{Y|X}(x) > \xi_Y$ for some x?
4. Are there bivariate distributions with simple forms such that $\xi_{Y|X}(x)$ is non-constant over x?

The copulas in (1) and (2) are related through

$$
\widehat{C}(u,v) = u + v - 1 + C(1-u, 1-v). \tag{3}
$$

Or stochastically, if $(U,V) \sim C$, then with reflected $U(0,1)$ random variables, $(1-U, 1-V) \sim \widehat{C}$. It turns out that C in (1) has upper tail dependence but not lower tail dependence, so that the reflected copula (2) has lower tail dependence but not upper tail dependence.

In copula families where we can compute $\xi_{Y|X}(x)$, a general observation is that upper tail dependence is linked to $\sup_x \xi_{Y|X}(x) < \xi_Y$. However, a proof of this as a general result does not appear tractable.

The definitions of upper and lower tail dependence for a bivariate continuous distribution $F_{X,Y}$ are as follows. See Section 2.13 of Joe (2014) for more details.

Definition (Tail Dependence Coefficients) Let $F_{X,Y}$ be the continuous bivariate cdf of a random vector (X,Y) with survival function $\overline{F}_{X,Y}$, univariate cdfs F_X and F_Y, and copula C. Let $\widehat{C}$ be defined as in (3). Provided the limits exist, the upper tail dependence coefficient is

$$\lambda_U = \lim_{u \to 0^+} \Pr\left(Y > F_Y^{-1}(1-u) \mid X > F_X^{-1}(1-u)\right)$$
$$= \lim_{u \to 0^+} u^{-1} \overline{F}_{X,Y}\left(F_X^{-1}(1-u), F_Y^{-1}(1-u)\right) = \lim_{u \to 0^+} u^{-1} \widehat{C}(u, u),$$

and the lower tail dependence coefficient is

$$\lambda_L = \lim_{u \to 0^+} \Pr\left(Y < F_Y^{-1}(u) \mid X < F_X^{-1}(u)\right)$$
$$= \lim_{u \to 0^+} u^{-1} F_{X,Y}\left(F_X^{-1}(u), F_Y^{-1}(u)\right) = \lim_{u \to 0^+} u^{-1} C(u, u).$$

3 Constructions of Pareto Mixtures

In this section, we consider constructions from mixtures of Pareto distributions of type I or type II. That is, $F_{Y|X}(\cdot|x)$ is Pareto with the scale parameter and/or tail parameter varying with x, and F_X has conveniently chosen distribution so that the joint distribution $F_{X,Y}$ is tractable for obtaining some tail and dependence properties.

Sometimes we take Pareto of type I and sometimes Pareto of type II depending on what is mathematically more convenient. Tail and dependence properties are not affected by the choice. With constant scale parameter and varying tail parameter, it is simpler to use the type I form $\overline{F}_{Y|X}(y|x) = (y\sigma)^{-\alpha(x)}$ for $y > \sigma$. With varying scale parameter and constant or varying tail parameter, the above type I form would have varying lower end point of support, so it is better to use Pareto of type II with $\overline{F}_{Y|X}(y|x) = (1 + y/\sigma(x))^{-\alpha(x)}$ for $y > 0$.

We would like to have the resulting bivariate distribution $F_{X,Y}$ to have positive dependence. For a tractable form of positive dependence, $F_{Y|X}(\cdot|x)$ can be stochastically increasing in x or $\overline{F}_{Y|X}(y|x)$ increasing in x for all $y > 0$; this implies that Y tends to be increasing as X increases. This condition requires $\alpha(x)$ to be decreasing in x and $\sigma(x)$ to be increasing in x. Negative dependence could be obtained by reversing the direction of monotonicity of these two functions. For dependence properties such as positive quadrant dependence and stochastic increasingness, detailed explanations are given in Chapter 2 of Joe (2014).

The bivariate survival function is

$$\overline{F}_{X,Y}(x, y) = \int_x^\infty \overline{F}_{Y|X}(y|z)\, f_X(z)\, \mathrm{d}z, \tag{4}$$

from which we can derive $\overline{F}_Y(y) = \overline{F}_{X,Y}(-\infty, y)$ and compute ξ_Y to compare with $\xi_{Y|X}(x) = 1/\alpha(x)$. We can also compute the other set of conditional distributions $\{F_{X|Y}(\cdot|y)\}$ to determine $\xi_{X|Y}(y)$ to compare with ξ_X.

In Sects. 3.1 and 3.2, we consider some cases so that the integration results in closed-form expressions, and as a consequence, tail and dependence properties can more easily be studied. These provide insights into how to generalize to get a wider range of dependence. The tail and dependence properties depend only on the copula, so when a parameter of the conditional distributions is constant, we can fix it at a convenient value for simpler derivations.

3.1 $X \sim$ Pareto(1, 1) on $[1, \infty)$ and $\sigma(x) = 1$

Suppose $\sigma(x)$ is constant and without loss of generality set to 1. Let $X \sim$ Pareto$(1, \gamma)$ on $[1, \infty)$ with scale parameter 1 and tail parameter γ. We can assume $\gamma = 1$ without loss of generality in terms of the resulting copula. Then, the density of X is $f_X(x) = x^{-2}$ for $x > 1$. From (4), we have

$$\overline{F}_{X,Y}(x, y) = \int_x^\infty y^{-\alpha(z)} z^{-2} \mathrm{d}z = \int_x^\infty \exp\{-\alpha(z)\log(y)\} z^{-2} \mathrm{d}z. \tag{5}$$

To obtain a closed-form integral, $-\alpha(z)\log(y)$ should be linear in z^{-1}. A possibility with constant scale is to choose $\alpha(z) = a_1 + a_2/z$ for $z \geq 1$, with $a_1 > 0$ and $a_2 > 0$ (so that $\alpha(z)$ is decreasing). Then, $\alpha(x)$ goes from $a_1 + a_2$ to a_1 as x increases from 1 to ∞.

For $x > 1$ and $y > 1$,

$$\begin{aligned}
\overline{F}_{X,Y}(x, y) &= \int_x^\infty \exp\{-(a_1 + a_2/z)\log(y)\} z^{-2} \mathrm{d}z \\
&= [a_2 \log y]^{-1} \exp\{-(a_1 + a_2/z)\log(y)\} \Big|_x^\infty \\
&= [a_2 \log y]^{-1} \{y^{-a_1} - y^{-(a_1 + a_2/x)}\} \\
&= [a_2 \log y]^{-1} y^{-a_1} \{1 - y^{-a_2/x}\}, && (6) \\
\overline{F}_Y(y) &= \overline{F}_{X,Y}(1, y) = [a_2 \log y]^{-1} y^{-a_1} \{1 - y^{-a_2}\}, && (7) \\
\overline{F}_Y(y) &\sim [a_2 \log y]^{-1} y^{-a_1}, \quad y \to \infty, \\
\overline{F}_Y(1) &= \lim_{y \to 1^+} \frac{1 - y^{-a_2}}{a_2 \log y} = \lim_{y \to 1^+} \frac{a_2 y^{-a_2 - 1}}{a_2 y^{-1}} = 1.
\end{aligned}$$

Hence, $\xi_Y = a_1^{-1}$ and $\xi_{Y|X}(x) = (a_1 + a_2/x)^{-1} < \xi_Y$ for $x > 1$, but $\sup_x \xi_{Y|X}(x) = a_1^{-1} = \xi_Y$.

For $\eta > 0$, let $H(w; \eta) = [\eta w \log w]^{-1}(1 - w^{-\eta})$ for $w > 1$. With $\theta = a_2/a_1$ and $w = y^{a_1}$, $\overline{F}_Y(y) = H(w; \theta)$, so that $H(1; \theta) = 1$, $H(\infty; \theta) = 0$, and H is decreasing; that is, it is a survival function on $[1, \infty)$. Furthermore, with $w = y^{a_1}$ and $\theta = a_2/a_1$,

$$\overline{F}(x, y) = [\theta \log w]^{-1} w^{-1} \{1 - w^{-\theta/x}\} = x^{-1} H(w; \theta/x).$$

Since $\overline{F}_X(x) = x^{-1}$ for $x > 1$ by construction, the copula of (6) is obtained by substituting $u = \overline{F}_X(x) = x^{-1}$ and $v = H(w; \theta)$ or $w = H^{-1}(v; \theta)$ to get

$$C(u, v; \theta) = \overline{F}_{X,Y}\big(\overline{F}_X^{-1}(u), \overline{F}_X^{-1}(v)\big) = uH\big(H^{-1}(v; \theta); \theta u\big), \quad 0 < u, v < 1. \tag{8}$$

That is, the copula depends on a_1, a_2 only through $\theta = a_2/a_1$. The above is a construction in Section 6.1.1 of Coia (2017) with a slightly different derivation.

Properties include the following:

- Positive quadrant dependence ($C(u, v; \theta) \geq uv$ for $0 < u, v < 1$) follows from the stochastic increasingness property.
- Concordance (or monotone dependence) increases as θ increases; this follows from results in Sect. 4.
- A boundary case is independence as $\alpha_2 \to 0$ or $\theta \to 0$ for the copula. However, the comonotonicity copula or perfect positive dependence cannot be achieved as $\theta \to \infty$.
- Spearman's rank correlation ρ_S increases in the concordance ordering, so there is an upper limit of $\rho_S(C(\cdot; \theta))$ for family (8). It can be shown numerically that the maximum dependence obtained is $\rho_S = 0.47$ (i.e., Cor (U, V) for $(U, V) \sim C(\cdot; \theta)$ as $\theta \to \infty$).

We can also study the other set of conditional distributions $\{F_{X|Y}(\cdot|y)\}$:

$$\begin{aligned}
f_Y(y) &= \frac{-\partial \overline{F}_Y(y)}{\partial y} \\
&= \frac{y^{-a_1-1}}{a_2 \log y}\Big\{(\log y)^{-1}(1 - y^{-a_2}) + a_1(1 - y^{-a_2}) - a_2 y^{-a_2}\Big\}, \\
\frac{-\partial \overline{F}_{X,Y}(x, y)}{\partial y} &= \frac{y^{-a_1-1}}{a_2 \log y}\Big\{(\log y)^{-1}(1 - y^{-a_2/x}) \\
&\quad + a_1(1 - y^{-a_2/x}) - a_2 x^{-1} y^{-a_2/x}\Big\}, \\
\overline{F}_{X|Y}(x|y) &= \frac{-\frac{\partial \overline{F}_{X,Y}(x,y)}{\partial y}}{f_Y(y)} \\
&= \frac{(\log y)^{-1}(1 - y^{-a_2/x}) + a_1(1 - y^{-a_2/x}) - a_2 x^{-1} y^{-a_2/x}}{(\log y)^{-1}(1 - y^{-a_2}) + a_1(1 - y^{-a_2}) - a_2 y^{-a_2}}.
\end{aligned}$$

For fixed y, as $x \to \infty$,

$$\overline{F}_{X|Y}(x|y) \sim \frac{a_2 x^{-1} + a_1 a_2 x^{-1} \log y - a_2 x^{-1}(1 - a_2 x^{-1} \log y)}{(\log y)^{-1}(1 - y^{-a_2}) + a_1(1 - y^{-a_2}) - a_2 y^{-a_2}}$$

$$\sim \frac{a_1 a_2 x^{-1} \log y + O(x^{-2})}{(\log y)^{-1}(1 - y^{-a_2}) + a_1(1 - y^{-a_2}) - a_2 y^{-a_2}}.$$

Hence, $\xi_{X|Y}(y) = 1 = \xi_X$, for all $y > 1$.

Notice that the choice of Pareto$(1, \gamma)$ with $\gamma = 1$ for the distribution of X is without loss of generality if we are interested in the dependence property (via the copula) and the relation of $\xi_{Y|X}(x)$ and ξ_Y. If we start with $\overline{F}_X(x) = x^{-\gamma}$ and $f_X(x) = \gamma x^{-\gamma-1}$, for $x > 1$ and $\gamma > 0$, then to get a closed-form bivariate survival function, we would choose $\alpha(x) = a_1 + a_2 x^{-\gamma}$, and the resulting copula is as above in (8).

However, we can choose other mixture distributions in order to get a family covering a wider range of dependence. These are shown in subsequent subsections.

3.2 $X \sim$ Fréchet(1) on $(0, \infty)$ and $\sigma(x) = 1$

Tractable results are also obtained if the Pareto distribution for F_X is replaced with the Fréchet distribution. It turns out that a wider range of dependence is obtained compared with the preceding subsection, and the intuition is due to a wide range of $\alpha(x)$ decreasing from ∞ to a positive constant.

Suppose $F_X(x) = 1 - \mathrm{e}^{-1/x}$ for $x > 0$, so that $f_X(x) = x^{-2}\mathrm{e}^{-1/x}$. This has the same upper tail behavior as Pareto(1,1) with $\xi_X = 1$. Let $\alpha(x) = a_1 + a_2/x$ be decreasing in $x > 0$, where $a_1, a_2 > 0$. Then, $\alpha(x)$ goes from ∞ to a_1 as x goes from 0 to ∞.

For $x > 0$ and $y > 1$, (4) becomes

$$\begin{aligned}
\overline{F}_{X,Y}(x, y) &= \int_x^\infty y^{-\alpha(z)} z^{-2} \mathrm{e}^{-1/z} \mathrm{d}z \\
&= \int_x^\infty \exp\{-(\log y)(a_1 + a_2/z) - z^{-1}\} z^{-2} \mathrm{d}z \\
&= [a_2 \log y + 1]^{-1} \{y^{-a_1} - y^{-a_1 - a_2/x} \mathrm{e}^{-1/x}\} \\
&= [a_2 \log y + 1]^{-1} y^{-a_1} (1 - y^{-a_2/x} \mathrm{e}^{-1/x}); \qquad (9) \\
\overline{F}_Y(y) &= \overline{F}_{X,Y}(0, y) = [a_2 \log y + 1]^{-1} y^{-a_1}, \quad \overline{F}_Y(1) = 1.
\end{aligned}$$

Hence, $\xi_Y = a_1^{-1}$ and $\xi_{Y|X}(x) = (a_1 + a_2/x)^{-1} < \xi_Y$ for $x > 1$, but $\sup_x \xi_{Y|X}(x) = a_1^{-1} = \xi_Y$.

Let $w = y^{a_1}$, $\theta = a_2/a_1 > 0$, and let

$$G(w; \theta) = [\theta \log w + 1]^{-1} w^{-1}, \quad w \geq 1, \theta > 0$$

be a survival function on $[1, \infty)$. Then, $\overline{F}_Y(y) = G(y^{a_1}; \theta) = G(w; \theta)$ and

$$\overline{F}_{X,Y}(x,y) = [\theta \log w + 1]^{-1} w^{-1}(1 - w^{-\theta/x}\mathrm{e}^{-1/x}) = G(w;\theta)(1 - w^{-\theta/x}\mathrm{e}^{-1/x}).$$

To get the copula based on survival functions, let $u = 1 - \mathrm{e}^{-1/x}$, $v = \overline{F}_Y(y) = G(w;\theta)$. Then,

$$C(u,v;\theta) = v\{1 - (1-u)[G^{-1}(v;\theta)]^{\theta \log(1-u)}\}, \quad 0 < u, v < 1. \tag{10}$$

We can also study the other set of conditional distributions $F_{X|Y}(\cdot|y)$:

$$\begin{aligned}
f_Y(y) &= [a_2 \log y + 1]^{-2} y^{-a_1-1}\{a_2 + a_1(a_2 \log y + 1)\};\\
-\frac{\partial F_{X,Y}}{\partial y} &= [a_2 \log y + 1]^{-2} y^{-a_1-1} \times \{a_2(1 - y^{-a_2/x}\mathrm{e}^{-1/x})\\
&\quad + a_1(a_2 \log y + 1)(1 - y^{-a_2/x}\mathrm{e}^{-1/x})\\
&\quad - a_2 x^{-1} y^{-a_2/x}\mathrm{e}^{-1/x}(a_2 \log y + 1)\};\\
\overline{F}_{X|Y}(x|y) &= \{a_2(1 - y^{-a_2/x}\mathrm{e}^{-1/x}) + a_1(a_2 \log y + 1)(1 - y^{-a_2/x}\mathrm{e}^{-1/x})\\
&\quad - a_2 x^{-1} y^{-a_2/x}\mathrm{e}^{-1/x}(a_2 \log y + 1)\} \,/\, \{a_2 + a_1(a_2 \log y + 1)\}.
\end{aligned}$$

Since $1 - y^{-a_2/x}\mathrm{e}^{-1/x} \sim x^{-1}(a_2 \log y + 1)$ as $x \to \infty$,

$$\begin{aligned}
&\overline{F}_{X|Y}(x|y)\\
&\sim \frac{a_2 x^{-1}(a_2 \log y + 1) + a_1 x^{-1}(a_2 \log y + 1)^2 - a_2 x^{-1}(a_2 \log y + 1) + O(x^{-2})}{a_2 + a_1(a_2 \log y + 1)}\\
&\sim \frac{a_1 x^{-1}(a_2 \log y + 1)^2}{a_2 + a_1(a_2 \log y + 1)}, \qquad x \to \infty.
\end{aligned}$$

Hence, $\xi_{X|Y}(y) = 1$ for all $y > 0$ and $\xi_X = 1$.

The properties of the copula family (10) are similar to those of copula family (8), except that there is a wider range of dependence. Numerically from simulations, the Spearman's rank correlation $\rho_S(C(\cdot;\theta))$ for (10) increases from 0 to about 0.68 as θ increases from 0 to ∞.

3.3 Other Pareto Mixtures

In this section, we consider more general Pareto mixtures that do not lead to closed-form cdfs as in the preceding two subsections. However, these constructions lead to a wider range of dependence as well as more flexible tail properties. The properties can be shown analytically and also be seen from scatterplots of simulated data.

Let the density of X be Fréchet(1) with $f_X(x) = x^{-2}e^{1/x}$. As an extension of the preceding section, we consider

$$\overline{F}_{X,Y}(x, y) = \int_x^\infty y^{-\alpha(z)} z^{-2} e^{-1/z} dz, \quad x > 0, y > 1. \tag{11}$$

Now, suppose $\alpha(x) = a_1 + a_2 x^{-\beta}$, where $a_1 \geq 0$, $a_2 > 0$, and $\beta > 0$. The bivariate distribution $F_{X,Y}$ is not tractable, but dependence properties can be obtained. Numerically for large values of a_2/a_1 and β, one can get Spearman's rank correlation approaching 1. Other parametric families of $\alpha(x)$ can also be considered to get this conclusion; the important property is that the family covers a wide range of derivatives of the decreasing function. Negative dependence can be obtained with families of $\alpha(x)$ consisting of increasing functions. Explanations are given in Sect. 4.

The joint distribution in (11) becomes

$$\overline{F}_{X,Y}(x, y) = \int_x^\infty \exp\{-(\log y)(a_1 + a_2 z^{-\beta})\} \cdot z^{-2} e^{-1/z} dz,$$

and this and its copula density can be evaluated with one-dimensional numerical integration. This distribution approaches comonotonicity as β increases because for large values of a_2/a_1 and β, the conditional tail parameter $\alpha(x)$ can decrease from ∞ to a_1 at a fast rate as x goes from 0 to ∞.

For another Pareto mixture, we allow the scale parameter to vary. In this case, we use Pareto distributions of type II in order that the support of Y conditional on x is always $(0, \infty)$. The most general form has f_X with support on $(0, \infty)$ combined with $\overline{F}_{Y|X}(y|x) = [1 + y/\sigma(x)]^{-\alpha(x)}$ for $y > 0$. The conditional scale parameter is $\sigma(x)$, and the conditional tail parameter is $\alpha(x)$. Assume that $\sigma(x)$ is constant or increasing in x and $\alpha(x)$ is constant or decreasing in x in order that $\overline{F}_{Y|X}(\cdot|x)$ is stochastically increasing as x increases. The resulting joint survival function is

$$\overline{F}_{X,Y}(x, y) = \int_x^\infty [1 + y/\sigma(z)]^{-\alpha(z)} f_X(z) \, dz, \quad x > 0, y > 0. \tag{12}$$

For f_X to have regularly varying tail, X can have Fréchet distribution or Pareto of type II. Some properties of (12) are given in Sects. 5 and 6 in special cases.

4 Concordance Ordering for Copulas from Different Pareto Mixtures

In this section, we show how to verify some concordance properties of the constructions in Sect. 3 for different $\alpha(x)$.

Definition (Bivariate Concordance) Let (W, Z) and (W', Z') be two dependent continuous random vectors such that $F_W = F_{W'}$ and $F_Z = F_{Z'}$. Then, (W', Z') is more concordant than (W, Z) if $F_{W',Z'}(w, z) \geq F_{W,Z}(w, z)$ for all $(w, z) \in \Re^2$.

Because of invariance to strictly increasing transformations, (W, Z) and (W', Z') are ordered by concordance if and only if their respective copulas $C_{W,Z}$ and $C_{W',Z'}$ are such that $C_{W',Z'}(u, v) \geq C_{W,Z}(u, v)$ for all $0 \leq u, v \leq 1$.

We next state conditions and results on the conditional distributions so that the copulas $C_{X,Y}$ and C_{X,Y^*} of $F_{X,Y}$ and F_{X,Y^*}, respectively, are ordered by concordance when Y and Y^* have different distributions.

Let X be a continuous random variable with cdf F_X. Let $\{F_{Y|X}(\cdot|x) : x \in \Re\}$ and $\{F_{Y^*|X}(\cdot|x) : x \in \Re\}$ be two sets of continuous conditional distributions leading to marginal cdfs F_Y and F_{Y^*}, respectively. Then, $V = F_Y(Y)$ and $V^* = F_{Y^*}(Y^*)$ are $U(0, 1)$ random variables, so that (X, V) and (X, V^*) can be compared with the concordance ordering.

A condition on the conditional distributions $F_{V|X}(\cdot|x)$ and $F_{V^*|X}(\cdot|x)$ leading to the concordance ordering is that

$$F_{V^*|X}^{-1}\big[F_{V|X}(v|x)|x\big] \uparrow x \text{ (increasing in } x\text{)}, \quad \forall v. \tag{13}$$

See Section 2.2.4 of Joe (1997) for details of this stochastic increasing ordering.

Note that

$$F_{V|X}(v|x) = \Pr\big(F_Y(Y) \leq v|X = x\big) = F_{Y|X}\big[F_Y^{-1}(v)|x\big],$$

and similarly $F_{V^*|X}(v|x) = F_{Y^*|X}(F_{Y^*}^{-1}(v)|x)$. We next convert (13) to a condition on $\{F_{Y|X}(\cdot|x)\}$ and $\{F_{Y^*|X}(\cdot|x)\}$. The left-hand side of (13) is

$$F_{Y^*}\big[F_{Y^*|X}^{-1}\big(F_{Y|X}[F_Y^{-1}(v)|x] \mid x\big)\big]. \tag{14}$$

With $y = F_Y^{-1}(v)$, (14) is increasing in x for all v if

$$F_{Y^*|X}^{-1}\big(F_{Y|X}[y|x] \mid x\big) \uparrow x, \quad \forall y. \tag{15}$$

Condition (15) is straightforward to check if $\{F_{Y|X}(\cdot|x)\}$ and $\{F_{Y^*|X}(\cdot|x)\}$ are Pareto distributions with different tail parameters as in Sect. 3.

Because the resulting copulas depend on a_1, a_2 only through $\theta = a_2/a_1$, it suffices to consider $\alpha(x) = 1 + \theta/x$ and $\alpha^*(x) = 1 + \theta^*/x$ with $0 < \theta < \theta^*$. We would like to show that the copula in (8) or (10) with parameter θ^* is more concordant than that with parameter θ.

The conditional distributions and inverses are

$$F_{Y|X}(y|x) = 1-y^{-\alpha(x)}, \; F_{Y^*|X}(y|x) = 1-y^{-\alpha^*(x)}, \; F_{Y^*|X}^{-1}(p|x) = (1-p)^{-1/\alpha^*(x)},$$

with $y > 1, x > 0, 0 < p < 1$. The left-hand side of (15) is

$$(1 - F_{Y|X}(y|x))^{-1/\alpha^*(x)} = y^{\alpha(x)/\alpha^*(x)};$$

this is increasing in x for all $y > 1$ if

$$\frac{\alpha(x)}{\alpha^*(x)} = \frac{1 + \theta/x}{1 + \theta^*/x} = 1 - \frac{\theta^* - \theta}{x + \theta^*}$$

is increasing in x. This holds if $\theta^* > \theta > 0$.

In Sect. 3.3, the conditional Pareto tail parameter is $\alpha(x) = a_1 + a_2 x^{-\beta}$ for $x > 0$, with $a_1 \geq 0$, $a_2 > 0$, and $\beta > 0$. Cases of ordered by concordance are listed below based on the triplets (a_1, a_2, β) for $\alpha(x)$ and (a_1^*, a_2^*, β^*) for $\alpha^*(x)$; this requires showing that $\alpha(x)/\alpha^*(x)$ is increasing in $x > 0$.

1. $(a_1^*, a_2^*, \beta^*) = (1, a_2/a_1, \beta)$ lead to the same copula, because $\alpha(x)/\alpha^*(x) = a^{-1}$ is constant over x.
2. $(a_1, a_2, \beta) = (1, \theta, \beta)$ and $(a_1^*, a_2^*, \beta^*) = (1, \theta^*, \beta)$ with $\theta^* > \theta > 0$. Then,

$$\frac{\alpha(x)}{\alpha^*(x)} = 1 - \frac{\theta^* - \theta}{x^\beta + \theta^*} \uparrow x.$$

3. $(a_1^*, a_2^*, \beta^*) = (0, 1, \beta)$. Then,

$$\frac{\alpha(x)}{\alpha^*(x)} = a_1 x^\beta + a_2 \uparrow x.$$

4. $(a_1, a_2, \beta) = (0, 1, \beta)$ and $(a_1^*, a_2^*, \beta^*) = (0, 1, \beta^*)$ with $\beta^* > \beta > 0$. Then,

$$\frac{\alpha(x)}{\alpha^*(x)} = x^{\beta^* - \beta} \uparrow x.$$

For $(a_1, a_2, \beta) = (0, 1, \beta)$, the explanation for comonotonicity as $\beta \to \infty$ is as follows. Suppose data are simulated conditionally with Pareto$(1, \alpha(x) = x^{-\beta})$. Let $x_1, \ldots, x_n$ be realizations of a Pareto(1,1) random sample with support on $(0, \infty)$, and let $u_1, \ldots, u_n$ be a $U(0, 1)$ random sample. Let $y_i = u_i^{-1/\alpha(x_i)} = u_i^{-x_i^\beta}$. Suppose β is large. Then, for $x_i > 1$, y_i is large, and for $x_i < 1$, y_i is near 1. Hence, Spearman's rank correlation of $(x_1, y_1), \ldots, (x_n, y_n)$, as a random sample from the Pareto mixture model, approaches 1 as $\beta \to \infty$. See Fig. 1 for an illustration.

With a similar analysis for (12), consider $F_{Y|X}$ based on $\alpha(x), \sigma(x)$ and $F_{Y^*|X}$ based on $\alpha^*(x), \sigma^*(x)$. Then, F_{X,Y^*} is more concordant than $F_{X,Y}$ if $\alpha(x) = \alpha^*(x)$ and $\sigma^*(x)/\sigma(x)$ is increasing. No general concordance result can be proved with $\sigma(x) = \sigma^*(x)$ and $\alpha(x)/\alpha^*(x)$ increasing. However, (12) includes comonotonicity as $\beta \to \infty$ from the case of constant $\sigma(x)$. As shown in Sect. 6, $\sigma(x)$ increasing at a sufficiently fast rate is needed for (12) to have upper tail dependence.

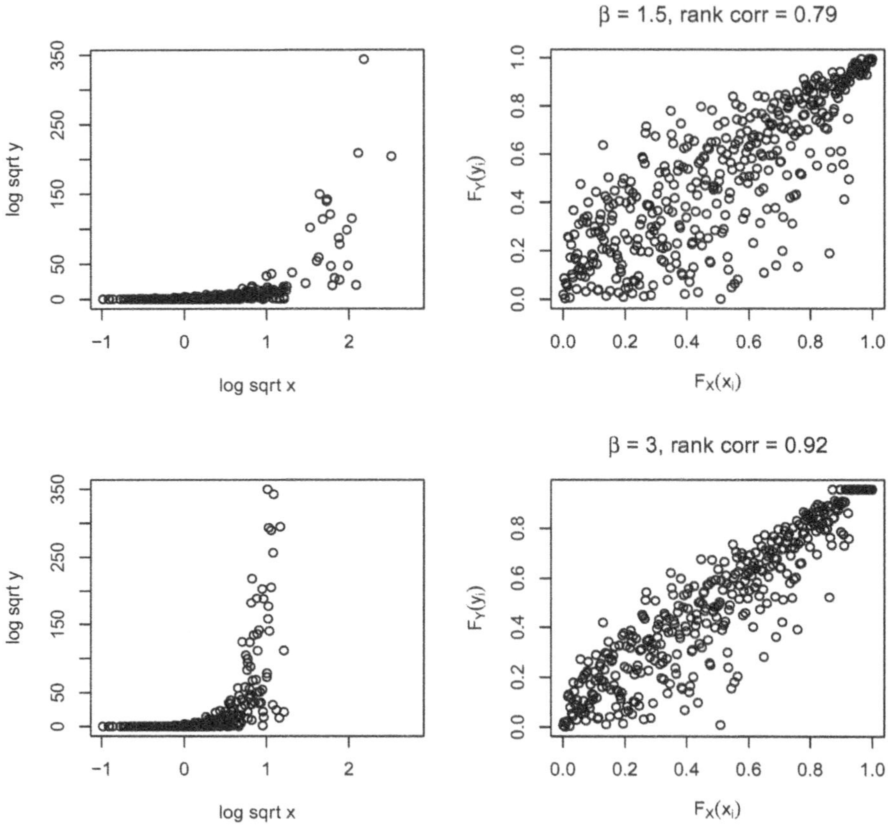

Fig. 1 Plots of simulated data from (11) with $\alpha(x) = x^{-\beta}$, $\beta = 1.5$ and 3. The plots on the right-hand side include the empirical Spearman's rank correlation values

5 $\xi_{Y|X}(x)$ Versus ξ_Y for Pareto Mixtures

In this section, we elaborate on a question from the end of Sect. 2 concerning conditions for $\sup_x \xi_{Y|X}(x) < \xi_Y$.

If $\xi_{Y|X}(x)$ is non-constant and the conditional Pareto scale parameter is constant, the examples in Sect. 3 have $\sup_x \xi_{Y|X}(x) = \xi_Y$. Proposition 2.5.1 in Coia (2017) establishes that under some regularity and continuity conditions, $\xi_{Y|X}(x) \leq \xi_Y$ for all x.

To get some initial insight, we analyze a special case of (12) with $\alpha(x) = \alpha > 0$ for which $\xi_{Y|X}(x) = \alpha^{-1}$ is constant. We consider conditions on the conditional scale parameter $\sigma(x)$ of the Pareto type II distributions $\overline{F}_{Y|X}(y|x) = (1 + y/\sigma(x))^{-\alpha}$ in order that $\xi_{Y|X}(x) = \alpha^{-1} < \xi_Y$.

For Y to be stochastically increasing in X, assume that $\sigma(x)$ is strictly increasing in x. For an assumption that leads to more tractable integrals, suppose $X \sim$ Pareto$(1, \gamma)$ with survival function $\overline{F}_X(x) = (1+x)^{-\gamma}$. The resulting joint distribution is

$$\overline{F}_{X,Y}(x, y) = \int_x^{\infty} [1 + y/\sigma(z)]^{-\alpha} \gamma (1+z)^{-\gamma-1} \mathrm{d}z, \quad x > 0, y > 0. \tag{16}$$

Without loss of generality, we can assume $\gamma = 1$ for study of dependence and tail properties.

Several cases are outlined below:

(a) Suppose $\sigma(x)$ is a smooth bounded function in the interval $[b_1, b_2]$, with $0 < b_1 < b_2 < \infty$. Then,

$$\begin{aligned}(1 + y/b_1)^{-\alpha} &= \int_0^{\infty} (1 + y/b_1)^{-\alpha} \gamma (1+x)^{-\gamma-1} \mathrm{d}x \\ &\leq \overline{F}_Y(y) = \int_0^{\infty} (1 + y/\sigma(x))^{-\alpha} \gamma (1+x)^{-\gamma-1} \mathrm{d}x \\ &\leq \int_0^{\infty} (1 + y/b_2)^{-\alpha} \gamma (1+x)^{-\gamma-1} \mathrm{d}x = (1 + y/b_2)^{-\alpha}.\end{aligned}$$

Assuming that $\overline{F}_Y$ has regularly varying tail, $\xi_Y = 1/\alpha = \xi_{Y|X}(x)$.

(b) Therefore, in order to have $\xi_{Y|X} < \xi_Y$, $\sigma(x)$ should be unbounded. Note that in the example in Sect. 2 based on Mardia's bivariate Pareto, $\sigma(x)$ ranges from 1 to ∞ and $\xi_{Y|X} < \xi_Y$. We show below with examples that if $\sigma(x)$ increases from b_1 to $b_2 = \infty$ at a fast enough rate, then $\xi_{Y|X} < \xi_Y$ holds.

We take $\gamma = 1$ and $\sigma(x) = (1+x)^a$ for different $a > 0$ for a concrete illustration of this claim. In this case, $\sigma(x)$ increases from 1 to ∞ as x goes from 0 to ∞. The comparison of $\xi_{Y|X}$ and ξ_Y will depend on the relative magnitudes of a and α. If $\gamma \neq 1$, a result will follow from the same steps as below.

Under the above assumptions, we have

$$\overline{F}_Y(y) = \int_0^{\infty} \left[1 + y/(1+x)^a\right]^{-\alpha} (1+x)^{-2} \mathrm{d}x.$$

To get approximations to this integral, we transform with $(1+x) = \mathrm{e}^z$ or $x = \mathrm{e}^z - 1$ for $z > 0$. Then,

$$\overline{F}_Y(y) = \int_0^{\infty} (1 + y\mathrm{e}^{-az})^{-\alpha} \mathrm{e}^{-z} \mathrm{d}z = \int_0^{\infty} \mathrm{e}^{-g(z)} \mathrm{d}z, \tag{17}$$

where $g(z; y) = \alpha \log(1 + y\mathrm{e}^{-az}) + z$. Then,

$$g'(z;y) = 1 - \alpha a y/(\mathrm{e}^{az} + y),$$
$$g''(z;y) = \alpha a^2 y\,\mathrm{e}^{az}/(\mathrm{e}^{az} + y)^2 > 0,$$

so that $g' > 0$ if $\alpha a \leq 1$ and $g(z;y)$ has a global minimum at $z^* = z^*(y) = a^{-1}\log[y(\alpha a - 1)]$ or $\mathrm{e}^{az^*} = y(\alpha a - 1)$ if $\alpha a > 1$. In the latter case, $g''(z^*;y) = (\alpha a - 1)/\alpha > 0$.

We consider three subcases: (i) $\alpha a < 1$, (ii) $\alpha a = 1$, and (iii) $\alpha a > 1$.

Case (i) For large y, (17) becomes

$$\overline{F}_Y(y) = y^{-\alpha}\int_0^\infty (y^{-1} + \mathrm{e}^{-az})^{-\alpha}\mathrm{e}^{-z}\mathrm{d}z = O(y^{-\alpha})$$

because

$$\lim_{y\to\infty}\int_0^\infty (y^{-1} + \mathrm{e}^{-az})^{-\alpha}\mathrm{e}^{-z}\mathrm{d}z = \int_0^\infty \mathrm{e}^{-z(1-\alpha a)}\mathrm{d}z = (1-\alpha a)^{-1},$$

by the dominated convergence theorem. Hence, $\xi_Y = \alpha^{-1} = \xi_{Y|X}(x)$.

Case (ii) Let $w = z/(\alpha\log y)$ so that (17) becomes

$$\overline{F}_Y(y) = y^{-\alpha}\int_0^\infty (1 + y^{-1}\mathrm{e}^{z/\alpha})^{-\alpha}\mathrm{d}z = \alpha y^{-\alpha}\log y\int_0^\infty (1 + y^{-1}\mathrm{e}^{w\log y})^{-\alpha}\mathrm{d}w$$
$$= \alpha y^{-\alpha}\log y\int_0^1 (1 + y^{-1+w})^{-\alpha}\mathrm{d}w + \alpha y^{-\alpha}\log y\int_1^\infty (1 + y^{-1+w})^{-\alpha}\mathrm{d}w.$$

For the first term, by the dominated convergence theorem,

$$\lim_{y\to\infty}\int_0^1 (1 + y^{-1+w})^{-\alpha}\mathrm{d}w = 1.$$

For the second term,

$$\int_1^\infty (1 + y^{-1+w})^{-\alpha}\mathrm{d}w \leq \int_1^\infty y^{-\alpha(w-1)}\mathrm{d}w = \int_1^\infty \exp\{-\alpha(\log y)(w-1)\}\mathrm{d}w$$
$$= \int_0^\infty \exp\{-\alpha(\log y)w'\}\mathrm{d}w' = \alpha^{-1}(\log y)^{-1}.$$

Hence, as $y \to \infty$,

$$\overline{F}_Y(y) = O(y^{-\alpha}\log y) + O(y^{-\alpha}) = O(y^{-\alpha}\log y).$$

Hence, $\xi_Y = \alpha^{-1} = \xi_{Y|X}(x)$, but the marginal distribution has slightly heavier tail because of the slowly varying $\log y$ term with a positive power.

Case (iii) For large y, apply Laplace's approximation (see Breitung 1994) to get

$$\begin{aligned}\overline{F}_Y(y) &\approx \int_0^\infty \exp\{-g(z^*;y) - \tfrac{1}{2}g''(z^*;y)(z-z^*)^2\}dz\\ &\approx \exp\{-g(z^*;y)\}[g''(z^*;y)]^{-1/2}\\ &= [1+1/(\alpha a-1)]^{-\alpha} y^{-1/a}(\alpha a-1)^{-1/a}\sqrt{\frac{\alpha}{\alpha a-1}}.\end{aligned}$$

Hence, $\xi_Y = a > \alpha^{-1} = \xi_{Y|X}(x)$.

The third case (iii) extends to (12) with a non-constant $\alpha(x)$; for some tractable approximations, we assume that the tail parameter is $\alpha(x) = a_1 + a_2 x^{-\beta}$ and f_X is Pareto(1,1) on $(0,\infty)$. The joint survival function is

$$\overline{F}_{X,Y}(x,y) = \int_x^\infty [1+y/\sigma(z)]^{-\alpha(x)}(1+z)^{-2}dz, \quad x>0, y>0. \tag{18}$$

The marginal survival function is

$$\overline{F}_Y(y) = \int_0^\infty (1+ye^{-az})^{-\alpha(z)}e^{-z}dz = \int_0^\infty e^{-g(z)}dz, \tag{19}$$

if $g(z;y) = \alpha(z)\log(1+ye^{-az}) + z$. For Laplace's approximation, $g'(z;y) = 1-\alpha(z)ay/(e^{az}+y) + \alpha'(z)\log(1+ye^{-az})$ and

$$g''(z;y) = \alpha(z)a^2ye^{az}/(e^{az}+y)^2 - 2\alpha'(z)ay/(e^{az}+y) + \alpha''(z)\log(1+ye^{-az}) > 0,$$

where $\alpha'(z) = -a_2\beta z^{-\beta-1} < 0$ and $\alpha''(z) = a_2\beta(1+\beta)z^{-\beta-2} > 0$.

Consider the case of $\alpha(z)a > 1$ for all $z > 0$ with $a_1 a > 1$. For large y, $g'(z;y)$ has a global minimum at $z^* = z^*(y)$ satisfying $g'(z^*;y) = 0$. With a tail expansion and $\delta = a_1 a - 1 > 0$, one gets

$$\begin{aligned}e^{az^*(y)} &= \delta y + r_y, \quad r_y = O(y(\log y)^{-\beta}),\\ z^*(y) &= a^{-1}\log(\delta y) + a^{-1}r_y(\delta y)^{-1} = a^{-1}\log(\delta y) + O((\log y)^{-\beta}).\end{aligned}$$

Now, substitute into $g(z^*)$ and $g''(z^*)$, to get, as $y \to \infty$,

$$\begin{aligned}g(z^*;y) &\sim [a_1 + a_2(a^{-1}\log(\delta y))^{-\beta}]\log(1+\delta^{-1}) + a^{-1}\log(\delta y) + O((\log y)^{-\beta})\\ &\sim \log(1+\delta^{-1})\cdot[a_1 + O((\log y)^{-\beta}] + a^{-1}\log(\delta y) + O((\log y)^{-\beta})\\ &\sim a^{-1}\log(\delta y) + \log(1+\delta^{-1}),\end{aligned}$$

$$
\begin{aligned}
\mathrm{e}^{-g(z^*;y)} &= O(y^{-1/a}),\\
g''(z^*;y) &\sim \alpha(z^*)a^2 y\mathrm{e}^{az^*}/(\mathrm{e}^{az^*}+y)^2 - 2\alpha'(z^*)ay/(\mathrm{e}^{az^*}+y)\\
&\quad +\alpha''(z^*)\log(1+y\mathrm{e}^{-az^*})\\
&= (aa_1-1)a_1^{-1} + O((z^*)^{-\beta}).
\end{aligned}
$$

For large y, Laplace's approximation yields

$$
\begin{aligned}
\overline{F}_Y(y) &\approx \int_0^\infty \exp\{-g(z^*;y) - \tfrac{1}{2}g''(z^*;y)(z-z^*)^2\}\mathrm{d}z\\
&\approx \exp\{-g(z^*;y)\}[g''(z^*;y)]^{-1/2} = O(y^{-1/a}).
\end{aligned}
$$

Hence, $\xi_Y = a > a_1^{-1} \geq \xi_{Y|X}(x) = (a_1 + a_2 x^{-\beta})^{-1}$, and $\xi_Y > \sup_x \xi_{Y|X}(x) = a_1^{-1}$.

6 Upper Tail Dependence for Pareto Mixtures

This section provides details on the result mentioned in Sect. 2 on the link between upper tail dependence and the property of $\xi_{Y|X}(x) < \xi_Y$, for the Pareto mixtures.

We first consider the case of constant $\alpha(x)$ in the conditional Pareto distribution and show that there is upper tail dependence when the scale function $\sigma(x)$ is increasing at a fast enough rate. We then show that there is no upper tail dependence for the constructions in Sects. 3.1 and 3.2 with constant $\sigma(x)$ and non-constant $\alpha(x)$. To achieve increasing $\xi_{Y|X}(x)$ with $\sup_x \xi_{Y|X}(x) < \xi_Y$ and upper tail dependence, we need $\sigma(x)$ increasing at a fast enough rate and non-constant $\alpha(x)$. The details are given below.

Let $\sigma(x)$ be increasing as in Sect. 5, and let $\gamma = 1$ and $\alpha > 0$. We show for the case of $\sigma(x)$ bounded in $[b_1, b_2]$ or $\sigma(x) = (1+x)^a$ with $\alpha a < 1$ (and $\alpha > 0$, $a > 0$) that the upper tail dependence coefficient is 0; for $\sigma(x) = (1+x)^a$ with $\alpha a > 1$, the upper tail dependence coefficient is in the interval (0, 1).

If $(X, Y) \sim F_{X,Y}$ is a continuous random vector, the upper tail dependence coefficient, defined in Sect. 2, is equivalent to

$$
\lambda_U = \lim_{u\to 0} u^{-1}\Pr\left(X > \overline{F}_X^{-1}(u), Y > \overline{F}_Y^{-1}(u)\right) = \lim_{u\to 0} u^{-1}\overline{F}_{X,Y}\left(\overline{F}_X^{-1}(u), \overline{F}_Y^{-1}(u)\right).
$$

If X is Pareto(1,1) on $(0,\infty)$, then $\overline{F}_X^{-1}(u) = u^{-1} - 1 \sim u^{-1}$ as $u \to 0^+$. For the Pareto scale mixture,

$$
\overline{F}_{X,Y}(x, y) = \int_x^\infty [1 + y/\sigma(z)]^{-\alpha}(1+z)^{-2}\mathrm{d}z,
$$

$$u^{-1}\overline{F}_{X,Y}\big(\overline{F}_X^{-1}(u), \overline{F}_Y^{-1}(u)\big) \sim u^{-1}\int_{u^{-1}}^{\infty}[1+\overline{F}_Y^{-1}(u)/\sigma(z)]^{-\alpha}(1+z)^{-2}\mathrm{d}z$$
$$= u^{-2}\int_{1}^{\infty}[1+\overline{F}_Y^{-1}(u)/\sigma(w/u)]^{-\alpha}(1+w/u)^{-2}\mathrm{d}w$$
$$\sim \int_{1}^{\infty}[1+\overline{F}_Y^{-1}(u)/\sigma(w/u)]^{-\alpha}w^{-2}\mathrm{d}w,$$

as $u \to 0$. Next, we consider several cases:

(a) $\sigma(x)$ bounded in $[b_1, b_2]$ with $0 < b_1 < b_2 < \infty$. From Sect. 5, $\overline{F}_Y^{-1}(u) \sim bu^{-1/\alpha}$ as $u \to 0$ for some $b > 0$, and $\sigma(w/u) \to b_2$ as $u \to 0$. Hence,

$$\lambda_U = \lim_{u\to 0}\int_{1}^{\infty}[1+\overline{F}_Y^{-1}(u)/\sigma(w/u)]^{-\alpha}w^{-2}\mathrm{d}w$$
$$= \lim_{u\to 0}\int_{1}^{\infty}[1+bu^{-1/\alpha}/b_2)]^{-\alpha}w^{-2}\mathrm{d}w = \lim_{u\to 0}\int_{1}^{\infty}ub^{-\alpha}b_2^{\alpha}w^{-2}\mathrm{d}w = 0.$$

(b) $\sigma(x) = (1+x)^a$ with $\alpha a < 1$. From Sect. 5, $\overline{F}_Y^{-1}(u) \sim (u/k)^{-1/\alpha}$ as $u \to 0$, for some $k > 0$. Hence,

$$\lambda_U = \lim_{u\to 0}\int_{1}^{\infty}[1+k^{1/\alpha}u^{-1/\alpha}/(1+(w/u))^{a}]^{-\alpha}w^{-2}\mathrm{d}w$$
$$= \lim_{u\to 0}\int_{1}^{\infty}[1+k^{1/\alpha}u^{a-1/\alpha}/w^{a}]^{-\alpha}w^{-2}\mathrm{d}w$$
$$= \lim_{u\to 0}u^{1-\alpha a}k^{-1}\int_{1}^{\infty}w^{-2+\alpha a}\mathrm{d}w$$
$$= \lim_{u\to 0}u^{1-\alpha a}k^{-1}(1-\alpha a)^{-1} = 0.$$

(c) $\sigma(x) = (1+x)^a$ with $\alpha a > 1$. From Sect. 5, $\overline{F}_Y^{-1}(u) \sim (u/k)^{-a}$ as $u \to 0$, for some $k > 0$. Hence,

$$\lambda_U = \lim_{u\to 0}\int_{1}^{\infty}[1+\overline{F}_Y^{-1}(u)/\sigma(w/u)]^{-\alpha}w^{-2}\mathrm{d}w \qquad (20)$$
$$= \lim_{u\to 0}\int_{1}^{\infty}[1+k^{a}u^{-a}/(1+(w/u))^{a}]^{-\alpha}w^{-2}\mathrm{d}w$$
$$= \lim_{u\to 0}\int_{1}^{\infty}[1+k^{a}/w^{a}]^{-\alpha}w^{-2}\mathrm{d}w \in (0,1).$$

For comparisons, next consider the copulas derived from the constructions in Sects. 3.1 and 3.2. Because the copula in (8) was obtained from the survival functions, it will have lower tail dependence if the original $\overline{F}_{X,Y}$ has upper tail dependence. It can be shown analytically (and numerically) that (8) does not have lower tail dependence; this is based on $H^{-1}(u;\eta) \sim [-\eta u \log u]^{-1}$ as $u \to 0$. With similar techniques, (10) also does not have lower tail dependence, based on $G^{-1}(u;\theta) \sim [-\theta u \log u]^{-1}$ as $u \to 0$. After substituting in $C(u,u)/u$ in the two cases, one makes use of $[-\theta u \log u]^{\theta u} \to 1$ as $u \to 0$.

To have non-constant $\xi_{Y|X}(x)$ and upper tail dependence, we consider (12) with appropriate non-constant $\sigma(x)$ and $\alpha(x)$. Consider the case at the end of Sect. 5 with $\alpha(x) = a_1 + a_2 x^{-\beta}$ with $a_1 > 0$, $a_2 > 0$, and $\beta > 0$, and $\sigma(x) = (1+x)^a$. Also, assume $aa_1 > 1$. Then, the expression and derivation for $\lambda_U > 0$ are similar to those in (20), making use of $\overline{F}_Y(y) = O(y^{-1/a})$ as $y \to \infty$.

7 Discussion

We have studied some properties of bivariate distributions based on Pareto mixtures. In this section, we give a big picture viewpoint of when the theory is relevant for data analysis and conditional tail inferences.

With bivariate data (x_i, y_i), $i = 1, \ldots, n$, from a random sample, different approaches, depending on sample size, can be used to assess if conditional extreme value index function is non-constant. One method is to apply the peaks over threshold method (Coles 2001) or fit generalized Pareto distributions to moving windows of x-values to evaluate if the estimation of $\xi_{Y|X}(x)$ is monotone or non-constant. Another method involves non-parametric estimation of conditional extreme quantiles such as in Gardes et al. (2010). Tail dependence properties can be assessed with bivariate plots after data have been transformed to $N(0,1)$ or with tail-weighted dependence measures (Krupskii and Joe 2015). The models in this chapter can be used if a monotone conditional extreme value index function is suggested, with or without tail dependence.

The constructions in the first two subsections of Sect. 3 have monotone $\xi_{Y|X}(x)$ approaching ξ_Y as $x \to \infty$ and constant $\xi_{X|Y}(y)$ and do not have tail dependence. The results in Sects. 5 and 6 suggest that the Pareto scale parameter must be increasing at a fast enough rate to achieve both $\sup_x \xi_{Y|X}(x) < \xi_Y$ and upper tail dependence.

We summarize the main results in Sects. 3–6 in order to discuss some results in Arnold et al. (1999) and possible future research. Consider $[Y|X = x] \sim \text{Pareto}(\sigma(x), \alpha(x))$ and $X > 0$ with regularly varying tail. For positive dependence, we have $\alpha(x)$ decreasing and $\sigma(x)$ increasing:

(a) With $\alpha(x)$ decreasing in x and $\sigma(x)$ constant, we can get families with positive dependence and $\xi_{Y|X}(x) < \xi_Y$. The range of dependence depends on the flexibility of the parametric family $\alpha(x)$. The specific examples in Sect. 3 do not have upper tail dependence.

(b) With $\alpha(x)$ constant and $\sigma(x)$ increasing and bounded, $\xi_{Y|X}(x) = \xi_Y$ and there is no upper tail dependence.
(c) With $\alpha(x)$ constant and $\sigma(x)$ unbounded and increasing at a fast enough rate, it is possible that $\xi_{Y|X}(x) < \xi_Y$ and upper tail dependence exists.
(d) With $\alpha(x)$ decreasing in x and $\sigma(x)$ unbounded and increasing at a fast enough rate, $\sup_x \xi_{Y|X}(x) < \xi_Y$ and upper tail dependence exists.

Qualitatively, these results should hold for more general Pareto families because they just concern a tail parameter and a scale parameter.

With conditionally specified Pareto or generalized Pareto distributions for $\{F_{Y|X}(\cdot|x)\}$ and $\{F_{X|Y}(\cdot|y)\}$, Arnold (1987) and Arnold et al. (1993) (see also Chapter 5 of Arnold et al. 1999) have a few closed-form joint densities that satisfy the functional equations from the compatibility constraints. However, these distributions do not have flexible ranges of dependence. With the generalized Pareto(σ, δ, α) or Burr family defined by $F_{\mathrm{GP}}(z; \sigma, \delta, \alpha) = 1 - [1 + (z/\sigma)^{\delta}]^{-\alpha}$ for $z > 0$, Arnold et al. (1993) consider the conditional specifications:

$$[X|Y = y] \sim F_{\mathrm{GP}}(\cdot; \sigma(y), \delta(y), \alpha(y)), \quad y > 0,$$

$$[Y|X = x] \sim F_{\mathrm{GP}}(\cdot; \tau(x), \gamma(x), \beta(x)), \quad x > 0.$$

They assume constant inner power parameters $\delta(y) = \delta$ and $\gamma(x) = \gamma$ and find examples of densities satisfying the compatibility constraints when the outer power parameters α and β are constants or when the scale parameters σ and τ are constants. Neither class of resulting densities has much range of dependence, and it can be shown that $\xi_{Y|X}(x) = \xi_Y$ and $\xi_{X|Y}(y) = \xi_X$, so that the conditional tail index functions are the same as their respective marginal tail indices. Also, there is no upper tail dependence, and the upper tail behaves like tail quadrant independence.

It is an open problem on how to construct bivariate models and copulas with simpler parametric forms that have non-constant $\xi_{Y|X}(x)$ and $\xi_{X|Y}(y)$, with possible tail dependence. One would have to relax the assumption that conditional distributions are Pareto throughout the whole domain and instead assume that the conditional tails are regularly varying. The results of this chapter suggest that the conditional tail indices for $\{F_{Y|X}(\cdot|x)\}$ and $\{F_{X|Y}(\cdot|y)\}$ should have a wide range of decreasing functions and that the scale functions for $\{F_{Y|X}(\cdot|x)\}$ and $\{F_{X|Y}(\cdot|y)\}$ should have a wide range of increasing functions.

The investigation here is mainly bivariate and is focused on getting bivariate copula families with properties that are not satisfied by commonly used copula families. If multivariate distributions with non-constant conditional extreme value index functions are needed, the bivariate copula constructions developed here can be used within vine copulas. Vine copulas (Czado 2019; Joe 2014) have flexible dependence structures and are composed from a sequence of bivariate copulas, most of which are used to summarize conditional dependence.

Acknowledgments The research has been supported by NSERC Discovery grants. The authors thank a referee for a careful reading and suggestions for improvement.

References

Arnold, B. C. (1987). Bivariate distributions with Pareto conditionals. *Statistics & Probability Letters, 5*, 263–266.
Arnold, B. C. (2015). *Pareto distributions* (2nd ed.). Roca Baton, FL: Chapman & Hall/CRC.
Arnold, B. C., Castillo, E., & Sarabia, J. M. (1993). Multivariate distributions with generalized Pareto conditionals. *Statistics & Probability Letters, 17*, 361–368.
Arnold, B. C., Castillo, E., & Sarabia, J. M. (1999). *Conditional specification of statistical models*. New York: Springer.
Balakrishnan, N., & Lai, C. D. (2009). *Continuous bivariate distributions* (2nd ed.). Dordrecht: Springer.
Breitung, K. W. (1994). *Asymptotic approximations for probability integrals*. Berlin: Springer.
Chavez-Demoulin, V., Embrechts, P., & Hobert, M. (2016). An extreme value approach for modeling operational risk losses depending on covariates. *Journal of Risk and Insurance, 83*(3), 735–776.
Coia, V. (2017). *Forecasting of Nonlinear Extreme Quantiles Using Copula Models*. PhD thesis, University of British Columbia.
Coles, S. (2001). *An introduction to statistical modeling of extreme values*. London: Springer.
Czado, C. (2019). *Analyzing dependent data with vine copulas. A practical guide with R*. Cham: Springer.
Gardes, L., Girard, S., & Lekina, A. (2010). Functional nonparametric estimation of conditional extreme quantiles. *Journal of Multivariate Analysis, 101*(2), 419–433.
Joe, H. (1997). *Multivariate models and dependence concepts*. London: Chapman & Hall.
Joe, H. (2014). *Dependence modeling with copulas*. Boca Raton, FL: Chapman & Hall/CRC.
Krupskii, P., & Joe, H. (2015). Tail-weighted measures of dependence. *Journal of Applied Statistics, 42*(3), 614–629.
Mardia, K. V. (1962). Multivariate Pareto distributions. *Annals of Mathematical Statistics, 33*(3), 1008–1015.
Rezaul, K., & Grout, V. (2007). A comparison of methods for estimating the tail index of heavy-tailed internet traffic. In T. Sobh, K. Elleithy, A. Mahmood, & M. Karim (Eds.), *Innovative algorithms and techniques in automation, industrial electronics and telecommunications* (pp. 219–222). Dordrecht: Springer.
Sklar, A. (1959). Fonctions de répartition à *n* dimensions et leurs marges. *Publications de l'Institut de Statistique de l'Université de Paris, 8*, 229–231.
Takahasi, K. (1965). Note on the multivariate Burr's distribution. *Annals of the Institute of Statistical Mathematics, 17*(2), 257–260.

Part IV
General

How and Why Did Probability Theory Come About?

Nozer D. Singpurwalla and Boya Lai

Abstract This paper is a top down historical perspective on the several phases in the development of probability from its prehistoric origins to its modern day evolution, as one of the key methodologies in artificial intelligence, data science, and machine learning.

It is written in honor of Barry Arnold's birthday for his many contributions to statistical theory and methodology. Despite the fact that much of Barry's work is technical, a descriptive document to mark his achievements should not be viewed as being out of line. Barry's dissertation adviser at Stanford (he received a Ph.D. in Statistics there) was a philosopher of Science, who dug deep in the foundations and roots of probability, and it is this breadth of perspective is what Barry has inherent. The paper is based on lecture materials compiled by the first author from various published sources, and over a long period of time. The material below gives a limited list of references because the cast of characters is many, and their contributions are a part of the historical heritage of those of us who are interested in probability, statistics, and the many topics they have spawned.

1 Overview

The material here attempts to give a top down historical perspective on the several phases in the evolution of probability, from its prehistoric origins for imperial needs, to its current state as a branch of mathematics. As a branch of the mathematical sciences, probability evolved in five stages, not counting a period of stagnation between the second and third stages, when doubts were cast about its relevance as a mathematical discipline. Also pointed out are paradoxes in probability, spawned

N. D. Singpurwalla (✉)
The George Washington University, Washington, DC, USA
e-mail: nozer@gwu.edu

B. Lai
The City University of Hong Kong, Kowloon, Hong Kong
e-mail: boyalai2-c@my.cityu.edu.hk

I. Ghosh et al. (eds.), *Advances in Statistics - Theory and Applications*, Emerging Topics in Statistics and Biostatistics, https://doi.org/10.1007/978-3-030-62900-7_11

by the absence of its precise definition, leading to its last two phases, namely, an axiomatic and a subjective view of probability.

2 The Prehistoric Phase

The rulers of ancient Egypt, Greece, and Rome collected census data for taxes, grain distribution, and other matters of administration; this activity certainty had an impact on the origins of probability.

Next to come was the "Doomsday" list of William the Norman (1027–1087), which was so exhaustive an economic survey that it reminded one of the final and the last judgment by God in the Christian faith. Following this were the "London Bills of Mortality," published since 1517, and notions such as the *chance of death* in a given time period, the *chance of survival* to a certain age, and the like, originated, around about 1535, almost a century before John Graunt's celebrated mortality table. Another impetus to the origins of probability came from marine insurance in the 1300s, and also during the renaissance, wherein an emphasis was placed on observation and experiments in the natural sciences—especially, on errors of observation.

From a philosophical angle, the interrelations between chance and causality have been on the philosopher's agenda since the ancient times. These too had an impact on the origins of probability. In 1292, a treatise on the theory of the logical ideas of *Syadvada* (which is the basis of India's Jaina religion) lists seven predications of which the fourth supplies a foundation for modern probability.

Another influential angle was the famous dictum of Thomas Hobbs (1588–1679), whose thesis was that no matter for how long we observe a phenomenon, this is not sufficient grounds for its absolute and definitive knowledge.

To summarize, the prehistoric impact on probability came from: census, commerce, renaissance, scientific observation, and philosophy.

3 Was Probability Not Spawned by Gambling?

Apart from the discussion above, there is another belief that probability theory owes its birth to gambling. To some, this is a questionable issue. They claim that since gambling has been practiced since 5000 BC, it could not have taken 6000 years for it to influence probability. Their view is that it was commerce that really influenced the development of probability.

Nonetheless, gambling has had an impact on probability, and its earliest traces are in the literature, such as "*De Vetula*" of Richard de Fournival (1200–1250) and Dante's "*Divine Comedy*" (1307–1321), wherein combinatorial arguments pertaining to outcomes of games of chance were mentioned.

Paccioli (1445–1514) published in 1487 "*Summa de Arithmetica, Geometria, Proportioni et Proportionalita*," which was an encyclopedia of the mathematical knowledge of his period in Venice, and in the section labeled "unusual problems," he discussed the question of the fair division of stakes when a match is stopped in advance of an agreed termination of the game. Paccioli's solution embeds notions of probability. This is also called the "*problem of points*" and was a trigger point of the famous Pascal Fermat correspondence.

Cardano (1501–1576) and Tartagalia (1499–1557) contributed much to the connection between probability and gambling. Cardano developed probabilistic notions in "The Book on Games of Chance," written in 1526, as "*Liber de Ludo Aleae*." In this book, Cardano enumerates possibilities, permutations, deviations of frequencies from "portion," introduces the notions of fair games and expectation, equally likely events, and uses the addition and multiplication rules of probability for independent events. He even came close to inventing the law of large numbers. However, Cardano was an ardent gambler who restricted his writings, only to games of chance. All the same, as one can surmise, he set the stage for much that was to follow.

Tartagalia (1499–1557) published in Venice in 1556, his treatise on "Number and Measure" in which he related problems of probability to those of combinatorics, and offered correct solutions to the problems posed by Paccioli, in particular, the problem of the division of stakes (or the problem of points). Following Cardano and Tartagalia, was Galileo (1564–1642), who posited that errors of measurement are inevitable; they are symmetric and clustered around a true value. He in fact revealed many of the characteristics of the normal probability distribution.

The above developments perhaps mark the end of the phase of the earliest writings on probability, subsequent to its prehistoric phase.

4 Development of Probability as a Science

This phase can be categorized into five stages and includes a phase called "the period of stagnation," between the second and third stage, when concerns were raised about probability as a branch of mathematics. Also included is a phase labeled "paradoxes in probability," which can be seen as the doorstep to the development of the last two stages in the evolution of probability as a mathematical discipline.

Within the five stages alluded to above, are also some milestones in the evolution of statistics, which evolved as a way to reason with numbers.

4.1 Stage I: *Of the Development of Probability as a Science*

Up until the middle of the seventeenth century, there were no general methods for solving probabilistic problems. Specific problems had been solved, and a substantial amount of knowledge was accumulated. The term probability (nor its disposition as a number) was not a part of the lexicon in the solution of such problems.

In the middle of the seventeenth century, some prominent mathematicians like Pascal, Fermat, and Huygens became involved in the development of probability, even without mentioning the term. These individuals were familiar with Cardano's addition and the multiplication rules, the notion of independence, and put to practice the notion of expectation using combinatorics. They developed new methods for solving problems, determined the realm of problems to which this new science is applicable, and in so doing were on the verge of transforming probability to a bona fide science.

Two very important and key individuals need to be mentioned in Stage I. They were Chevalier de Mére and Christian Huygens. They brought probability into a new stage as a science. Chevalier de Mére (1607–1684) was a philosopher and a man of letters; he wrote to Pascal about the division of stakes (considered by Paccioli but per Shafer (2019)) solved in the 1400s by two Italian abacus masters, and his (de Mére's) solution to it. With Pascal and Fermat, he had authored in 1662 "*Ars Cognitandi*" (Art of Thinking) as a part of the Arnold - Nicole (who were abbots at the Port Royal Monastry), a book on "*Port RoyaleLogic*." de Mére's letter to Pascal triggered a correspondence between Pascal and Fermat in 1654, and thus originated the founding document on mathematical probability.

Even though many mathematicians of that period devoted much attention to the solution of games of chance, actual gambling was condemned. Thus, the myth that Chevalier de Mere was a fervent gambler. Rather, he was a man of letters who viewed probability only as a "useless curiosity." By contrast, Cardano, who was an ardent gambler, used mathematics for gambling but in 1526 did not quite hit upon the notion of probability as a number.

Christian Huygens (1629–1695), a Dutchman from Holland, visited Paris in 1655 to receive a doctorate in law. He was impressed with the problems on gambling of Pascal and Fermat and undertook further work on it. He was told of the solutions but not the methods (which were published posthumously, because both Pascal and Fermat posed problems to each other but hid their methods of solution). The correspondence between Pascal and Fermat was published only in 1679.

Huygens returned to Holland and begun work on solving the problems posed by Pascal and Fermat. Huygens solutions, independent of the methods of Pascal and Fermat, but identical to those of Pascal and Fermat, were published in his book (written in Latin) called "*About Dice Games*." This book appeared in 1657 wherein Huygens says "...we are dealing not only with games but rather with a foundation of a new theory, both deep and interesting." His reasons for writing this book was the absence of methods used by Pascal and Fermat.

This book is viewed as the first published treatise on mathematical probability. Huygens's book can be viewed as being the first formal document on the introduction of mathematical probability, until Bernoulli's famous "*Ars Conjectandi*" (a possible imitation of the Pascal–Fermat–de Mere's, Ars Cognitandi). Huygens' book was also the first to introduce and to apply the notion of expectation in commercial and industrial problems. Huygens' terminology was commercial.

Subsequent to the above, more and more works on probability began to appear, most notable being the birth to a new discipline, now called "*Data Science*." In 1662, at about the same time as Huygens' book, John Graunt, an Englishman, published a tiny book devoted to problems of vital statistics. Huygens was asked to comment on this landmark book, which he did favorably. Indeed, in 1669, using Graunt's work Huygens constructed a mortality curve and initiated the application of probability to demography, and to annuities. In 1690, another Englishman, by the name of William Petty, published his treaties on "*Political Arithmetic*," which was about a method of reasoning on matters of government, via the use of numbers. This can now be seen as a founding document on Government Statistics.

Preceding Petty's treatise, was work on actuarial mathematics and the worth of annuities, due to deWitts in 1671, followed by that of Edmund Haley in 1693, who published the very first mortality table based on data from Breslau. Between 1791 and 1799, a Scotsman named John Sinclair published 21 volumes of his Statistical Account of Scotland and introduced the word "*Statistics*" to replace Petty's political arithmetic. Up until 1796, the word "statistics" was used in Germany to describe the political strength, happiness, and the improvement of a country, as a measure of its well-being. Statistics was an artificial word, with no evidential meaning, that is now used for anything having to do with data. Sinclair used it to garner attention over Petty's political arithmetic, which did not seemed to have gained traction (cf. von Collani 2014).

To summarize, Huygens recognized the role of probability as a science, wrote the first book on it, applied the notion of expectation to commerce and industry, and used probability for assessing demography and insurance. Huygens' Book played an important role in the history of probability. Jacob Bernoulli, who introduced the term "probability," based on the Latin "*probabilitas*," was greatly influenced by Huygens' book. Bernoulli's work established the foundations of mathematical probability.

Bernoulli's word probability is based on the term "*probabilitas*," which was a moral system of the Catholic Church. Probabilitas was formally introduced in 1577 by the Spanish Dominican, Bartolome de Medina, and was mainly applied by Jesuit priests. Bernoulli's aim in writing Ars Conjectandi was to introduce a new branch of science that he called Stochastics, or the science of prediction.

To Bernoulli, a relevant feature of "stochastics" was an event's ***readiness to occur***, and "probability," the ***degree of certainty*** of its occurrence, see von Collani (2014). Thus, to Bernoulli, stochastics was the art of measuring probability as exactly as is possible.

However, Bernoulli acknowledged that the determination of the true value of probability is impossible and labeled as "mad" any attempt at doing so. This motivated him to develop his law of large numbers, as an empirical method to determine a lower and an upper limit for an unknown probability. Note that Bernoulli's notion of probability was devoid of any mathematical basis.

Given below in Fig. 1 is a graphic of the evolution of mathematical probability, up until the beginning of Stage II that established it as a mathematical science.

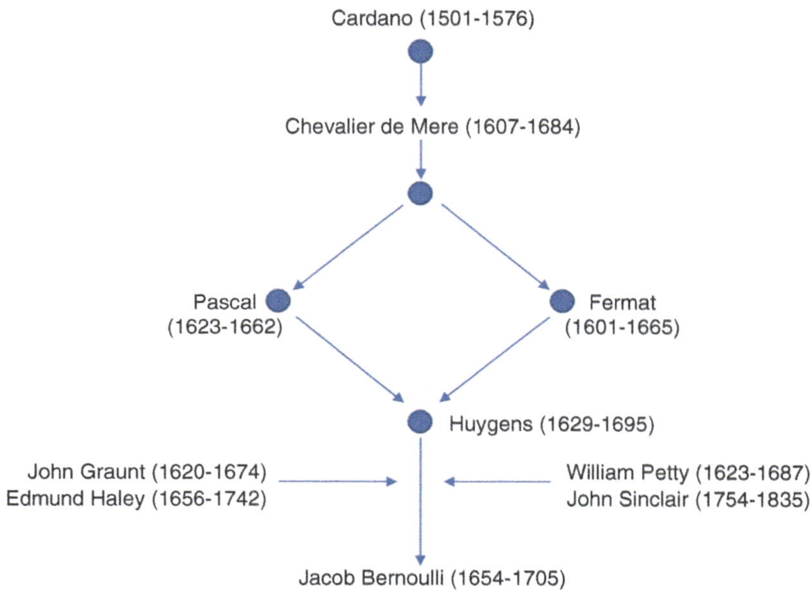

Fig. 1 Evolution of mathematical probability

4.2 Stage II: *Bernoulli Makes Probability a Bona Fide Mathematical Science*

James (Jacques) Bernoulli (1654–1705) in his 1713 "Ars Conjectandi" proved the first limit theorem and, in so doing, raised the status of probability to that of a formal mathematical science. This book was published posthumously by his nephew Nichols (1) Bernoulli (who also applied probability to matters of jurisprudence, like the credibility of a witness).

The contribution of Bernoulli to make probability a bona fide mathematical science is that he interpreted propositions in Huygens' book, showed inapplicability of the addition law to non-disjoint events, gave the binomial formula, and used Leibnitz's combinatorics for solving probability problems.

He proved the weak law of large numbers as a way to bound a "true" probability and interpreted probability as the degree of certainty of an event's occurrence. Bernoulli was a metaphysical determinist; that is, if we know the position of a dice, its speed, its distance from the board, etc., we can exactly predict its outcome. Thus, to Bernoulli, probability, or chance, the terms he used interchangeably, depends on our state of knowledge and is thus personal to the individual specifying it.

However, since all knowledge is not possible, we assume a statistical regularity in a large number of trials, say n, and conclude that for the tossing of coins, the deviation of m/n from p, as $n \to \infty$, is small with a large probability; m is the total number of heads in the n trials. Bernoulli also touched upon the philosophical problems connected with probability, and asserted probability should also be applied to situations outside games of chance.

Besides Bernoulli, there were others who worked on probability during the beginning of the eighteenth century. We name a few.

Pierre de Montmort (1678–1719), a mathematician, who was chosen by Leibnitz on the commission to inquire about the priority of inventing differential and integral calculus between him and Newton; de Montmort favored Newton; see Maistrov (1974). His basic work on probability entitled "*Essai d'Analyse sur les Jeux de Hazard*" was published in 1708 (5 years prior to Bernoulli's posthumously published work). It was in a letter to de Montmort that Nicholas (1) Bernoulli posed the St. Petersburg paradox. Montmort's main effort was the applications of probability to human behavior.

Abraham de Moivre's (1667–1754) principal work in probability was in "*The Doctrine of Chances*," 1718. Here, without addressing the matter of what probability is, de Moivre discusses topics connected to Bernoulli's theorem, and the problem of the duration of the play (first proposed by Huygens). de Moivre investigated the probabilities of various deviations between m/n and p, for $p = 1/2$. Laplace extended these to $p \in (0,1)$, and thus, the de Moivre–Laplace theorem is the second limit theorem in mathematical probability.

Thomas Bayes (1792–1761), speculated as being tutored by de Moivre, published his famous essay posthumously in 1763; it was entitled "*Thomas Bayes's Essay Towards* Solving *a Problem in the Doctrine of Chances*"; it addressed the following question: what is the chance that $p \in (a, b)$ given x and n? Bayes offered a solution to this problem using solely the calculus of probability. In so doing, he introduced the notion of what is referred to as "***probabilistic induction***."

To obtain his solution, Bayes used what is now called Bayes formula (which is really an alternative form of the well-known, by then, multiplication rule), interpreted conditional probability and its subtleties, and assumed a uniform distribution on p (via eliciting priors on the observables—i.e., the predictive distribution). It was Laplace who coined the term "Bayes Theorem" and set in notion this terminology—Bayes did not invent Bayes Theorem.

Daniel Bernoulli (1700–1782) introduced the idea of probability curves, applied differential calculus to problems of probability theory and, in so doing, simplified many of the cumbersome combinatoric formulas used before. However, his most important contribution is the introduction of the notion of "*utility*" or "*moral* expectation" and its use in solving the St. Petersburg paradox, posed by Nicholas (1) Bernoulli.

Condorcet [Jean Antoine de Caritat, Marquis de Condorcet] (1743–1794) was a well-known sociologist and economist during the period of the French Revolution. His main contribution is his introduction of the notion of "*probabilite' propre*," which is a subjective, or personal, probability. His ideas were rejected as being beyond the scope of mathematical probability theory.

After Bernoulli, one of the great minds who came to wrestle with probability was Pierre Simon, de Laplace. His main technical contribution is the de Moivre–Laplace central limit theorem, for Bernoulli trials. His contribution to larger issues is extending the realm of applicability of probability to social phenomena, and his reinforcement of Condorcet's notion of subjective probability. That is "probability is relative in part to ignorance, and our knowledge." If a coin is asymmetrical, but we do not know which side, then its probability of head is 1/2. Laplace also played a role in developing statistics.

Stage II of the development of probability ends with Gauss (1777–1855), who derived the normal law for the distribution of errors. [This was also done by Robert Adrian (1755–1843) an obscure American mathematician.]

Poisson (1781–1840) did much work on technical and practical aspects of probability. He subscribed to the subjective view of probability and like Laplace felt that probability can also be applied to jurisprudence. Poisson's main contribution is a generalization of Bernoulli's theorem when the probability of an event changes from trial to trial, so that if $\tilde{p}$ is the arithmetic mean of these probabilities, then

$$\lim_{n\to\infty} P\left(\left|\frac{m}{n} - \tilde{p}\right| < \epsilon\right) = 1, \tag{1}$$

and his proof that as $p_n \to 0$, then as $n \to \infty$, $P(m/n) = \frac{e^{-n}}{m!}e^{-\lambda}$, where $\lambda = np_n$, the famous Poisson formula; recall that m is the number of events in n Bernoulli trials.

4.3 The Period of Stagnation

The period (1860–1900) is also viewed as one of stagnation in the development of probability. Many felt that its application to social problems was a compromise in the mathematical sciences.

The areas of application being not clearly defined there was much controversy about the subject. There was much criticism of the early developers, like Pascal, Bernoulli, Laplace, and Poisson for their subjectivist inklings via metaphysical determinism. The period of stagnation terminated with the emergence of the now famous Russian School of probability.

4.4 **Stage III:** *Creation of the Russian School*

The originators of the Russian School of probability were Ostrogradski (1801–1862) and Bunyakovsky (1804–1889). Ostrogradski, influenced by Laplace, was a proponent of the principle of insufficient reason and applied the theory of probability to moral problems. He too subscribed to the notion that probability is a measure of our ignorance and is thus subjective. Bunyakovsky wrote the first Russian book in probability and introduced the needed terminology; he too was a determinist in the spirit of Bernoulli and Laplace.

Chebyshev (1821–1894), influenced by Ostrogradski and Bunyakovsky, is credited with the creation of the Russian School of probability. His students Markov, Voroni, Lyapunov, and Steklov pushed frontiers of the subject to the modern era. In effect, Chebyshev and his followers broke the period of stagnation and impasse in probability, as a mathematical science. Chebyshev defined the subject matter of probability theory as the mathematical science of constructing probabilities of an event based on probabilities of other events. He did not discuss how initial probabilities are to be obtained. Chebyshev introduced mathematical rigor in the theorems and obtained exact estimates or inequalities of derivations from limiting laws that arise when the number of trials is large but finite.

Philosophically, Chebyshev and his followers were materialists through the natural sciences, mechanics, and mathematics. They were guided by the opinion that only those investigations initiated by applications are of value, and only theories that arise from a consideration of particular cases are useful. The materialist philosophy is founded on the belief that nothing exists but matter itself and its manifestations.

Markov (1856–1922) was Chebyshev's closest disciples and his most colorful spokesperson. He transformed probability, with clarity and rigor, to one of the most perfect field in mathematics. His noteworthy works are on the limit theorems for sums of independent and dependent random variables using the method of moments. Markov introduced the famous chain named after him, for analyzing Pushkin's poem "*Eugene Onegnin*."

Lyapunov (1857–1918) improvised on the proofs of Markov's theorems using characteristic functions; the central limit theorem is named after him. Lindberg and Feller later improved on Lyapunov's theorems.

4.5 Probability in Physics

The evolution of probability as a mathematical science would not complete without a mention of its impact in physics, one of the most basic of all the sciences. In 1827, Robert Brown, an English botanist, detected the movement of minute suspended particles in an unpredictable manner. This movement is due to random bombardments of chaotically moving molecules in suspension. Using probabilistic arguments, Albert Einstein in 1905 was able to develop a sound theory for such motions. It was observed that every sufficiently small grain suspended in a fluid constantly moves in an unpredictable manner.

If before the second half of the nineteenth century, the basic areas of application of probability were in the processing of observations, and the second half was in physics. This was prompted by the work of Ludwig Boltzmann (1844–1906), an Austrian, and Josiah Willard Gibbs (1839–1903), an American.

Boltzmann is credited with the initiation of statistical physics, and the probabilistic interpretation of entropy. His work paved the way for quantum theory. Boltzmann was preceded by Maxwell who thought of molecules as elastic solids, whose behavior can be studied through the methods of probability.

In 1902, Gibbs, who was occupied with problems of mechanics, published his famous book "*Basic Principles of Statistical Mechanics*." This book was an influential development for the enhancement of probabilistic notions in physics.

4.6 *Paradoxes in Probability*

Toward the beginning of the twentieth century, great inroads were made in probability as a mathematical discipline by Chebyshev, Markov, and Lyapunov, and into its inroads in physics by Maxwell, Boltmann, and Gibbs. However, mathematicians were repeatedly pointing out concerns regarding the need for a precise meaning of probability.

Indeed Bertrand (of Bertrand's Paradox, of which is Borel's Paradox, and the three envelope problem are examples), and Henri Poincare, via their paradoxes, tried to emphasize the inaccuracies and vaguenesses in the basic notions of interpreting probability.

Emil Borel (1871–1956) and Henri Poincare (1854–1912), both prominent French mathematicians, were determinists whose notion of probability was that it is a reflection of our ignorance. Both wrote two highly influential books on the subject and called for a rigorous definition of the meaning of probability. These can be seen as paving the path toward Stage IV and V on the axiomatic and the subjective development of probability.

4.7 Stage IV: *The Axiomatic Development*

The axiomatic method in science, particularly, the mathematical sciences, makes it possible to apply any theory to many areas. For example, Lobachevskii (1829) suggested the possibility of constructing geometry based on a system of axioms, different from those of Euclid, whereas Hilbert, Peano, and Kagan investigated such a possibility for geometry in the early part of the twentieth century; Hilbert and Peano also did this for arithmetic.

With probability, Laplace's classical definition using equiprobable events was a tautology because equiprobable $\Leftrightarrow$ equal probability. Also, the subjective interpretation of probability had, at the early part of the twentieth century, serious flaws having to do with a linear utility for money and state dependence. As a consequence, the need for axiomatization was becoming more and more pressing.

In 1917, S.N. Bernstein (1880–1968) published a paper hinting the axiomatization of probability. This marked a new stage in its development. Bernstein's axiomatization was based on the notion of qualitative comparisons of events in which larger and smaller probabilities serve as a foundation. Bernstein's ideas were further developed by Glivenko and, more recently, by Koopman (1940). Bernstein's notion of probability was also materialistic and was for applications to the natural sciences.

Richard von Mises (1883–1953) was a strong critic of both the equiprobable and the subjective theory of interpreting probability. His main contribution is the frequency approach; that is, probability is relevant only to mass phenomena. Approaches alternate to von Mises were due to Keynes, followed by Harold Jeffreys, who viewed probability as a degree of likelihood, wherein every proposition has a certain definite probability. It is said that later on, Keynes recanted this position.

Simultaneous with attempts to lay the foundations of probability were rapid new developments in the mathematical sciences, vis-a-vis the works of Khinchin, Borel, Cantelli, Hardy, Littlewood, and Hausdorff. These trends facilitated Kolmogorov to construct his axiomatization of probability and lay the foundation for a decisive stage in its development. In particular, Bernoulli's result on the weak law and Borel's on the strong law led Kolmogorov to notice the connection between probability and measure and thus began his work on axiomatization, resulting in the publication of his famous book, in 1933.

Kolmogorov's aim was not to clarify the meaning of probability but to establish a branch of mathematics in exactly the same way as algebra and geometry. To Kolmogorov, the concept of a theory of probability is a system of sets that satisfy certain conditions. He thus introduced the term probability in the above context, detached from any real world meaning.

Not all applied scenarios satisfy Kolmogorov's setup and architecture. Consequently, there are alternatives to probability like Zadeh's Possibility Theory for fuzzy sets, and the Dempster–Shafer Belief Function Theory.

4.8 Stage V: *Personal Probability*

Approaches at interpreting probability, alternate to the "classical" one of La Place, the "frequency" one of von Mises, the "logical" one of Keynes, as well as the axiomatics of Kolmogorov (that technically speaking are free of interpretation) were due to de Finetti, and Ramsey, who interpret probability as a subjective quantity, personal to each individual. Whereas de Finetti interprets probability as a two-sided bet assuming a linear utility for money, Savage motivated by Ramsey takes an axiomatic approach.

Savage's approach to personal probability was modeled after von-Neumann and Morgernstern's axiomatic development of utility theory. This approach is the most widely referenced approach to personal probability; it has as its foundation behavioristic axioms of choice. Perhaps, it is not too well recognized that these axioms appear to be rooted in Bernstein's qualitative comparison of events; save for the feature that they pertain to choices between actions in the face of uncertainty.

A striking feature of Savage's axioms is that their consequences lead to the simultaneous existence of both a subjective probability and a utility, and the maximization of expected utility as a recipe for decision making under uncertainty.

Savage's subjective probability conforms to the Kolmogorov axioms; however, in the latter's setup, conditional probability is a definition, whereas in the former, it is a consequence of the Savage axioms.

Acknowledgments The work reported here was supported by a grant from the City University of Hong Kong, Project Number 9380068, and by the Research Grants Council Theme-Based Research Scheme Grant T32-102/14N and T32-101/15R. Comments by Glen Shafer and Fabrizio Ruggeri have helped correct some inaccuracy in the original versions.

References

Koopman, B. O. (1940). The axioms and algebra of intuitive probability. *Annals of Mathematics*, 269–292.

Lobachevskii, N. L. (1829). On the foundation of geometry, III. Section, 12, 227–243.

Maistrov, L. E. (1974). *Probability theory: A historical sketch.* New York: Academic

Shafer, G. (2019). Pascal's and Huygens's game-theoretic foundations for probability. Sartoniana, 32(117–145), 9.

von Collani, E. (2014). Five turning points in the historical progress of statistics - My personal vision. *Serdica Journal of Computing, Bulgarian Academy of Sciences, 8*(3), 199–226.

Part V
Goodness-of-Fit Tests

Assessment of Distributional Goodness-of-Fit for Modeling the Superposition of Renewal Process Data

Wei Zhang and William Q. Meeker

Abstract Parametric maximum likelihood methods can be used to estimate the renewal distribution based on aggregate data from superpositions of a group of renewal processes (SRP). The traditional distributional assessment approaches are, however, unable to be applied to the SRP data directly as the actual locations where the renewal events occurred are unknown. In this paper, we present two graphical distributional assessment procedures to evaluate how well alternative parametric models fit the observed SRP data. The first procedure provides a flexible semi-parametric estimate of the renewal distribution which is based on a piecewise exponential (PEX) model. Corresponding nonparametric simultaneous confidence bands (NPSCBs) are given to assess the amount of statistical uncertainty of the semi-parametric estimate. The results show that the PEX model with NPSCBs provides a flexible framework for comparing different parametric distributions. The second procedure is based on a comparison of parametric and nonparametric estimates of the mean cumulative function (MCF) for the SRP recurrence data. These two procedures are illustrated by applications to both real and simulated SRP data.

1 Introduction

1.1 Background and Motivation

Certain applications result in data from a group of superpositions of renewal processes (SRP). For example, recurrence data from a collection of systems are of interest in maintenance and warranty applications. Often a system consists of multiple identical copies of certain components. If one component fails, it can be replaced by a new one, which will restore the system operation. Then the replacement history at each component location (socket) can be modeled as

---

W. Zhang · W. Q. Meeker (✉)
Department of Statistics, Iowa State University, Ames, IA, USA
e-mail: wqmeeker@iastate.edu

I. Ghosh et al. (eds.), *Advances in Statistics - Theory and Applications*, Emerging Topics in Statistics and Biostatistics, https://doi.org/10.1007/978-3-030-62900-7_12

a renewal process (RP), based on the assumption that all the components are assumed to be identical and independent. Examples in industrial applications include cylinders and valve seats in a locomotive engine, DIMM memory modules on a laptop computer motherboard, headlights and tires in an automobile, etc. For such systems, it is common that the recurrence data are available in a scenario, such as event times at the system level are available, but the socket identities for these events are unknown. The reason for this is that maintenance database systems were designed to capture financial information, not engineering information. This kind of data structure generates an SRP.

Zhang et al. (2017) described the maximum likelihood (ML) method for estimating the renewal distribution from SRP data. In their work, the renewal distribution is assumed to be a particular distribution from the log-location-scale family (e.g., Weibull or lognormal). Enumerating all possible allocations of the SRP recurrent events to sockets in the system allows computation of the likelihood function that can be maximized to obtain the ML estimates for the renewal distribution. The performance of the proposed ML estimator was investigated extensively in their simulation study.

One natural question arising from this work is how to determine whether the SRP data are consistent with the particular assumed renewal distribution. Due to lack of information about the positions of the events within each system, however, it is difficult to apply the traditional probability plotting method to the SRP data. In this paper, we propose two alternative graphical methods to assess the adequacy of a particular parametric model for modeling the SRP data. The first method is an extension of the traditional probability plotting method for complete and censored data. The other method is based on the comparison of the nonparametric estimate of the mean cumulative function (MCF) from the observed SRP data and the parametric fitted-model MCF computed from the ML estimates of renewal distribution parameters.

1.2 Related Work

In reliability data analysis, probability plots are commonly used as a graphical technique for assessing distributional assumptions. The idea is to plot the nonparametric estimate $\widehat{F}(t)$ on the linearizing probability scales and assess departure from a straight line. The linearity of the $\widehat{F}(t)$ on the probability paper serves as a measure of the agreement of the data with the candidate distribution. Much research related to the probability plotting has been done for complete and censored data. Details and additional references can be found, for example, in Chapter 6 of Meeker and Escobar (1998).

For commonly occurring multiply censored data, Kaplan and Meier (1958) proposed the nonparametric maximum likelihood estimator (also known as the product-limit estimator) to estimate the distribution $F(t)$ of lifetimes, and this estimator is commonly used in constructing probability plots. For the SRP data, however, the actual event times within each socket are unknown, and thus, the Kaplan–Meier (KM) estimation method cannot be used. Here we propose an extension of the traditional probability plotting method for the SRP data. A piecewise exponential (PEX) model is used to obtain a flexible semi-parametric estimate of the renewal (component lifetime) distribution $F(t)$ that can be used in place of the KM estimate. The PEX model is semi-parametric in the sense that unlike fitting a parametric distribution, the form of the cumulative distribution function (cdf) is not specified.

The PEX model was introduced by Grenander (1956) as a nonparametric model for estimating lifetime distribution for complete data. In his work, hazard jump points were assumed to occur at the observed failure times. Padgett and Wei (1980) generalized the PEX model to right-censored data. In this case, the PEX estimator can be viewed as a competitor to the Kaplan–Meier estimator. The performances of the two estimators were compared by Kitchin et al. (1983). Kim and Proschan (1991) used PEX model to estimate the life distribution from a set of right-censored data in a telecommunication application.

The PEX model can also be interpreted as a parametric model. Miller (1960) studied a special case where there is only one hazard jump point. Estimates of the two hazard levels and the jump point are obtained using maximum likelihood estimation. Prairie and Ostle (1961) extended Miller's method to the case of three hazard levels. For right-censored and nonoverlapping data, Colvert and Boardman (1976) provided the estimates of the piecewise constant hazard levels under PEX model using maximum likelihood estimation when the hazard jump points are pre-specified. Loubert (1986) extended the PEX model to the case of arbitrarily censored data with the constraint that the distribution has a monotone hazard function.

In addition to the nonparametric estimate $\widehat{F}(t)$, nonparametric simultaneous confidence bands (NPSCBs) are usually given on the probability plot to assess the amount of uncertainty of $\widehat{F}(t)$. Greenwood (1926) suggested a formula that gives an estimate of the variance of the Kaplan–Meier estimator. Nair (1981, 1984) showed how to extend the usual pointwise confidence intervals based on Greenwood's variance formula to large-sample simultaneous confidence bands. Nair called these "equal precision" (EP) bands because the replacement of the usual standard normal distribution $(1 - \alpha/2)$ quantile used to compute pointwise approximate confidence intervals with a larger factor that provides asymptotically correct simultaneous confidence bands. Nair compared the performance of the EP band with other existing confidence bands, such as the Hall–Wellner (HW) band and R band (a censored version of the Rényi band). In this paper, we extend the idea of Nair's EP band and derive a NPSCB for the SRP data based on a bootstrap resampling procedure given in Sect. 2.

The second tool to assess the distributional goodness-of-fit for the SRP data is based on comparing the nonparametric and parametric estimates of the MCF. The MCF, $M(t)$, as described by Nelson (2003, page 25) and Cook and Lawless (2007, page 9), is interpreted as the population expected cumulative number of events per system at time t. Thus, the MCF describes the average behavior of multiple systems. Nelson gives a nonparametric estimate of the MCF (also known as the empirical

MCF). The shape of the nonparametric MCF estimate can reveal important features about the behavior of the recurrent events. We propose also to use a comparison of the nonparametric and the parametric estimates of the MCF to assess the adequacy of a parametric fit for SRP data.

1.3 Overview

The rest of this paper is organized as follows. Section 2 illustrates an extension of the probability plotting method. We introduce the definition of the semi-parametric PEX estimator of the renewal distribution and show how to construct the NPSCB, followed by some illustrative examples. Section 3 illustrates the use of the MCF nonparametric and parametric comparison to assess the goodness-of-fit of the proposed parametric distributions. Section 4 describes an application of the probability plotting method and the MCF method to a locomotive maintenance data example. Section 5 gives concluding remarks and discussion of possible extensions of the proposed methods.

2 Probability Plotting Method

In this section, we show how to construct a probability plot for SRP data by plotting the semi-parametric PEX estimate $\widehat{F}(t)$ and the NPSCBs on a linearized probability scale. For a particular distribution, if it is possible to draw a straight line between the NPSCBs on the probability paper, then the distribution is consistent with the SRP data.

2.1 A Semi-Parametric Estimate of $F(t)$ Using the PEX Model

2.1.1 The PEX Model

The PEX model is characterized by a piecewise constant hazard function with specified jump points. We denote the PEX model as PEX($\boldsymbol{\gamma}, \boldsymbol{\omega}$), where $\boldsymbol{\omega}' = (\omega_1, \omega_2, \ldots, \omega_b)$ are the b pre-specified jump points of the hazard function, $0 < \omega_1 < \omega_2 < \cdots < \omega_b$, and $\omega_{b+1} = \infty$. The vector $\boldsymbol{\gamma}' = (\gamma_1, \gamma_2, \ldots, \gamma_b)$ denotes the values of the hazard function, where γ_p is the value of the hazard function in the pth hazard interval $[\omega_p, \omega_{p+1})$. Thus the PEX hazard function is

$$\gamma(t) = \sum_{p=1}^{b} \gamma_p \mathrm{I}_{[\omega_p, \omega_{p+1})}(t),$$

where $I_{[\omega_p,\omega_{p+1})} = 1$ if $t \in [\omega_p, \omega_{p+1})$, and 0 otherwise. In this study, the first jump point ω_1 is set as the smallest event time in the SRP data. Similar to the nonparametric KM estimate, because there are no events before the first event time, the probability to fail at any time before ω_1 is estimated to be 0. That is, $\widehat{\gamma}(t) = 0$ for $0 < t < \omega_1$. Thus, ω_1 serves as a threshold for the time t.

The PEX cumulative hazard function at time t is

$$\boldsymbol{\xi}_t'\boldsymbol{\gamma} = \int_0^t \gamma(u)du = -\log \mathrm{S}(t),$$

where $\boldsymbol{\xi}_t' = (\xi_{t,1}, \xi_{t,2}, \ldots, \xi_{t,b})$, $0 \le \xi_{t,p} \le \omega_{p+1} - \omega_p$, and $\mathrm{S}(t)$ is the survival function of the PEX model. We see that $\log \mathrm{S}(t)$ is a piecewise linear function of the elements in $\boldsymbol{\gamma}$. Figure 1 provides a plot of the PEX hazard and cumulative hazard functions for a simple example with seven jump points and a hazard function increasing at an increasing rate. Thus, the cdf of the PEX model is

$$\begin{aligned}\mathrm{F}(t) = 1 - \mathrm{S}(t) &= 1 - \exp(-\boldsymbol{\xi}_t'\boldsymbol{\gamma})\\ &= 1 - \exp\left[-\gamma_1(t - \omega_1)\right] \mathrm{I}_{[\omega_1,\omega_2)}\\ &\quad - \sum_{p=2}^{b+1} \exp\left[-\sum_{q=1}^{p-1} \gamma_q(\omega_{q+1} - \omega_q) - \gamma_p(t - \omega_p)\right] \mathrm{I}_{[\omega_p,\omega_{p+1})},\end{aligned} \tag{1}$$

and the density of the PEX model is

$$\begin{aligned}f(t) &= \mathrm{S}(t)\gamma(t) = \exp(-\boldsymbol{\xi}_t'\boldsymbol{\gamma})\gamma(t)\\ &= \gamma_1 \exp\left[-\gamma_1(t - \omega_1)\right] \mathrm{I}_{[\omega_1,\omega_2)}\\ &\quad + \sum_{p=2}^{b+1} \gamma_p \exp\left[-\sum_{q=1}^{p-1} \gamma_q(\omega_{q+1} - \omega_q) - \gamma_p(t - \omega_p)\right] \mathrm{I}_{[\omega_p,\omega_{p+1})}.\end{aligned} \tag{2}$$

2.1.2 Choosing the Number and Locations of Hazard Jump Points

Note that the PEX model is completely determined by the specification of the locations of the hazard jump points and the values of the hazard function between each pair of jump points. Therefore, one of the key challenges of working with the PEX model is how to properly specify a sequence of jump points which provides a good approximation for the lifetime distribution. The adequacy of the approximation depends on the size of the data set as well as the number and locations of the hazard jump points.

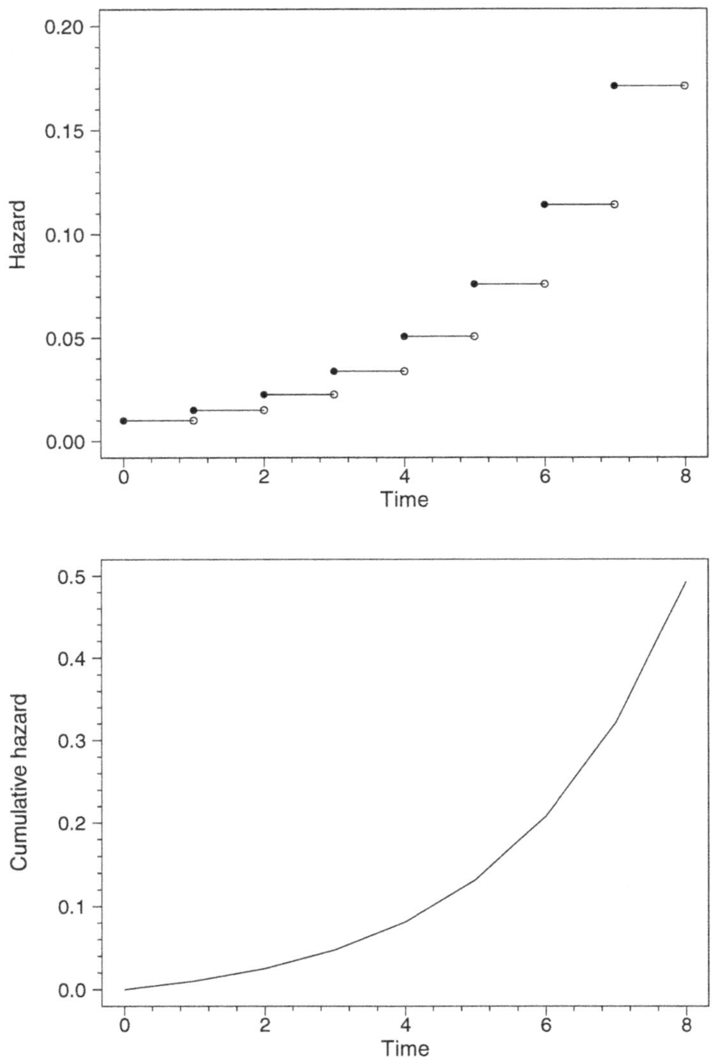

Fig. 1 A PEX hazard function (top) and cumulative hazard function (bottom)

For some of the earlier work related to the PEX model, the hazard jump points were defined at the observed failure times, which is not feasible for the SRP data as the exact component failure times are unknown within each system. To overcome this difficulty, we first focus on the data for the first replacement time within each system, and use this information as a guideline to specify the number of locations of the hazard jump points. The observed first failures from the collection of systems are a sample from the distribution of the minimum of the m sockets in each system.

Although the PEX model allows flexibility for the number of jump points, it is important to point out that there is a tradeoff. If one specifies a number of jump points that is too large, the procedure is more computationally intensive. In addition, due to potential identifiability problems, unstable estimates for the hazard values may result unless there is a large amount of data. In other words, the resulting PEX parameters are not clearly identifiable. On the other hand, a hazard function based on just a few jump points may produce a poor approximation for the true lifetime distribution. Based on some numerical studies (an example is given in Appendix 1), we found that using 6–10 jump points (possibly 4 for a small set of SRP data) for the hazard function ensures sufficient flexibility of the model, and does not require too much computer time.

Furthermore, the location of the jump points also plays a central role in using the PEX goodness-of-fit assessment. When choosing the locations of the hazard jump points, a key requirement is that there should be event times that fall within each of the different time intervals. If this is not the case, sensible estimates of the hazard values cannot be obtained by the optimization of the likelihood. In our approach, the quantiles of the distribution for the first replacement time within each system are used to determine the locations of the jump points. This will guarantee identifiability of the model.

Specifically, suppose there are n systems in a fleet and n^* of these systems contain events. Let $(\tau_1^1, \tau_1^2, \ldots, \tau_1^{n^*})$ denote the first replacement times in the n^* systems. Therefore, the desired number of hazard jump points b should be an integer that is less than n^*. According to the proposed algorithm, the hazard jump points $(\omega_1, \omega_2, \ldots, \omega_b)$ correspond to the

$$\left[\frac{0}{b}, \frac{1}{b}, \ldots, \frac{(b-1)}{b}\right] \tag{3}$$

sample quantiles of the sequence $(\tau_1^1, \tau_1^2, \ldots, \tau_1^{n^*})$. The sample quantiles are computed using the R function `quantiles()` with the default quantile algorithm (type = 7) discussed in Hyndman and Fan (1996).

It is worth noting that according to Drenick's theorem (Drenick 1960), an SRP behaves as a homogeneous Poisson process (HPP), irrespective of the underlying renewal distribution, when the combined number of systems and sockets is large, and the time of operation becomes long enough. Thus, most of the information allowing for discrimination among different parametric distributions will be in the early part of the probability plot. For this reason, our probability plotting procedure focuses on the lower tail of the renewal distribution by using the above algorithm to determine the hazard jump points.

2.1.3 PEX Likelihood for SRP Data

Zhang et al. (2017) showed how to compute the likelihood for SRP data for log-location-scale distributions. Their method extends to the PEX model without difficulty. For a group of independent SRPs, the log-likelihood can be expressed as the sum of the log-likelihoods for each individual SRP. Here we briefly review how to compute the likelihood for a single SRP as applied to the PEX model. See Zhang et al. (2017) for a more detailed description, examples, and other information.

Consider an SRP with m sockets and an observed event history $\mathscr{H}_{\tau_c} = (\tau_1, \tau_2, \ldots, \tau_r, \tau_c)$, where r is the number of events within the SRP, $\tau_1 < \cdots < \tau_r$, and the end-of-observation time τ_c with $\tau_c \geq \tau_r$. Therefore, there are h partitions of the integer r, where a partition $\mathscr{E}_i^r = (r_1, \cdots, r_{l_i})$ is a list of l_i nonincreasing positive integers that sum to r (see Hankin 2006). The partition suggests that l_i out of the m sockets contain events and how many events are assigned to each of these l_i sockets. For a given partition $\mathscr{E}_i^r$, the way of the observed event times are allocated to the l_i sockets is defined as the unique-likelihood configuration, which corresponds to the set partition of an integer partition, as described by Hankin and West (2007). Within each partition, the number of ways that one can choose l_i sockets from the m sockets in an SRP is given by the number of permutations k_i (see more details in Zhang et al. 2017). To write down the likelihood of a particular SRP, we consider all possible data configurations that could have led to the observed r events. The data configurations can be enumerated by considering all possible partitions of r and then enumerating all possible unique-likelihood configurations within each partition. Therefore, the likelihood $L\left(\boldsymbol{\gamma}; \mathscr{H}_{\tau_c}\right)$ for the observed SRP is defined as

$$L\left(\boldsymbol{\gamma}; \mathscr{H}_{\tau_c}\right) = \sum_{i=1}^{h} k_i \sum_{j=1}^{s_i} L_{i,j}\left(\boldsymbol{\gamma}; \mathscr{H}_{\tau_c}\right), \tag{4}$$

where $L_{i,j}\left(\boldsymbol{\gamma}; \mathscr{H}_{\tau_c}\right)$ is the likelihood for jth unique-likelihood configuration $[j = (1, \cdots, s_i)]$ within the ith partition $\mathscr{E}_i^r = (r_1, r_2, \ldots, r_{l_i})$, and k_i is the number of permutations of the socket labels. Based on (1) and (2), and the corresponding unique-likelihood configuration, $L_{i,j}\left(\boldsymbol{\gamma}; \mathscr{H}_{\tau_c}\right)$ in (4) can be expressed as a function of the unknown parameters given by the hazard values $\boldsymbol{\gamma}$ for the PEX model.

For a fleet of n independent systems, suppose that there are m_k sockets and r_k events in system k, $k = 1, 2, \ldots, n$. Let $\mathscr{H}_{\tau_c^k}^k = (\tau_1^k, \tau_2^k, \ldots, \tau_{r_k}^k, \tau_c^k)$ denote the observed event history of system k, where observed failure times $\tau_1^k < \cdots < \tau_{r_k}^k$, and end-of-observation time $\tau_c^k \geq \tau_{r_k}^k$. Then the total log-likelihood for the fleet is

$$\begin{aligned}\mathscr{L}\left[\boldsymbol{\gamma}; (\mathscr{H}^1_{\tau^1_c}, \mathscr{H}^2_{\tau^2_c}, \ldots, \mathscr{H}^n_{\tau^n_c})\right] &= \sum_{k=1}^{n} \mathscr{L}_k\left(\boldsymbol{\gamma}; \mathscr{H}^k_{\tau^k_c}\right) \\ &= \sum_{k=1}^{n} \log\left[L_k\left(\boldsymbol{\gamma}; \mathscr{H}^k_{\tau^k_c}\right)\right].\end{aligned} \tag{5}$$

2.1.4 Constrained Optimization of the Likelihood

The PEX ML estimates $\widehat{\boldsymbol{\gamma}}$ are obtained by maximizing the sum of the log-likelihoods for all of the SRPs in the data, set subject to: $\gamma_p \geq 0, \quad p = 1, \ldots, b$. Note that we constrain the hazard levels $\boldsymbol{\gamma}$ such that they are all nonnegative. Hence, this ML problem is expressed as a constrained nonlinear optimization problem. The optimization is done by using the R function `constrOptim()`. Based on the resulting estimates $\widehat{\boldsymbol{\gamma}}$ of the hazard levels, the PEX semi-parametric estimate $\widehat{F}(t)$ for the cdf of the renewal distribution is obtained by evaluating (1) at $\widehat{\boldsymbol{\gamma}}$.

2.2 *Probability Plot for a Specified Distribution*

A probability plot presents the nonparametric estimate $\widehat{F}(t)$ using particular plotting scales that linearize the candidate probability distribution. The plotting scales vary from distribution to distribution, as described in Chapter 6 of Meeker and Escobar (1998). Following Zhang et al. (2017), we mainly use the log-location-scale family to model the renewal distribution. A probability plot for a pre-specified distribution is constructed by linearizing the cdf $F(t)$. That is, by finding appropriate transformations of $F(t)$ and t such that the relationship between the two transformed variables is linear. The resulting probability axis is nonlinear and is called the probability scale.

Here we illustrate this idea with a Weibull distribution. For the common parameterization of the Weibull (β, η) distribution, the cdf is

$$F(t) = \Pr(T \leq t) = 1 - \exp\left[-(t/\eta)^{\beta}\right],$$

where β and η are the shape and scale parameters, respectively. The corresponding quantile function can be expressed as $t_p = \eta[-\log(1-p)]^{1/\beta}$. Therefore, we have

$$\log(t_p) = \log(\eta) + \log[-\log(1-p)]\frac{1}{\beta}.$$

The above equation suggests that plotting $\log[-\log(1-p)]$ against $\log(t_p)$ generates a straight line, defining the Weibull probability plot axes.

In our probability plot procedure, the semi-parametric PEX estimate $\widehat{F}(t)$ is plotted on the probability axes and we assess the fit by comparing with a straight line. Departure from this straight line indicates departure from the specified distribution.

2.3 Assessing Sampling Variability Using Nonparametric Simultaneous Confidence Bands

In addition to the PEX-based $\widehat{F}(t)$, nonparametric simultaneous confidence bands (NPSCBs) are often used to indicate the amount of sampling variability that one might expect to see in the probability plot, as described by Nair (1981, 1984). In this section, we describe how to construct PEX-based NPSCBs for $F(t)$ over the time span of interest $[t_l, t_u]$, based on a bootstrap resampling procedure.

For time $t_l < t < t_u$, a two-sided $100(1-\alpha)\%$ NPSCBs for $F(t)$ is defined as

$$\Pr\left\{F(t) \in \left[\widehat{F}(t) - e_l\widehat{SE}_{\widehat{F}}(t), \widehat{F}(t) + e_u\widehat{SE}_{\widehat{F}}(t)\right], t \in [t_l, t_u]\right\} = 1 - \alpha, \tag{6}$$

where $\widehat{SE}_{\widehat{F}}(t)$ is the standard error of $\widehat{F}(t)$, which can be obtained by using the observed Fisher information matrix $I(\widehat{\boldsymbol{\gamma}})$ for the PEX model, evaluated at the ML estimates $\widehat{\boldsymbol{\gamma}}$. Let

$$\triangledown(\boldsymbol{\gamma}) = \left[\frac{\partial}{\partial\gamma_1}F(\boldsymbol{\gamma}), \frac{\partial}{\partial\gamma_2}F(\boldsymbol{\gamma}), \ldots, \frac{\partial}{\partial\gamma_b}F(\boldsymbol{\gamma})\right]$$

denote the first-order derivatives of $F(\boldsymbol{\gamma})$ and $\triangledown(\widehat{\boldsymbol{\gamma}})$ is the estimate of $\triangledown(\boldsymbol{\gamma})$. Then according to the delta method, the standard error of $\widehat{F}(t)$ is computed as

$$\widehat{SE}_{\widehat{F}}(t) = \sqrt{\triangledown(\widehat{\boldsymbol{\gamma}})I(\widehat{\boldsymbol{\gamma}})^{-1}\triangledown(\widehat{\boldsymbol{\gamma}})'}. \tag{7}$$

In many reliability applications, it is desirable to obtain NPSCBs with approximately equal error probabilities in each tail. For this purpose, we use the constraint

$$\begin{aligned}&\Pr\left\{F(t) \in \left[\widehat{F}(t) - e_l\widehat{SE}_{\widehat{F}}(t), \infty\right), t \in [t_l, t_u]\right\}\\ &= \Pr\left\{F(t) \in \left(-\infty, \widehat{F}(t) + e_u\widehat{SE}_{\widehat{F}}(t)\right], t \in [t_l, t_u]\right\}\end{aligned}$$

for the NPSCBs. Unlike the confidence interval for a single parameter, it is known that combining a one-sided lower and upper $100(1-\alpha/2)\%$ NPSCBs will not generate two-sided $100(1-\alpha)\%$ NPSCBs. Thus, to find the solution to (6), we used a numerical procedure for constructing two-sided NPSCBs with equal error probabilities in both tails. More specifically, we first re-express the two-sided coverage probability of NPSCBs as a function of the coverage probability of the one-sided NPSCBs to reduce the dimension of root-finding, and then find the error probability that gives the desired two-sided coverage probability.

A bootstrap method is used to determine the critical values e_l, e_u for a given α. The procedure is described below.

Bootstrap NPSCBs for $F(t)$

1. Determine the hazard jump points according to (3) and use this set of jump points for all of the bootstrap samples.
2. Determine the upper bound t_u of the time range of interest for the NPSCB. First, calculate the average number of events per socket in the fleet $\bar{r} = \sum_{k=1}^{n} r_k / \sum_{k=1}^{n} m_k$. Then let $\tau_{c,\max}$ denote the maximum end-of-observation time for all of the systems, and set the upper bound to be $t_u = \tau_{c,\max}/\bar{r}$.
3. Determine the lower bound t_l of the time range of interest for the NPSCB. First generate the ℓ-th bootstrap SRP data by resampling from the systems with replacement. Then find the smallest recurrence time $\tau_{(1),\ell}$ in resample ℓ. Repeat the procedure for $\ell = 1, \ldots, B$, and determine the maximum $\tau_{(1),\max}$ of $[\tau_{(1),1}, \tau_{(1),2}, \ldots, \tau_{(1),B}]$. Set the lower bound to be $t_l = \tau_{(1),\max}$.
4. For the ℓ-th bootstrap SRP data set, compute the PEX estimate $\widehat{F}(t)^{\ell}$ and the $\widehat{SE}(t)^{\ell}$ for $t \in [t_l, t_u]$, $\ell = 1, \ldots, B$.
5. Based on the B bootstrap estimates, calculate the values e_l, e_u that give the two-sided $100(1-\alpha)\%$ NPSCBs with equal coverage probability in the two tails.
6. For the original SRP data, compute the PEX estimate $\widehat{F}(t)$ and the $\widehat{SE}(t)$ for $t \in [t_l, t_u]$.
7. Compute the NPSCBs by using

$$\widehat{F}(t) - e_l \widehat{SE}_{\widehat{F}}(t)$$
$$\widehat{F}(t) + e_u \widehat{SE}_{\widehat{F}}(t)$$

for $t \in [t_l, t_u]$.

Note that this bootstrap procedure is computationally intensive as it requires the PEX estimation for each bootstrap sample. Thus, computation time goes up linearly with the number of bootstrap resamples. However, for purposes of a graphical assessment of goodness-of-fit (as opposed to reporting numerical confidence bounds), a high degree of precision is not needed. A simulation study showed that $B = 200$ is sufficient to generate NPSCBs because even with this small number of bootstrap trials, the amount of Monte Carlo error is small relative to the width of the NPSCBs. Appendix 2 gives an example.

2.4 Illustrative Examples

In this section, we illustrate the use of the PEX semi-parametric estimate of $F(t)$ and NPSCBs for two sets of simulated SRP data. Both of the data sets were simulated from a Weibull renewal distribution ($\eta = 3378$ h and $\beta = 4$), with $n = 50$ systems and the expected number of events $E(R) = 4$ per system. The two data sets only differ in the number of sockets, corresponding to $m = 2$ (Case 1) and $m = 16$ (Case 2) sockets, respectively.

For the Case 1 SRP data, the top and bottom plots in Fig. 2 show, respectively, the Weibull and Fréchet probability plots. The dot-dash curve corresponds to the semi-parametric PEX estimate of $F(t)$ with the number of jump points $b = 10$, and the two dashed curves correspond to the approximate 95% NPSCBs. The time range of interest is $(t_l, t_u) = (1574, 3743)$ h. The bootstrap procedure gives the critical values $e_l = 2.70$ and $e_u = 3.60$ for the NPSCBs over (t_l, t_u). The idML estimation method from Zhang et al. (2017) was used to estimate the Weibull distribution parameters (the solid straight line corresponding to the idMLE_Weibull in the top plot) and the Fréchet distribution parameters (the solid straight line corresponding to the idMLE_Fréchet in the bottom plot), respectively. Figure 2 indicates that the Weibull distribution provides a good fit to the SRP data, which is not surprising because the data were simulated from a Weibull distribution. The Fréchet estimate has a larger departure from the PEX estimate. It is not possible to draw a straight line through the NPSCB bands, indicating the Fréchet distribution is not consistent with the Case 1 SRP data (see Nair 1981).

Similarly, Fig. 3 shows the Weibull and Fréchet probability plots for the Case 2 SRP data, including the semi-parametric PEX estimate of $F(t)$ (with number of jump points $b = 5$), the approximate 95% NPSCBs for $t \in (t_l, t_u) = (1034, 2443)$ h, and the parametric idMLE fit. The critical values for the NPSCBs are $e_l = 2.40$ and $e_u = 3.17$. One can see that the Weibull distribution appears to provide a better description of the simulated SRP data as the PEX estimate has a better agreement with the straight line on the Weibull probability plot. In this case, however, we cannot rule out the Fréchet distribution because it is possible to draw a straight line through the NPSCBs. Note that in the Case 2 data, the fraction of sockets with events is approximately $E(R)/m = 4/16 = 0.25$; therefore, we expect to have a good estimation of quantiles up to $t_{0.25}$. This explains the relatively low power of the probability plots in detecting the lack of fit because the data are apparently only from the lower tail of the renewal distribution, providing less information to discriminate among candidate probability distributions.

3 MCF Method

In this section, we describe another goodness-of-fit procedure based on the MCF plot of the SRP data.

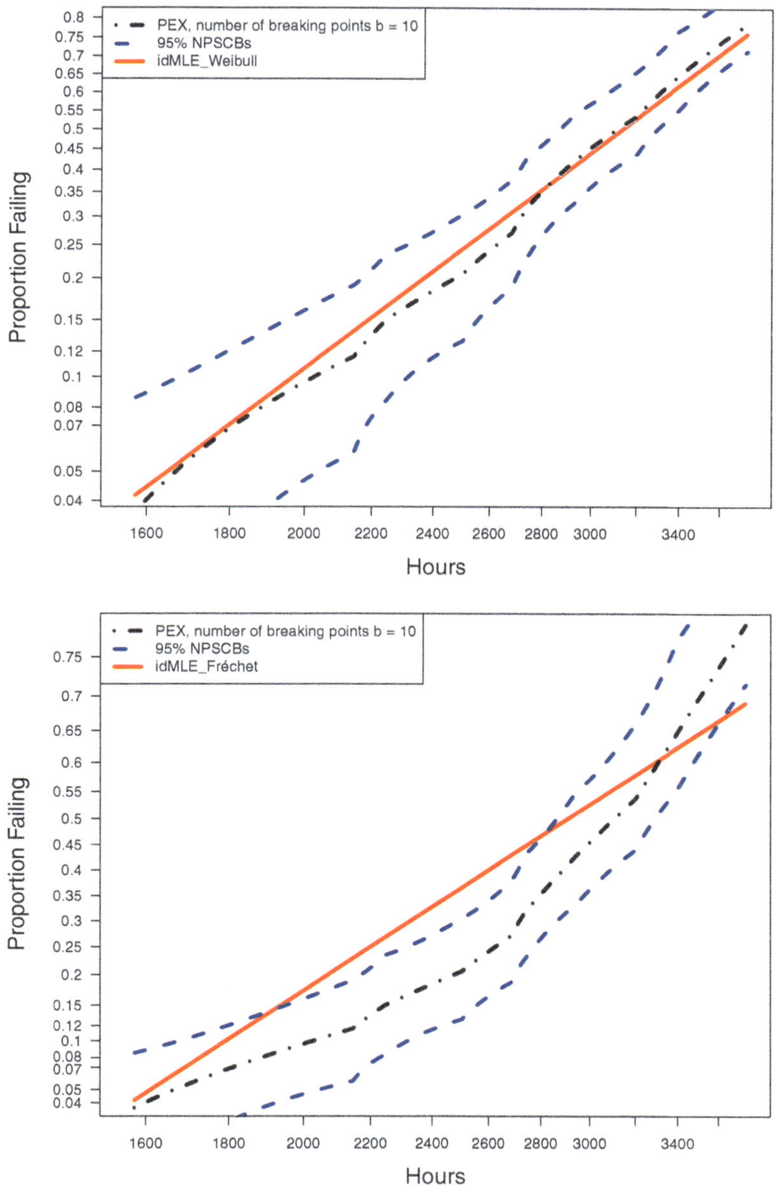

Fig. 2 Weibull (top) and Fréchet (bottom) probability plots for the Case 1 SRP data ($n = 50$ systems, $m = 2$ sockets, $E(R) = 4$ events from a Weibull distribution)

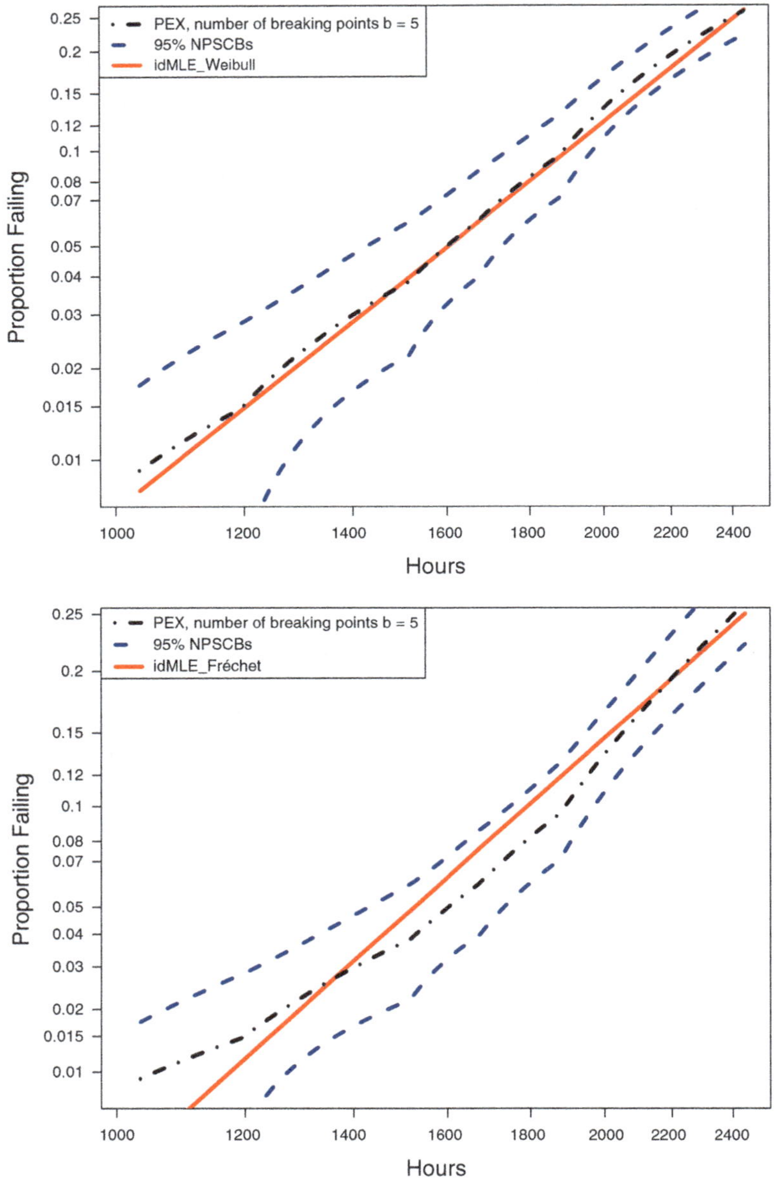

Fig. 3 Weibull (top) and Fréchet (bottom) probability plots for the Case 2 SRP data ($n = 50$ systems, $m = 16$ sockets, $E(R) = 4$ events from a Weibull distribution)

3.1 Nonparametric MCF Estimate and Its Variance

First, the nonparametric graphical estimate of the MCF is computed by using the following algorithm, as described, for example, in Lawless and Nadeau (1995) and Nelson (2003).

1. Among all of the n systems, find all the V unique event times and order them from t_1 to t_V.
2. For $v = 1, 2, \ldots, V$, compute the total number of events $d_k(t_v)$ for system k at t_v.
3. Let $\delta_k(t_v) = 1$ if system k is still being observed at time t_v and $\delta_k(t_v) = 0$ otherwise.
4. The nonparametric estimate of the MCF $M(t_j)$ at time t_v, $j = 1, 2, \ldots, V$, is computed as

$$\widehat{M}(t_j) = \sum_{u=1}^{j} \left[\frac{\sum_{k=1}^{n} \delta_k(t_v) d_k(t_v)}{\sum_{k=1}^{n} \delta_k(t_v)} \right] = \sum_{v=1}^{j} \frac{d_{.}(t_v)}{\delta_{.}(t_v)} = \sum_{v=1}^{j} \bar{d}(t_v), \tag{8}$$

where $d_{.}(t_v)$ is the total number of system events at time t_v, $\delta_{.}(t_v)$ is the number of systems at risk at t_v, and $\bar{d}(t_v)$ is the average number of events per system at time t_v.

Thus, the nonparametric MCF estimate $\widehat{M}(t)$ at time t is a step function, which is constant between the unique event times $t_1 < t_2 < \cdots < t_V$. These estimates do not impose any underlying assumption for the recurrence process; therefore, serves as a reference for the parametric fit.

To compute an estimate of the variance of $\widehat{M}(t_j)$, Lawless and Nadeau (1995) suggested

$$\widehat{\text{Var}}\left[\widehat{M}(t_j)\right] = \sum_{k=1}^{n} \left\{ \sum_{v=1}^{j} \frac{\delta_k(t_v)}{\delta_{.}(t_v)} \left[d_k(t_v) - \bar{d}(t_v) \right] \right\}^2. \tag{9}$$

3.2 Parametric MCF Estimate

Zhang et al. (2017) showed how to compute a parametric estimate of the MCF (fitted-model MCF) from a large number simulated realizations of the SRP data from the ML estimate of the renewal distribution. By displaying both of the fitted-model MCF and the nonparametric MCF on the same plot, the MCF plot can be used as a graphical tool for checking deviations between the two estimates of MCF. Suppose there is deviation detected from the MCF plot, one question arises whether the deviation comes from random noise or there is a lack of fit for the specified parametric distribution.

3.3 Assessing Sampling Variability Using Nonparametric Simultaneous Confidence Bands

Similar to the probability plotting method, we can also construct NPSCBs to assess the sampling variability of the MCF estimate over a specified time range $[t_l, t_u]$ based on a bootstrap resampling procedure. For time $t_l < t < t_u$, a two-sided $100(1-\alpha)\%$ NPSCBs for the MCF $M(t)$ is defined as

$$\Pr\left\{M(t) \in \left[\widehat{M}(t) - e_l \widehat{SE}_{\widehat{M}}(t), \widehat{M}(t) + e_u \widehat{SE}_{\widehat{M}}(t)\right], t \in [t_l, t_u]\right\} = 1 - \alpha, \tag{10}$$

where $\widehat{SE}_{\widehat{M}}(t)$ is the standard error of $\widehat{M}(t)$, which can be computed using (9). The following constraint

$$\begin{aligned}
&\Pr\left\{M(t) \in \left[\widehat{M}(t) - e_l \widehat{SE}_{\widehat{M}}(t), \infty\right), t \in [t_l, t_u]\right\} \\
&\quad = \Pr\left\{M(t) \in \left(-\infty, \widehat{M}(t) + e_u \widehat{SE}_{\widehat{M}}(t)\right], t \in [t_l, t_u]\right\}
\end{aligned}$$

is used to obtain NPSCBs with approximately equal coverage probabilities in each tail.

Here we propose a bootstrap resampling method to obtain the NPSCBs for a specified time range $[t_l, t_u]$. The method is described as below. *Bootstrap NPSCBs for $M(t)$*

1. Generate the ℓ-th bootstrap SRP data by resampling from the systems with replacement. Then find the range of t values $[\tau_{(1),\ell}, \tau_{c,\max,\ell}]$, where $\tau_{(1),\ell}$ is the smallest recurrence time and $\tau_{c,\max,\ell}$ is the largest end-of-observation time.
2. Repeat step 1 for $\ell = 1, \ldots, B$, and determine the intersection $[t_l, t_u]$ of all the ranges $[\tau_{(1),\ell}, \tau_{c,\max,\ell}]$. $[t_l, t_u]$ will be the time range of interest for the NPSCBs.
3. For the ℓ-th bootstrap SRP data set, compute the nonparametric MCF estimates and their variances within the time range $t \in [t_l, t_u]$, $\ell = 1, 2, \ldots, B$.
4. Calculate the values e_l, e_u that give the two-sided $100(1-\alpha)\%$ NPSCBs with equal coverage probability in two tails.
5. For the original SRP data, compute the nonparametric MCF estimate $\widehat{M}(t)$ and the $\widehat{SE}(t)$ for $t \in [t_l, t_u]$.
6. Construct the NPSCBs by using

$$\widehat{M}(t) - e_l \widehat{SE}_{\widehat{M}}(t)$$
$$\widehat{M}(t) + e_u \widehat{SE}_{\widehat{M}}(t)$$

for $t \in [t_l, t_u]$.

For a particular distribution from log-location-scale family whose cdf can be expressed as

$$F(t; \mu, \sigma) = \Phi\left(\frac{\log(t) - \mu}{\sigma}\right),$$

first obtain the idML estimates $\widehat{\mu}$ and $\widehat{\sigma}$ for the shape and location parameters, respectively. Compute the corresponding MCF based on $\widehat{\boldsymbol{\theta}} = (\widehat{\mu}, \widehat{\sigma})$, which is the parametric MCF estimate described in Sect. 3.2. Then display the parametric MCF estimates on the same plot with the nonparametric MCF estimates and NPSCBs.

3.4 *Illustrative Examples*

In this section, we use the same Cases 1 and 2 Weibull data examples in Sect. 2.4 to illustrate how the above simulation procedure is used to check the adequacy of the assumed parametric model for the SRP data. Two parametric distributions, Weibull and Fréchet, were fit to the Case 1 SRP data, respectively. The nonparametric MCF estimates and the two parametric MCF estimates, Weibull and Fréchet, are shown in Fig. 4. The results show, as expected, that Weibull parametric MCF estimates have a better agreement with the nonparametric MCF estimates. Thus, compared to the Fréchet distribution, the Weibull distribution gives a better fit, which is consistent with the fact that the data set was simulated from a Weibull distribution. As described in Sect. 2.1.2, Drenick's theorem suggests that an SRP behaves as

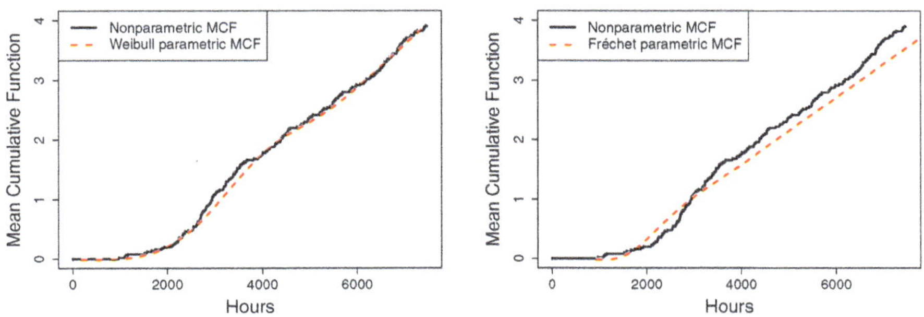

Fig. 4 Weibull (left) and Frećhet (right) fitted MCF plots for Case 1 Weibull data. The solid and dashed curves correspond to the nonparametric and parametric MCF estimates, respectively

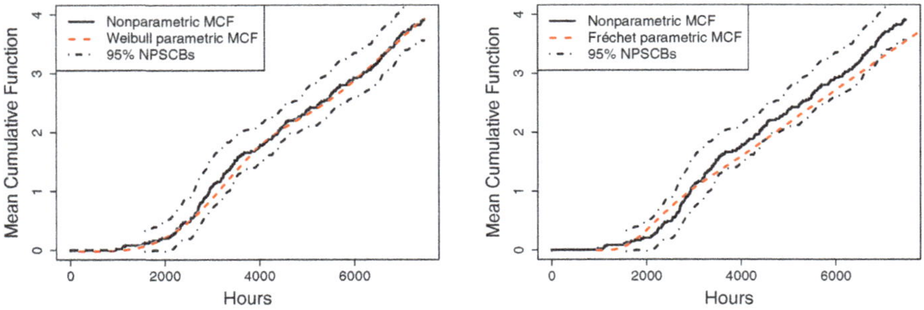

Fig. 5 Weibull (left) and Frećhet (right) fitted MCF plots for Case 1 Weibull SRP data. The solid, dashed, and dot-dash curves correspond to the nonparametric, parametric MCF estimates, and 95% NPSCBs, respectively

a HPP when the number of systems and the operation times are large enough. Furthermore, it is known that the MCF of an HPP is linear. These facts provide an explanation for why the nonparametric MCF estimates are nearly linear after $t = 4000\,\text{h}$.

To assess the amount of sampling variability and check the lack of fit, the approximate 95% NPSCBs over $(t_l, t_u) = (1574, 7485)$ h were obtained (according to Sect. 3.3) and presented on the plots of Fig. 5 (dot-dash curves around the two MCF estimates). The critical values are $e_l = 3.20$ and $e_u = 4.40$, respectively. The Weibull and Fréchet parametric MCF estimates are presented on the left and right plots, respectively. The results indicate that Weibull distribution is consistent with the Case 1 SRP data. The deviation between the nonparametric and Weibull parametric MCF estimates is due to natural variability and there is no statistical evidence for a departure from the Weibull distribution. The right-hand plot in Fig. 5 suggests, however, Fréchet parametric MCF estimate has a large departure from the nonparametric MCF estimate; thus, it is not a good candidate in describing the Case 1 SRP data, based on the fact that the parametric MCF estimate almost falls outside the 95% NPSCBs.

For the Case 2 data example, the nonparametric and parametric MCF estimates, along with the 95% NPSCBs for $t \in (t_l, t_u) = (1034, 2443)$ h, are presented in Fig. 6. The NPSCB critical values are $e_l = 2.75$ and $e_u = 5.05$, respectively. Note that in this case, again due to Drenick's theorem, most of the information for distinguishing among different parametric distributions is in the early times of the renewal processes (the fraction of sockets with events in this example is 0.25). One can see that both the Weibull and the Fréchet parametric estimates stay within the NPSCBs, indicating that both distributions are consistent with the Case 2 SRP data. The Weibull distribution, however, fits better in the sense that the Weibull parametric MCF estimate has a better agreement with the nonparametric MCF estimate, which is consistent with the observations from the probability plot in Fig. 3.

The above examples show how much sampling variability one can expect in the MCF estimates if a parametric distribution is specified correctly. If the parametric

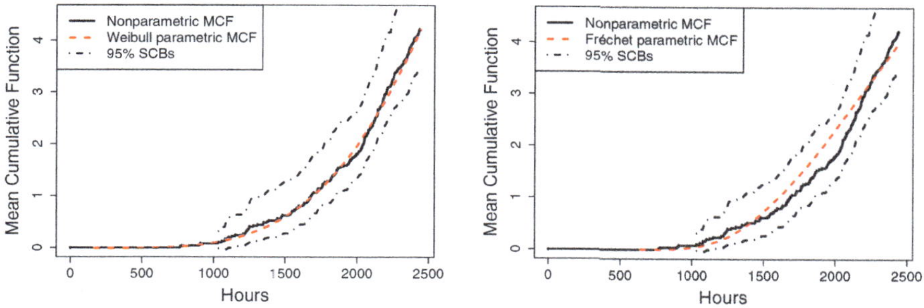

Fig. 6 Weibull (left) and Frećhet (right) fitted MCF plots for Case 2 Weibull SRP data. The solid, dashed, and dot-dash curves correspond to the nonparametric, parametric MCF estimates, and 95% NPSCBs, respectively

MCF estimate has a large deviation from the nonparametric MCF estimate, and it falls outside the NPSCBs, then the proposed parametric distribution is not consistent with the SRP data.

4 Application to the Cylinder Data

In the work of Zhang et al. (2017), the idML estimation was performed on the locomotive cylinder data that first appeared in Nelson and Doganaksoy (1989) and was subsequently given in Meeker and Escobar (1998). The data includes $n = 120$ systems, $m = 16$ sockets per system, and a total of 156 events in the fleet. Both the Weibull and Fréchet distributions were fit to the data. In this section, we apply both goodness-of-fit methods to the data to check the adequacy of the parametric distributions.

4.1 Probability Plotting Method

The PEX semi-parametric estimate of the cdf $F(t)$ with the number of breaking points $b = 8$ were obtained and presented in Fig. 7 (the dot-dash curves). The bootstrap procedure gives the critical values $e_l = 2.71$ and $e_u = 3.86$, and 95% NPSCBs over the time range $(t_l, t_u) = (910, 1719)$ days were presented using the dashed curves in Fig. 7. The results showed that Fréchet distribution gives a better fit to the cylinder data than the Weibull distribution, as the PEX estimate roughly follows a straight line on the Fréchet probability plot. The Weibull distribution does not fit as well, but cannot be ruled out for the cylinder data because it is possible to draw a straight line within the 95% NPSCBs.

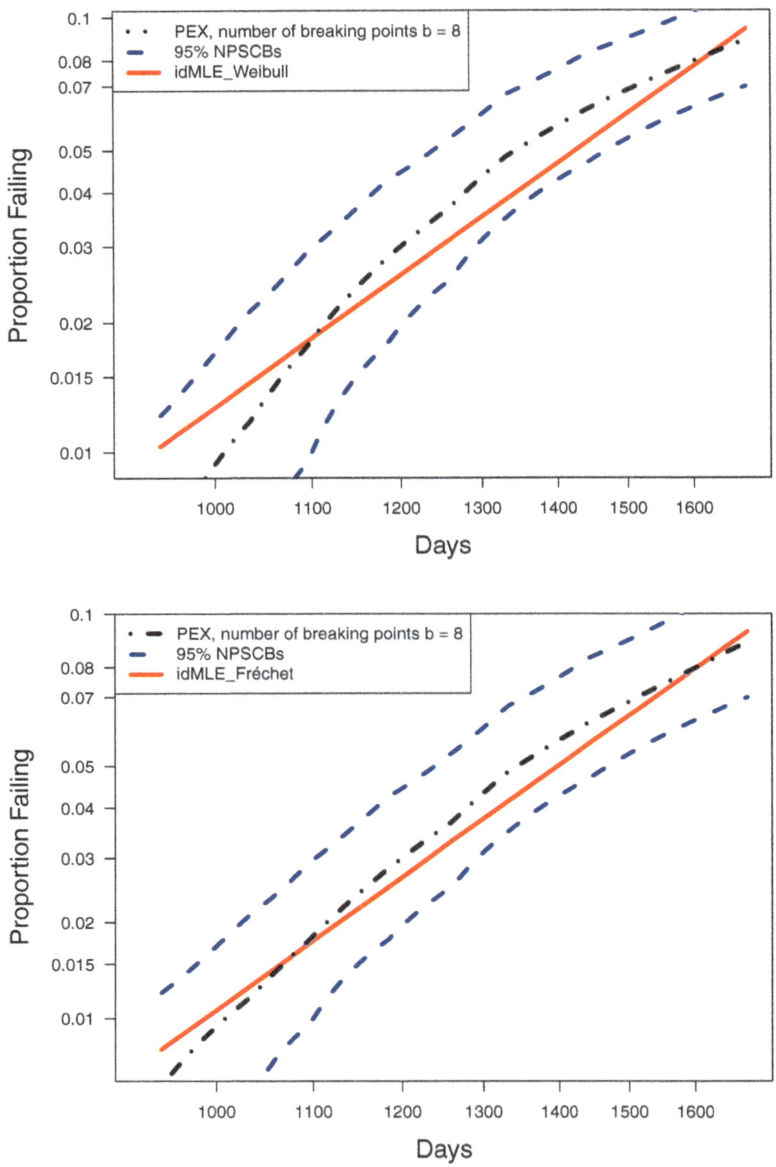

Fig. 7 Weibull (top) and Fréchet (bottom) probability plots for the cylinder data

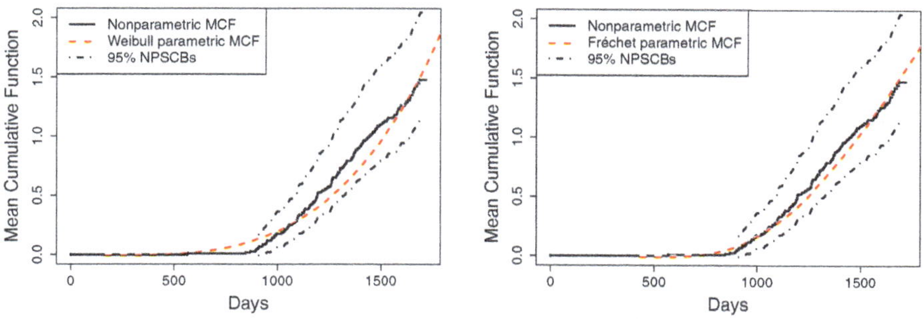

Fig. 8 Weibull (left) and Frećhet (right) fitted MCF plots for the cylinder data. The solid, dashed, and dot-dash curves correspond to the nonparametric, parametric MCF estimates, and 95% NPSCBs, respectively

4.2 MCF Method

The nonparametric MCF estimates and parametric MCF estimates for the Weibull and Fréchet distributions are shown in Fig. 8. We see that, as with the probability plotting method, the Fréchet distribution has a better agreement with the data compared to the Weibull distribution. However, there is still some deviation between the two estimates of MCF. Following the simulation procedure described in Sect. 3, we obtained the 95% NPSCBs of the MCF over the time range $(t_l, t_u) = (910, 1704)$ days (the dot-dash curves in Fig. 8). The bootstrap procedure gives the critical values $e_l = 2.68$ and $e_u = 4.50$. Based on the results, we draw the conclusion that the Weibull distribution does not provide an adequate description of the renewal distribution for the locomotive cylinder data. The deviation in the right-hand MCF plot in Fig. 8 is due to natural variability and there is no statistical evidence of a departure from the Fréchet distribution. These observations are consistent with the conclusions from using the probability plotting method.

5 Concluding Remarks and Areas for Future Research

In this paper, we developed two graphical diagnostic approaches to examine the fit of a distributional model to SRP data detect and assess departures from a fitted distribution. The two methods were based on probability plotting and MCF estimation, respectively. The probability plotting method for detecting overall lack of fit is a modification and extension of the traditional probability plotting method. For the probability plotting method, the PEX model provides graphical semi-parametric estimate of the cdf $F(t)$ and the NPSCBs quantify statistical uncertainty. If a straight line cannot be drawn within the bands, then data are not consistent with the proposed distributional model. Thus, the probability plot method performs insightful graphical tests of goodness-of-fit hypotheses. The MCF graphical test of goodness-of-fit, requires a comparison of the nonparametric MCF estimate with the parametric MCF estimate for a particular distribution. The amount of sampling error can, again, be judged by using NPSCBs, which show the underlying structure and helps point out the departures from the fitted model.

We did an informal study to investigate the effect that the number of jump points in the PEX model has on the graphical goodness-of-fit method described in Sect. 2. The purpose of this appendix is to outline how we did that study and to explain why we suggest between 6 and 10 jumps.

Some possible areas for future research include:

- It would be useful to develop alternative methods to determine the number and location of hazard jump points. For example, Gamerman (1991, 1994) and Demarqui et al. (2014, 2008, 2012) proposed a Bayesian approach for the PEX model in which the hazard jump points are a random quantity, and further introduced a flexible class of prior distributions for modeling jointly the hazard jump points and the corresponding hazard levels.
- The NPSCBs used in the paper are based on the idea of Nair's EP band. Our bootstrap procedure is, however, computationally intensive. Alternative techniques for generating the NPSCBs are needed for situations involving large data sets.
- It would be useful to extend the goodness-of-fit method to applications where different systems are operated in different environments. In such applications, system-level covariates can be used and the methods in this paper can be extended to provide a tool to help identify a baseline renewal distribution.

Appendix 1: Choosing the Number of PEX Jump Points

Starting with the cylinder SRP data, we applied the PEX probability plotting goodness-of-fit procedure described in Sect. 2. The plots in Fig. 9 show the PEX point estimates (solid piecewise linear curve) and the NPSCBs from bootstrapping, using $b = 3, \ldots, 8$ jump points (similar plots were made also for $b = 9$ and 10, but are not shown here). The results were plotted on Fréchet probability scales (the distribution that provides the best fit for the cylinder SRP data, as shown in Sect. 4). Also shown on the plots are ML estimates for the Fréchet (straight dashed line) and the Weibull (dash-dot curve) distributions. The PEX and Fréchet distribution estimates agree well for $b \geq 4$ and the conclusions from visual assessment are not sensitive to the choice of b. That is, the cylinder SRP data are consistent with the Fréchet distribution.

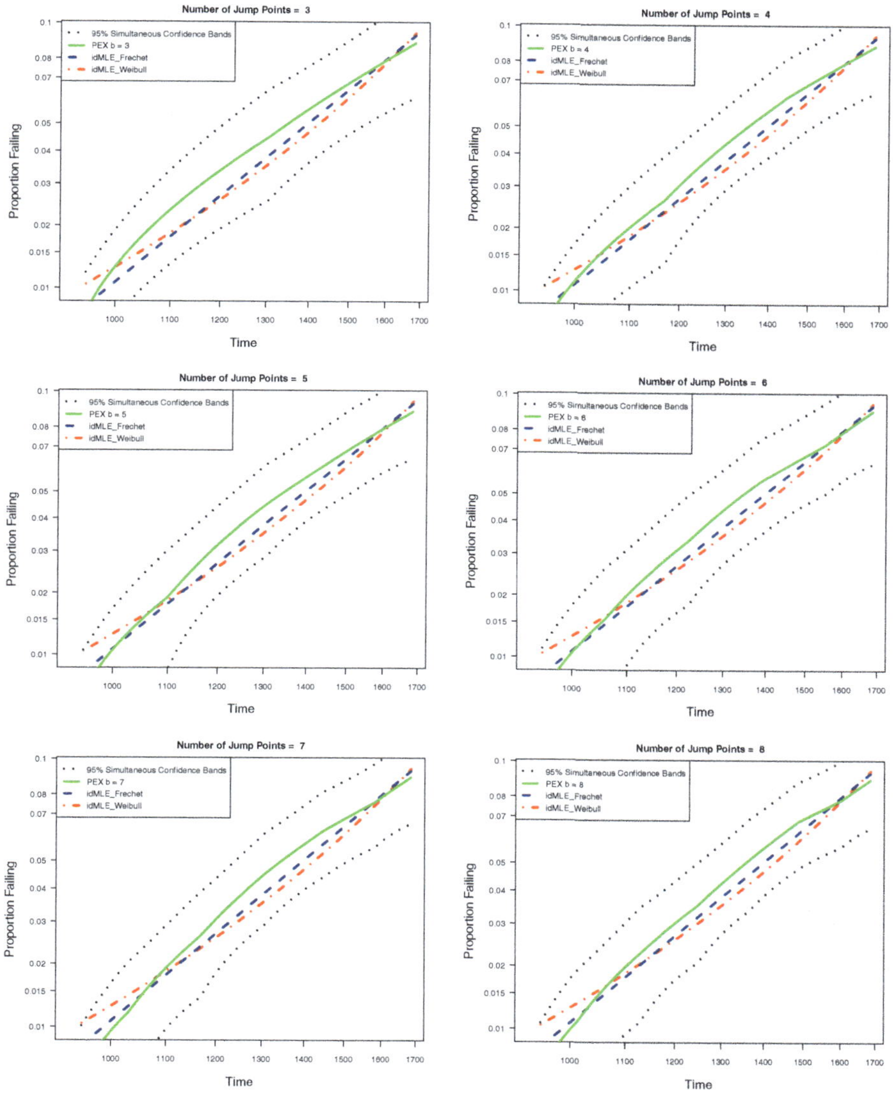

Fig. 9 Fréchet probability plots showing application of the PEX probability plot procedure for $b = 3, \ldots, 8$ jump points

Appendix 2: Choosing the Number of Bootstrap Samples

We did an informal simulation study to investigate the effect that bootstrap sample size has on the graphical goodness-of-fit method for the PEX model. The purpose of this appendix is to outline how we did that study and to explain why the bootstrap sample size $B = 200$ is sufficiently large. We simulated $B = 200$ bootstrap SRP data sets, as described in Sect. 2.3 (simulations were also done with other distributions with similar results). For each bootstrap SRP data set, we computed the PEX estimates with $b = 7$ jump points and the corresponding standard errors. Then, given pre-specified nominal values of e_l and e_u, a pair of SCBs was generated for each bootstrap SRP data set. In Fig. 10, the solid gray curves (above) and the dashed gray curves (below) show these upper bounds and lower bounds, respectively, plotted on Fréchet distribution probability scales. Based on the 200 bootstrap confidence-bound pairs, we calculated new calibrated values e_l and e_u that have equal simultaneous coverage probability in the two tails. Then the calibrated values e_l, e_u were used to construct the two-sided 95% NPSCBs for the original SRP data set using the PEX point estimate and standard errors at a large number of time points. When the bootstrap procedure was repeated, the resulting NPSCBs were,

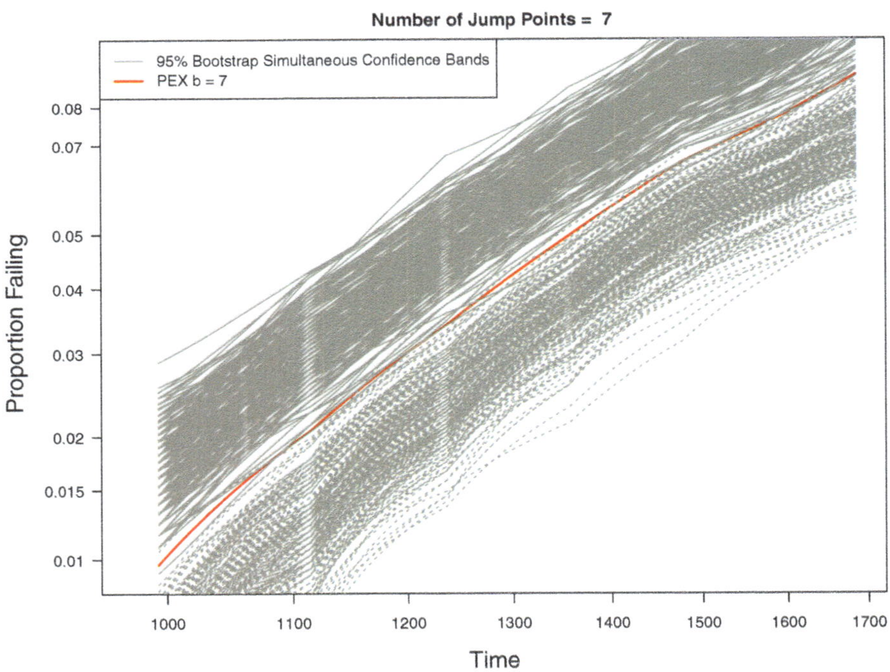

Fig. 10 Upper and lower simultaneous approximate one-sided 97.5% confidence bounds generated from $B = 200$ bootstrap samples

visually, reasonably stable. With only $B = 200$ bootstrap the confidence bounds will not have three (or even two) digits of accuracy, but such is not necessary for the graphical goodness-of-fit application.

References

Colvert, R. E., & Boardman, T. J. (1976). Estimation in the piece-wise constant hazard rate model. *Communications in Statistics: Theory and Methods, 5*, 1013–1029.

Cook, R., & Lawless, J. F. (2007). *The statistical analysis of recurrent events*. Statistics for biology and health. Berlin: Springer.

Demarqui, F. N., Dey, D. K., Loschi, R. H., & Colosimo, E. A. (2014). Fully semiparametric Bayesian approach for modeling survival data with cure fraction. *Biometrical Journal, 56*, 198–218.

Demarqui, F. N., Loschi, R. H., & Colosimo, E. A. (2008). Estimating the grid of time-points for the piecewise exponential model. *Lifetime Data Analysis, 14*, 333–356.

Demarqui, F. N., Loschi, R. H., Dey, D. K., & Colosimo, E. A. (2012). A class of dynamic piecewise exponential models with random time grid. *Journal of Statistical Planning and Inference, 142*, 728–742.

Drenick, R. F. (1960). The failure law of complex equipment. *Journal of the Society for Industrial and Applied Mathematics, 8*, 680–690.

Gamerman, D. (1991). Dynamic Bayesian models for survival data. *Journal of the Royal Statistical Society. Series C (Applied Statistics), 40*, 63–79.

Gamerman, D. (1994). Bayes estimation of the piece-wise exponential distribution. *IEEE Transactions on Reliability, 43*, 128–131.

Greenwood, M. (1926). *A Report on the Natural Duration of Cancer*. Number 33 in Reports on public health and medical subjects. Her Majesty's Stationery Office.

Grenander, U. (1956). On the theory of mortality measurement. *Scandinavian Actuarial Journal, 1956*, 125–153.

Hankin, R. K., & West, L. J. (2007). Set partitions in R. *Journal of Statistical Software, 23*, 1–12.

Hankin, R. K. S. (2006). Additive integer partitions in R. *Journal of Statistical Software, 16*, 1–3.

Hyndman, R. J., & Fan, Y. (1996). Sample quantiles in statistical packages. *The American Statistician, 50*, 361–365.

Kaplan, E. L., & Meier, P. (1958). Nonparametric estimation from incomplete observations. *Journal of the American Statistical Association, 53*, 457–481.

Kim, J. S., & Proschan, F. (1991). Piecewise exponential estimator of the survivor function. *IEEE Transactions on Reliability, 40*, 134–139.

Kitchin, J., Naftali, A. L., & Proschan, F. (1983). A new-method for estimating life distributions from incomplete data. *Statistics & Risk Modeling, 1*, 241–256.

Lawless, J. F., & Nadeau, C. (1995). Some simple robust methods for the analysis of recurrent events. *Technometrics, 37*, 158–168.

Loubert, S. K. (1986). *Inference procedures for the piecewise exponential model when the data are arbitrarily censored*. PhD thesis, Iowa State University.

Meeker, W. Q., & Escobar, L. A. (1998). *Statistical methods for reliability data*. London: Wiley.

Miller, R. G. (1960). Early failures in life testing. *Journal of the American Statistical Association, 55*, 491–502.

Nair, V. N. (1981). Plots and tests for goodness of fit with randomly censored data. *Biometrika, 68*, 99–103.

Nair, V. N. (1984). Confidence bands for survival functions with censored data: A comparative study. *Technometrics, 26*, 265–275.

Nelson, W. (2003). *Recurrent events data analysis for product repairs, disease recurrences, and other applications*. ASA-SIAM Series on Statistics and Applied Probability. Philadelphia, PA: Society for Industrial and Applied Mathematics.

Nelson, W., & Doganaksoy, N. (1989). A computer program for an estimate and confidence limits for the mean cumulative function for cost or number of repairs of repairable products. TIS report 89CRD239, General Electric Company Research and Development, Schenectady, NY.

Padgett, W. J., & Wei, L. J. (1980). Maximum likelihood estimation of a distribution function with increasing failure rate based on censored observations. *Biometrika, 67*, 470–474.

Prairie, R. R., & Ostle, B. (1961). An analysis of some relay failure data from a composite exponential population. *Technometrics, 3*, 423–428.

Zhang, W., Tian, Y., Escobar, L. A., & Meeker, W. Q. (2017). Estimating a parametric component lifetime distribution from a collection of superimposed renewal processes. *Technometrics, 59*, 202–214.

Goodness-of-Fit Tests for Cauchy Distributions Using Data Transformations

J. A. Villaseñor and E. González-Estrada

Abstract The Cauchy distribution is commonly used for modeling symmetric data sets with heavy tails in the areas of finance and economics, among others. In the last two decades, several authors have addressed the problem of testing the null hypothesis of the Cauchy distribution. Here, for testing this hypothesis based on a random sample, it is proposed to transform the sample to approximately exponential random variables and then to test for exponentiality. A power simulation study to compare this test against other tests for the same problem provides evidence that this test is competitive in terms of power versus several types of alternative distributions included in the study. As an application, the returns of daily closing prices for the period September 1st, 2018 to February 28th, 2019 of the German Stock Index (DAX) are analyzed, where the sample size is 122. The studied tests reject the Cauchy distribution hypothesis at the level $\alpha = 0.05$.

1 Introduction

A random variable X follows the Cauchy distribution with location and scale parameters $-\infty < \lambda < \infty$ and $\kappa > 0$, denoted by $X \sim C(\lambda, \kappa)$, while the cdf of X is given by

$$F_0(x; \lambda, \kappa) = \frac{1}{2} + \frac{1}{\pi} \arctan\left(\frac{x-\lambda}{\kappa}\right), \quad -\infty < x < \infty. \tag{1}$$

The Cauchy distribution is commonly used for modeling symmetric data sets with heavy tails in the areas of finance, economics, etc. (Johnson et al. 1994). Williams et al. (2015) argue that the distribution of firm growth rates is best approximated by the Cauchy distribution than by lighter tail distributions like

J. A. Villaseñor (✉) · E. González-Estrada
Colegio de Postgraduados, México, México
e-mail: jvillasr@colpos.mx; egonzalez@colpos.mx

I. Ghosh et al. (eds.), *Advances in Statistics - Theory and Applications*, Emerging Topics in Statistics and Biostatistics, https://doi.org/10.1007/978-3-030-62900-7_13

Laplace. Mahdizadeh and Zamanzade (2017) conclude that the closing prices of the German Stock Index follow a Cauchy distribution.

In the last two decades, several authors have addressed the problem of testing the composite null hypothesis

$$H_0 : X_1, \ldots, X_n \sim C(\lambda, \kappa), \text{ where } \lambda \text{ and } \kappa \text{ are unknown,} \tag{2}$$

versus the alternative hypothesis $H_1 : X_1, \ldots, X_n \nsim C(\lambda, \kappa)$, where $X_1, \ldots, X_n$ are a random sample from a given population with continuous cdf F. Gürtler and Henze (2000), and Matsui and Takemura (2005) consider tests for H_0 based on certain differences between the empirical characteristic function of the standardized data and the characteristic function of the standard Cauchy distribution. Onen et al. (2001) present several modified EDF goodness-of-fit tests. Litvinova (2005) constructs two EDF tests for Cauchy distributions based on characterizations due to Arnold (1979) and Ramachandran and Rao (1970). Morris and Szynal (2013) give tests using characterization conditions of continuous distributions in terms of moments of the k-th record values. Mahdizadeh and Zamanzade (2017) propose three tests based on the likelihood ratio statistic and a test based on the Kullback–Leibler information criterion. Gürtler and Henze (2000)'s tests overpower the classical EDF goodness-of-fit tests, and Mahdizadeh and Zamanzade (2017)'s tests are more powerful than the existing tests, especially for small sample sizes versus light-tailed symmetric alternatives.

Data transformations have proved to be useful for testing goodness of fit of distributions with tails heavier than the normal distribution. For instance, for testing the Generalized Pareto distribution hypothesis, Meintanis and Bassiakos (2007) used a data transformation to approximately exponentially distributed random variables. Simulation results provided by González-Estrada and Villaseñor (2016) show that for testing the Laplace distribution hypothesis, it is better to use Anderson–Darling test based on a sample of transformed data to approximately exponentially distributed random variables than Anderson–Darling test without using such transformation.

Chen and Balakrishnan (1995) proposed a general goodness-of-fit test procedure based on a data transformation to approximately normal random variables. Following the spirit of Chen and Balakrishnan's approach, a procedure for testing goodness of fit of the Cauchy family of distributions is proposed here. The random sample is transformed to approximately exponential random variables, and then Anderson and Darling's (1952) test is used for testing exponentiality.

This manuscript is organized as follows. Two parameter estimation methods for the Cauchy distribution are reviewed in Sect. 2. The proposed testing procedure is presented in Sect. 3. The results of a simulation study on the power of the test are presented in Sect. 4. Daily price's returns of the German stock index are analyzed in Sect. 5. Some conclusions are given in Sect. 6.

2 Parameter Estimation

Let $X_1, \ldots, X_n$ be a random sample from the $C(\lambda, \kappa)$ distribution. The maximum likelihood estimators (MLE) of λ and κ, denoted by $\hat{\lambda}$ and $\hat{\kappa}$, are obtained as the solution to the following system of equations, which is solved by using numerical algorithms like Newton–Raphson.

$$\sum_{i=1}^{n} \frac{x_i - \lambda}{\kappa^2 + (x_i - \lambda)^2} = 0,$$

$$\sum_{i=1}^{n} \frac{\kappa^2}{\kappa^2 + (x_i - \lambda)^2} = \frac{1}{2}n.$$

In general, the likelihood function has a unique root, except in some cases where samples are of size 2 and for any arbitrary sample size n when half of the observations are at some point x_1 (Copas 1975).

Let ξ_p $(0 < p < 1)$ denote the p-quantile of F_0, and let $\tilde{\xi}_{pn}$ denote the sample p-quantile of $X_1, \ldots, X_n$. The unbiased sample median and the sample half-interquartile range are also estimators for λ and κ, which are defined as follows:

$$\tilde{\lambda} = \begin{cases} \frac{1}{2}\left(X_{(n/2)} + X_{(n/2+1)}\right), & \text{if } n \text{ is even} \\ X_{(\lfloor n/2 \rfloor + 1)}, & \text{otherwise} \end{cases} \tag{3}$$

and

$$\tilde{\kappa} = \frac{1}{2}\left(\tilde{\xi}_{(3/4)n} - \tilde{\xi}_{(1/4)n}\right), \tag{4}$$

where $X_{(1)} < \cdots < X_{(n)}$ denote the order statistics of $X_1, \ldots, X_n$, and $\lfloor x \rfloor$ denotes the largest integer not greater than x.

3 The New Test

It is well known that if $X_1, \ldots, X_n$ are iid random variables with continuous cdf $F(\cdot; \theta)$, then the random variables $V_1, \ldots, V_n$ are iid with $Exp(1)$ distribution, where $V_i = -\log F(X_i; \theta)$, $i = 1, \ldots, n$. $Exp(1)$ denotes the standard exponential distribution with cdf $1 - e^{-v}$, $v > 0$.

Therefore, based on this result, for testing H_0 in (2), the following test procedure is proposed:

1. Estimate $\theta' = (\lambda, \kappa)$ by its MLE $\hat{\theta}_n$.
2. Calculate $v_i = -\log(F_0(x_i; \hat{\theta}_n))$, $i = 1, \ldots, n$.

3. Calculate $p_i = 1 - \exp(-v_{(i)}/\bar{v})$, $i = 1, \ldots, n$, where $v_{(1)} < \cdots < v_{(n)}$ are the ordered values corresponding to $v_1, \ldots, v_n$ and $\bar{v} = \sum_{i=1}^{n} v_i/n$.
4. Compute Anderson–Darling test statistic by using the formula

$$A^2 = -n - \frac{1}{n}\sum_{i=1}^{n}\left[(2i-1)\log p_i + (2n+1-2i)\log(1-p_i)\right]. \qquad (5)$$

5. Reject H_0 at the significance level $\alpha \in (0, 1)$ if $A^2 > k_{1-\alpha}$, where $k_{1-\alpha}$ is such that $\alpha = P(A^2 > k_{1-\alpha}|H_0)$, that is, $k_{1-\alpha}$ is the $1-\alpha$ quantile of the distribution of A^2 under H_0. This critical value can be obtained by Monte Carlo simulation for any finite sample size n.

For completeness, a brief description of Anderson–Darling test is provided in the next subsection.

3.1 Anderson–Darling Test

Let $Y_1, \ldots, Y_n$ be a random sample of size n from a continuous population. Anderson–Darling test for $H_0^* : Y_1, \ldots, Y_n \sim G(\cdot; \theta_1)$ vs. $H_1^* : Y_1, \ldots, Y_n \nsim G(\cdot; \theta_1)$, where $G(\cdot; \theta_1)$ is some continuous cdf and θ_1 is an unknown parameter, is based on the test statistic

$$A^2 = n\int_{-\infty}^{\infty}\frac{\left[G_n(y) - G(y;\hat{\theta}_1)\right]^2}{G(y;\hat{\theta}_1)\left[1 - G(y;\hat{\theta}_1)\right]}dG(y;\hat{\theta}_1), \qquad (6)$$

where G_n is the EDF of the $Y_i^{\prime}s$ and $\hat{\theta}_1$ is an efficient estimator of θ_1 (typically, $\hat{\theta}_1$ is the maximum likelihood estimator of θ_1). H_0^* is rejected for large values of A^2. The formula to compute A^2 is given in (5), where $p_i = G(y_{(i)}; \hat{\theta}_1)$ and $y_{(1)} < \cdots < y_{(n)}$ are the ordered values of the observed sample $y_1, \ldots, y_n$.

4 Power Study

A Monte Carlo simulation study was conducted in order to assess the power performance of the proposed test in comparison to the tests presented in Sect. 4.1.

4.1 *Other Tests for the Cauchy Distribution*

As before, let $X_1, \ldots, X_n$ be a random sample of size n from a population with continuous cdf F.

4.1.1 Chen–Balakrishnan Test

For testing $H_0' : X_1, \ldots, X_n \sim F_0'$, where F_0' is the cdf of some skew pdf, Chen and Balakrishnan (1995) proposed a testing procedure that consists in transforming the observations to approximately normally distributed random variables and then testing normality. The procedure is intended to facilitate the computation of critical values when F_0' is the cdf of some skew pdf; however, it can also be used for testing goodness of fit of location-scale families of distributions. Here, we use it for testing H_0 in (2). To our knowledge, this procedure has not been used previously for testing H_0. The test procedure is as follows:

1. Estimate $\theta' = (\lambda, \kappa)'$ by its MLE $\hat{\theta}$.
2. Compute $u_i = F_0(x_i; \hat{\theta})$, $i = 1, \ldots, n$.
3. Calculate $v_i' = \Phi^{-1}(u_i)$, $i = 1, \ldots, n$, where Φ^{-1} is the inverse function of Φ, the standard normal cdf.
4. Compute $p_i = \Phi\left((v_{(i)}' - \bar{v}')/s\right)$, $i = 1, \ldots, n$, where $\bar{v}'$ and s are the sample mean and standard deviation of $v_1', \ldots, v_n'$.
5. Calculate Anderson–Darling test statistic (A^2) by using formula (5).
6. Reject H_0 at the significance level $\alpha \in (0, 1)$ if $A^2 > k_{1-\alpha}$, where $k_{1-\alpha}$ is such that $\alpha = P(A^2 > k_{1-\alpha} | H_0)$ and it can be obtained by Monte Carlo simulation.

4.1.2 An Empirical Characteristic Function Test

Gürtler and Henze (2000) proposed a test for the Cauchy distribution based on the empirical characteristic function $\Psi_n(t)$ of the standardized observations $Y_j = (X_j - \tilde{\lambda})/\tilde{\kappa}$, $j = 1, \ldots, n$, which has the following definition: $\Psi_n(t) = \frac{1}{n}\sum_{j=1}^{n} \exp(itY_j)$, where $\tilde{\lambda}$ and $\tilde{\kappa}$ are given in (3) and (4). The test statistic is $D_{n,a} = n\int_{-\infty}^{\infty} |\Psi_n(t) - e^{-|t|}|^2 e^{-a|t|} dt$, where $a > 0$ is a fixed weighting parameter. H_0 is rejected for large values of $D_{n,a}$. Critical values are provided in Tables 1 and 2 of the same reference for different values of parameter a, as suggested by the same authors. Here, a was fixed at 5.

For testing H_0, Gürtler and Henze (2000) considered a version of Anderson–Darling test described in Sect. 3.1 based on the parameter estimators given in (3) and (4).

4.1.3 Kullback–Leibler Test

Mahdizadeh and Zamanzade (2017) proposed a test for H_0 based on the Kullback–Leibler distance. The test statistic is

$$\tilde{D}_{inf} = \exp\left\{-H_{m,n} - \frac{1}{n}\sum_{i=1}^{n} \log f_0(X_i; \tilde{\lambda}, \tilde{\kappa})\right\},$$

where f_0 is the Cauchy density function and $H_{m,n}=\frac{1}{n}\sum_{i=1}^{n} \log\left\{\frac{n}{2m}\left(X_{(i+m)} - X_{(i-m)}\right)\right\}$. Parameter m (window size) is such that $0 < m \leq n/2$. H_0 is rejected for large values of $\tilde{D}_{inf}$. Critical values are provided by the authors for different sample sizes.

4.2 *Simulation Experiment*

The powers of the proposed test and the tests described in Sect. 4.1 were estimated at a test size $\alpha = 0.05$ by simulating 10,000 pseudo random samples of sizes $n = 20, 35$, and 50 of each considered alternative distribution, which belongs to the following families of probability distributions:

1. Stable(a, b): four parameter stable distributions with stability index $a \in (0, 2]$ and skewness parameter $b \in [-1, 1]$. The location and scale parameters were fixed at 0 and 1 because all tests under comparison are location-scale invariant. This family includes the Cauchy ($a = 1, b = 0$) and normal ($a = 2, b = 0$) distributions as particular cases. When $a < 1$ ($a > 1$), the stable distributions have heavier (lighter) tails than the Cauchy distribution.
2. DoubleGP(ξ): double generalized Pareto distributions with shape parameter $\xi \geq 0$. The DoubleGP distribution reduces to the standard Laplace distribution when $\xi = 0$.
3. $t(\nu)$: Student's t with ν degrees of freedom. This family of distributions includes the Cauchy distribution as a particular case when $\nu = 1$. When $\nu > 1$, the tails of these distributions are lighter than those of Cauchy's.
4. st(a, ν): skew-t distributions with slant parameter $a \in (-\infty, \infty)$ and $\nu > 0$ degrees of freedom. Reduces to the $t(\nu)$ distribution when $a = 0$.
5. Logistic: standard logistic distribution.
6. LN(0,σ): lognormal distributions with parameters (0,σ). The tails of these distributions become fatter as the value of σ increases.
7. GP(ξ): generalized Pareto distributions with shape parameter ξ. GP distributions with parameter $\xi > 0.5$ are heavy tailed.

Computations were carried out in R (R Core Team 2019). Packages `sn` (Azzalini 2017) and `stable` (Wuertz et al. 2016) were used to simulate random numbers from the skew-t and stable distributions.

Table 1 Estimated power of the tests with $n = 20$ and $\alpha = 0.05$

Tail	Skew	Support	Alternative	A^2_{Exp}	A^2_{Norm}	A^2	$\tilde{D}_{inf}$	D_n
Heavy	0	R	DoubleGP(2)	0.75	0.51	0.60	0.02	0.53
Heavy	0	R	DoubleGP(1.5)	0.48	0.24	0.35	0.02	0.33
Heavy	0	R	DoubleGP(1)	0.17	0.08	0.14	0.03	0.15
	0	R	DoubleGP(0.75)	0.07	0.05	0.07	0.04	0.08
	0	R	DoubleGP(0)	0.06	0.14	0.03	0.31	0.06
Heavy	0	R	Stable(0.5, 0)	0.74	0.50	0.60	0.02	0.53
Heavy	0	R	Stable(0.75, 0)	0.24	0.11	0.17	0.02	0.18
Heavy	0	R	Stable(1, 0)	0.05	0.05	0.05	0.05	0.05
	0	R	Stable(1.25, 0)	0.04	0.08	0.03	0.13	0.03
	0	R	Stable(1.5, 0)	0.08	0.16	0.03	0.27	0.06
	0	R	Stable(1.75, 0)	0.15	0.29	0.04	0.47	0.12
	0	R	Stable(2, 0)	0.25	0.42	0.06	0.72	0.22
	0	R	t(2)	0.05	0.11	0.03	0.21	0.04
	0	R	t4)	0.12	0.23	0.04	0.42	0.10
	0	R	t(6)	0.15	0.29	0.04	0.53	0.13
	0	R	t(12)	0.20	0.35	0.05	0.62	0.17
	0	R	logistic	0.16	0.30	0.04	0.55	0.14
Heavy	+	R	st(1, 0.75)	0.37	0.19	0.33	0.09	0.14
Heavy	+	R	st(1, 1)	0.18	0.13	0.18	0.12	0.07
Heavy	+	R	st(2, 0.75)	0.55	0.40	0.52	0.22	0.16
Heavy	+	R	st(2, 1)	0.32	0.30	0.34	0.23	0.09
Heavy	+	R	Stable(0.5, 0.5)	0.88	0.66	0.77	0.08	0.53
Heavy	+	R	Stable(0.75, 0.5)	0.44	0.26	0.35	0.08	0.19
	+	R	Stable(1.25, 0.5)	0.06	0.14	0.06	0.19	0.04
	+	R	Stable(1.5, 0.5)	0.08	0.20	0.04	0.31	0.07
	+	R	Stable(1.75, 0.5)	0.16	0.30	0.04	0.49	0.12
	+	R	Stable(2, 0.5)	0.25	0.42	0.06	0.72	0.22
	+	R+	GP(−0.25)	0.45	0.77	0.26	0.95	0.35
	+	R+	GP(0.25)	0.52	0.76	0.44	0.87	0.22
	+	R+	GP(0.5)	0.63	0.80	0.56	0.81	0.20
Heavy	+	R+	GP(0.75)	0.76	0.86	0.68	0.78	0.20
Heavy	+	R+	GP(1)	0.85	0.91	0.78	0.74	0.23
	+	R+	LN(0, 0.5)	0.22	0.49	0.13	0.73	0.18
	+	R+	LN(0, 1)	0.43	0.69	0.38	0.80	0.19
Heavy	+	R+	LN(0, 2)	0.94	0.97	0.89	0.87	0.33
Heavy	+	R+	LN(0, 3)	1.00	1.00	0.98	0.91	0.56

4.3 Results

Tables 1, 2, and 3 contain the estimated powers of the tests rounded to two decimal positions, where A^2_{Exp} denotes the proposed test, A^2_{Norm} denotes Chen–

Table 2 Estimated power of the tests with $n = 35$ and $\alpha = 0.05$

Tail	Skew	Support	Alternative	A^2_{Exp}	A^2_{Norm}	A^2	$\tilde{D}_{inf}$	D_n
Heavy	0	R	DoubleGP(2)	0.93	0.80	0.78	0.00	0.70
Heavy	0	R	DoubleGP(1.5)	0.68	0.45	0.45	0.00	0.44
Heavy	0	R	DoubleGP(1)	0.24	0.11	0.15	0.01	0.16
	0	R	DoubleGP(.75)	0.08	0.05	0.08	0.04	0.07
	0	R	DoubleGP(0)	0.20	0.29	0.07	0.72	0.30
Heavy	0	R	Stable(0.5, 0)	0.93	0.83	0.76	0.00	0.69
Heavy	0	R	Stable(0.75, 0)	0.33	0.19	0.19	0.01	0.21
Heavy	0	R	Stable(1, 0)	0.05	0.06	0.05	0.05	0.05
	0	R	Stable(1.25, 0)	0.08	0.13	0.04	0.18	0.10
	0	R	Stable(1.5, 0)	0.24	0.34	0.07	0.43	0.27
	0	R	Stable(1.75, 0)	0.48	0.61	0.14	0.73	0.53
	0	R	Stable(2, 0)	0.71	0.84	0.26	0.99	0.79
	0	R	t(2)	0.14	0.22	0.05	0.39	0.17
	0	R	t4)	0.39	0.53	0.11	0.77	0.45
	0	R	t(6)	0.51	0.64	0.15	0.90	0.58
	0	R	t(12)	0.61	0.76	0.20	0.96	0.70
	0	R	logistic	0.52	0.64	0.16	0.93	0.61
Heavy	+	R	st(1, 0.75)	0.54	0.27	0.49	0.05	0.21
Heavy	+	R	st(1, 1)	0.27	0.19	0.30	0.11	0.11
Heavy	+	R	st(2, 0.75)	0.79	0.58	0.78	0.17	0.33
Heavy	+	R	st(2, 1)	0.57	0.48	0.59	0.24	0.22
Heavy	+	R	Stable(0.5, 0.5)	0.98	0.91	0.94	0.02	0.77
Heavy	+	R	Stable(0.75, 0.5)	0.63	0.44	0.53	0.04	0.28
	+	R	Stable(1.25, 0.5)	0.14	0.25	0.11	0.26	0.13
	+	R	Stable(1.5, 0.5)	0.25	0.39	0.10	0.49	0.29
	+	R	Stable(1.75, 0.5)	0.47	0.58	0.15	0.77	0.54
	+	R	Stable(2, 0.5)	0.70	0.81	0.25	0.99	0.79
	+	R+	GP(−0.25)	0.93	0.99	0.69	1.00	0.89
	+	R+	GP(0.25)	0.96	1.00	0.83	0.98	0.66
	+	R+	GP(0.5)	0.98	1.00	0.91	0.94	0.59
Heavy	+	R+	GP(0.75)	0.99	1.00	0.96	0.87	0.59
Heavy	+	R+	GP(1)	1.00	1.00	0.98	0.79	0.62
	+	R+	LN(0.5)	0.68	0.91	0.39	0.98	0.67
	+	R+	LN(0, 1)	0.91	0.99	0.78	0.96	0.59
Heavy	+	R+	LN(0, 2)	1.00	1.00	0.99	0.92	0.77
Heavy	+	R+	LN(0, 3)	1.00	1.00	1.00	0.90	0.94

Balakrishnan test, and A^2 denotes Gürtler and Henze (2000)'s version of Anderson–Darling test based on estimators (3) and (4). Notations D_n and $\tilde{D}_{inf}$ are defined in Sect. 4.1. The power of the tests versus the Stable(1,0) distribution provides the

Table 3 Estimated power of the tests with $n = 50$ and $\alpha = 0.05$

Tail	Skew	Support	Alternative	A^2_{Exp}	A^2_{Norm}	A^2	$\tilde{D}_{inf}$	D_n
Heavy	0	R	DoubleGP(2)	0.98	0.94	0.92	0.00	0.88
Heavy	0	R	DoubleGP(1.5)	0.83	0.65	0.64	0.00	0.63
Heavy	0	R	DoubleGP(1)	0.31	0.17	0.20	0.01	0.24
	0	R	DoubleGP(0.75)	0.09	0.06	0.09	0.04	0.10
	0	R	DoubleGP(0)	0.37	0.49	0.11	0.94	0.39
Heavy	0	R	Stable(0.5, 0)	0.98	0.95	0.92	0.00	0.87
Heavy	0	R	Stable(0.75, 0)	0.42	0.29	0.25	0.00	0.31
Heavy	0	R	Stable(1, 0)	0.05	0.06	0.05	0.05	0.04
	0	R	Stable(1.25, 0)	0.13	0.19	0.05	0.23	0.10
	0	R	Stable(1.5, 0)	0.41	0.51	0.12	0.53	0.37
	0	R	Stable(1.75, 0)	0.74	0.83	0.29	0.83	0.71
	0	R	Stable(2, 0)	0.93	0.98	0.54	1.00	0.93
	0	R	t(2)	0.26	0.35	0.07	0.51	0.22
	0	R	t4)	0.65	0.77	0.22	0.93	0.61
	0	R	t(6)	0.79	0.88	0.31	0.98	0.76
	0	R	t(12)	0.87	0.95	0.42	1.00	0.86
	0	R	logistic	0.81	0.88	0.33	1.00	0.79
Heavy	+	R	st(1, 0.75)	0.69	0.35	0.69	0.02	0.28
Heavy	+	R	st(1, 1)	0.36	0.25	0.47	0.10	0.14
Heavy	+	R	st(2, 0.75)	0.91	0.72	0.93	0.07	0.47
Heavy	+	R	st(2, 1)	0.74	0.63	0.81	0.18	0.34
Heavy	+	R	Stable(0.5, 0.5)	1.00	0.98	0.99	0.00	0.91
Heavy	+	R	Stable(0.75, 0.5)	0.76	0.59	0.73	0.01	0.38
	+	R	Stable(1.25, 0.5)	0.22	0.38	0.20	0.30	0.18
	+	R	Stable(1.5, 0.5)	0.44	0.59	0.20	0.60	0.40
	+	R	Stable(1.75, 0.5)	0.73	0.82	0.32	0.85	0.71
	+	R	Stable(2, 0.5)	0.93	0.97	0.53	1.00	0.93
	+	R+	GP(−0.25)	1.00	1.00	0.95	1.00	0.99
	+	R+	GP(0.25)	1.00	1.00	0.99	0.98	0.90
	+	R+	GP(0.5)	1.00	1.00	0.99	0.85	0.86
Heavy	+	R+	GP(0.75)	1.00	1.00	1.00	0.67	0.86
Heavy	+	R+	GP(1)	1.00	1.00	1.00	0.49	0.88
	+	R+	LN(0.5)	0.94	0.99	0.72	1.00	0.88
	+	R+	LN(0, 1)	1.00	1.00	0.98	0.96	0.85
Heavy	+	R+	LN(0, 2)	1.00	1.00	1.00	0.62	0.95
Heavy	+	R+	LN(0, 3)	1.00	1.00	1.00	0.31	1.00

estimated size of the tests since a Stable(1,0) distribution is the standard Cauchy distribution. The tests preserve the nominal size, in general.

The power results indicate that A^2_{Exp} test is more powerful than the rest of the tests under comparison versus the considered symmetric alternative distributions with tails heavier than Cauchy's distribution. On the other hand, when the alternative has tails lighter than Cauchy's, A^2_{Exp} is competitive with D_n test.

$\tilde{D}_{inf}$ test is powerful versus alternative distributions with light tail; however, its power is zero or close to zero versus heavy-tailed alternatives for all sample sizes considered and, in some cases, its power decreases as the sample size increases (see, for instance, the cases of st and GP(1) alternatives).

A^2 is a competitive test for this problem against heavy-tailed alternatives; however, this test has low power versus light-tailed alternative distributions with support in the whole real line.

Notice that A^2_{Norm} test is in general more powerful than A^2_{Exp}, A^2 and D_n tests versus both symmetric and skew alternatives with light tail. Furthermore, this test turns out to be the best among these three tests versus the considered skew alternatives with support on R^+.

The powers of A^2_{Exp}, A^2_{Norm}, and D_n tests increase as the skewness of the alternative increases, the tail of the alternative becomes either fatter or lighter than Cauchy's, both the skewness and the weight of the tail differ from those of Cauchy's distribution, and the sample size increases.

5 A Financial Data Set

Mahdizadeh and Zamanzade (2017) consider 30 returns of the closing prices of the German Stock Index (DAX), observed daily from January 1st, 1991, excluding weekends and public holidays. They apply 8 tests for the Cauchy distribution hypothesis to this data set. By using any of these tests, the null hypothesis is not rejected with a test size $\alpha = 0.05$.

Here, the returns of the closing prices of the DAX index observed daily in the semester from September 1st, 2018 to February 28th, 2019 are considered.[1] Figure 1 shows a histogram of these 122 values. The five tests compared in Sect. 4 are applied to these observations. Opposite to Mahdizadeh and Zamanzade (2017)'s results, according to four of the considered tests, this data set with a larger sample size does not support the null hypothesis that the Cauchy distribution is a plausible model for the returns because this hypothesis is rejected by such tests with $\alpha = 0.05$. A^2 does not reject H_0. The calculated p-values are the following:

A^2_{Exp}	A^2_{Norm}	A^2	$\tilde{D}_{inf}$	D_n
0.00214	0.00018	0.05386	2e-05	0.00102

[1]Data downloaded from Yahoo Finance website https://finance.yahoo.com.

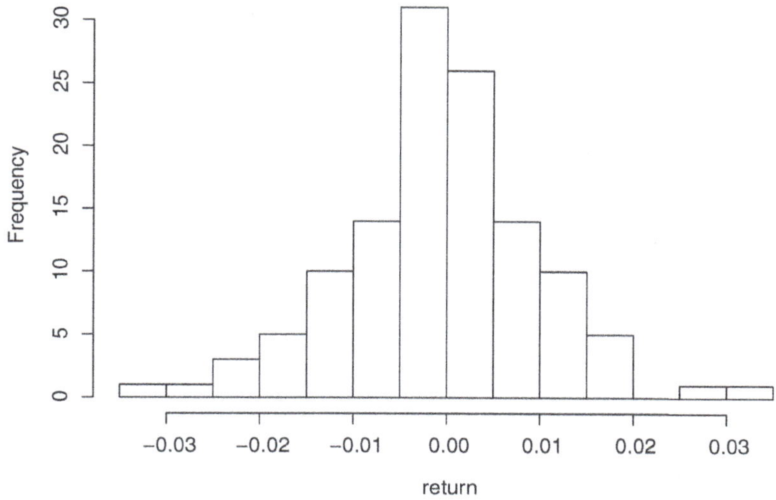

Fig. 1 Histogram of the returns

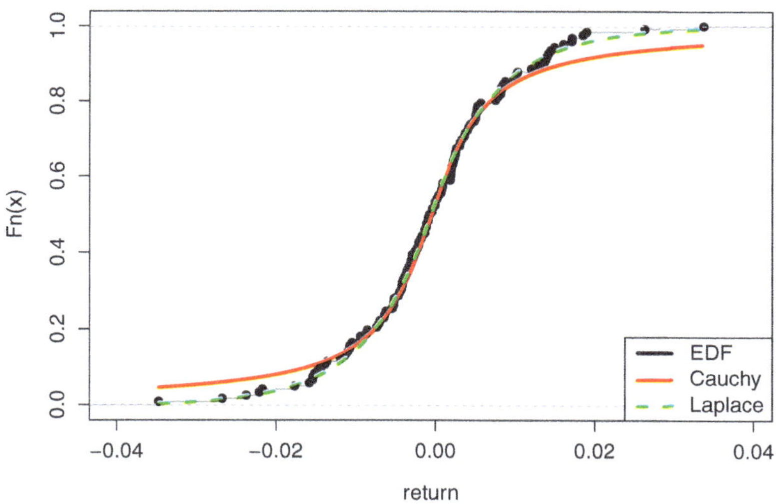

Fig. 2 EDF, fitted Cauchy and Laplace distributions to the returns

The conclusion of rejecting H_0 is supported by Fig. 2, which shows a significant disagreement between the EDF of the observations and the MLE fitted Cauchy distribution. Figure 2 also shows that the Laplace (or double exponential) distribution provides a better fit to this data set. This observation agrees with the result of the test for the Laplace distribution hypothesis based on a transformation to exponentiality proposed by González-Estrada and Villaseñor (2016), which produces a p-value = 0.5831.

6 Conclusions

A goodness-of-fit test procedure (A^2_{Exp}) is proposed in this manuscript for testing the Cauchy distribution hypothesis. Monte Carlo simulation results on the power of the test provide evidence that this test is competitive with respect to most of the groups of alternative distributions studied. Also notice that, against the considered heavy-tailed symmetric alternatives, A^2_{Exp} is in general the most powerful test.

References

Arnold, B. C. (1979). Some characterizations of the Cauchy distribution. *Australian Journal of Statistics, 21*, 166–169.

Azzalini, A. (2017). The R package 'sn': The skew-normal and related distributions such as the skew-t (version 1.5–1). Retrieved from http://azzalini.stat.unipd.it/SN

Chen, G., & Balakrishnan, N. (1995). A general purpose approximate goodness of fit test. *Journal of Quality Technology, 27*(2), 154–161.

Copas, J. B. (1975). On the unimodality of the likelihood for the Cauchy distribution. *Biometrica, 62*, 701–704.

González-Estrada, E., & Villaseñor, J. A. (2016). A ratio goodness of fit test for the Laplace distribution. *Statistics & Probability Letters, 119*, 30–35.

Gürtler, N., & Henze, N. (2000). Goodness-of-fit tests for the Cauchy distribution based on the empirical characteristic function. *Annals of the Institute of Statistical Mathematics, 52*(2), 267–286.

Johnson, N. L., Kotz, S., & Balakrishnan, N. (1994). Continuous univariate distributions (vol. 1, 2nd edn.). Hoboken: Wiley.

Litvinova, V. V. (2005). Two criteria of goodness-of-fit for Cauchy distributions based on characterizations. *Journal of Mathematical Sciences, 127*(1), 1752–1756.

Mahdizadeh, M., & Zamanzade, E. (2017). New goodness of fit tests for the Cauchy distribution. *Journal of Applied Statistics, 44*(6), 1106–1121.

Matsui, M., & Takemura, A. (2005). Empirical characteristic function approach to goodness-of-fit tests for the Cauchy distribution with parameters estimated by MLE or EISE. *Annals of the Institute of Statistical Mathematics, 57*(1), 183–199.

Meintanis, S. G., & Bassiakos, Y. (2007). Data transformation and test of fit for the generalized Pareto hypothesis. *Communications in Statistics: Theory and Methods, 36*(4), 833–849.

Morris, K. W., & Szynal, D. (2013). Goodness-of-fit tests via characterizations. Special cases. *Journal of Mathematical Sciences, 191*(4), 550–567.

Onen, B. H., Dietz, D. C., Yen, V. C., & Moore, A. H. (2001). Goodness-of-fit tests for the Cauchy distribution. *Computational Statistics, 16*(1), 97–107.

R Core Team. (2019). R: A language and environment for statistical computing. Vienna, Austria. Retrieved from https://www.R-project.org/

Ramachandran, B., & Rao, C. R. (1970). Solutions of functional equations arising in some regression problems and a characterization of the Cauchy law. *Sankhya, Series A, 32*(1), 1–30.

Williams, M. A., Pinto, B. J., & Park, D. (2015). Global evidence on the distribution of firm growth rates. *Physica A: Statistical Mechanics and its Applications, 432*, 102–107.

Wuertz, D., Maechler, M., & Rmetrics Core Team Members. (2016). Stabledist: Stable distribution functions. R package version 0.7-1. Retrieved from https://CRAN.R-project.org/package=stabledist

Part VI
Statistical Inference

A Bayesian Approach to Cluster Sampling Under Simple Random Sampling

Michael Soma and Glen Meeden

Abstract Two-stage cluster sampling arises when units in the population belong to groups or clusters, and drawing a sample must proceed in two stages. First, a subset of the clusters is chosen, and then within the selected clusters, a subset of the units within a cluster is selected. When there is little available prior information about the population, simple random sampling without replacement is often used at both stages, and the ratio estimate is used to estimate the population total. Here, we will compare this estimate with two Bayesian alternatives and see that the Bayesian estimators are a slight improvement over the standard method.

1 Introduction

Two-stage cluster sampling arises when the units in the population (secondary) come in groups or clusters (primary), and drawing a sample must proceed in two stages. First, a subset of the primary units is chosen, and then within the selected clusters, a subset of the secondary units within a cluster is selected. An important special case is when there is little available prior information about the clusters or units within the clusters. In such cases, simple random sampling without replacement is used in both stages. In this note, we will assume that the quantity of interest associated with each secondary unit can take on just two values, zero or one.

For this setup, Nandram and Sedransk (1993) introduced a Bayesian hierarchical model. A limitation of their approach was that their prior distribution on the hyperparameter assumed a particular simple form. In this note, we will we show that a non-informative prior suggested in Gelman et al. (2004) works better for this problem. In the special case when all the clusters are of the same size and the

M. Soma
Department of Statistics, Iowa State University, Ames, IA, USA

G. Meeden (✉)
School of Statistics, University of Minnesota, Minneapolis, MN, USA
e-mail: gmeeden@umn.edu

I. Ghosh et al. (eds.), *Advances in Statistics - Theory and Applications*, Emerging Topics in Statistics and Biostatistics, https://doi.org/10.1007/978-3-030-62900-7_14

same number of secondary units are take from each sample cluster, Meeden (1999) showed that a stepwise Bayes approach based on the Polya posterior essentially agrees with standard methods. Here, we will consider a modification to this approach which allows for different cluster sizes and different sample sizes within clusters. We will see that both Bayesian approaches can give slightly better results that the standard frequentist estimator.

In Sect. 2, we describe in detail the two Bayesian approaches, and in Sect. 3, we present some simulation results that compare the Bayesian approaches with the ratio estimator.

2 Existing Bayesian Methods for Two-Stage Cluster Sampling

We begin by setting the notation. Let N be the number of clusters or the number of primary sampling units. For a given cluster i, let M_i be the number of secondary sampling units in the cluster. For a given cluster i, let y_{ij} be the value of the quantity of interest for unit j in cluster i. That is, y_{ij} is the value of the jth secondary unit in the ith primary unit. We assume that the every y_{ij} has either the value one or the value zero. Let y_i be the cluster total for the ith cluster. Let $y = (y_1, \ldots, y_N)$ be the vector of cluster totals.

Let n denote the number of clusters in the first stage of sampling. Let s be the indices of the clusters in the sample and s' be the indices of the clusters not in the sample. For a given i, let m_i be the size of the sample taken from cluster i. Given s, M_s will denote the sizes of the clusters in the sample, and $M_{s'}$ will denote the sizes of the clusters not in s. Similarly, y_s and $y_{s'}$ will denote the cluster totals for the clusters in the sample and those not in the sample, respectively.

2.1 A Proper Bayesian Approach

In the absence of an informative prior, a Bayesian approach desires exchangeability between the sampled and unsampled units. Exchangeability for a Bayesian approach is analogous to independent and identically distributed random variables for a frequentist. If a sequence of random variables has a joint distribution that is invariant under all permutations of the indices, it is said to be finitely exchangeable. For predictive inference, exchangeability ensures that the probability distribution on the population y does not depend on the order units were drawn or which units were sampled and unsampled.

For a two-stage cluster sample, we desire exchangeability not only between sampled and unsampled units within a cluster but also between sampled and unsampled clusters.

Nandram and Sedransk (1993) propose a fully Bayesian approach for binary y. Their model assumes that given a θ_i, the $\{y_{ij} : j = 1, 2, \ldots, M_i\}$ are independent with

$$Pr(y_{ij} = 1|\theta_i) = \theta_i \quad \text{and} \quad Pr(y_{ij} = 0|\theta_i) = 1 - \theta_i.$$

Here, given θ_i, the probability distribution of y_i is the binomial distribution with parameters θ_i and M_i. That is,

$$f(y_i|\theta_i) = \binom{M_i}{y_i}\theta_i^{y_i}(1-\theta_i)^{M_i-y_i}.$$

If we take as the prior for the θ_i's a Beta(α_1, α_2) distribution, where the parameters α_1 and α_2 are fixed and known, then the posterior distribution for the θ_i's is independent, and given y_i, the distribution for θ_i is a Beta distribution with parameters $y_i + \alpha_1$ and $M_i - y_i + \alpha_2$.

If, however, we place a hyperprior on $\alpha = (\alpha_1, \alpha_2)$, we are able to derive a posterior for α conditional on the observed data which can be used to better understand how the θ_i's are distributed for the unobserved clusters. This allows for a more flexible Bayesian model than specifying an exact pair of values for α. Nandram and Sedransk propose a prior on θ_i that limits α_1 to take on only a finite set of possible values and fixes $\alpha_2 = \tau - \alpha_1$ for some fixed τ. More formally, they assume that

$$\alpha_1 \in \{a_r : 0 < a_1 < a_2 < \cdots < a_R < \tau\}$$

$$Pr(\alpha_1 = a_r) = \omega_r \quad \text{and} \quad \sum_{r=1}^{R} \omega_r = 1,$$

where the a_i's and the ω's must be specified by the statistician.

Given the current methods in Bayesian computing, we can now extend the approach of Nandram and Sedransk (1993) to the case where we specify a continuous probability function on the set of α's, where α_1 and α_2 can range from zero to infinity.

Let $h(\alpha)$ denote a prior density for α, and consider the joint distribution of y, θ, and α:

$$p(y, \theta, \alpha) = h(\alpha)\prod_{i=1}^{N} f(y_i|\theta_i)g(\theta_i|\alpha).$$

Since we are assuming that given the θ_i's, the cluster totals are independent, this joint distribution can be rewritten as the product of the sampled and unsampled units. That is, ignoring $h(\alpha)$ for a moment, we have

$$\prod_{i=1}^{N} f(y_i|\theta_i)g(\theta_i|\alpha) = \prod_{i\in s} f(y_{s_i}|\theta_{s_i})g(\theta_{s_i}|\alpha)\prod_{i\in s'} f(y_{s'_i}|\theta_{s'_i})g(\theta_{s'_i}|\alpha). \tag{1}$$

A similar argument can be applied to the sampled and unsampled secondary sampling units for the partially observed clusters:

$$\prod_{i\in s} f(y_{s_i}|\theta_{s_i})g(\theta_{s_i}|\alpha) = \prod_{i\in s} f(z_{s_i}, z_{s'_i}|\theta_{s_i})g(\theta_{s_i}|\alpha). \tag{2}$$

Now, our joint density can be expressed in terms of the observed data. Using (1) and (2), our joint density is now

$$\begin{aligned} p(y,\theta,\alpha) &= p(z_s,\ z_{s'},\ y_{s'},\ \theta_s,\ \theta_{s'},\ \alpha) \\ &= h(\alpha)\prod_{i\in s} f(z_{s_i}, z_{s'_i}|\theta_{s_i})g(\theta_{s_i}|\alpha)\prod_{i\in s'} f(y_{s'_i}|\theta_{s'_i})g(\theta_{s'_i}|\alpha). \end{aligned} \tag{3}$$

Using (3), the joint density conditional on the observed data is

$$p(z_{s'},\ y_{s'},\ \theta_s,\ \theta_{s'},\ \alpha|\ z_s) = \frac{p(y,\theta,\alpha)}{p(z_s)}.$$

By integrating out θ_s, we have the joint density of $z_{s'},\ y_{s'},\ \theta_{s'}$, and α given the observed data is

$$p(z_{s'},\ y_{s'},\ \theta_{s'},\ \alpha|\ z_s) = \frac{h(\alpha)\prod_{i\in s} f(z_{s_i}, z_{s'_i}|\alpha)\prod_{i\in s'} f(y_{s'_i}|\theta_{s'_i})g(\theta_{s'_i}|\alpha)}{p(z_s)}.$$

Using the fact that we can rewrite the conditional distribution of z_{s_i} and $z_{s'_i}$ given α as

$$\begin{aligned} f(z_{s_i}, z_{s'_i}|\alpha) &= \frac{p(z_{s_i}, z_{s'_i}, \alpha)}{p(\alpha)} \\ &= \frac{p(z_{s_i}, z_{s'_i}, \alpha)}{p(z_{s_i}, \alpha)}\frac{p(z_{s_i}, \alpha)}{p(\alpha)} \\ &= p(z_{s'_i}|z_{s_i}, \alpha)p(z_{s_i}|\alpha). \end{aligned}$$

We can now write the joint distribution of $z_{s'_i},\ y_{s'_i},\ \theta_{s'_i}$, and α conditional on the observed clusters as

$$
\begin{aligned}
&p(z_{s'},\ y_{s'},\ \theta_{s'},\ \alpha|\ z_s) \\
&= \left(\frac{h(\alpha)\prod_{i\in s} p(z_{s_i}|\alpha)}{p(z_s)}\right)\prod_{i\in s} p(z_{s_i'}|z_{s_i},\ \alpha)\prod_{i\in s'} f(y_{s_i'}|\theta_{s_i'})g(\theta_{s_i'}|\alpha) \\
&= p(\alpha|z_{s_i})\prod_{i\in s} p(z_{s_i'}|z_{s_i},\ \alpha)\prod_{i\in s'} f(y_{s_i'}|\theta_{s_i'})g(\theta_{s_i'}|\alpha).
\end{aligned}
$$

Next, we need to choose a prior distribution for α. Since we want our prior to be "non-informative," we need one that puts most of its mass close to (0, 0). We have found that the prior discussed in Gelman et al. (2004),

$$
h(\alpha_1, \alpha_2) \propto (\alpha_1 + \alpha_2)^{-5/2} \quad \text{for} \quad \alpha_1 > 0 \ \text{ and } \ \alpha_2 > 0,
$$

works well for our problem. Now, we evaluate Eq. (2.1) for this choice of the prior h. For the rest of the discussion for notational simplicity, we will assume that the clusters selected in the first stage where primary units $i = 1, \ldots, n$. In this case, we can write the joint distribution as

$$
\begin{aligned}
p(z_{s_i},\ \theta_{s_i},\ \alpha) &= h(\alpha)\prod_{i=1}^{n} f(z_{s_i}|\theta_{s_i})g(\theta_{s_i}|\alpha) \\
&\propto (\alpha_1+\alpha_2)^{-5/2}\prod_{i=1}^{n}\binom{m_{s_i}}{z_{s_i}}\theta_{s_i}{}^{z_{s_i}}(1-\theta_{s_i})^{(m_{s_i}-z_{s_i})}\frac{\Gamma(\sum_{l=1}^{2}\alpha_l)}{\prod_{l=1}^{2}\Gamma(\alpha_l)}\theta_{s_i}{}^{\alpha_1-1}(1-\theta_{s_i})^{\alpha_2-1} \\
&\propto (\alpha_1+\alpha_2)^{-5/2}\left(\frac{\Gamma(\sum_{l=1}^{2}\alpha_l)}{\prod_{l=1}^{2}\Gamma(\alpha_l)}\right)^{n}\prod_{i=1}^{n}\binom{m_{s_i}}{z_{s_i}}\prod_{i=1}^{n}\theta_{s_i}{}^{(z_{s_i}+\alpha_1-1)}(1-\theta_{s_i})^{(m_{s_i}-z_{s_i}+\alpha_2-1)} \\
&\propto (\alpha_1+\alpha_2)^{-5/2}\prod_{i=1}^{n}\theta_{s_i}{}^{(z_{s_i}+\alpha_1-1)}(1-\theta_{s_i})^{(m_{s_i}-z_{s_i}+\alpha_2-1)}.
\end{aligned}
$$

Integrating out θ_{s_i}, we find

$$
\begin{aligned}
&p(z_{s_i},\ \alpha) \\
&\propto (\alpha_1+\alpha_2)^{-5/2}\int_{\theta_{s_1}}\cdots\int_{\theta_{sn}}\prod_{i=1}^{n}\theta_{s_i}{}^{(z_{s_i}+\alpha_1-1)}(1-\theta_{s_i})^{(m_{s_i}-z_{s_i}+\alpha_2-1)}d\theta_{s_1}\ldots d\theta_{s_n} \\
&\propto (\alpha_1+\alpha_2)^{-5/2}\prod_{i=1}^{n}\frac{\Gamma(z_{s_i}+\alpha_1)\Gamma(m_{s_i}-z_{s_i}+\alpha_2)}{\Gamma(m_{s_i}+\alpha_1+\alpha_2)},
\end{aligned}
$$

and so we have

$$p(\alpha|z_{s_i}) \propto (\alpha_1+\alpha_2)^{-5/2}\left(\frac{\Gamma(\sum_{l=1}^{2}\alpha_l)}{\prod_{l=1}^{2}\Gamma(\alpha_l)}\right)^n \prod_{i=1}^{n}\frac{\Gamma(z_{s_i}+\alpha_1)\Gamma(m_{s_i}-z_{s_i}+\alpha_2)}{\Gamma(m_{s_i}+\alpha_1+\alpha_2)}.$$

Thus, we have the log posterior:

$$\log p(\alpha|z_s) \propto \frac{-5}{2}\log(\alpha_1+\alpha_2)+n\left(\log(\Gamma(\sum_{l=1}^{2}\alpha_l))-\log(\Gamma(\alpha_1))-\log(\Gamma(\alpha_2))\right)$$
$$+\sum_{i=1}^{n}\left[\log(\Gamma(z_{s_i}+\alpha_1))+\log(\Gamma(m_{s_i}-z_{s_i}+\alpha_2))-\log(\Gamma(m_{s_i}+\alpha_1+\alpha_2))\right].$$

We can easily use the Metropolis algorithm to simulate from this posterior for α. We can generate roughly independent draws from the posterior distribution by saving every rth draw (Geyer 2011, Section 1.12.9.). In the examples that follow, we use $r = 1000$, but the length required for roughly independent draws is always unknown but can be estimated from the output of the algorithm if the Markov chain has been run long enough. When computing the Bayes estimator, acceptance rates for the Metropolis algorithm were tuned to have a roughly 20% acceptance (Geyer 2011, Section 1.13 and references cited therein). All simulations were done in the R programming language (R Core Team 2020).

Putting this all together, given a sample, we can now simulate complete copies of the full population for our Bayesian model. First, we get an "independent" draw from $P(\alpha|z_s)$. Then, for an unobserved cluster, $i \in s'$, we

1. generate $\theta_{s'_i}$ from $g(\theta_{s'_i}|\alpha) \sim \text{Beta}(\alpha)$ and
2. generate $y_{s'_i}$ from $f(y_{s'_i}|\theta_{s'_i}) \sim \text{Binomial}(\theta_{s'_i}, M_{s_i'})$.

Similarly, we can simulate the remaining $M_i - m_i$ values for the observed clusters $i \in s$ by

1. Generate θ_{s_i} from $P(\theta_{s_i} \mid z_{s_i}, \alpha) \sim \text{Beta}\left(z_{s_i}+\alpha_1, M_{s_i}-z_{s_i}+\alpha_2\right)$ and
2. Generate $z_{s'_i}$ from $P(z_{s'_i}|\theta_{s_i}) \sim \text{Binomial}(\theta_{s_i}, M_{s_i})$.

2.2 A Stepwise Bayes Approach

The Polya posterior is related to the Polya urn distribution. For a finite population y, no clusters for now, assume that we have a sample y_s of size n. We write the observed y_i values on n pieces of paper which are then placed in an urn. The first step in generating a complete simulated copy of a population is to select a piece of paper at random from the urn. If the paper selected has the value y_i, it is returned to the urn along with another piece of paper which also has the value y_i. So now the urn contains $n+1$ pieces of paper. The next step is to repeat the process, copying the new y_i value onto another blank piece of paper and placing both pieces of paper back into the urn. The process is repeated until the urn contains N pieces of paper, where N is the size of the population y. The set of numbers written on the N pieces of paper represents on simulated copy of the population under the Polya posterior. By simulating many such complete copies of the population, one can make inferences about the finite population y in the usual Bayesian manor.

When estimating the population mean, the sample mean is the posterior expectation of the population mean under the Polya posterior, and its posterior variance is $(n-1)/(n+1)$ times the design-based estimate of variance when the sampling design is simple random sampling without replacement. From the Bayesian point of view, the Polya posterior is appropriate when the sampler's beliefs about the sampled and unsampled units are exchangeable and little else is known about the population. Lo (1988) showed that asymptotic distribution of the Polya posterior is normal. Moreover, the Polya posterior is just the Bayesian bootstrap of Rubin (1981) applied to finite population sampling. The Polya posterior is not a true Bayesian posterior since it does not arise from a single prior distribution. But it does have a stepwise Bayesian justification, a notion introduced in Hsuan (1979). Using this idea, one can prove the admissibility of the sample mean when estimating the population mean. A detailed exposition of this story is given in Ghosh and Meeden (1997).

Meeden (1999) proposed a Polya posterior approach to two-stage cluster sampling given that simple random sampling without replacement was used in both stages. He also assumed that the clusters were all of the same size and that the sample size at the second stage was the same for all selected clusters. To simulate complete copies of the population of clusters given the sample, he proceeded as follows. In the first stage, he treated the cluster labels as single units and assigned sampled clusters to unsampled clusters using the Polya posterior for the primary sampling units. Assume for simplicity the sample clusters $s = \{1, 2, \ldots, n\}$. After this first step, the $N - n$ unobserved clusters now have a label $i \in \{1, 2, \ldots, n\}$ assigned using the Polya posterior. In this way, there are z_{s_i} ones and $m - z_{s_i}$ zeros copied onto an unobserved cluster according to the label derived from the Polya posterior. Meeden suggests using the Polya posterior again within each cluster to generate the remaining $M - m$ values to give one complete simulated copy of the population. As usual, we calculate the desired statistic and repeat this process many times. It is shown that when the number of clusters N is large compared to the number of sampled clusters n, the usual design-based and Polya estimates of the population total are almost the same and have approximately the same variance.

The condition of equal m_i's and M_i's is a very strong one, but we now suggest a simple modification that will work for our setup with different m_i's and M_i's. A problem arises when in the first stage of Polya sampling, a sampled cluster, say i, is assigned to an unsampled cluster, say j, where $m_i > M_j$. In this case, we will select a random sample of size M_j from the observed sample of m_i values. In the second stage of Polya sampling, we will consider this cluster "complete," and no further Polya sampling will be done.

3 Simulation Studies

For two-stage cluster sampling, when simple random sampling is used in both stages, the standard frequentist method is to use the ratio estimator. In our simulations, we wish to compare it with the Bayes estimator and the stepwise Bayes estimator described in the previous section. For our simulations, we constructed four populations with 30 different clusters of various sizes ranging from 13 to 28. Then, for each cluster, we generated its y vector of 0's and 1's. Figure 1 shows the plot of the cluster total, y_i against the cluster size, M_i for the four populations.

From each of these four fixed populations, we took 500 samples of 18 clusters and between 50 and 80% of the secondary sampling units within these sampled

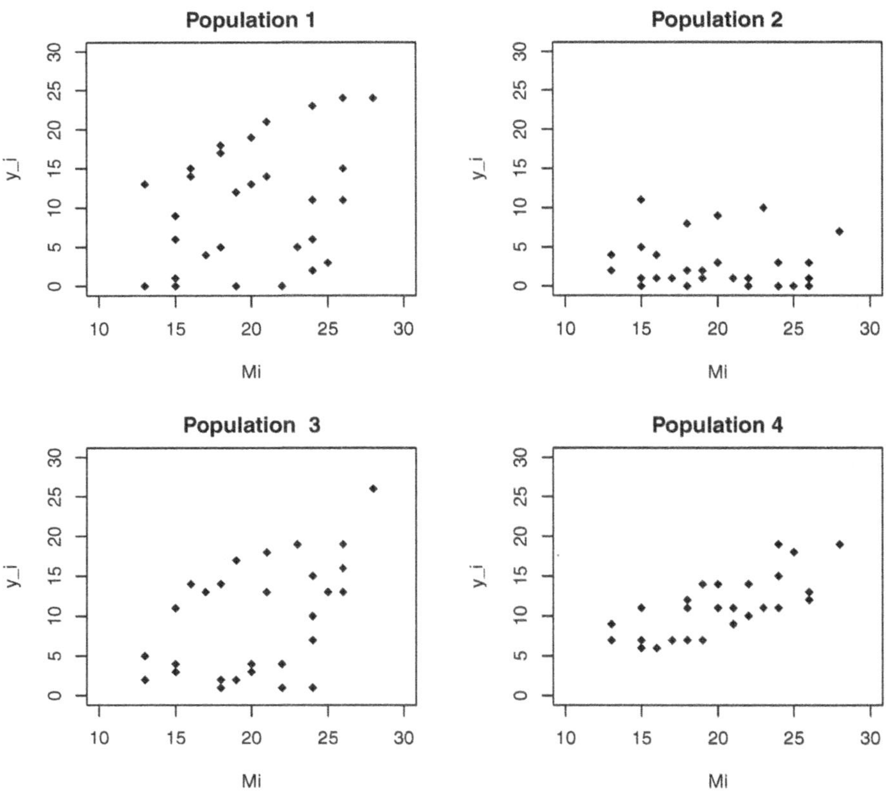

Fig. 1 For the four test populations, a plot of the cluster totals against the cluster sizes

clusters. In these simulations, we are assuming that M_i is known for all clusters, and thus M_0 is known. The summary of the results over these 500 samples is given in the tables. Each table gives with the average estimate for the total and its average absolute error. The average lower bound and the average length of the 95% confidence interval and its frequency of containing the true population total are also given. We considered three different estimators: the ratio, the Polya posterior, and the Bayes. They are denoted by t_{rat}, t_{pp}, and t_b, respectively. The simulation results for the four populations are given in Tables 1, 2, 3, and 4.

In all four cases, the ratio estimator had the biggest average absolute error. Although our estimators did not perform dramatically better, for the first population, our Bayes estimator did approximately 7% better. There is evidence that a Bayesian posterior can be a better alternative for interval estimates than the traditional design-based confidence intervals. For all four populations considered, the design-based estimate never dominated either the Polya posterior or the Gelman prior in terms of better coverage and shorter interval estimates. In all four populations, the Gelman prior had better coverage than the design-based interval, and in two of the populations, they also had shorter intervals. The Polya posterior had a shorter interval than the design-based interval for all four populations, and for two of the populations, it also had better coverage.

Table 1 Results for estimating the true total, 618, for the first population

	$\hat{t}$	$\lvert t - \hat{t}\rvert$	$\hat{t}_{0.025}$	$\hat{t}_{0.975} - \hat{t}_{0.025}$	$t \in [\hat{t}_{0.025}, \hat{t}_{0.975}]$
t_{rat}	615.6	64.15	469	293	0.926
t_{pp}	615.9	62.54	480	278	0.930
t_b	615.8	59.55	479	284	0.948

Table 2 Results for estimating the true total, 334, for the second population

	$\hat{t}$	$\lvert t - \hat{t}\rvert$	$\hat{t}_{0.025}$	$\hat{t}_{0.975} - \hat{t}_{0.025}$	$t \in [\hat{t}_{0.025}, \hat{t}_{0.975}]$
t_{rat}	333.1	47.74	219	228	0.924
t_{pp}	333.0	45.73	241	211	0.928
t_b	343.9	45.08	245	229	0.956

Table 3 Results for estimating the true total, 749, for the third population

	$\hat{t}$	$\lvert t - \hat{t}\rvert$	$\hat{t}_{0.025}$	$\hat{t}_{0.975} - \hat{t}_{0.025}$	$t \in [\hat{t}_{0.025}, \hat{t}_{0.975}]$
t_{rat}	747.1	55.36	616	263	0.942
t_{pp}	748.2	53.10	628	242	0.936
t_b	753.6	52.38	626	252	0.956

Table 4 Results for estimating the true total, 750, for the fourth population

	$\hat{t}$	$\lvert t - \hat{t}\rvert$	$\hat{t}_{0.025}$	$\hat{t}_{0.975} - \hat{t}_{0.025}$	$t \in [\hat{t}_{0.025}, \hat{t}_{0.975}]$
t_{rat}	751.1	27.56	691	120	0.910
t_{pp}	750.2	24.06	689	119	0.938
t_b	750.0	26.93	677	145	0.972

4 Final Remarks

Here, we have focused on the situation where the secondary units can take on only two values. But the methods easily generalize to the case where they can take on only some finite set of values.

Sometimes, one has additional information about the population, for example, the value of an auxiliary variable for either the primary or the secondary units in the population. In other situations, one could be interested in estimating other population parameters, say the population median. Soma (2012) discusses how the methods given here and some other Bayesian approaches can be used in for such problems.

References

Gelman, A., Carlin, J., Stern, S., & Rubin, D. (2004). *Bayesian data analysis*. London: Chapman and Hall.

Geyer, C. (2011). Introduction to Markov chain Monte Carlo. In S. Brooks, A. Gelman, G. Jones, & X.-L. Meng (Eds.), Chapter 1, *Handbook of Markov chain Monte Carlo* (pp. 3–48). Boca Raton, FL: Chapman & Hall/CRC.

Ghosh, M., & Meeden, G. (1997). *Bayesian methods for finite population sampling*. New York, NY: Chapman and Hall.

Hsuan, F. C. (1979). A stepwise Bayesian procedure. *Annals of Statistics, 7*, 860–868.

Lo, A. (1988). A Bayesian bootstrap for a finite population. *Annals of Statistics, 16*, 1684–1695.

Meeden, G. (1999). A noninformative Bayesian approach for two-stage cluster sampling. *Sankhya. Series A, 61*, 133–144.

Nandram, B., & Sedransk, J. (1993). Predictive inference for a finite population proportion two-stage cluster sampling. *Journal of the Royal Statistical Society. Series B (Methodological), 55*(2), 399–408.

R Core Team. (2020). *R: A language and environment for statistical computing*. Vienna: R Foundation for Statistical Computing. http://www.R-project.org/

Rubin, D. (1981). The Bayesian bootstrap. *Annals of Statistics, 9*, 130–134.

Soma, M. (2012). *A Bayesian approach to cluster sampling*. Ph.D. thesis, University of Minnesota.

Bayesian Model Assessment and Selection Using Bregman Divergence

Gyuhyeong Goh and Dipak K. Dey

Abstract One of the fundamental steps in statistical modeling is to select the best-fitting model from a set of candidate models for given data. In this paper, based on Bayesian decision theory, we introduce a new model selection criterion, called Bregman divergence criterion (BDC). The proposed criterion improves many existing Bayesian model selection methods such as Bayes factor, intrinsic Bayes factor, pseudo-Bayes factor, etc. In addition, using a Monte Carlo approach, we develop an efficient estimator that significantly eases the computational burden associated with our approach and prove its consistency. The versatility of our methodology is demonstrated on both simulated and real data; to this end, some illustrative examples are provided for linear regression models and longitudinal data models.

1 Introduction

In a Bayesian framework, various predictive densities have been utilized as essential ingredients for developing Bayesian model selection criteria. For instance, the Bayes factor is a ratio of prior predictive densities for two candidate models and represents an intuitively appealing tool for selecting a better model. Stone (1974) and Geisser (1975) proposed the pseudo-Bayes factor based on posterior predictive densities coupled with the idea of leave-one-out cross-validation. In similar spirit, Berger and Pericchi (1996b) introduced the intrinsic Bayes factor based on posterior predictive densities characterized by the notion of minimal training samples to ensure the existence of posterior predictive densities.

G. Goh
Department of Statistics, Kansas State University, Manhattan, KS, USA
e-mail: ggoh@k-state.edu

D. K. Dey (✉)
Department of Statistics, University of Connecticut, Storrs, CT, USA
e-mail: dipak.dey@uconn.edu

I. Ghosh et al. (eds.), *Advances in Statistics - Theory and Applications*, Emerging Topics in Statistics and Biostatistics, https://doi.org/10.1007/978-3-030-62900-7_15

In this paper, our primary goal is to develop a general tool for Bayesian model selection and assessment. To unify and extend many existing predictive model selection and assessment procedures, we consider a general conditioning scheme for predictive density and introduce a fairly general summary measure for observed predictive densities. Our summary measure is analogous to a scoring rule which assigns a numerical score for the observed data based on their predictive densities. In general, there are many kinds of scoring rules available such as logarithmic score, quadratic score, and ranked probability score (Gneiting and Raftery 2007). From a Bayesian perspective, we adopt the Bregman divergence scoring rule (Grünwald and Dawid 2004). This rule offers a general scoring method in the sense that the Bregman divergence (Bregman 1967) includes, as a special case, many well-known loss functions such as squared error loss, Kullback–Leibler divergence, and Mahalanobis distance.

In a frequentist framework, the predictive density approach for model selection produces a convenient tool because a predictive density can be easily calculated by plugging the maximum likelihood estimate into the predictive density function. However, the calculation of Bayesian predictive density is a challenge due to the fact that, in many cases, the predictive density function cannot be expressed in a closed form. Several attempts have been made to address this problem. Gelfand and Dey (1994) proposed a Monte Carlo estimator for several types of conditional predictive densities. Chen (1994) developed a relatively accurate estimation method for the prior predictive (or marginal) density. As an extension of Gelfand and Dey (1994) and Chen (1994), we introduce a general Monte Carlo estimator to calculate various predictive densities.

Some remarks are due on notation and assumptions used in this paper. We use $f(\mathbf{y}|\boldsymbol{\theta})$, $m(\mathbf{y})$, $p(\mathbf{y}_1|\mathbf{y}_2)$, $\pi(\boldsymbol{\theta})$, and $\pi(\boldsymbol{\theta}|\mathbf{y})$ to denote, respectively, the likelihood function, the marginal density (or prior predictive density), conditional predictive density (or posterior predictive density), the prior, and the posterior, where $\mathbf{y} = (y_1, \ldots, y_n)$ is the observed data set, $\mathbf{y}_1$ and $\mathbf{y}_2$ are sub-vectors of $\mathbf{y}$, and $\boldsymbol{\theta} = (\theta_1, \ldots, \theta_q)$ represents a vector of parameters such that $\boldsymbol{\theta} \in \Theta$ for a suitable parameter space Θ. We remark here that there is no restriction on the nature of the posterior, i.e., the posterior can be a density with respect to the Lebesgue measure or with respect to a counting measure or can also be a mixture of densities. For notational convenience, the distributions, normal, inverse-gamma, inverse-Wishart, and uniform are, respectively, denoted as N, IG, IW, and U.

The outline of the remainder of the paper is as follows. In Sect. 2, we introduce our main construct and result. Section 3 details the calculation of Bayesian predictive density with some examples. Simulation studies are conducted with a linear regression model and a longitudinal data model in Sect. 4. Section 5 offers some concluding remarks.

2 Model Selection Using Bregman Divergence

2.1 Predictive Model Selection and Bayesian Decision-Making

A predictive model selection problem can be considered as a decision-making problem; see Bernardo and Smith (2000) and the references therein. In other words, the best model among candidate models is the one whose prediction performance is most similar to the true model's. To formalize this idea, let M^{true} be the true model and $\mathscr{M} = \{M^1, M^2, \ldots, M^K\}$ be a collection of candidate models, where the number of candidate models, K, is assumed to be known, and further there is no preferred model. Suppose that $\mathbf{y}_{\text{new}}$ is a future observation after $\mathbf{y}_{\text{old}}$ is observed. Let $p(\mathbf{y}_{\text{new}}|\mathbf{y}_{\text{old}}, M^{\text{true}})$ be the true conditional predictive density of $\mathbf{y}_{\text{new}}$ given $\mathbf{y}_{\text{old}}$, that is,

$$p(\mathbf{y}_{\text{new}}|\mathbf{y}_{\text{old}}, M^{\text{true}}) = \int f(\mathbf{y}_{\text{new}}|\boldsymbol{\theta}, \mathbf{y}_{\text{old}}, M^{\text{true}})\pi(\boldsymbol{\theta}|\mathbf{y}_{\text{old}}, M^{\text{true}})d\boldsymbol{\theta}.$$

For model M^k, we denote the conditional predictive density by $p(\mathbf{y}_{\text{new}}|\mathbf{y}_{\text{old}}, M^k)$. Then, predictive model selection can be formulated as finding a model that has the *minimum dissimilarity* between $p(\mathbf{y}_{\text{new}}|\mathbf{y}_{\text{old}}, M^{\text{true}})$ and $p(\mathbf{y}_{\text{new}}|\mathbf{y}_{\text{old}}, M^k)$ as follows:

$$M^* = \arg\min_{M^k \in \mathscr{M}} d\left(p(\mathbf{y}_{\text{new}}|\mathbf{y}_{\text{old}}, M^{\text{true}}), p(\mathbf{y}_{\text{new}}|\mathbf{y}_{\text{old}}, M^k)\right), \tag{1}$$

where $d(\cdot, \cdot)$ is an appropriate functional divergence measure between two density functions satisfying

$$d(f, g) \geq 0, \quad \text{and} \quad d(f, g) = 0 \text{ if and only if } f = g, \ a.e.$$

For example, if we define $d(\cdot, \cdot)$ as the Kullback–Leibler divergence, then we reduce (1) to

$$M^* = \arg\min_{M^k \in \mathscr{M}} \int \log\left\{\frac{p(\mathbf{y}_{\text{new}}|\mathbf{y}_{\text{old}}, M^{\text{true}})}{p(\mathbf{y}_{\text{new}}|\mathbf{y}_{\text{old}}, M^k)}\right\} p(\mathbf{y}_{\text{new}}|\mathbf{y}_{\text{old}}, M^{\text{true}})d\mathbf{y}_{\text{new}}.$$

The proposed method in (1) looks straightforward and reasonable, but two serious problems occur in practice. First, since the true model M^{true} is unknown, then the true predictive density $p(\mathbf{y}_{\text{new}}|\mathbf{y}_{\text{old}}, M^{\text{true}})$ is unknown. Second, the calculation of functional divergence between M^{true} and M^k over $\mathbf{y}_{\text{new}}$ may not have an analytical solution.

To address the first challenge, following Bernardo and Smith (2000), Gelfand and Ghosh (1998), Gutierrez-Pena and Walker (2001), Laud and Ibrahim (1995), and San Martini and Spezzaferri (1984), we employ Bayesian decision theory as follows. Define $\mathscr{S}$ to represent a collection of all possible models. Let M $(\in \mathscr{S})$ be the unknown true model (*the unknown state of nature*) and $\mathscr{M}$ be a collection of candidate models under consideration (*the decision space*). We define the loss function by $L(M, a) = d\left(p(\mathbf{y}_{\text{new}}|\mathbf{y}_{\text{old}}, M), p(\mathbf{y}_{\text{new}}|\mathbf{y}_{\text{old}}, a)\right)$, where $M \in \mathscr{S}$ and $a \in \mathscr{M}$. The posterior expected loss is given as

$$\rho\left(\pi(M|\mathbf{y}_{\text{old}}), a\right) = \int_{M\in\mathscr{S}} L(M, a)\pi(M|\mathbf{y}_{\text{old}})dM, \tag{2}$$

where

$$\pi(M|\mathbf{y}_{\text{old}}) = \frac{m(\mathbf{y}_{\text{old}}|M)\pi(M)}{\int_{M\in\mathscr{S}} m(\mathbf{y}_{\text{old}}|M)\pi(M)dM},$$

and the prior $\pi(M)$ reflects our prior information or belief about the true model. Hence, the Bayes rule is given as

$$\tilde{M} = \arg\min_{a\in\mathscr{M}} \rho\left(\pi(M|\mathbf{y}_{\text{old}}), a\right). \tag{3}$$

Based on the aforementioned Bayesian decision theory, we can estimate the best model M^* in (1) by $\tilde{M}$. We further assume that $M \in \mathscr{M}$, that is, one of the candidate models is the true model, often referred to as the $\mathscr{M}$-closed framework (Bernardo and Smith 2000). Since we consider $\mathscr{M} = \{M^1, M^2, \ldots, M^K\}$ as a pool of candidate models for the true model with no preference, we naturally define

$$\pi(M) = \begin{cases} \frac{1}{K}, & M \in \mathscr{M} \\ 0, & M \notin \mathscr{M} \end{cases}, \quad M \in \mathscr{S}.$$

Under this prior, the posterior expected loss (2) can be explicitly expressed as

$$\rho\left(\pi(M|\mathbf{y}_{\text{old}}), a\right) = \frac{\sum_{l=1}^{K} d\left(p(\mathbf{y}_{\text{new}}|\mathbf{y}_{\text{old}}, M^l), p(\mathbf{y}_{\text{new}}|\mathbf{y}_{\text{old}}, a)\right) m(\mathbf{y}_{\text{old}}|M^l)}{\sum_{k=1}^{K} m(\mathbf{y}_{\text{old}}|M^k)}. \tag{4}$$

For the second issue, we propose to use the cross-validation approach as in Stone (1974), Geisser (1975), Geisser and Eddy (1979), and Dawid (1984). In this paper, we consider a similar strategy used in Gelfand and Dey (1994) in order to provide more flexible grouping and conditioning schemes than the classical cross-validation methods. Suppose that $\mathbf{y} = (y_1, \ldots, y_n)$ is observed. Let $\mathbf{y}_{s_1}, \mathbf{y}_{s_2}, \ldots, \mathbf{y}_{s_m}$ be $m(\leq n)$ subsets of $\mathbf{y}$ such that $\mathbf{y} = (\mathbf{y}_{s_1}, \mathbf{y}_{s_2}, \ldots \mathbf{y}_{s_m})$. Define $\mathbf{y}_{-s_i}$ as a complement of $\mathbf{y}_{s_i}$, that is, $\mathbf{y}_{-s_i} = \mathbf{y} \setminus \mathbf{y}_{s_i}$ for $i = 1, 2, \ldots, m$. Now, we treat $\mathbf{y}_{s_i}$ and $\mathbf{y}_{-s_i}$ as the future data and the observed data, respectively. The determination of sub-sample $\mathbf{y}_{s_i}$ should depend on the nature of data. In practice, the leave-one-out approach (i.e., $y_{s_i} = y_i$) is commonly used for small- or moderate-sized data. For large data, tenfold cross-validation (or 10% of data) is generally preferred to define the subsample because the leave-one-out approach is computationally inefficient in this case. For each observed $\mathbf{y}_{s_i}$, the posterior expected loss (4) reduces to

$$\rho^*\left(\pi(M|\mathbf{y}_{-s_i}), a\right) = \frac{\sum_{l=1}^{K} D\left(p(\mathbf{y}_{s_i}|\mathbf{y}_{-s_i}, M^l), p(\mathbf{y}_{s_i}|\mathbf{y}_{-s_i}, a)\right) m(\mathbf{y}_{-s_i}|M^l)}{\sum_{k=1}^{K} m(\mathbf{y}_{-s_i}|M^k)},$$

where $D(\cdot,\cdot)$ denotes a divergence measure between two vectors (or scalars). Inspired by (3), we define our best model as follows:

$$\hat{M} = \arg\min_{a \in \mathcal{M}} \sum_{i=1}^{m} \rho^*\left(\pi(M|\mathbf{y}_{-s_i}), a\right). \tag{5}$$

2.2 *Bregman Divergence Criterion*

To employ our minimum divergence approach in (5), a valid divergence measure between two vectors should be determined. We consider a general class of divergence measures, called Bregman divergence.

Definition 1 Let $\psi : \Omega \to \mathbb{R}$ be a strictly convex and differentiable function on a nonempty convex set $\Omega \subseteq \mathbb{R}^m$. Then, the Bregman divergence BD_ψ is defined as

$$\mathrm{BD}_\psi(\mathbf{x}, \mathbf{y}) = \psi(\mathbf{x}) - \psi(\mathbf{y}) - \langle \mathbf{x} - \mathbf{y}, \nabla\psi(\mathbf{y})\rangle,$$

where $\nabla\psi$ represents the gradient vector of ψ.

It is worthwhile to note that Bregman divergences reduce to various divergence measures according to the choice of the convex function ψ; few illuminating examples are enumerated below.

Example 1 Let $\mathbf{x} = (x_1, \ldots, x_m)^{\mathrm{T}}$ and $\mathbf{y} = (y_1, \ldots, y_m)^{\mathrm{T}}$. Suppose $\psi(\mathbf{x}) = \sum_{i=1}^{m}\{x_i \log x_i\}$, then the Bregman divergence is given as

$$\begin{aligned}\mathrm{BD}_\psi(\mathbf{x}, \mathbf{y}) &= \sum_{i=1}^{m}\{x_i \log x_i\} - \sum_{i=1}^{m}\{y_i \log y_i\} - \sum_{i=1}^{m}\{(x_i - y_i)(\log y_i + 1)\} \\ &= \sum_{i=1}^{m}\left\{x_i \log \frac{x_i}{y_i} - x_i + y_i\right\},\end{aligned}$$

which is the generalized Kullback–Leibler divergence between $\mathbf{x}$ and $\mathbf{y}$.

Example 2 Suppose $\psi(\mathbf{x}) = \sum_{i=1}^{m}\{-\log x_i\}$, then the Bregman divergence is written as

$$\mathrm{BD}_\psi(\mathbf{x},\mathbf{y}) = \sum_{i=1}^{m}\{-\log x_i\} - \sum_{i=1}^{m}\{-\log y_i\} - \sum_{i=1}^{m}\{(x_i - y_i)(-1/y_i)\}$$
$$= \sum_{i=1}^{m}\left\{\frac{x_i}{y_i} - \log\frac{x_i}{y_i} - 1\right\},$$

which is called Itakura–Saito distance (Itakura and Saito 1970) between $\mathbf{x}$ and $\mathbf{y}$.

Example 3 Suppose $\psi(\mathbf{x}) = \mathbf{x}^{\mathrm{T}}\mathbf{A}\mathbf{x}$, where $\mathbf{A}$ is a positive definite matrix, then the Bregman divergence is given as

$$BD_\psi(\mathbf{x},\mathbf{y}) = \mathbf{x}^{\mathrm{T}}\mathbf{A}\mathbf{x} - \mathbf{y}^{\mathrm{T}}\mathbf{A}\mathbf{y} - \langle \mathbf{x}-\mathbf{y}, 2\mathbf{A}\mathbf{y}\rangle$$
$$= (\mathbf{x}-\mathbf{y})^{\mathrm{T}}\mathbf{A}(\mathbf{x}-\mathbf{y}).$$

If $\mathbf{A}$ is assumed to be an inverse covariance matrix, then the Bregman divergence becomes the Mahalanobis distance between $\mathbf{x}$ and $\mathbf{y}$. If we assume that $\mathbf{A}$ is the identity matrix, then the Bregman divergence reduces to the squared Euclidean distance between $\mathbf{x}$ and $\mathbf{y}$ such that $BD_\psi(\mathbf{x},\mathbf{y}) = \|\mathbf{x}-\mathbf{y}\|^2$, where $\|\mathbf{x}\| = \sqrt{\mathbf{x}^{\mathrm{T}}\mathbf{x}}$.

Another important feature of Bregman divergence is that under the Bregman divergence loss, the proposed model selection criterion in (5) can be viewed as Bregman divergence.

Theorem 1 *Let* $\bar{p}_i = \sum_{l=1}^{K} \frac{m(\mathbf{y}_{-s_i}|M^l)}{\sum_{k=1}^{K} m(\mathbf{y}_{-s_i}|M^k)} p(\mathbf{y}_{s_i}|\mathbf{y}_{-s_i}, M^l)$ *and* $p_i^{(a)} = p(\mathbf{y}_{s_i}|\mathbf{y}_{-s_i}, a)$ *for* $i = 1, 2, \ldots, m$ *and* $m \le n$. *If* $D(\cdot,\cdot) = BD_\psi(\cdot,\cdot)$, *we have*

$$\arg\min_{a\in\mathcal{M}} \sum_{i=1}^{m} \rho^*\left(\pi(M|\mathbf{y}_{-s_i}), a\right) = \arg\min_{a\in\mathcal{M}} BD_\psi\left(\bar{\mathbf{p}}, \mathbf{p}^{(a)}\right),$$

where $\bar{\mathbf{p}} = (\bar{p}_1, \bar{p}_2, \ldots, \bar{p}_m)$ *and* $\mathbf{p}^{(a)} = (p_1^{(a)}, p_2^{(a)}, \ldots, p_m^{(a)})$. *Note that this holds for any strictly convex and differentiable function* ψ.

From Theorem 1, we now define a new Bayesian model selection criterion, called Bregman divergence criterion (BDC).

Definition 2 (Bregman Divergence Criterion)

$$\mathrm{BDC}_\psi(k) = \mathrm{BD}_\psi\left(\bar{\mathbf{p}}, \mathbf{p}^{(M^k)}\right), \tag{6}$$

where $\mathbf{p}^{(M^k)} = (p_1^{(M^k)}, p_2^{(M^k)}, \ldots, p_m^{(M^k)})$ with $p_i^{(M^k)} = m(\mathbf{y}|M^k)/m(\mathbf{y}_{-s_i}|M^k)$ and $\bar{\mathbf{p}} = (\bar{p}_1, \bar{p}_2, \ldots, \bar{p}_m)$ with $\bar{p}_i = \{\sum_{l=1}^{K} m(\mathbf{y}|M^l)\}/\{\sum_{t=1}^{K} m(\mathbf{y}_{-s_i}|M^t)\}$.

The BDC defined in (6) measures the dissimilarity in the Bregman divergence sense between the predictive density vector of model M^k and the average vector of predictive densities under each of the models considered. Hence, the model with the smallest BDC is preferred. In Sect. 4.1, using simulation studies, we show that our model selection with BDC is more powerful than the existing Bayesian model selection methods.

3 Calculation of BDC

For calculation of BDC, it suffices to compute $m(\mathbf{y}_s|M^k)$ for an arbitrary subset $\mathbf{y}_s$ and $k \in \{1, 2, \ldots, K\}$. Therefore, in this section, we mainly discuss the calculation of the marginal density. Our approach relies on a Monte Carlo method with a single set of posterior samples, which is computationally efficient. For simplicity of notation, we omit to indicate the given model M^k. Hence, $m(\mathbf{y}_s|M^k)$ will be denoted by $m(\mathbf{y}_s)$ throughout this section.

In some cases, one may be fortunate enough to obtain $m(\mathbf{y}_s)$ in a closed form. The following example illustrates the abovementioned scenario in the case of the linear regression model with independent errors.

Example 4 (Linear Regression Model) Consider the linear model given in Berger and Pericchi (1996a). Suppose that model M is given as

$$M : \mathbf{y} = \mathbf{X}\boldsymbol{\beta} + \boldsymbol{\epsilon}, \quad \boldsymbol{\epsilon} \sim \mathrm{N}(\mathbf{0}, \sigma^2\mathbf{I}_n),$$

where $\boldsymbol{\beta} = (\beta_1, \ldots, \beta_q)^{\mathrm{T}}$ and σ^2 are unknown, $\mathbf{y} = (y_1, \ldots, y_n)^{\mathrm{T}}$ is the data vector, $\mathbf{X}$ is the $(n \times q)$ design matrix with rank $q(< n)$, and $\mathbf{x}_i$ is the ith row of $\mathbf{X}$. Consider the objective prior $\pi(\boldsymbol{\beta}, \sigma^2) = 1/\sigma^2$. Let n_s be the number of observations in $\mathbf{y}_s(\subseteq \mathbf{y})$. With a straightforward calculation, the marginal density is explicitly expressed as follows. If $n_s \geq q$, then

$$m(\mathbf{y}_s) = \frac{(\pi)^{-\frac{n_s-q}{2}}\Gamma\left(\frac{n_s-q}{2}\right)}{\left|\mathbf{X}_s^{\mathrm{T}}\mathbf{X}_s\right|^{1/2}\left[(\mathbf{y}_s - \hat{\mathbf{y}}_s)^{\mathrm{T}}(\mathbf{y}_s - \hat{\mathbf{y}}_s)\right]^{\frac{n_s-q}{2}}},$$

where $\hat{\mathbf{y}}_s = \mathbf{X}_s(\mathbf{X}_s^{\mathrm{T}}\mathbf{X}_s)^{-1}\mathbf{X}_s^{\mathrm{T}}\mathbf{y}_s$. If $n_s < q$, then $m(\mathbf{y}_s)$ is undefined (improper).

Example 4 represents a special case where the marginal density can be expressed in a closed form. However, in general, the calculation of marginal density is not an easy task within a Bayesian framework; pertinently, even if it is amenable to calculation via numerical methods, the huge computational burden associated with the task creates a significant obstacle; this is so since the marginal density needs to be calculated for each sub-sample $\mathbf{y}_{s_i}$, $i = 1, \ldots, m$. In view of that, we propose a Monte Carlo estimator of the marginal density based on a single set of Markov Chain Monte Carlo (MCMC) samples from the stationary full posterior distribution. In this approach, all the required marginal densities can be simultaneously computed by the single set of MCMC samples. In addition, our method considerably mitigates the burden of Bayesian computation since the posterior sample should be already generated for the inference procedure in the first place. We formalize the preceding discussion with the following theorem.

Theorem 2 *Suppose that $g(\cdot)$ is a probability density function satisfying supp$(g) \subset$ supp(π). Let $1(A)$ be the indicator function for a set A and $f(\mathbf{y}|\boldsymbol{\theta})$ be the likelihood function. If $\{\boldsymbol{\theta}^j\}_{j=1}^N$ is a set of MCMC samples from the full posterior distribution $\pi(\boldsymbol{\theta}|\mathbf{y})$ and $p(\mathbf{y}_s|\mathbf{y}_{-s}) < \infty$, where $\mathbf{y}_{-s} = \mathbf{y} \setminus \mathbf{y}_s$, then*

$$\lim_{N\to\infty}\left[\frac{1}{N}\sum_{j=1}^{N}\left\{\frac{1}{f(\mathbf{y}_s|\mathbf{y}_{-s},\boldsymbol{\theta}^j)}\left(\frac{g(\boldsymbol{\theta}^j)}{\pi(\boldsymbol{\theta}^j)}\right)^{1(\{\mathbf{y}_{-s}\}=\emptyset)}\right\}\right]^{-1} \overset{a.s.}{=} p(\mathbf{y}_s|\mathbf{y}_{-s}). \quad (7)$$

It is easy to check that the marginal density can be expressed as

$$m(\mathbf{y}_s) = m(\mathbf{y})/p(\mathbf{y}_{-s}|\mathbf{y}_s). \quad (8)$$

From Theorem 2 and (8), a Monte Carlo estimator of marginal density is given by

$$\hat{m}(\mathbf{y}_s) = \left\{\sum_{j=1}^{N}\frac{f(\mathbf{y}_s|\boldsymbol{\theta}^j)}{f(\mathbf{y}|\boldsymbol{\theta}^j)}\right\}\left\{\sum_{j=1}^{N}\frac{g(\boldsymbol{\theta}^j)}{f(\mathbf{y}|\boldsymbol{\theta}^j)\pi(\boldsymbol{\theta}^j)}\right\}^{-1}, \quad (9)$$

for $i = 1, \ldots, m$, where $g(\cdot)$ is a probability density function, $\pi(\cdot)$ is a prior density function, and $\{\boldsymbol{\theta}^j\}_{j=1}^N$ is a set of MCMC samples from the full posterior density $\pi(\boldsymbol{\theta}|\mathbf{y})$. Note that using Theorem 2 and (8), the following argument can be easily shown:

$$\hat{m}(\mathbf{y}_s) \overset{\text{a.s.}}{=} m(\mathbf{y}_s).$$

To minimize the variance of our Monte Carlo estimator, the weight function $g(\cdot)$ should be chosen to be close to the target function $f(\mathbf{y}|\cdot)\pi(\cdot)$. Chen (1994) proposed to use a density function such that its mean and variance match the posterior mean and variance. Later, Goh and Dey (2014) showed that if $g(\cdot)$ is a normal density function, then the mean and variance matching density minimizes the Kullback–Leibler divergence between $g(\cdot)$ and $f(\mathbf{y}|\cdot)\pi(\cdot)$. Let $\phi(\cdot;\boldsymbol{\mu},\Sigma)$ be a density function of $\mathrm{N}(\boldsymbol{\mu},\Sigma)$. Here, we define $g(\cdot) = \phi(\cdot;\boldsymbol{\mu}_\theta,\Sigma_\theta)$ with

$$\boldsymbol{\mu}_\theta = \frac{1}{N}\sum_{j=1}^{N}\boldsymbol{\theta}^j \quad \text{and} \quad \Sigma_\theta = \frac{1}{N-1}\sum_{j=1}^{N}(\boldsymbol{\theta}^j - \boldsymbol{\mu}_\theta)(\boldsymbol{\theta}^j - \boldsymbol{\mu}_\theta)^{\mathrm{T}},$$

where $\{\boldsymbol{\theta}^j\}_{j=1}^N$ is a set of MCMC samples from the full posterior density $\pi(\boldsymbol{\theta}|\mathbf{y})$. In addition, a suitable burn-in length and a large number of MCMC draws are necessary to improve the precision of the Monte Carlo estimate. Liu et al. (2016) and the references therein provide useful guidance on the number of MCMC draws and the burn-in length.

The following example describes the utility of our Monte Carlo estimator in generalized linear models.

Example 5 (Generalized Linear Model) Suppose that $\mathbf{y} = (y_1, \ldots, y_n)^{\mathrm{T}}$ is a vector of independent observations such that the density of the observation y_j belongs to the natural exponential family, that is,

$$f(y_j|\theta_j) = \exp\left\{\theta_j y_j - a(\theta_j) + b(y_j)\right\}, \tag{10}$$

where $a(\cdot)$ and $b(\cdot)$ are known functions. Let θ_j be related to the regression coefficients such that

$$\theta_j = h(\mathbf{x}_j^{\mathrm{T}}\boldsymbol{\beta}). \tag{11}$$

Then, the model determined by (10) and (11) is called the generalized linear model (GLM). Let $\pi(\boldsymbol{\beta})$ be a prior density. From (10) and (11), the posterior density of $\boldsymbol{\beta}$ is given by

$$\pi(\boldsymbol{\beta}|\mathbf{y}) \propto \exp\left[\sum_{j=1}^{n}\left\{y_j h(\mathbf{x}_j^{\mathrm{T}}\boldsymbol{\beta}) - a\left(h(\mathbf{x}_j^{\mathrm{T}}\boldsymbol{\beta})\right)\right\}\right]\pi(\boldsymbol{\beta}). \tag{12}$$

Let $\left\{\boldsymbol{\beta}^l\right\}_{l=1}^{N}$ be a set of MCMC samples from the full posterior density in (12). The Monte Carlo estimator in (9) is written as

$$\begin{aligned}\hat{m}(\mathbf{y}_s) = &\left[\sum_{l=1}^{N}\exp\left\{\sum_{j=1}^{n} d_j\left\{a\left(h(\mathbf{x}_j^{\mathrm{T}}\boldsymbol{\beta}^l)\right) - y_j h(\mathbf{x}_j^{\mathrm{T}}\boldsymbol{\beta}^l) - b(y_j)\right\}\right\}\right]\\ &\times\left[\sum_{l=1}^{N}\exp\left\{\sum_{j=1}^{n}\left\{a\left(h(\mathbf{x}_j^{\mathrm{T}}\boldsymbol{\beta}^l)\right) - y_j h(\mathbf{x}_j^{\mathrm{T}}\boldsymbol{\beta}^l) - b(y_j)\right\}\right\}\right.\\ &\left.\times\frac{\phi(\boldsymbol{\beta}^l;\boldsymbol{\mu}_\beta,\Sigma_\beta)}{\pi(\boldsymbol{\beta}^l)}\right]^{-1},\end{aligned}$$

where $d_j = \mathbf{1}\left(y_j \notin \mathbf{y}_s\right)$, $\boldsymbol{\mu}_\beta = \frac{1}{N}\sum_{l=1}^{N}\boldsymbol{\beta}^l$, and $\Sigma_\beta = \frac{1}{N-1}\sum_{l=1}^{N}(\boldsymbol{\beta}^l - \boldsymbol{\mu}_\beta)(\boldsymbol{\beta}^l - \boldsymbol{\mu}_\beta)^{\mathrm{T}}$.

Remark 1 In this paper, our computation of the BDC relies on an importance sampling approach, but this may fail if the proposal distribution does not sufficiently well approximate the target. To improve the accuracy, using *Truncated Importance*

Sampling (Ionides 2008), (9) can be replaced by

$$\hat{m}(\mathbf{y}_s) = \left[\sum_{j=1}^{N} \min\{W_1(\boldsymbol{\theta}^j), \sqrt{N}\bar{W}_1\}\right]\left[\sum_{j=1}^{N} \min\{W_2(\boldsymbol{\theta}^j), \sqrt{N}\bar{W}_2\}\right]^{-1},$$

where $W_1(\boldsymbol{\theta}^j) = \frac{f(\mathbf{y}_s|\boldsymbol{\theta}^j)}{f(\mathbf{y}|\boldsymbol{\theta}^j)}$, $W_2(\boldsymbol{\theta}^j) = \frac{g(\boldsymbol{\theta}^j)}{f(\mathbf{y}|\boldsymbol{\theta}^j)\pi(\boldsymbol{\theta}^j)}$, and $\bar{W}_i = \sum_{j=1}^{N} W_i(\boldsymbol{\theta}^j)/N$ for $i = 1, 2$.

4 Illustrative Examples

To show the applicability and reliability of BDC for variable selection and determination of covariance matrix, we discuss some illustrative examples via simulation studies and real data analysis.

4.1 Linear Regression Models

In this section, we conduct some simulation studies to compare the variable selection performance with existing Bayesian model selection methods under a linear regression model setup, which are the most popular statistical models in practical application. To define the predictive density, we use the leave-one-out cross-validation approach, also known as the Conditional Predictive Ordinate (CPO) approach, i.e., $\mathbf{y}_{s_i} = y_i$. To define BDC, we need to specify a Bregman divergence. As in Goh and Dey (2014), we consider a subclass of Bregman divergence, called Beta-divergence, rather than choosing one specific Bregman divergence.

$$\mathrm{BDC}_{\psi_\gamma}(k) = \begin{cases} \sum_{i=1}^{m} \left\{\bar{p}_i/p_i^{(M^k)} - \log\left(\bar{p}_i/p_i^{(M^k)}\right) - 1\right\}, & \gamma = 0 \\ \sum_{i=1}^{m} \left\{\bar{p}_i \log\left(\bar{p}_i/p_i^{(M^k)}\right) - \bar{p}_i + p_i^{(M^k)}\right\}, & \gamma = 1 \\ \sum_{i=1}^{m} \frac{(\bar{p}_i)^\gamma + (\gamma-1)\left(p_i^{(M^k)}\right)^\gamma - \gamma\bar{p}_i\left(p_i^{(M^k)}\right)^{\gamma-1}}{\gamma(\gamma-1)}, & \gamma \in \mathbb{R}\setminus\{0,1\} \end{cases},$$

where

$$\psi_\gamma(\mathbf{x}) = \begin{cases} \sum_{i=1}^{m} \{-\log x_i + x_i - 1\}, & \gamma = 0 \\ \sum_{i=1}^{m} \{x_i \log x_i - x_i + 1\}, & \gamma = 1 \\ \frac{1}{\gamma(\gamma-1)} \sum_{i=1}^{m} \left\{x_i^\gamma - \gamma x_i + (\gamma - 1)\right\}, & \gamma \in \mathbb{R}\setminus\{0,1\} \end{cases}.$$

Note that ψ_γ is continuous with respect to γ (Hennequin et al. 2011).

Consider three models M^1, M^2, and M^3 such that

$$M^k : \mathbf{y} = \mathbf{X}\boldsymbol{\beta}_k + \boldsymbol{\epsilon}, \quad k = 1, 2, 3,$$

where $\boldsymbol{\beta}_1 = (\beta_0, \beta_1, \beta_2, \beta_3)^{\mathrm{T}}$, $\boldsymbol{\beta}_2 = (\beta_0, \beta_1, \beta_2, 0)^{\mathrm{T}}$, $\boldsymbol{\beta}_3 = (\beta_0, \beta_1, 0, 0)^{\mathrm{T}}$, $\boldsymbol{\epsilon} \sim \mathrm{N}(\mathbf{0}, \sigma_k^2 \mathbf{I}_n)$ (σ_k^2 is unknown), $\mathbf{y} = (y_1, \ldots, y_n)^{\mathrm{T}}$, and $\mathbf{X} = [\mathbf{1}_n, X_1, X_2, X_3]$ is the $(n \times 4)$ design matrix with full column rank. Define $\mathbf{X}_1 = [\mathbf{1}_n, X_1, X_2, X_3]$, $\mathbf{X}_2 = [\mathbf{1}_n, X_1, X_2]$, and $\mathbf{X}_3 = [\mathbf{1}_n, X_1]$. Consider the objective prior $\pi_k(\boldsymbol{\beta}_k, \sigma_k) = 1/\sigma_k^2$ for $k = 1, 2, 3$, then for given k, the posterior distribution is

$$\pi(\boldsymbol{\beta}_k, \sigma_k^2 | \mathbf{y}) \propto (\sigma_k^2)^{-(\frac{n}{2}+1)} \exp\left\{ -\frac{1}{2\sigma_k^2} \left(\mathbf{y} - \mathbf{X}_k \boldsymbol{\beta}_k\right)^{\mathrm{T}} \left(\mathbf{y} - \mathbf{X}_k \boldsymbol{\beta}_k\right) \right\}. \tag{13}$$

From (13), we can easily determine that

$$\sigma_k^2 | \mathbf{y} \sim \mathrm{IG}\left(\frac{n - q_k}{2}, \frac{(\mathbf{y} - \hat{\mathbf{y}}_k)^{\mathrm{T}} (\mathbf{y} - \hat{\mathbf{y}}_k)}{2} \right), \tag{14}$$

$$\boldsymbol{\beta}_k | \sigma_k^2, \mathbf{y} \sim \mathrm{N}\left(\hat{\boldsymbol{\beta}}_k, \sigma_k^2 (\mathbf{X}_k^{\mathrm{T}} \mathbf{X}_k)^{-1} \right), \tag{15}$$

where $\hat{\mathbf{y}}_k = \mathbf{X}_k (\mathbf{X}_k^{\mathrm{T}} \mathbf{X}_k)^{-1} \mathbf{X}_k^{\mathrm{T}} \mathbf{y}$, $\hat{\boldsymbol{\beta}}_k = (\mathbf{X}_k^{\mathrm{T}} \mathbf{X}_k)^{-1} \mathbf{X}_k^{\mathrm{T}} \mathbf{y}$, and q_k is the dimension of $\boldsymbol{\beta}_k$ for $k = 1, 2, 3$. Therefore, the full posterior sample, $\left\{(\boldsymbol{\beta}_k^l, \sigma_k^{2l})\right\}_{l=1}^N$, can be directly generated from (14) and (15).

We simulate 2000 data sets under the following setting: for given $n = 100$, we set $\boldsymbol{\beta} = (2, -2, 2.5, 0)^{\mathrm{T}}$, $\mathbf{X} = [\mathbf{1}_n, X_1, X_2, X_3]$ with $x_{ij} \overset{iid}{\sim} \mathrm{N}(0, 1)$, where x_{ij} indicates ith element of a vector X_j, and $\sigma^2 = 1$. In this setting, the true model is M^2. The models M^1 and M^3 are over-fitting and under-fitting, respectively. The size of full posterior samples is $N = 3000$ in each simulation. Note that since our sampling procedure generates an independently and identically distributed (i.i.d.) sample from the posterior distribution, the burn-in period is not needed.

Table 1 summarizes the variable selection performance of $\mathrm{BDC}_{\psi_\gamma}$ for $\gamma = 0, 0.2, \ldots, 2.0$. For comparison purposes, Deviance Information Criterion (DIC) and pseudo-Bayes factor (PSBF) are also computed. Note that PSBF evaluates proposed models based on CPOs, which are also used in BDC, but PSBF summarizes the obtained CPOs simply by the log sum, or equivalently, the geometric mean. Table 1 shows that the percentage of true model ($= M^2$) selected by BDCs is about 90% across the 2000 Monte Carlo replicates, while about 85% of the true model has been selected by PSBF and DIC. This result demonstrates that BDC is more powerful than DIC and PSBF. In addition, the percentage of selecting the true model is constantly about 90% for any value of γ. This shows that BDC is robust to the choice of convex function.

To check the accuracy of our Monte Carlo estimator in (9), we fit a simple linear regression model for the true CPOs as a linear function of estimated CPOs in which

Table 1 Summary of model selection rates (%)

	Model		
Criterion	M^1	M^2	M^3
$\text{BDC}_{\psi_{0.0}}$	9.10	90.90	0.00
$\text{BDC}_{\psi_{0.2}}$	9.15	90.85	0.00
$\text{BDC}_{\psi_{0.4}}$	9.15	90.85	0.00
$\text{BDC}_{\psi_{0.6}}$	9.25	90.75	0.00
$\text{BDC}_{\psi_{0.8}}$	9.30	90.70	0.00
$\text{BDC}_{\psi_{1.0}}$	9.30	90.70	0.00
$\text{BDC}_{\psi_{1.2}}$	9.35	90.65	0.00
$\text{BDC}_{\psi_{1.4}}$	9.20	90.80	0.00
$\text{BDC}_{\psi_{1.6}}$	9.20	90.80	0.00
$\text{BDC}_{\psi_{1.8}}$	9.30	90.70	0.00
$\text{BDC}_{\psi_{2.0}}$	9.35	90.65	0.00
PSBF	15.00	85.00	0.00
DIC	15.35	84.65	0.00

Table 2 True CPOs versus estimated CPOs

Comparison	Coef. est.	s.e.	MSE	R^2
$p(y_i \mid \mathbf{y}_{-i}, M^1)$ vs $\hat{p}(y_i \mid \mathbf{y}_{-i}, M^1)$	1	1.304×10^{-6}	3.009828×10^{-8}	1
$p(y_i \mid \mathbf{y}_{-i}, M^2)$ vs $\hat{p}(y_i \mid \mathbf{y}_{-i}, M^2)$	1	1.046×10^{-6}	1.956894×10^{-8}	1
$p(y_i \mid \mathbf{y}_{-i}, M^3)$ vs $\hat{p}(y_i \mid \mathbf{y}_{-i}, M^3)$	1	9.171×10^{-7}	2.099638×10^{-9}	1
$p(y_i \mid \mathbf{y}_{-i}, \hat{M}^{\text{true}})$ vs $\hat{p}(y_i \mid \mathbf{y}_{-i}, \hat{M}^{\text{true}})$	1	1.026×10^{-6}	1.877235×10^{-8}	1

we assume that the regression line passes through the origin, that is, the intercept is assumed to be zero. The results are shown in Table 2. All the estimated coefficients (i.e., slopes) are one with extremely small standard errors. Furthermore, R^2 is one, and mean squared error (MSE) is extremely small for all the models. Therefore, we conclude that the proposed Monte Carlo estimator is very accurate in this simulation study.

4.2 Bayesian Longitudinal Data Models

Many biological experiments are conducted under a longitudinal study setup, where the measurements on subjects are repeatedly measured over time. Due to the experimental scheme, a correlation between measurements on the given subject naturally occurs, so the determination of correlation structure requires a special care in the statistical modeling for longitudinal data models. In this section, we assume that every individual has the same number of observations, but unequal size of observations can occur due to missing data in practice. Suppose that y_{ij} denotes the jth measurement on the ith subject and $\mathbf{X}_i$ is an $(T \times q)$ design matrix of covariates for ith subject in the longitudinal study for $i = 1, 2, \ldots, n$ and $j = 1, 2, \ldots, T$.

Then, the following linear model can be used to fit the longitudinal data:

$$\mathbf{y}_i = \mathbf{X}_i \boldsymbol{\beta} + \boldsymbol{\epsilon}_i, \tag{16}$$

where $\mathbf{y}_i = (y_{i1}, y_{i2}, \ldots, y_{iT})^{\mathrm{T}}$, $\boldsymbol{\beta} = (\beta_0, \beta_1, \ldots, \beta_{q-1})^{\mathrm{T}}$ is a q-dimensional parameter vector, and $\boldsymbol{\epsilon}_i$ is the random error vector with $E(\boldsymbol{\epsilon}_i) = 0$ and $Cov(\boldsymbol{\epsilon}_i, \boldsymbol{\epsilon}_j) = \mathbf{V}_i$ if $i = j$ and $Cov(\boldsymbol{\epsilon}_i, \boldsymbol{\epsilon}_j) = 0$ if $i \neq j$ for $i, j = 1, 2, \ldots, n$. In general, the normality is assumed for the error vector $\boldsymbol{\epsilon}_i$ with the homogeneity, i.e., $\mathbf{V}_i = \mathbf{V}$ for all i, and then we can write (16) as

$$\mathbf{y} \sim \mathrm{N}(\mathbf{Z}\boldsymbol{\beta}, \mathbf{I}_n \otimes \mathbf{V}), \tag{17}$$

where $\mathbf{y} = (\mathbf{y}_1^{\mathrm{T}}, \mathbf{y}_2^{\mathrm{T}}, \ldots, \mathbf{y}_n^{\mathrm{T}})^{\mathrm{T}}$, $\mathbf{Z} = \left[\mathbf{X}_1^{\mathrm{T}}, \mathbf{X}_2^{\mathrm{T}}, \ldots, \mathbf{X}_n^{\mathrm{T}}\right]^{\mathrm{T}}$, $\mathbf{I}_n$ is the $(n \times n)$ identity matrix, and $\mathbf{I}_n \otimes \mathbf{V}$ denotes the Kronecker product of $\mathbf{I}_n$ and $\mathbf{V}$. In model (17), the correlation between measurements is determined by the covariance matrix $\mathbf{V}$. In this section, we exemplify the determination of covariance matrix using BDC with rat population growth data (Gelfand et al. 1990). The data consist of the weights of 30 young rats ($n = 30$) that were measured weekly for 5 weeks ($T = 5$). Define that y_{ij} is the weight of the ith rat at time point j and the jth row of $\mathbf{X}_i$ is $\mathbf{x}_{ij}^{\mathrm{T}} = (1, x_{ij})$, where x_{ij} is the age in days at the point j for $i = 1, 2, \ldots, 30$ and $j = 1, 2, \ldots, 5$. In many cases, a uniform correlation between measurements (called compound symmetry) on the individual subject is assumed on the covariance matrix $\mathbf{V}$ such that

$$\mathbf{V} = \sigma^2 \mathbf{V}^1(\rho) = \sigma^2 \begin{bmatrix} 1 & \rho & \rho & \rho & \rho \\ \rho & 1 & \rho & \rho & \rho \\ \rho & \rho & 1 & \rho & \rho \\ \rho & \rho & \rho & 1 & \rho \\ \rho & \rho & \rho & \rho & 1 \end{bmatrix},$$

where $0 < \rho < 1$. If the correlation between any two measurements on the same subject dramatically decreases toward zero as the time distance between the measurements increases, then the exponential correlation function can be considered as follows:

$$\rho(l, k) = \exp\left(-b|t_l - t_k|\right), \tag{18}$$

where b is an unknown constant, and t_l and t_k indicate the time points of lth and kth measurements, respectively. Since the weights were measured once every week, i.e., $|t_l - t_k| \propto |l - t|$, then (18) can be rewritten as

$$\rho(l, k) = \rho^{|l-k|}, \tag{19}$$

where $\rho = \exp(-b)$, and a common constant in $|t_l - t_k|$ is absorbed into the unknown constant b for $l, k = 1, 2, \ldots, 5$. According to (19), the covariance matrix $\mathbf{V}$ is given as

$$\mathbf{V} = \sigma^2 \mathbf{V}^2(\rho) = \sigma^2 \begin{bmatrix} 1 & \rho & \rho^2 & \rho^3 & \rho^4 \\ \rho & 1 & \rho & \rho^2 & \rho^3 \\ \rho^2 & \rho & 1 & \rho & \rho^2 \\ \rho^3 & \rho^2 & \rho & 1 & \rho \\ \rho^4 & \rho^3 & \rho^2 & \rho & 1 \end{bmatrix},$$

where $0 < \rho < 1$. Now, we compare the following four models: (1) model M^1 (uniform correlation) with $\mathbf{V} = \sigma^2 \mathbf{V}^1(\rho)$, (2) model M^2 (exponential correlation) with $\mathbf{V} = \sigma^2 \mathbf{V}^2(\rho)$, (3) model M^3 (no correlation) with $\mathbf{V} = \sigma^2 \mathbf{I}_5$, and (4) model M^4 (unspecified dependence structure) with $\mathbf{V} = \boldsymbol{\Sigma}$. Let us consider the following priors:

$$\pi(\boldsymbol{\beta}, \sigma^2, \rho) \propto \sigma^{-2} \qquad \text{for model } M^1, M^2, M^3, \tag{20}$$

$$(\boldsymbol{\beta}, \boldsymbol{\Sigma}) \sim \mathrm{IW}(v_0, \boldsymbol{\Sigma}_0) \qquad \text{for model } M^4, \tag{21}$$

where $v_0 = 5$ and $\boldsymbol{\Sigma}_0 = 0.001\mathbf{I}_5$. After some calculations with (17), (20), and (21), we obtain the following full conditionals for each model:
For models M^1 and M^2,

$$\boldsymbol{\beta}|\sigma^2, \rho, \mathbf{y}, M^k \sim \mathrm{N}\left(\tilde{\boldsymbol{\beta}}^k, \sigma^2 \left[\mathbf{Z}^{\mathrm{T}} \tilde{\mathbf{V}}^k(\rho)^{-1} \mathbf{Z}\right]^{-1}\right),$$

$$\sigma^2|\rho, \boldsymbol{\beta}, \mathbf{y}, M^k \sim \mathrm{IG}\left(\frac{nT}{2}, \frac{(\mathbf{y} - \mathbf{Z}\boldsymbol{\beta})^{\mathrm{T}} \tilde{\mathbf{V}}^k(\rho)^{-1} (\mathbf{y} - \mathbf{Z}\boldsymbol{\beta})}{2}\right),$$

$$\pi(\rho|\boldsymbol{\beta}, \sigma^2, \mathbf{y}, M^k) \propto \left|\mathbf{V}^k(\rho)\right|^{-\frac{n}{2}} \exp\left\{-\frac{(\mathbf{y} - \mathbf{Z}\boldsymbol{\beta})^{\mathrm{T}} \tilde{\mathbf{V}}^k(\rho)^{-1} (\mathbf{y} - \mathbf{Z}\boldsymbol{\beta})}{2\sigma^2}\right\},$$

where $\tilde{\boldsymbol{\beta}}^k = \left(\mathbf{Z}^{\mathrm{T}} \tilde{\mathbf{V}}^k(\rho)^{-1} \mathbf{Z}\right)^{-1} \mathbf{Z}^{\mathrm{T}} \tilde{\mathbf{V}}^k(\rho)^{-1} \mathbf{y}$ and $\tilde{\mathbf{V}}^k(\rho)^{-1} = \mathbf{I}_n \otimes \mathbf{V}^k(\rho)^{-1}$ for $k = 1, 2$. For model M^3,

$$\boldsymbol{\beta}|\sigma^2, \mathbf{y}, M^3 \sim \mathrm{N}\left(\hat{\boldsymbol{\beta}}, \sigma^2 \left(\mathbf{Z}^{\mathrm{T}}\mathbf{Z}\right)^{-1}\right),$$

$$\sigma^2|\boldsymbol{\beta}, \mathbf{y}, M^3 \sim \mathrm{IG}\left(\frac{nT}{2}, \frac{(\mathbf{y} - \mathbf{Z}\boldsymbol{\beta})^{\mathrm{T}} (\mathbf{y} - \mathbf{Z}\boldsymbol{\beta})}{2}\right),$$

where $\hat{\boldsymbol{\beta}} = \left(\mathbf{Z}^{\mathrm{T}}\mathbf{Z}\right)^{-1} \mathbf{Z}^{\mathrm{T}}\mathbf{y}$. For model M^4,

$$\boldsymbol{\beta}|\boldsymbol{\Sigma}, \mathbf{y}, M^4 \sim \mathrm{N}\left(\tilde{\boldsymbol{\beta}}^4, \left[\mathbf{Z}^{\mathrm{T}}\tilde{\boldsymbol{\Sigma}}^{-1}\mathbf{Z}\right]^{-1}\right),$$

$$\boldsymbol{\Sigma}|\boldsymbol{\beta}, \mathbf{y}, M^4 \sim \mathrm{IW}\left(v_0 + n, \boldsymbol{\Sigma}_0 + \sum_{i=1}^{n}(\mathbf{y}_i - \mathbf{X}_i\boldsymbol{\beta})(\mathbf{y}_i - \mathbf{X}_i\boldsymbol{\beta})^{\mathrm{T}}\right),$$

where $\tilde{\boldsymbol{\beta}}^4 = \left(\mathbf{Z}^{\mathrm{T}}\tilde{\boldsymbol{\Sigma}}^{-1}\mathbf{Z}\right)^{-1}\mathbf{Z}^{\mathrm{T}}\tilde{\boldsymbol{\Sigma}}^{-1}\mathbf{y}$, $\tilde{\boldsymbol{\Sigma}}^{-1} = \mathbf{I}_n \otimes \boldsymbol{\Sigma}^{-1}$. Using the full conditionals, we generate 10,000 samples from the full posterior (after 5000 burn-in iterations) using Gibbs sampler in each model. In models M^1 and M^2, we use Metropolis–Hastings algorithm within the Gibbs chain in order to generate samples from ρ. For the proposal distribution, we approximate the conditional distribution of ρ given posterior mean of $(\boldsymbol{\beta}, \sigma^2)$ (obtained from M^3) using Gaussian approximation and then truncate the distribution with lower tail 0 and upper tail 1. Since the data have the dependency within the subject, we define $\mathbf{y}_{s_i} = \mathbf{y}_{i.} = (y_{i1}, y_{i2}, \ldots, y_{i5})$ for $i = 1, 2, \ldots, 30$. The Monte Carlo estimators of $m(\mathbf{y}_{s_i}|M^k)$ and $m(\mathbf{y}|M^k)$ are, respectively, given as

$$\hat{m}(\mathbf{y}_{s_i}|M^k) = \left\{\sum_{l=1}^{N}\frac{f(\mathbf{y}_{i.}|\boldsymbol{\theta}_k^l, M^k)}{f(\mathbf{y}|\boldsymbol{\theta}_k^l, M^k)}\right\}\left\{\sum_{l=1}^{N}\frac{g^k(\boldsymbol{\theta}_k^l)}{f(\mathbf{y}|\boldsymbol{\theta}_k^l, M^k)\pi(\boldsymbol{\theta}_k^l)}\right\}^{-1}, \tag{22}$$

$$\hat{m}(\mathbf{y}|M^k) = \left\{\frac{1}{N}\sum_{l=1}^{N}\frac{g^k(\boldsymbol{\theta}_k^l)}{f(\mathbf{y}|\boldsymbol{\theta}_k^l, M^k)\pi(\boldsymbol{\theta}_k^l)}\right\}^{-1}, \tag{23}$$

where $\left\{\boldsymbol{\theta}_1^l = (\boldsymbol{\beta}_1^l, \sigma_1^{2l}, \rho_1^l)\right\}_{l=1}^N$, $\left\{\boldsymbol{\theta}_2^l = (\boldsymbol{\beta}_2^l, \sigma_2^{2l}, \rho_2^l)\right\}_{l=1}^N$, $\left\{\boldsymbol{\theta}_3^l = (\boldsymbol{\beta}_3^l, \sigma_3^{2l})\right\}_{l=1}^N$, and $\left\{\boldsymbol{\theta}_4^l = (\boldsymbol{\beta}_4^l, \boldsymbol{\Sigma}_4^l)\right\}_{l=1}^N$, respectively, indicate sets of MCMC samples of full posterior distributions under models M^1, M^2, M^3, and M^4. Note that the likelihood functions in (22) and (23) can be easily obtained from (17).

We compare $\mathrm{BDC}_{\psi_\gamma}$ ($\gamma = 0, 1, 2$) with DIC and PSBF. The result is shown in Table 3. All the BDCs and DIC select M^4 as the best model, while PSBF chooses M^2. Hence, we conclude that model M^4 is the best model for the rat population growth data.

Table 3 BDCs, DIC, and PSBF for M_1, M_2, M_3, and M_4

	Model			
Criterion	M^1	M^2	M^3	M^4
$\mathrm{BDC}_{\psi_{0.0}}$	2.429×10^2	1.350×10^1	4.207×10^5	7.382×10^{-3}
$\mathrm{BDC}_{\psi_{1.0}}$	3.650×10^{-7}	3.832×10^{-7}	2.423×10^{-6}	7.806×10^{-11}
$\mathrm{BDC}_{\psi_{2.0}}$	1.027×10^{-14}	7.176×10^{-14}	3.517×10^{-14}	3.314×10^{-18}
PSBF	−557.684	−522.710	−649.105	−525.991
DIC	1125.526	1052.211	1309.100	1031.423

Table 4 Summary of model selection rates (%)

	Model			
Criterion	M^1	M^2	M^3	M^4
$\text{BDC}_{\psi_{0.0}}$	100	0	0	0
$\text{BDC}_{\psi_{1.0}}$	100	0	0	0
$\text{BDC}_{\psi_{2.0}}$	100	0	0	0
LPML	100	0	0	0
DIC	100	0	0	0

Note that one may suspect that BDC supports the more highly parameterized model rather than the true model for the determination of covariance matrix. To deal with this contention, we conduct a small simulation study as follows. Let $\hat{\mathbf{V}}_1$ and $\hat{\boldsymbol{\beta}}_1$ be the obtained Bayes estimates (i.e., posterior means) for $\mathbf{V}$ and $\boldsymbol{\beta}$ under M^1, respectively. For given $\mathbf{Z}$, $\hat{\mathbf{V}}_1$, and $\hat{\boldsymbol{\beta}}$, we generate $\mathbf{y}$ from (17). Based on 100 replicates, we compute the selection rate (%) for BDCs, DIC, and PSBF. The result in Table 4 shows that all model selection criteria always select the true model ($= M^1$) rather than over-parameterized model ($= M^4$). This experiment demonstrates the reliability of our real data analysis conducted in this section.

5 Concluding Remarks

We have introduced a new Bayesian model selection criterion, named BDC. In order to calculate BDC, we have proposed a Monte Carlo method that requires only a single set of MCMC samples from the full posterior distribution. It is worth noting that the proposed Monte Carlo estimator can be directly applied to computing many Bayes factors such as BF, PSBF, and IBF.

In this paper, we have used the Bregman divergence between two vectors with the cross-validation approach in order to avoid the calculation of functional divergence over the new observation space in the posterior expected loss (2). A possible extension of BDC can be made by using the following functional Bregman divergence (Goh and Dey 2014; Grünwald and Dawid 2004):

$$\text{fDB}_\xi(f, g) = \int \xi(f(y)) - \xi(g(y)) - \{f(y) - g(y)\}\xi'(g(y))dy,$$

where $\xi : (0, \infty) \to \mathbb{R}$ is a strictly convex and differentiable function, and ξ' represents the first derivative of ξ. Then, under the functional Bregman divergence loss, the Bayes rule in (3) can be obtained by

$$\tilde{M} = \arg\min_{a \in \mathscr{M}} \text{fBD}_\xi\left(\bar{p}(\mathbf{y}_{\text{new}}|\mathbf{y}_{\text{old}}), p(\mathbf{y}_{\text{new}}|\mathbf{y}_{\text{old}}, a)\right),$$

where $\bar{p}(\mathbf{y}_{\text{new}}|\mathbf{y}_{\text{old}}) = \int p(\mathbf{y}_{\text{new}}|\mathbf{y}_{\text{old}}, M)\pi(M|\mathbf{y}_{\text{old}})dM$. If we can find the analytical or numerical solution, this criterion can be considered as a general extension of BDC.

6 Proofs

6.1 Proof of Theorem 1

Let $w_{li} = \frac{m(\mathbf{y}_{-s_i}|M^l)}{\sum_{k=1}^K m(\mathbf{y}_{-s_i}|M^k)}$. By the fact that $\sum_{l=1}^K w_{li} = 1$, we have

$$\rho^*\left(\pi(M|\mathbf{y}_{-s_i}), a\right) = \sum_{l=1}^K w_{li}\text{BD}_\psi\left(p(\mathbf{y}_{s_i}|\mathbf{y}_{-s_i}, M^l), p(\mathbf{y}_{s_i}|\mathbf{y}_{-s_i}, a)\right)$$

$$= \sum_{l=1}^K w_{li}\psi\left(p(\mathbf{y}_{s_i}|\mathbf{y}_{-s_i}, M^l)\right) - \psi\left(p(\mathbf{y}_{s_i}|\mathbf{y}_{-s_i}, a)\right)$$

$$- \left\{\bar{p}_i - p(\mathbf{y}_{s_i}|\mathbf{y}_{-s_i}, a)\right\}\psi'\left(p(\mathbf{y}_{s_i}|\mathbf{y}_{-s_i}, a)\right)$$

$$= \sum_{l=1}^K w_{li}\psi\left(p(\mathbf{y}_{s_i}|\mathbf{y}_{-s_i}, M^l)\right) - \psi\left(\bar{p}_i\right) + \text{BD}_\psi\left(\bar{p}_i, p(\mathbf{y}_{s_i}|\mathbf{y}_{-s_i}, a)\right),$$

where $\bar{p}_i = \sum_{l=1}^K w_{li}p(\mathbf{y}_{s_i}|\mathbf{y}_{-s_i}, M^l)$. This implies that

$$\arg\min_{a\in\mathcal{M}}\sum_{i=1}^m \rho^*\left(\pi(M|\mathbf{y}_{-s_i}), a\right) = \arg\min_{a\in\mathcal{M}}\sum_{i=1}^m \text{BD}_\psi\left(\bar{p}_i, p(\mathbf{y}_{s_i}|\mathbf{y}_{-s_i}, a)\right)$$

$$= \arg\min_{a\in\mathcal{M}}\text{BD}_\psi\left(\bar{\mathbf{p}}, \mathbf{p}^{(a)}\right).$$

6.2 Proof of Theorem 2

When $\{\mathbf{y}_{-s}\} = \emptyset$, the left-hand side of (7) is

$$\left[\frac{1}{N}\sum_{j=1}^N \frac{g(\boldsymbol{\theta}^j)}{f(\mathbf{y}|\boldsymbol{\theta}^j)\pi(\boldsymbol{\theta}^j)}\right]^{-1},$$

which converges, as $N \to \infty$, to $m(\mathbf{y})$ almost surely (Chen 1994). Assume $\{\mathbf{y}_{-s}\} \neq \emptyset$, and then

$$
\begin{aligned}
p(\mathbf{y}_s|\mathbf{y}_{-s}) &= \frac{m(\mathbf{y})}{m(\mathbf{y}_{-s})} \\
&= \frac{m(\mathbf{y})}{\int_\Theta f(\mathbf{y}_{-s}|\boldsymbol{\theta})\pi(\boldsymbol{\theta})d\boldsymbol{\theta}} \\
&= \frac{m(\mathbf{y})}{\int_\Theta \frac{f(\mathbf{y}|\boldsymbol{\theta})}{f(\mathbf{y}_s|\mathbf{y}_{-s},\boldsymbol{\theta})}\pi(\boldsymbol{\theta})d\boldsymbol{\theta}} \\
&= \left[\int_\Theta \frac{\pi(\boldsymbol{\theta}|\mathbf{y})}{f(\mathbf{y}_s|\mathbf{y}_{-s},\boldsymbol{\theta})}d\boldsymbol{\theta}\right]^{-1} \\
&\overset{\text{a.s.}}{=} \lim_{N\to\infty}\left[\frac{1}{N}\sum_{j=1}^{N}\frac{1}{f(\mathbf{y}_s|\mathbf{y}_{-s},\boldsymbol{\theta}^j)}\right]^{-1},
\end{aligned}
$$

where the last part of proof can be done by the pointwise ergodic theorem.

References

Berger, J. O., & Pericchi, L. R. (1996a). The intrinsic Bayes factor for linear models. In J. M. Bernardo, J. O. Berger, A. P. Dawid, & A. F. M. Smith (Eds.), *Bayesian statistics* (vol. 5, pp. 25–44). Oxford: Oxford University Press.

Berger, J. O., & Pericchi, L. R. (1996b). The intrinsic Bayes factor for model selection and prediction. *Journal of the American Statistical Association, 91*, 109–122.

Bernardo, J. M., & Smith, A. F. M. (2000). *Bayesian theory*. Chichester: Wiley.

Bregman, L. M. (1967). The relaxation method of finding the common points of convex sets and its application to the solution of problems in convex programming. *USSR Computational Mathematics and Mathematical Physics, 7*, 200–217.

Chen, M. H. (1994). Importance-weighted marginal Bayesian posterior density estimation. *Journal of the American Statistical Association, 89*, 818–824.

Dawid, A. P. (1984). Statistical theory: The prequential approach. *Journal of the Royal Statistical Society, Series B, 147*, 278–292.

Geisser, S. (1975). The predictive sample reuse method with applications. *Journal of the American Statistical Association, 70*, 320–328.

Geisser, S., & Eddy, W. (1979). A predictive approach to model selection. *Journal of the American Statistical Association, 74*, 153–160.

Gelfand, A. E., & Dey, D. K. (1994). Bayesian model choice: Asymptotics and exact calculations. *Journal of the Royal Statistical Society, Series B, 56*, 501–514.

Gelfand, A. E., & Ghosh, S. K. (1998). Model choice: A minimum posterior predictive loss approach. *Biometrika, 85*, 1–11.

Gelfand, A. E., Hills, S. E., Racine-Poon, A., & Smith, A. F. M. (1990). Illustration of Bayesian inference in normal data models using Gibbs sampling. *Journal of the American Statistical Association, 85*, 972–985.

Gneiting, T., & Raftery, A. E. (2007). Strictly proper scoring rules, prediction, and estimation. *Journal of the American statistical Association, 102*(477), 359–378.

Goh, G., & Dey, D. K. (2014). Bayesian model diagnostics using functional Bregman divergence. *Journal of Multivariate Analysis, 124*, 371–383.

Grünwald, P. D., & Dawid, A. P. (2004). Game theory, maximum entropy, minimum discrepancy and robust Bayesian decision theory. *Annals of Statistics, 32*, 1367–1433.

Gutierrez-Pena, E., & Walker, S. G. (2001). A Bayesian predictive approach to model selection. *Journal of Statistical Planning and Inference, 93*, 259–276.

Hennequin, R., David, B., & Badeau, R. (2011). Beta-divergence as a subclass of Bregman divergence. *IEEE Signal Processing Letters, 18*, 83–86.

Ionides, E. L. (2008). Truncated importance sampling. *Journal of Computational and Graphical Statistics, 17*, 295–311.

Itakura, F., & Saito, S. (1970). A statistical method for estimation of speech spectral density and formant frequencies. *Electronics and Communications in Japan, 53*, 36–43.

Laud, P. W., & Ibrahim, J. G. (1995). Predictive model selection. *Journal of the Royal Statistical Society, Series B, 57*, 247–262.

Liu, J., Nordman, D. J., & Meeker, W. Q. (2016). The number of MCMC draws needed to compute Bayesian credible bounds. *The American Statistician, 70*(3), 275–284.

San Martini, A., & Spezzaferri, F. (1984). A predictive model selection criterion. *Journal of the Royal Statistical Society, Series B, 46*, 296–303.

Stone, M. (1974). Cross-validation choice and assessment of statistical predictions (with discussion). *Journal of the Royal Statistical Society, Series B, 36*, 111–147.

A Simple Step-Stress Model for Lehmann Family of Distributions

Ayan Pal, Debashis Samanta, Sharmishtha Mitra, and Debasis Kundu

Abstract In this chapter, we consider a flexible simple step-stress model for the Lehmann family of distributions, also known as the exponentiated distributions, when the data are Type-II censored. At each stress level, we assume that the lifetime distribution of the experimental units follows a member of the Lehmann family of distributions with different shape and scale parameters. The distribution under each stress level is connected through a failure rate-based step-stress accelerated life testing (SSALT) model. We obtain the maximum likelihood estimators (MLEs) of the unknown model parameters. It is observed that the MLEs of the unknown parameters do not always exist, and whenever they exist, they are not in closed form. However, the failure rate-based SSALT model assumption simplifies the inference problem to a significant extent. It is not possible to obtain the exact distribution of the MLEs, and hence, we have constructed the asymptotic confidence intervals (CIs) based on the observed Fisher information matrix. We have also obtained the bootstrap CIs for model parameters. Extensive simulation study is carried out when the lifetime distribution is a two-parameter generalized exponential (GE) distribution, an important member of the Lehmann family. A real data set has been analyzed assuming that the lifetimes follow a few important members of the Lehmann family for illustration purposes.

1 Introduction

Industrial products nowadays are highly reliable due to advancement in science and technology, and one of the major recent challenges in reliability analysis is to conduct their life testing experiments. Mean time to failure is quite high

A. Pal · S. Mitra · D. Kundu (✉)
Department of Mathematics and Statistics, Indian Institute of Technology, Kanpur, India
e-mail: ayanpal@iitk.ac.in; smitra@iitk.ac.in; kundu@iitk.ac.in

D. Samanta
Department of Mathematics and Statistics, Aliah University, Kolkata, West Bengal, India

I. Ghosh et al. (eds.), *Advances in Statistics - Theory and Applications*, Emerging Topics in Statistics and Biostatistics, https://doi.org/10.1007/978-3-030-62900-7_16

in industries like VLSI (very large-scale integrated) electronic devices, computer equipment, missiles, automobile parts, etc. Performing life tests under normal operating condition (NOC) often turns out to be impractical, expensive, and time intensive.

Censoring is a well-known statistical technique to truncate the life testing experiment in a well-planned manner before all the items fail. But censoring of a life testing experiment under NOC will not resolve the issue of insufficient number of failures for proper statistical analysis. To address this problem, accelerated life testing (ALT) experiment has been introduced, which ensures a faster rate of failure. The step-stress accelerated life testing (SSALT) experiment is a special class of the ALT experiment in which the experimenter has the flexibility to perform the experiment under one or more stress levels. In a multiple step-stress model setup, n identical units are placed on a life testing experiment at an initial stress level s_1 and then the stress level is gradually increased to $s_2 < s_3 < \cdots < s_{m+1}$ at pre-fixed times $\tau_1 < \tau_2 < \cdots < \tau_m$, respectively. If $m = 1$, the corresponding model is called a simple step-stress model. One way to truncate the life testing experiment is to fix some positive integer $1 \leq r \leq n$, and then the experiment is allowed to stop as soon as the rth failure occurs. This is the usual Type-II censoring case, and total time of experimental duration here is random. The successive failure times thus recorded may then be extrapolated to estimate the failure time distribution under NOC. If there are only two stress levels, the model is called a simple step-stress model. To analyze the failure time data from any SSALT experiment, we need a model that relates the distributions under different stress levels. The popular model in the literature is the cumulative exposure model (CEM), introduced by Sedyakin (1966) and later generalized by Bagdonavičius (1978) and Nelson (1980). Here, if $F_1(.)$ and $F_2(.)$ are the cumulative distribution functions (CDFs) of lifetimes under the constant stress levels s_1 and s_2, respectively, the CDF of the lifetime of the experimental unit under the CEM is given by

$$F_{CEM}(t) = \begin{cases} F_1(t) & \text{if} \quad 0 < t \leq \tau \\ F_2(t + \tau - \tau^*) & \text{if} \quad \tau < t < \infty. \end{cases} \tag{1}$$

Here, τ^* is the solution of the equation $F_2(\tau^*) = F_1(\tau)$ and τ is the stress-changing time. Another widely used model is the proportional hazards model (PHM) introduced by Cox (1992). It describes the impact of the covariates on the lifetime distribution. Later, as a variation of Cox's PHM, Bhattacharyya and Soejoeti (1989) introduced the tampered failure rate model (TFRM). The assumption here is that the effect of increasing the stress level from s_1 to s_2 is equivalent to multiply the initial failure rate function at stress level s_1 by an unknown factor $\alpha > 0$. Therefore, the hazard function (HF) of the lifetime of the experimental unit under the TFRM is given by

$$h_{\mathrm{TFRM}}(t) = \begin{cases} h_1(t) & \text{if} \quad 0 < t \le \tau \\ \alpha h_1(t) & \text{if} \quad \tau < t < \infty, \end{cases} \tag{2}$$

where $h_1(.)$ is the HF at the stress level s_1. It may be mentioned that Madi (1993) used the TFRM for the multiple SSALT model ($m \ge 2$) when the lifetime distribution across the stress levels is Weibull with common shape parameter and different scale parameters. Under a similar setup, Khamis and Higgins (1998) derived the MLEs of the common shape parameter and different scale parameters using a log-link model. Their model is well known as the Khamis–Higgins model (KHM).

In this chapter, we work with a flexible failure rate based SSALT model with pre-fixed but arbitrarily chosen failure rates at different stress levels. If s_1 and s_2 are the two stress levels and τ is the stress-changing time point, it is assumed that the hazard rate of the distribution under the step-stress pattern is as follows:

$$h(t) = \begin{cases} h_1(t) & \text{if} \quad 0 < t \le \tau \\ h_2(t) & \text{if} \quad \tau < t < \infty, \end{cases} \tag{3}$$

where $h_i(t)$ is the HF corresponding to the CDF $F_i(t)$, $i = 1, 2$. On simplifying, one can obtain the distribution function corresponding to $h(t)$ as follows:

$$F(t) = \begin{cases} F_1(t) & \text{if} \quad 0 < t \le \tau \\ 1 - \dfrac{1 - F_1(\tau)}{1 - F_2(\tau)}(1 - F_2(t)) & \text{if} \quad \tau < t < \infty. \end{cases} \tag{4}$$

In fact, the CEM, TFRM, and the failure rate-based SSALT model coincide when the underlying distributions at the two stress levels are exponential. The flexibility of this model allows us to assume difference in both shape and scale parameters of the underlying failure distribution in the different stress levels. This assumption will take prior information about the failure situations under different stress levels into account. For the probabilistic interpretation, flexibility, and application of this model, readers are referred to Kateri and Kamps (2015, 2017).

A family of distributions is said to belong to Lehmann family if the CDF is given by

$$F^*(t; \alpha, \lambda) = \begin{cases} [G_0(t; \lambda)]^\alpha & \text{if} \quad t > 0, \\ 0 & \text{otherwise.} \end{cases} \tag{5}$$

Here, $G_0(t; \lambda)$ is some baseline absolutely continuous CDF assumed to be completely specified except for the unknown parameter λ, and depending on $G_0(.)$, $\alpha > 0$ and $\lambda > 0$ can be shape, scale, or location parameters. In general, a standard form of the baseline CDF is assumed to take the following form:

$$G_0(t;\lambda) = 1 - e^{-\lambda Q(t)}, \tag{6}$$

where $Q(t)$ is a strictly increasing function, differentiable on $(0, \infty)$ with $Q(0) = 0$ and $Q(\infty) = \infty$. The Lehmann family of distributions discussed in this chapter is also known as the exponentiated distributions. This model is quite flexible in reliability analysis in the sense that one can obtain the various well-known lifetime distributions as special cases for different choices of $Q(.)$. For example,

- $Q(t) = t$ gives the exponentiated (generalized) exponential (GE) distribution (see Gupta and Kundu 1999).
- $Q(t) = t^2$ leads to the generalized Rayleigh (GR) distribution. It is also known as Burr type-X distribution (see Surles and Padgett 2005).
- $Q(t) = \ln(1 + t)$ gives the exponentiated Pareto (EP) distribution (see Gupta et al. 1998; Shawky and Abu-Zinadah 2009).
- $Q(t) = \frac{a}{\lambda}t + \frac{b}{2\lambda}t^2$ leads to the generalized failure rate distribution with parameters a, b, α and will be denoted by GFRD(a, b, α) (see Sarhan and Kundu 2009).

Not many authors focus on inferential procedures in SSALT setup, when the lifetime distribution is a member or belongs to the Lehmann family of distributions. It may be mentioned that Abdel-Hamid and Al-Hussaini (2009) considered the inference of parameters of a GE distribution for simple SSALT model for Type-I censored data based on the CEM assumptions. The lifetime distribution at each of the two stress levels is assumed to have the common shape parameter, and the only difference lies in the scale parameters across the stress levels. El-Monem and Jaheen (2015) considered the problem of maximum likelihood estimation for a simple step-stress accelerated GE distribution with Type II censored data based on the CEM assumptions and keeping shape parameters fixed at both the stress levels. Ismail (2014) considered the maximum likelihood estimation of the GE distribution parameters and the acceleration factor under step-stress partially accelerated life testing (SSPALT) when the data are Type-II censored and the underlying model is the tampered random variable model (TRVM). Recently Samanta and Kundu (2018) provided an order-restricted inference of the multiple step-stress model when the lifetime distribution at the different stress levels is GE distribution with common shape parameter and different scale parameters. However, a flexible SSALT experiment with difference in both the shape and scale parameters is yet to be addressed.

The main intent of this chapter is to consider the likelihood inference of a simple step-stress model for the Lehmann family of distributions based on Type-II censoring under failure rate-based SSALT model assumptions.

It is assumed that the lifetime distribution of the experimental units at each of the stress levels belongs to the Lehmann family with difference in shape and scale parameters. In particular, the CDF, probability density function (PDF), and the HF of the lifetime distribution at the ith stress level for $i = 1, 2$ are given by

$$F_i^*(t) = \begin{cases} [G_0(t;\lambda_i)]^{\alpha_i} & \text{if} \quad t > 0 \\ 0 & \text{otherwise,} \end{cases} \tag{7}$$

$$f_i^*(t) = \begin{cases} \alpha_i [G_0(t;\lambda_i)]^{\alpha_i - 1} [g_0(t;\lambda_i)] & \text{if} \quad t > 0 \\ 0 & \text{otherwise,} \end{cases} \tag{8}$$

and

$$h_i^*(t) = \begin{cases} \dfrac{\alpha_i [G_0(t;\lambda_i)]^{\alpha_i - 1} g_0(t;\lambda_i)}{1 - [G_0(t;\lambda_i)]^{\alpha_i}} & \text{if} \quad t > 0 \\ 0 & \text{otherwise.} \end{cases} \tag{9}$$

The existence of MLEs of the unknown model parameters depends on the number of failures at the two stress levels s_1 and s_2. However, given that they exist, the MLEs cannot be obtained in closed form but can be obtained by solving a four-dimensional optimization problem. The assumption of the failure rate-based SSALT model simplifies the optimization problem in terms of dimension reduction. The MLEs can then be obtained by solving a one-dimensional and a two-dimensional optimization problems. In the complete sample ($r = n$) case, the optimization problem gets even more simplified. The MLEs can then be obtained by solving two one-dimensional optimization problems.

It is not possible to obtain the exact distributions of the MLEs, as they are not in closed forms. We suggest to use the observed Fisher information matrix to construct the asymptotic CIs of the unknown model parameters assuming the asymptotic normality of the MLEs. The parametric bootstrap CIs are also proposed as an alternative as they are easy to implement in practice.

The rest of the chapter is organized as follows. In Sect. 2, we provide the model description, likelihood function, and MLEs of the unknown model parameters. For illustration purpose, some specific results for the GE distribution are demonstrated. The construction of both asymptotic and bootstrap CIs is discussed in Sect. 3. To see the effectiveness of the proposed methods, an extensive simulation experiment is carried out in Sect. 4 for different sample sizes, censoring proportions, and stress-changing time points. We have analyzed a real-life data set for illustrative purpose, assuming that the lifetime distribution follows different important members of the Lehmann family. Finally we conclude the chapter in Sect. 5.

2 Model Description, Likelihood Function, and MLEs

2.1 Model Description

We consider a simple step-stress model with two stress levels s_1 and s_2 under Type-II censoring scheme. Initially n identical units are placed on the life testing experiment at the stress level s_1. The stress level is changed to a higher level s_2 at the pre-fixed time τ $(0 < \tau < \infty)$, and the experiment terminates as soon as the r-th failure occurs (r is a prefixed integer less than or equal to n). Let n_i be the number of units that fail at stress level s_i $(i = 1, 2)$. With this notation, we observe the following ordered failure time data:

$$\mathcal{D} = \left\{t_{1:n} < \cdots < t_{n_1:n} < \tau < t_{n_1+1:n} < \cdots < t_{r:n}\right\}, \tag{10}$$

where $r = n_1 + n_2$.

Suppose that the lifetime distributions of the experimental units at stress levels s_1 and s_2 belong to the Lehmann family of distributions with difference in both the shape and scale parameters. To relate the CDFs of lifetime distributions at two consecutive stress levels to the CDF of the lifetime under the used conditions, we follow the failure rate-based SSALT model assumptions. Under the assumption of the failure rate-based SSALT model to analyze the failure time data, the HF $h(t)$, the corresponding CDF $G(t)$ and the associated PDF $g(t)$ of the lifetime of an experimental unit are, respectively, given by

$$h(t) = \begin{cases} \dfrac{\alpha_1[G_0(t;\lambda_1)]^{\alpha_1-1}g_0(t;\lambda_1)}{1-[G_0(t;\lambda_1)]^{\alpha_1}} & \text{if} \quad 0 < t \leq \tau \\ \\ \dfrac{\alpha_2[G_0(t;\lambda_2)]^{\alpha_2-1}g_0(t;\lambda_2)}{1-[G_0(t;\lambda_2)]^{\alpha_2}} & \text{if} \quad \tau < t < \infty, \end{cases}$$

$$G(t) = \begin{cases} [G_0(t;\lambda_1)]^{\alpha_1} & \text{if} \quad 0 < t \leq \tau \\ 1 - \dfrac{\left\{1-[G_0(\tau;\lambda_1)]^{\alpha_1}\right\}}{\left\{1-[G_0(\tau;\lambda_2)]^{\alpha_2}\right\}}\left\{1-[G_0(t;\lambda_2)]^{\alpha_2}\right\} & \text{if} \quad \tau < t < \infty, \end{cases}$$

$$g(t) = \begin{cases} \alpha_1[G_0(t;\lambda_1)]^{\alpha_1-1}[g_0(t;\lambda_1)] & \text{if} \quad 0 < t \leq \tau \\ \alpha_2\dfrac{\left\{1-[G_0(\tau;\lambda_1)]^{\alpha_1}\right\}}{\left\{1-[G_0(\tau;\lambda_2)]^{\alpha_2}\right\}}[G_0(t;\lambda_2)]^{\alpha_2-1}[g_0(t;\lambda_2)] & \text{if} \quad \tau < t < \infty. \end{cases}$$

2.2 Likelihood Function and MLEs

2.2.1 Type-II Censoring Case

In this subsection, we consider the likelihood function based on the observed Type-II censored data in (10) and obtain the MLEs of the unknown model parameters $\alpha_1, \lambda_1, \alpha_2$, and λ_2.

If $T_{1:n} < \cdots < T_{r:n}$ denote the ordered Type-II censored sample from any absolutely continuous CDF $F_T(.)$, PDF $f_T(.)$, then the likelihood function of this censored sample (see Arnold et al. 1992) can be written as

$$L(\boldsymbol{\theta} \mid \text{Data}) = \frac{n!}{(n-r)!}\left\{\prod_{k=1}^{r} f_T(t_{k:n})\right\}\{1 - F_T(t_{r:n})\}^{n-r},$$
$$0 < t_{1:n} < \cdots < t_{r:n} < \infty, \tag{11}$$

where $\boldsymbol{\theta}$ is the vector of model parameters.

Let $\boldsymbol{\theta} = (\alpha_1, \lambda_1, \alpha_2, \lambda_2)$ be the set of unknown model parameters of interest. Based on the observed Type-II censored data in (10) of failure time from the Lehmann family of distributions with difference in both the shape and scale parameters at each of the two stress levels and assuming a failure rate-based simple SSALT model, we obtain the likelihood function $L^{II}(\boldsymbol{\theta} \mid \mathcal{D})$ as

$$L^{\text{II}}(\boldsymbol{\theta} \mid \mathcal{D}) = \frac{n!}{(n-r)!}\, \alpha_1^{n_1}\, \alpha_2^{n_2} \prod_{k=1}^{n_1} [G_0(t_{k:n}; \lambda_1)]^{\alpha_1 - 1}$$
$$\times \prod_{k=n_1+1}^{r} [G_0(t_{k:n}; \lambda_2)]^{\alpha_2 - 1} \prod_{k=1}^{n_1} [g_0(t_{k:n}; \lambda_1)] \prod_{k=n_1+1}^{r} [g_0(t_{k:n}; \lambda_2)]$$
$$\times \left\{1 - [G_0(t_{r:n}; \lambda_2)]^{\alpha_2}\right\}^{n-r} \left[\frac{1 - [G_0(\tau; \lambda_1)]^{\alpha_1}}{1 - [G_0(\tau; \lambda_2)]^{\alpha_2}}\right]^{n-n_1},$$
$$0 < t_{1:n} < \cdots < t_{n_1:n} < \tau < t_{n_1+1:n} < \cdots < t_{r:n} < \infty. \tag{12}$$

The MLE of $\boldsymbol{\theta}$, say $\widehat{\boldsymbol{\theta}} = (\widehat{\alpha}_1, \widehat{\lambda}_1, \widehat{\alpha}_2, \widehat{\lambda}_2)$, can be obtained by maximizing (12) over the region $\Theta = (0, \infty) \times (0, \infty) \times (0, \infty) \times (0, \infty)$. The associated log-likelihood function $l^{\text{II}}(\boldsymbol{\theta} \mid \mathcal{D})$ of the observed data without additive constants is given by

$$l^{\text{II}}(\boldsymbol{\theta} \mid \mathcal{D}) = g_1(\alpha_1, \lambda_1) + g_2(\alpha_2, \lambda_2), \tag{13}$$

where

$$g_1(\alpha_1, \lambda_1) = n_1 \ln \alpha_1 + (\alpha_1 - 1) \sum_{k=1}^{n_1} \ln G_0(t_{k:n}; \lambda_1) + \sum_{k=1}^{n_1} \ln g_0(t_{k:n}; \lambda_1)$$
$$+ (n - n_1) \ln\{1 - [G_0(\tau; \lambda_1)]^{\alpha_1}\}, \tag{14}$$

$$
\begin{aligned}
g_2(\alpha_2, \lambda_2) = \; & n_2 \ln \alpha_2 + (\alpha_2 - 1) \sum_{k=n_1+1}^{r} \ln G_0(t_{k:n}; \lambda_2) \\
& + \sum_{k=n_1+1}^{r} \ln g_0(t_{k:n}; \lambda_2) + (n-r) \ln\{1 - [G_0(t_{r:n}; \lambda_2)]^{\alpha_2}\} \\
& -(n-n_1) \ln\{1 - [G_0(\tau; \lambda_2)]^{\alpha_2}\}.
\end{aligned} \tag{15}
$$

Hence, $\widehat{\boldsymbol{\theta}}$ can be obtained by maximizing the log-likelihood function (13) over the region Θ. The log-likelihood function (13) can be written as the sum of two terms $g_1(\alpha_1, \lambda_1)$ and $g_2(\alpha_2, \lambda_2)$. Differentiating the log-likelihood function (13) with respect to $\alpha_1, \lambda_1, \alpha_2$ and λ_2, respectively, and equating them to zero, the four normal equations are obtained (see Appendix section "Normal Equations for the Type-II Censoring Case"). $\widehat{\boldsymbol{\theta}}$ can directly be obtained by solving the four normal equations. In this context, it is to note that the assumption of the failure rate-based SSALT model yields the simple representation of the log-likelihood function. It indicates that the separate maximization of the constituent functions $g_1(\alpha_1, \lambda_1)$ and $g_2(\alpha_2, \lambda_2)$ is sufficient to obtain $(\widehat{\alpha}_1, \widehat{\lambda}_1)$, $(\widehat{\alpha}_2, \widehat{\lambda}_2)$, and hence $\widehat{\boldsymbol{\theta}}$, provided that the log-likelihood function (13) is unimodal. Additionally, from the normal equations associated with $g_1(\alpha_1, \lambda_1)$, it can be easily seen that $\widehat{\alpha}_1(\lambda_1)$ maximizes $g_1(\alpha_1, \lambda_1)$ for a given λ_1, where $\widehat{\alpha}_1(\lambda_1)$ is

$$
\frac{\ln[G_0(\tau; \lambda_1)] \sum_{k=1}^{n_1} \dfrac{n_o(t_{k:n}; \lambda_1)}{g_0(t_{k:n}; \lambda_1)} - \dfrac{n_1 m_0(\tau; \lambda_1)}{G_0(\tau; \lambda_1)} - \ln[G_0(\tau; \lambda_1)] \sum_{k=1}^{n_1} \dfrac{m_0(t_{k:n}; \lambda_1)}{G_0(t_{k:n}; \lambda_1)}}{\dfrac{m_0(\tau; \lambda_1)}{G_0(\tau; \lambda_1)} - \ln[G_0(\tau; \lambda_1)] \sum_{k=1}^{n_1} \dfrac{m_0(t_{k:n}; \lambda_1)}{G_0(t_{k:n}; \lambda_1)}}. \tag{16}
$$

For details of the calculation and expressions for $m_0(.; \lambda_1)$ and $n_0(.; \lambda_1)$, the readers are referred to Appendix section "Normal Equations for the Type-II Censoring Case". This provides an extra edge over solving the usual four-dimensional optimization problem in the sense that we are now maximizing a single one-dimensional nonlinear function for estimating λ_1 and a single two-dimensional nonlinear function $g_2(\alpha_2, \lambda_2)$ for estimating α_2 and λ_2. Note that once we obtain $\widehat{\lambda}_1$ by maximizing $g_1(\widehat{\alpha}_1(\lambda_1), \lambda_1)$, we can obtain $\widehat{\alpha}_1 = \widehat{\alpha}_1(\widehat{\lambda}_1)$. Next, we address the complete sample ($r = n$) scenario, a particular case of Type-II censoring. In fact, inference becomes simplified to a large extent in the complete sample case.

2.2.2 Complete Sample ($r = n$) Case

The likelihood function $L^c(\boldsymbol{\theta} \mid \mathcal{D})$ of the observed complete data is given by

$$L^c(\boldsymbol{\theta} \mid \mathcal{D}) = n!\, \alpha_1^{n_1}\, \alpha_2^{n_2} \prod_{k=1}^{n_1} [G_0(t_{k:n}; \lambda_1)]^{\alpha_1 - 1} \prod_{k=n_1+1}^{n} [G_0(t_{k:n}; \lambda_2)]^{\alpha_2 - 1}$$
$$\times \prod_{k=1}^{n_1} [g_0(t_{k:n}; \lambda_1)] \prod_{k=n_1+1}^{n} [g_0(t_{k:n}; \lambda_2)] \left[\frac{1 - [G_0(\tau; \lambda_1)]^{\alpha_1}}{1 - [G_0(\tau; \lambda_2)]^{\alpha_2}} \right]^{n-n_1}. \tag{17}$$

The MLE of $\boldsymbol{\theta}$, say $\widehat{\boldsymbol{\theta}} = (\widehat{\alpha}_1, \widehat{\lambda}_1, \widehat{\alpha}_2, \widehat{\lambda}_2)$, can be obtained by maximizing (17) over the region $\Theta = (0, \infty) \times (0, \infty) \times (0, \infty) \times (0, \infty)$. The associated log-likelihood function $l^c(\boldsymbol{\theta} \mid \mathcal{D})$ of the observed complete data without additive constants is given by

$$l^c(\boldsymbol{\theta} \mid \mathcal{D}) = m_1(\alpha_1, \lambda_1) + m_2(\alpha_2, \lambda_2), \tag{18}$$

where

$$m_1(\alpha_1, \lambda_1) = n_1 \ln \alpha_1 + (\alpha_1 - 1) \sum_{k=1}^{n_1} \ln G_0(t_{k:n}; \lambda_1) + \sum_{k=1}^{n_1} \ln g_0(t_{k:n}; \lambda_1)$$
$$+ (n - n_1) \ln\{1 - [G_0(\tau; \lambda_1)]^{\alpha_1}\}, \tag{19}$$

$$m_2(\alpha_2, \lambda_2) = n_2 \ln \alpha_2 + (\alpha_2 - 1) \sum_{k=n_1+1}^{r} \ln G_0(t_{k:n}; \lambda_2) + \sum_{k=n_1+1}^{r} \ln g_0(t_{k:n}; \lambda_2)$$
$$- (n - n_1) \ln\{1 - [G_0(\tau; \lambda_2)]^{\alpha_2}\}. \tag{20}$$

Hence, $\widehat{\boldsymbol{\theta}}$ can be obtained by maximizing the log-likelihood function (18) over the region Θ. In this case, also the log-likelihood function (18) can be written as the sum of two terms $m_1(\alpha_1, \lambda_1)$ and $m_2(\alpha_2, \lambda_2)$. Differentiating the log-likelihood function (18) with respect to α_1, λ_1, α_2 and λ_2, respectively, and equating them to zero, the four normal equations are obtained (see Appendix section "Normal Equations for the Complete Sample Case"). It is to note that $m_1(\alpha_1, \lambda_1) = g_1(\alpha_1, \lambda_1)$. Hence, from the normal equations associated with $g_1(\alpha_1, \lambda_1)$, it is obvious that $\widehat{\alpha}_1(\lambda_1)$ maximizes $m_1(\alpha_1, \lambda_1)$ for a given λ_1, where $\widehat{\alpha}_1(\lambda_1)$ is given by Eq. (16). Once we obtain $\widehat{\lambda}_1$ by maximizing $m_1(\widehat{\alpha}_1(\lambda_1), \lambda_1)$, we can obtain $\widehat{\alpha}_1 = \widehat{\alpha}_1(\widehat{\lambda}_1)$. Unlike the Type-II censoring case, the inference associated with $m_2(\alpha_2, \lambda_2)$ is much simplified for obtaining $\widehat{\alpha}_2$ and $\widehat{\lambda}_2$ in the complete sample case.

From the normal equations associated with $m_2(\alpha_2, \lambda_2)$ and proceeding along the same lines as in Appendix section "Normal Equations for the Type-II Censoring

Case", it can be easily seen that $\widehat{\alpha}_2(\lambda_2)$ maximizes $m_2(\alpha_2, \lambda_2)$ for a given λ_2, where $\widehat{\alpha}_2(\lambda_2)$ is

$$\frac{\ln[G_0(\tau;\lambda_2)] \sum\limits_{k=n_1+1}^{n} \frac{n_0(t_{k:n};\lambda_2)}{g_0(t_{k:n};\lambda_2)} - \frac{n_1 m_0(\tau;\lambda_2)}{G_0(\tau;\lambda_2)} - \ln[G_0(\tau;\lambda_2)] \sum\limits_{k=n_1+1}^{n} \frac{m_0(t_{k:n};\lambda_2)}{G_0(t_{k:n};\lambda_2)}}{\frac{m_0(\tau;\lambda_2)}{G_0(\tau;\lambda_2)} - \ln[G_0(\tau;\lambda_2)] \sum\limits_{k=n_1+1}^{n} \frac{m_0(t_{k:n};\lambda_2)}{G_0(t_{k:n};\lambda_2)}}. \tag{21}$$

For details of the calculation and expressions for $m_0(.;\lambda_2)$ and $n_0(.;\lambda_2)$, the readers are referred to Appendix section "Normal Equations for the Type-II Censoring Case". Note that once we obtain $\widehat{\lambda}_2$ by maximizing $m_2(\widehat{\alpha}_2(\lambda_2), \lambda_2)$, we can obtain $\widehat{\alpha}_2 = \widehat{\alpha}_2(\widehat{\lambda}_2)$. The four-dimensional optimization problem now thus boils down to maximizing two one-dimensional nonlinear functions, one for each one of the scale parameters.

Remarks

1. The MLEs of $\alpha_1, \lambda_1, \alpha_2$, and λ_2 exist only when $\{2 \le n_1, n_2 \le r-2,\ r \ge 4\}$.
2. In case of equality of shape or equality in scale parameters, dimension of the optimization problem cannot be reduced. We need to perform a three-dimensional optimization problem by using some numerical routines.

Special Case: Generalized Exponential (GE) Distribution $Q(t) = t$ in (6) gives rise to the two-parameter GE distribution with shape parameter α and scale parameter λ in (5). This distribution was first considered by Gupta and Kundu (1999) as an alternative to the well-known gamma or Weibull distribution. It has received considerable amount of attention in recent years. Interested readers are referred to a survey on this distribution by Nadarajah (2011), and a recent monograph by Al-Hussaini and Ahsnullah (2015).

Based on the observed Type-II censored data in (10) and assuming a failure rate-based simple SSALT model, we obtain the log-likelihood function of $\boldsymbol{\theta}$ as follows:

$$l_{\text{GE}}(\boldsymbol{\theta} \mid \mathcal{D}) = g_1(\alpha_1, \lambda_1) + g_2(\alpha_2, \lambda_2),$$

where

$$\begin{aligned} g_1(\alpha_1, \lambda_1) &= \ln n! - \ln(n-r)! + n_1 \ln \alpha_1 + n_1 \ln \lambda_1 - \lambda_1 \sum_{k=1}^{n_1} t_{k:n} \\ &\quad + (\alpha_1 - 1) \sum_{k=1}^{n_1} \ln\left(1 - e^{-\lambda_1 t_{k:n}}\right) \\ &\quad + (n - n_1) \ln\{1 - \left(1 - e^{-\lambda_1 \tau}\right)^{\alpha_1}\}, \end{aligned} \tag{22}$$

$$g_2(\alpha_2, \lambda_2) = n_2 \ln \alpha_2 + n_2 \ln \lambda_2 - (n - n_1) \ln \left\{1 - \left(1 - e^{-\lambda_2 \tau}\right)^{\alpha_2}\right\}$$
$$+ (\alpha_2 - 1) \sum_{k=n_1+1}^{r} \ln \left(1 - e^{-\lambda_2 t_{k:n}}\right) - \lambda_2 \sum_{k=n_1+1}^{r} t_{k:n}$$
$$+ (n - r) \ln \left\{1 - \left(1 - e^{-\lambda_2 t_{r:n}}\right)^{\alpha_2}\right\}. \tag{23}$$

Differentiating the log-likelihood function $l_{GE}(\boldsymbol{\theta} \mid \mathcal{D})$ with respect to $\alpha_1, \lambda_1, \alpha_2$ and λ_2, respectively, the normal equations are obtained in Appendix section "Normal Equations for the Type-II Censoring Case." From the normal equations associated with $g_1(\alpha_1, \lambda_1)$ in (22), it can be easily seen that $\widehat{\alpha}_1(\lambda_1)$ maximizes $g_1(\alpha_1, \lambda_1)$ for a given λ_1, where

$$\widehat{\alpha}_1(\lambda_1) = \frac{\dfrac{n_1}{\lambda_1} \ln\left(1 - e^{-\lambda_1 \tau}\right) - \dfrac{n_1 \tau e^{-\lambda_1 \tau}}{1 - e^{-\lambda_1 \tau}} - \ln\left(1 - e^{-\lambda_1 \tau}\right) \sum\limits_{k=1}^{n_1} \dfrac{t_{k:n}}{1 - e^{-\lambda_1 t_{k:n}}}}{\dfrac{\tau e^{-\lambda_1 \tau}}{1 - e^{-\lambda_1 \tau}} \sum\limits_{k=1}^{n_1} \ln\left(1 - e^{-\lambda_1 t_{k:n}}\right) - \ln\left(1 - e^{-\lambda_1 \tau}\right) \sum\limits_{k=1}^{n_1} \dfrac{t_{k:n} e^{-\lambda_1 t_{k:n}}}{1 - e^{-\lambda_1 t_{k:n}}}}. \tag{24}$$

Once we obtain $\widehat{\lambda}_1$ by maximizing $g_1(\widehat{\alpha}_1(\lambda_1), \lambda_1)$, we can obtain $\widehat{\alpha}_1 = \widehat{\alpha}_1(\widehat{\lambda}_1)$.

Remarks

1. In Type-II censoring case, we need to maximize $g_2(\alpha_2, \lambda_2)$ to obtain $\widehat{\alpha}_2$ and $\widehat{\lambda}_2$.
2. Additionally, in the complete sample $(r = n)$ case, maximization of $g_2(\alpha_2, \lambda_2)$ becomes much simpler in the sense that from the normal equations associated with $g_2(\alpha_2, \lambda_2)$ in (23), it can be easily seen that $\widehat{\alpha}_2(\lambda_2)$ maximizes $g_2(\alpha_2, \lambda_2)$ for a given λ_2, where

$$\widehat{\alpha}_2(\lambda_2) = \frac{\dfrac{n_2}{\lambda_2} \ln(1 - e^{-\lambda_2 \tau}) - \dfrac{n_2 \tau e^{-\lambda_2 \tau}}{1 - e^{-\lambda_2 \tau}} - \ln(1 - e^{-\lambda_2 \tau}) \sum\limits_{k=n_1+1}^{n} \dfrac{t_{k:n}}{1 - e^{-\lambda_2 t_{k:n}}}}{\dfrac{\tau e^{-\lambda_2 \tau}}{1 - e^{-\lambda_2 \tau}} \sum\limits_{k=n_1+1}^{n} \ln(1 - e^{-\lambda_2 t_{k:n}}) - \ln(1 - e^{-\lambda_2 \tau}) \sum\limits_{k=n_1+1}^{n} \dfrac{t_{k:n} e^{-\lambda_2 t_{k:n}}}{1 - e^{-\lambda_2 t_{k:n}}}}. \tag{25}$$

Once we obtain $\widehat{\lambda}_2$ by maximizing $g_2(\widehat{\alpha}_2(\lambda_2), \lambda_2)$, we can obtain $\widehat{\alpha}_2 = \widehat{\alpha}_2(\widehat{\lambda}_2)$.

3 Interval Estimation

In this section, we present two different methods for construction of CIs of the unknown model parameters $\alpha_1, \lambda_1, \alpha_2$, and λ_2. Since the closed forms of the MLEs do not exist, we cannot obtain the exact CIs of the unknown model parameters.

First, we provide asymptotic CIs assuming the asymptotic normality of the MLEs and then the parametric bootstrap CIs.

3.1 Asymptotic Confidence Intervals

Here, we present a method that assumes asymptotic normality of the MLEs to obtain the CIs for $\alpha_1, \lambda_1, \alpha_2$, and λ_2, using the observed Fisher information matrix. This method is useful for its computational simplicity and provides good coverage probabilities (close to the nominal value) for large sample sizes.

At first, explicit expressions for elements of the Fisher information matrix $I(\boldsymbol{\theta})$ need to be obtained. Then, the $100(1-\gamma)\%$ asymptotic CIs for $\alpha_1,\ \lambda_1,\ \alpha_2,$ and λ_2 are, respectively,

$$\left(\widehat{\alpha}_1 \pm z_{1-\frac{\gamma}{2}}\sqrt{V_{11}}\right),\ \left(\widehat{\lambda}_1 \pm z_{1-\frac{\gamma}{2}}\sqrt{V_{22}}\right),\ \left(\widehat{\alpha}_2 \pm z_{1-\frac{\gamma}{2}}\sqrt{V_{33}}\right),\ \left(\widehat{\lambda}_2 \pm z_{1-\frac{\gamma}{2}}\sqrt{V_{44}}\right),$$

where z_q is the qth upper percentile of a standard normal distribution, V_{ij} is the (i, j)th element of the inverse of the Fisher information matrix $I(\boldsymbol{\theta})$.

3.2 Bootstrap Confidence Intervals

In this subsection, we obtain the parametric bootstrap CIs for $\alpha_1, \lambda_1, \alpha_2$, and λ_2. The following algorithm can be employed to construct the parametric bootstrap CIs.

Algorithm 1

Step 1: For given $n,\ r,$ and τ, the MLEs of $(\alpha_1, \lambda_1, \alpha_2, \lambda_2)$, say $(\widehat{\alpha}_1, \widehat{\lambda}_1, \widehat{\alpha}_2, \widehat{\lambda}_2)$, are computed based on the original sample $t = (t_1, \ldots, t_{n_1}, t_{n_1+1}, \ldots, t_r)$.

Step 2: To generate the bootstrap sample from the proposed model, first generate n observations from $U(0,1)$ distribution and sort them. Suppose that the ordered observations are $u_{1:n} < u_{2:n} < \cdots < u_{n:n}$.

Step 3: Find $n_1 = \max\{k : u_{k:n} \le G(\tau) \le u_{k+1:n}\}$, where $G(\tau) = \{1 - e^{-\widehat{\lambda}_1 Q(\tau)}\}^{\widehat{\alpha}_1}$.

Step 4: For $1 \le i \le n_1$, find t_i^* by solving $u_{i:n} = [G_0(t_i^*; \widehat{\lambda}_1)]^{\widehat{\alpha}_1}$ and for $n_1+1 \le i \le r$, find t_i^* by solving $u_{i:n} = 1 - \dfrac{\left\{1-[G_0(\tau;\widehat{\lambda}_1)]^{\widehat{\alpha}_1}\right\}}{\left\{1-[G_0(\tau;\widehat{\lambda}_2)]^{\widehat{\alpha}_2}\right\}}\left\{1 - [G_0(t_i^*; \widehat{\lambda}_2)]^{\widehat{\alpha}_2}\right\}$.

Step 5: Based on n, r, τ, and the bootstrap sample $\{t_1^*, t_2^*, \ldots, t_{n_1}^*, t_{n_1+1}^*, \ldots, t_r^*\}$, the MLEs of $\alpha_1, \lambda_1, \alpha_2,$ and λ_2 are computed, say $(\widehat{\alpha}_1^{(1)}, \widehat{\lambda}_1^{(1)}, \widehat{\alpha}_2^{(1)}, \widehat{\lambda}_2^{(1)})$.

Step 6: Suppose $\boldsymbol{\delta} = (\delta_1, \delta_2, \delta_3, \delta_4) = (\alpha_1, \lambda_1, \alpha_2, \lambda_2)$ and $\widehat{\boldsymbol{\delta}}^{(i)} = (\widehat{\delta}_1^{(i)}, \widehat{\delta}_2^{(i)}, \widehat{\delta}_3^{(i)}, \widehat{\delta}_4^{(i)}) = (\widehat{\alpha}_1^{(i)}, \widehat{\lambda}_1^{(i)}, \widehat{\alpha}_2^{(i)}, \widehat{\lambda}_2^{(i)})$. Repeat steps 2 − 5, B times to obtain B sets of MLE of $\boldsymbol{\delta}$, say $\widehat{\boldsymbol{\delta}}^{(i)}$, $i = 1, 2, \ldots, B$.

Step 7: Arrange $\widehat{\delta}_j^{(1)}, \widehat{\delta}_j^{(2)}, \ldots, \widehat{\delta}_j^{(B)}$ in ascending order and denote the ordered MLEs as $\widehat{\delta}_j^{[1]} < \widehat{\delta}_j^{[2]} < \cdots < \widehat{\delta}_j^{[B]}$, $j = 1, 2, 3, 4$.

A two-sided $100(1 - \alpha)\%$ bootstrap confidence interval of δ_j is then given by $(\widehat{\delta}_j^{[\frac{\alpha}{2}B]}, \widehat{\delta}_j^{[(1-\frac{\alpha}{2})B]})$, where $[x]$ denotes the largest integer less than or equal to x.

The performances of all these confidence intervals are evaluated through an extensive simulation study in Sect. 4.

4 Simulation Studies and Data Analysis

4.1 Simulation Studies

In this section, we perform extensive Monte Carlo simulation study to evaluate the performance of the proposed parameter estimation method in a simple step-stress setup. In the simulation study, we consider an important member of the Lehmann family—the GE distribution as the failure time distribution with difference in both the shape and scale parameters across the two stress levels. For analysis purpose, we have taken different sample sizes (n) ranging from moderate to large $(n = 40, 60, 80, 100)$, two different values of r $(r = 0.8n$ and $r = n)$. Associated with each of these choices of (n, r), we have considered different values of stress-changing time points $(\tau = 0.45, 0.50, 0.55)$. The parameter values are set as $\alpha_1 = 3.0$, $\lambda_1 = 1.0$, $\alpha_2 = 2.0$, and $\lambda_2 = 1.5$. The average biases and the associated mean squared errors (MSEs) of the MLEs are provided in Table 1.

For interval estimation, we resort to 95% asymptotic CIs and 95% parametric bootstrap CIs. The average lengths (ALs) and the associated coverage probabilities (CPs) of the two different CIs are reported in Tables 2 and 3, respectively. For computing the asymptotic CIs, the elements of the Fisher information matrix $I^{GE}(\alpha_1, \lambda_1, \alpha_2, \lambda_2)$ are provided in Appendix section "GE Distribution". All the results are based on 10,000 replications, and for bootstrap CIs, we have taken $B =$ 15,000.

Some of the observations are quite obvious from the above results. It can be observed from the biases in Table 1 that for fixed n and r, as τ increases, the estimates of α_1 and λ_1 approach toward the true values of α_1 and λ_1 and the corresponding MSEs decrease. On the other hand, as expected, one observes exactly the opposite behavior for the estimates of α_2 and λ_2. Again for fixed n, as r increases we can see the improved behavior of the estimates and MSEs of α_2 and λ_2. For fixed (r, τ), as the sample size grows, the MLEs approach the true values and the corresponding MSEs decrease. It indicates the asymptotic consistency property of the MLEs. The performances of both types of CIs are quite satisfactory in terms of CP. For fixed n and r, as τ increases, the average lengths of α_1 and λ_1 decrease, while under same conditions, the average lengths of α_2 and λ_2 increase. As the sample size increases, the average lengths of all the model parameters decrease, which is also quite expected.

Table 1 Biases and MSEs of MLEs of model parameters

			α_1		λ_1		α_2		λ_2	
n	r	τ	Bias	MSE	Bias	MSE	Bias	MSE	Bias	MSE
40	32	0.45	0.3364	1.8161	0.6881	0.8821	0.5698	2.5607	0.0904	0.1631
		0.50	0.2974	1.7611	0.5199	0.6048	0.6046	2.6813	0.0838	0.1714
		0.55	0.2884	1.7503	0.3981	0.4416	0.6178	2.7907	0.0767	0.1825
	40	0.45	0.3492	1.8072	0.6950	0.8885	0.4577	2.1413	0.0698	0.1033
		0.50	0.3063	1.7540	0.5242	0.6062	0.4952	2.2976	0.0681	0.1093
		0.55	0.3011	1.7650	0.4034	0.4483	0.5150	2.4648	0.0604	0.1095
60	48	0.45	0.3004	1.7216	0.4288	0.5312	0.4852	2.1975	0.0771	0.1302
		0.50	0.2643	1.6982	0.2949	0.3776	0.5103	2.3723	0.0722	0.1207
		0.55	0.2699	1.6887	0.2118	0.2942	0.5274	2.4894	0.0635	0.1217
	60	0.45	0.2734	1.6581	0.4184	0.5130	0.3825	1.7558	0.0602	0.0836
		0.50	0.2516	1.6376	0.2927	0.3695	0.4240	1.9755	0.0583	0.0847
		0.55	0.2210	1.6105	0.1925	0.2807	0.4320	2.1076	0.0516	0.0891
80	64	0.45	0.2606	1.6678	0.2821	0.3935	0.4099	1.8933	0.0619	0.1023
		0.50	0.2410	1.5942	0.1741	0.2883	0.4519	2.1073	0.0629	0.1030
		0.55	0.2325	1.5960	0.1143	0.2388	0.4848	2.2681	0.0607	0.0967
	80	0.45	0.2585	1.6335	0.2812	0.3882	0.2711	1.3723	0.0388	0.0668
		0.50	0.2302	1.6258	0.1780	0.2956	0.3177	1.5895	0.0397	0.0668
		0.55	0.2186	1.5247	0.1127	0.2325	0.3844	1.8279	0.0470	0.0670
100	80	0.45	0.2424	1.6052	0.1968	0.3290	0.3473	1.6198	0.0549	0.0935
		0.50	0.2196	1.5334	0.1175	0.2570	0.3990	1.8790	0.0544	0.0898
		0.55	0.2206	1.4764	0.0753	0.2129	0.4428	2.0723	0.0561	0.0848
	100	0.45	0.2315	1.5871	0.1937	0.3263	0.2379	1.1450	0.0348	0.0566
		0.50	0.2518	1.5701	0.1304	0.2626	0.2665	1.3618	0.0375	0.0569
		0.55	0.2381	1.5151	0.0793	0.2170	0.3118	1.5766	0.0375	0.0570

Table 2 CP and AL of 95% asymptotic CIs of the model parameters

			α_1		λ_1		α_2		λ_2	
n	r	τ	CP	AL	CP	AL	CP	AL	CP	AL
40	32	0.45	0.9549	8.3843	0.9980	4.0943	0.9997	8.8531	0.9955	2.1452
		0.50	0.9503	8.2463	0.9969	3.6549	0.9997	9.9223	0.9962	2.2166
		0.55	0.9496	8.1102	0.9942	3.2972	0.9998	9.9766	0.9974	2.2837
	40	0.45	0.9558	8.4811	0.9980	4.1150	0.9949	6.9413	0.9862	1.5422
		0.50	0.9570	8.2816	0.9961	3.6664	0.9991	7.8038	0.9886	1.5818
		0.55	0.9772	7.9878	0.9927	3.2748	0.9998	8.6274	0.9906	1.6057
60	48	0.45	0.9494	7.8394	0.9906	3.5575	0.9964	6.9265	0.9934	1.6912
		0.50	0.9465	7.6278	0.9839	3.1531	0.9988	7.8597	0.9963	1.7511
		0.55	0.9500	7.3855	0.9804	2.8270	0.9990	8.7875	0.9963	1.8054
	60	0.45	0.9491	7.7510	0.9912	3.5374	0.9822	5.5080	0.9834	1.2324
		0.50	0.9477	7.6035	0.9838	3.1512	0.9921	6.1893	0.9873	1.2606
		0.55	0.9393	7.3490	0.9772	2.8164	0.9973	6.8647	0.9874	1.2907
80	64	0.45	0.9468	7.3980	0.9798	3.2116	0.9899	5.8899	0.9899	1.4351
		0.50	0.9448	7.1114	0.9709	2.8329	0.9968	6.6501	0.9956	1.4868
		0.55	0.9467	6.8140	0.9665	2.5261	0.9995	7.5039	0.9966	1.5437
	80	0.45	0.9469	7.3705	0.9801	3.2015	0.9687	4.6845	0.9686	1.0560
		0.50	0.9472	7.1696	0.9731	2.8496	0.9817	5.2523	0.9819	1.0811
		0.55	0.9506	6.8342	0.9666	2.5317	0.9894	5.8523	0.9868	1.1048
100	80	0.45	0.9431	7.0682	0.9677	2.9701	0.9808	5.2058	0.9868	1.2756
		0.50	0.9455	6.6814	0.9609	2.6011	0.9918	5.8950	0.9941	1.3208
		0.55	0.9467	6.3581	0.9547	2.3077	0.9967	6.6584	0.9948	1.3736
	100	0.45	0.9484	7.0957	0.9702	2.9746	0.9664	4.1607	0.9646	0.9394
		0.50	0.9455	6.6820	0.9632	2.6017	0.9777	4.6742	0.9755	0.9626
		0.55	0.9458	6.3185	0.9568	2.3027	0.9812	5.1905	0.9795	0.9860

4.2 Data Analysis

4.2.1 Fish Data Set

In this section, we consider a real-life step-stress fish data set obtained from Greven et al. (2004). A sample of 15 fish were swum at initial flow rate of 15 cm/s. The time at which a fish could not maintain its position was recorded as its failure time. To ensure an early failure, the stress level was increased (flow rate by 5 cm/s) at time 110, 130, 150, and 170 min, respectively. The observed failure time data are presented in Table 4.

There are five stress levels, and the number of failures at each stress level is 4, 6, 0, 3, and 2, respectively. For our analysis purpose, we consider it as a simple step-stress data merging the first two stress levels into a single stress level and the remaining stress levels to another single stress level. For computational purpose, we have subtracted 80 from each data points, divided them by 150, and then analyzed

Table 3 CP and AL of 95% bootstrap CIs of the model parameters

			α_1		λ_1		α_2		λ_2	
n	r	τ	CP	AL	CP	AL	CP	AL	CP	AL
40	32	0.45	0.9993	5.6187	0.8156	2.7256	0.9976	6.7509	0.9843	1.6206
		0.50	0.9994	5.6028	0.8628	2.5029	0.9928	6.9105	0.9827	1.6209
		0.55	0.9996	5.5967	0.8700	2.2507	0.9996	7.0273	0.9906	1.6227
	40	0.45	0.9990	5.6346	0.8176	2.7304	0.9776	6.1875	0.9593	1.3525
		0.50	0.9996	5.6229	0.8330	2.4722	0.9923	6.4338	0.9700	1.3533
		0.55	0.9996	5.6046	0.8800	2.2555	0.9963	6.6588	0.9763	1.3675
60	48	0.45	0.9986	5.5270	0.8850	2.4634	0.9733	6.1632	0.9686	1.4139
		0.50	0.9993	5.5029	0.9400	2.2253	0.9876	6.4390	0.9820	1.4141
		0.55	0.9973	5.4828	0.9773	2.0406	0.9976	6.6909	0.9870	1.4210
	60	0.45	0.9993	5.5175	0.8810	2.4599	0.9536	5.4065	0.9490	1.1519
		0.50	0.9990	5.5080	0.9356	2.2284	0.9686	5.7482	0.9566	1.1545
		0.55	0.9996	5.4862	0.9763	2.0467	0.9786	6.0299	0.9636	1.1548
80	64	0.45	0.9996	5.4548	0.9486	2.2963	0.9696	5.6035	0.9636	1.2732
		0.50	0.9900	5.4083	0.9830	2.0855	0.9783	5.9800	0.9670	1.2742
		0.55	0.9976	5.3813	0.9900	1.9152	0.9866	6.3047	0.9763	1.2767
	80	0.45	0.9883	5.4617	0.9503	2.3050	0.9543	4.7643	0.9436	1.0108
		0.50	0.9890	5.4203	0.9810	2.0881	0.9560	5.2115	0.9510	1.0143
		0.55	0.9866	5.3690	0.9856	1.9179	0.9646	5.5305	0.9493	1.0800
100	80	0.45	0.9890	5.3960	0.9813	2.1937	0.9583	5.1345	0.9560	1.1724
		0.50	0.9883	5.3445	0.9893	1.9904	0.9650	5.5649	0.9586	1.1722
		0.55	0.9843	5.2703	0.9890	1.8300	0.9750	5.9379	0.9680	1.1726
	100	0.45	0.9890	5.3952	0.9826	2.1945	0.9560	4.2940	0.9530	0.9216
		0.50	0.9850	5.3325	0.9800	1.9885	0.9620	4.6512	0.9526	0.9217
		0.55	0.9833	5.2506	0.9866	1.8265	0.9613	5.0611	0.9453	0.9260

Table 4 Fish data set

Stress level	Failure times
s_1	91.00, 93.00, 94.00, 98.20
s_2	115.81, 116.00, 116.50, 117.25, 126.75, 127.50
s_3	No failures
s_4	154.33, 159.50, 164.00
s_5	184.14, 188.33

the data with $n = r = 15$, $\tau = 0.33$. Here, we consider the complete sample for analysis purpose and stop at the 15th failure to facilitate the Type-II censoring.

As a choice of the failure time distribution, we consider three members (GE, GR, and EP) of the Lehmann family of distributions. All these three distributions are fitted to the Fish data set assuming difference in both the shape and scale parameters at each of the two stress levels. MLEs of the model parameters are obtained by solving one-dimensional optimization problems. The MLEs of the

Table 5 MLEs, K-S statistics, and the corresponding p-values of the Fish data set

Model	MLEs		K-S statistics	p-Value
GE	$\widehat{\alpha}_1$	2.8304	0.1833	0.6437
	$\widehat{\lambda}_1$	5.8775		
	$\widehat{\alpha}_2$	2264.2688		
	$\widehat{\lambda}_2$	13.8730		
GR	$\widehat{\alpha}_1$	0.9459	0.1639	0.7776
	$\widehat{\lambda}_1$	9.2678		
	$\widehat{\alpha}_2$	35.1339		
	$\widehat{\lambda}_2$	11.3299		
EP	$\widehat{\alpha}_1$	3.3031	0.1901	0.6022
	$\widehat{\lambda}_1$	7.2645		
	$\widehat{\alpha}_2$	17,876.6484		
	$\widehat{\lambda}_2$	22.1745		

Table 6 Bootstrap CIs of parameters based on the Fish data set

		α_1		λ_1		α_2		λ_2	
Model	Level	LL	UL	LL	UL	LL	UL	LL	UL
GE	90%	1.4493	8.5005	2.9325	9.7810	976.3842	4129.729	11.7081	15.4846
	95%	1.2838	10.7785	2.4991	10.6449	938.3585	4315.795	11.4094	15.8299
	99%	1.0355	16.1782	1.6474	12.1417	907.2052	4460.666	10.7977	16.5033
GR	90%	0.5371	1.6997	3.1702	13.1903	12.3428	88.2046	7.6982	15.2679
	95%	0.4878	1.9145	2.3662	13.5989	11.1726	93.8493	7.2067	16.0640
	99%	0.4097	2.4103	1.5100	13.9127	10.2514	98.6554	6.4699	17.8533
EP	90%	1.6466	10.1209	3.7740	11.8878	12,572.91	28,660.54	20.2098	24.1174
	95%	1.4745	12.6201	3.2021	12.7611	12,284.68	29,350.65	19.7901	24.4845
	99%	1.1784	17.2071	2.0931	14.5229	12,052.65	29,883.83	18.9644	25.2057

model parameters, the Kolmogorov–Smirnov (K-S) distances between the fitted and the empirical distribution functions, and the p-values for the K-S test are presented in Table 5. 90%, 95%, and 99%, bootstrap CIs are presented in Table 6.

Examining the K-S statistics and the p-values, it is observed that although all the three distributions fit the data well, the GR distribution has a better fit than the other two distributions. The plot of the empirical CDF along with the fitted CDF based on the GR fit is provided in Fig. 1.

In Figs. 2 and 3, we have provided the plots for the profile likelihood functions of λ_1 and λ_2, respectively. It is observed that both the functions are unimodal functions of the respective parameters.

One may be interested to know whether we can analyze the same data assuming equality of the shape or equality of the scale parameters. For this purpose, we perform the corresponding likelihood ratio-based tests. First, we want to test the following hypotheses:

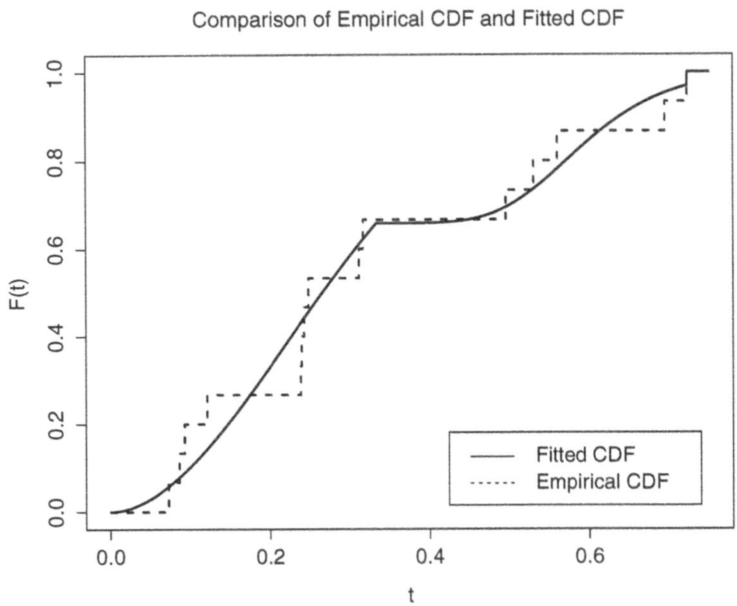

Fig. 1 Plot of empirical and fitted CDFs of Fish data set assuming GR distribution

A. $H_o : \alpha_1 = \alpha_2$ **vs** $H_1 : \alpha_1 \neq \alpha_2$.
Under H_o, the MLEs are $\widetilde{\alpha} = 1.0367$, $\widetilde{\lambda}_1 = 10.0857$, $\widetilde{\lambda}_2 = 3.9102$. The likelihood ratio test (LRT) statistic and $-2lnLRT$ are obtained as 0.0896 and 4.8245, respectively, and the corresponding p value is 0.0280. Thus, we reject the null hypothesis in this case at 5% level of significance.

Now we consider the following testing problem:

B. $H_o : \lambda_1 = \lambda_2$ **vs** $H_1 : \lambda_1 \neq \lambda_2$.
Under H_o, the MLEs are: $\widetilde{\alpha}_1 = 1.0125$, $\widetilde{\alpha}_2 = 26.6399$, $\widetilde{\lambda} = 10.3797$. The likelihood ratio test (LRT) statistic and $-2lnLRT$ are obtained as 0.9490 and 0.1045, respectively. The corresponding p value is 0.7464. Thus, in this case, we accept the null hypothesis.

The two testing procedures lead us to assume difference in shape parameters and equality in scale parameters and carry on the appropriate analysis assuming the GR distribution. Assuming different shape parameters and common scale parameters, the MLEs of the model parameters are obtained as $\widehat{\alpha}_1 = 1.0125$, $\widehat{\alpha}_2 = 26.6399$, $\widehat{\lambda} = 10.3797$. As a measure of the goodness of fit, we have computed the K-S statistics and the associated p-value. The K-S distance and the associated p-value are obtained as 0.1753 and 0.7023, respectively. It indicates a good fit of the given data. The plot of the empirical v/s the fitted CDFs is shown in Fig. 4. 90%, 95%, and 99% asymptotic and bootstrap CIs of the model parameters are given in Table 7. The elements of the associated Fisher information matrix $I_{sc}^{GR}(\alpha_1, \lambda, \alpha_2)$ are provided in

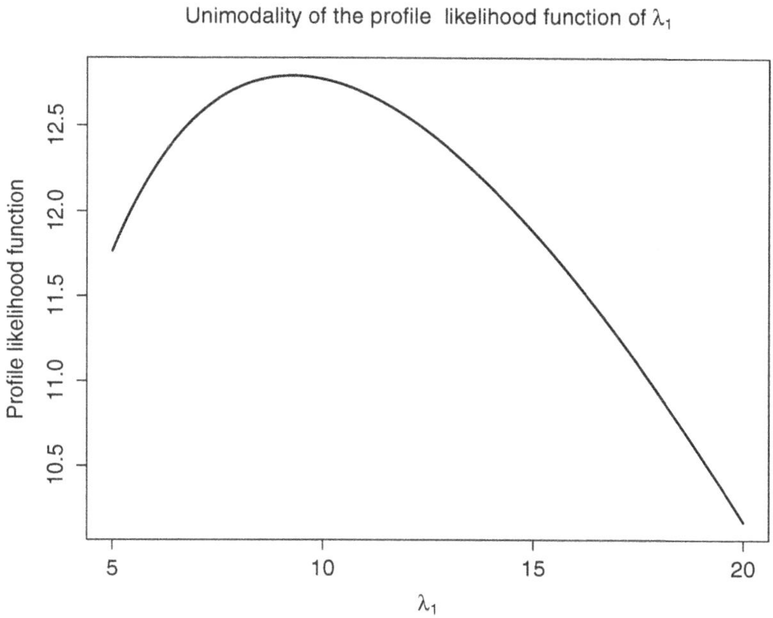

Fig. 2 Unimodality of the profile log-likelihood function of λ_1 for Fish data set assuming GR distribution

Appendix section "GR Distribution with Different Shape and Common Scale Parameter".

5 Conclusion

In this chapter, we have considered the likelihood inference of a simple-step stress model under Type-II censoring, when the lifetime distribution at each of the stress levels belongs to the Lehmann family of distributions. To relate the distributions at the two stress levels, a failure rate-based SSALT model is proposed. Further, all the underlying two parameters (especially the shape parameter) of the lifetime distribution are allowed to vary across the stress levels, which makes this model a flexible one. In case of Type-II censoring, the MLEs of the model parameters can be obtained by solving a one-dimensional and a two-dimensional optimization problems. Again, in the complete sample case, inference becomes much simplified in terms of dimension reduction, as expected. The MLEs can then be obtained by solving two one-dimensional optimization problems. Due to the absence of closed form solutions of the likelihood equations, the asymptotic and the bootstrap CIs have been obtained here. Performance of the proposed model for analyzing time to failure

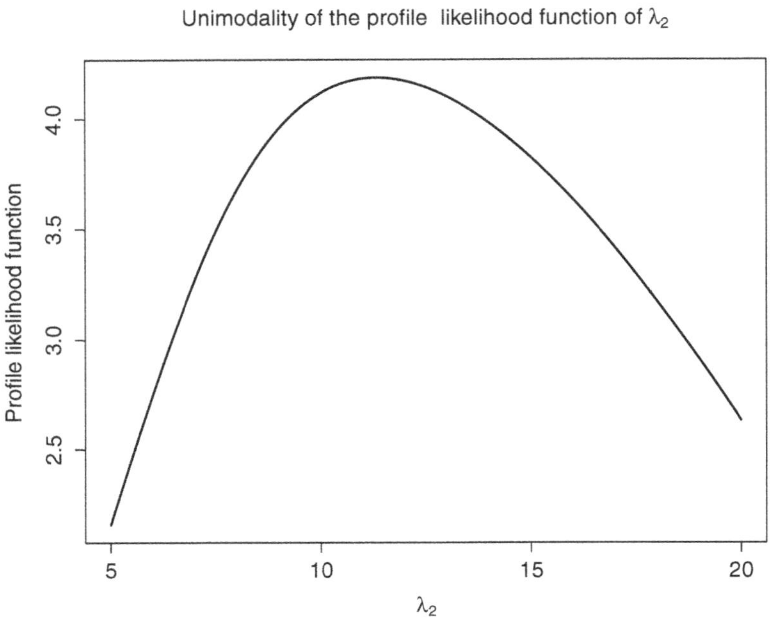

Fig. 3 Unimodality of the profile log-likelihood function of λ_2 for Fish data set assuming GR distribution

Table 7 Asymptotic and bootstrap CIs of Fish data set

		α_1		λ		α_2	
CI	Level	LL	UL	LL	UL	LL	UL
Asymptotic	90%	0.4807	1.5442	5.1565	15.6028	0	72.0466
	95%	0.3788	4.1556	16.6038	1.6461	0	80.7481
	99%	0.1796	1.8453	2.1995	18.5500	0	97.7535
Bootstrap	90%	0.6674	1.8023	6.8463	14.1895	8.3102	62.6906
	95%	0.6159	2.0243	6.2858	14.9762	6.7643	66.2360
	99%	0.5307	2.5515	5.3487	16.6555	4.3802	69.2758

data has been evaluated through an extensive simulation study considering GE distribution, an important distribution of the Lehmann family. From the simulation study, it has been observed that the estimators are consistent and the CPs of the different CIs are close to the nominal values.

A real data set is analyzed for illustrative purpose. It has been observed that different members of the general family fit the data set quite well.

Although we have only considered the Type-II censoring here, the data set from other censoring schemes can also be analyzed in a similar way. Again, not restricting to a simple step-stress model, the analysis can easily be extended to a multiple step-stress scenario. In this work, we have only considered the classical inference of the

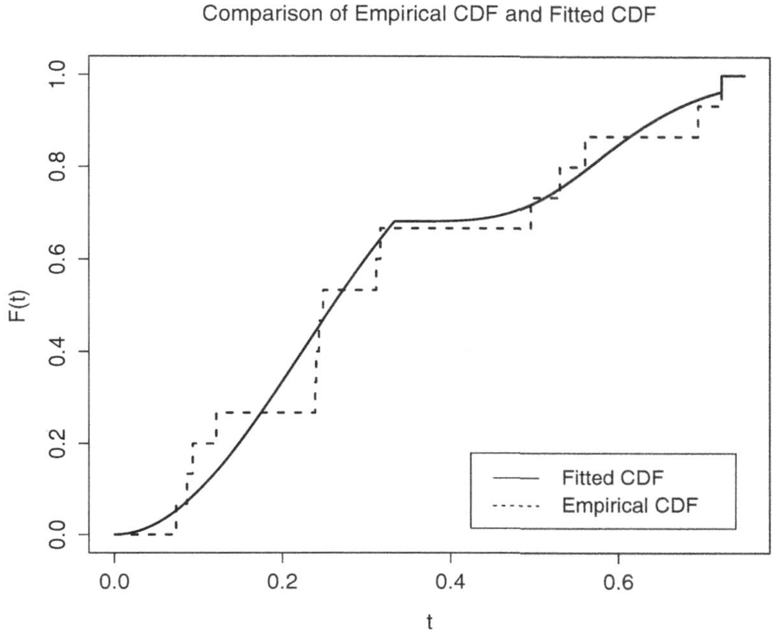

Fig. 4 Plot of empirical and fitted CDFs of Fish data set assuming GR distribution with different shape parameters and common scale parameter

proposed model. However, it would be interesting to work on the Bayesian analysis of the proposed model. The order-restricted inference can also be considered for this model. More work is needed along these directions.

Acknowledgments The authors would like to thank the reviewers for their constructive comments that had helped to improve the manuscript significantly.

Appendix

Lehmann Family of Distributions

Normal Equations for the Type-II Censoring Case

The normal equations associated with the log-likelihood function (13) are given by

$$\frac{\partial l^{II}}{\partial \alpha_1} = \frac{n_1}{\alpha_1} + \sum_{k=1}^{n_1} \ln G_0(t_{k:n}; \lambda_1) - \frac{(n-n_1)\{G_0(\tau; \lambda_1)\}^{\alpha_1} \ln G_0(\tau; \lambda_1)}{1 - \{G_0(\tau; \lambda_1)\}^{\alpha_1}} = 0, \tag{A.1}$$

$$\frac{\partial l^{II}}{\partial \lambda_1} = (\alpha_1 - 1) \sum_{k=1}^{n_1} \frac{m_0(t_{k:n}; \lambda_1)}{G_0(t_{k:n}; \lambda_1)} - \frac{(n-n_1)\alpha_1\{G_0(\tau; \lambda_1)\}^{\alpha_1 - 1} m_0(\tau; \lambda_1)}{1 - \{G_0(\tau; \lambda_1)\}^{\alpha_1}} + \sum_{k=1}^{n_1} \frac{n_0(t_{k:n}; \lambda_1)}{g_0(t_{k:n}; \lambda_1)} = 0, \tag{A.2}$$

$$\frac{\partial l^{II}}{\partial \alpha_2} = \frac{n_2}{\alpha_2} - \sum_{k=n_1+1}^{r} \ln G_0(t_{k:n}; \lambda_1) + \frac{(n-n_1)\{G_0(\tau; \lambda_2)\}^{\alpha_2} \ln G_0(\tau; \lambda_2)}{1 - \{G_0(\tau; \lambda_2)\}^{\alpha_2}} - \frac{(n-r)\{G_0(t_{r:n}; \lambda_2)\}^{\alpha_2} \ln G_0(t_{r:n}; \lambda_2)}{1 - \{G_0(t_{r:n}; \lambda_2)\}^{\alpha_2}} = 0, \tag{A.3}$$

$$\frac{\partial l^{II}}{\partial \lambda_2} = (\alpha_2 - 1) \sum_{k=n_1+1}^{r} \frac{m_0(t_{k:n}; \lambda_2)}{G_0(t_{k:n}; \lambda_2)} + \frac{(n-n_1)\alpha_2\{G_0(\tau; \lambda_2)\}^{\alpha_2 - 1} m_0(\tau; \lambda_2)}{1 - \{G_0(\tau; \lambda_2)\}^{\alpha_2}} + \sum_{k=n_1+1}^{r} \frac{n_0(t_{k:n}; \lambda_2)}{g_0(t_{k:n}; \lambda_2)} - \frac{(n-r)\alpha_2\{G_0(t_{r:n}; \lambda_2)\}^{\alpha_2 - 1} m_0(t_{r:n}; \lambda_2)}{1 - \{G_0(t_{r:n}; \lambda_2)\}^{\alpha_2}} = 0, \tag{A.4}$$

where

$$m_0(.; \lambda_1) = \frac{\partial}{\partial \lambda_1} G_0(.; \lambda_1), \quad n_0(.; \lambda_1) = \frac{\partial}{\partial \lambda_1} g_0(.; \lambda_1),$$
$$m_0(.; \lambda_2) = \frac{\partial}{\partial \lambda_2} G_0(.; \lambda_2), \quad n_0(.; \lambda_2) = \frac{\partial}{\partial \lambda_2} g_0(.; \lambda_2).$$

Now multiplying (A.1) by $\frac{\alpha_1 m_0(\tau; \lambda_1)}{G_0(\tau; \lambda_1)}$ and (A.2) by $\ln G_0(\tau; \lambda_1)$, respectively, we have

$$\frac{n_1 m_0(\tau; \lambda_1)}{G_0(\tau; \lambda_1)} - \frac{(n-n_1)\alpha_1\{G_0(\tau; \lambda_1)\}^{\alpha_1 - 1} m_0(\tau; \lambda_1) \ln G_0(\tau; \lambda_1)}{1 - \{G_0(\tau; \lambda_1)\}^{\alpha_1}} + \frac{\alpha_1 m_0(\tau; \lambda_1)}{G_0(\tau; \lambda_1)} \sum_{k=1}^{n_1} \ln G_0(t_{k:n}; \lambda_1) = 0, \tag{A.5}$$

$$
-\frac{(n-n_1)\alpha_1\{G_0(\tau;\lambda_1)\}^{\alpha_1-1}m_0(\tau;\lambda_1)\ln G_0(\tau;\lambda_1)}{1-\{G_0(\tau;\lambda_1)\}^{\alpha_1}}
$$

$$
+\ln G_0(\tau;\lambda_1)\sum_{k=1}^{n_1}\frac{n_0(t_{k:n};\lambda_1)}{g_0(t_{k:n};\lambda_1)}+(\alpha_1-1)\ln G_0(\tau;\lambda_1)\sum_{k=1}^{n_1}\frac{m_0(t_{k:n};\lambda_1)}{G_0(t_{k:n};\lambda_1)}=0. \tag{A.6}
$$

Subtracting (A.6) from (A.5), and after little simplification, finally we establish the following relation and $\widehat{\alpha}_1(\lambda_1)$ is

$$
\frac{\ln[G_0(\tau;\lambda_1)]\sum_{k=1}^{n_1}\frac{n_o(t_{k:n};\lambda_1)}{g_0(t_{k:n};\lambda_1)}-\frac{n_1 m_o(\tau;\lambda_1)}{G_0(\tau;\lambda_1)}-\ln[G_0(\tau;\lambda_1)]\sum_{k=1}^{n_1}\frac{m_o(t_{k:n};\lambda_1)}{G_0(t_{k:n};\lambda_1)}}{\frac{m_o(\tau;\lambda_1)}{G_0(\tau;\lambda_1)}-\ln[G_0(\tau;\lambda_1)]\sum_{k=1}^{n_1}\frac{m_o(t_{k:n};\lambda_1)}{G_0(t_{k:n};\lambda_1)}}. \tag{A.7}
$$

Normal Equations for the Complete Sample Case

$$
\frac{\partial l^c}{\partial \alpha_1}=\frac{n_1}{\alpha_1}+\sum_{k=1}^{n_1}\ln G_0(t_{k:n};\lambda_1)-\frac{(n-n_1)\{G_0(\tau;\lambda_1)\}^{\alpha_1}\ln G_0(\tau;\lambda_1)}{1-\{G_0(\tau;\lambda_1)\}^{\alpha_1}}=0,
$$

$$
\frac{\partial l^c}{\partial \lambda_1}=(\alpha_1-1)\sum_{k=1}^{n_1}\frac{m_o(t_{k:n};\lambda_1)}{G_0(t_{k:n};\lambda_1)}-\frac{(n-n_1)\alpha_1\{G_0(\tau;\lambda_1)\}^{\alpha_1-1}m_o(\tau;\lambda_1)}{1-\{G_0(\tau;\lambda_1)\}^{\alpha_1}}
$$

$$
+\sum_{k=1}^{n_1}\frac{n_o(t_{k:n};\lambda_1)}{g_0(t_{k:n};\lambda_1)}=0,
$$

$$
\frac{\partial l^c}{\partial \alpha_2}=\frac{n_2}{\alpha_2}-\sum_{k=n_1+1}^{r}\ln G_0(t_{k:n};\lambda_1)+\frac{(n-n_1)\{G_0(\tau;\lambda_2)\}^{\alpha_2}\ln G_0(\tau;\lambda_2)}{1-\{G_0(\tau;\lambda_2)\}^{\alpha_2}}=0,
$$

$$
\frac{\partial l^c}{\partial \lambda_2}=(\alpha_2-1)\sum_{k=n_1+1}^{r}\frac{m_o(t_{k:n};\lambda_2)}{G_0(t_{k:n};\lambda_2)}+\frac{(n-n_1)\alpha_2\{G_0(\tau;\lambda_2)\}^{\alpha_2-1}m_o(\tau;\lambda_2)}{1-\{G_0(\tau;\lambda_2)\}^{\alpha_2}}
$$

$$
+\sum_{k=n_1+1}^{r}\frac{n_o(t_{k:n};\lambda_2)}{g_0(t_{k:n};\lambda_2)}=0.
$$

Special Case: GE Distribution

Normal Equations for the Type-II Censoring Case

$$\frac{\partial l_{\text{GE}}}{\partial \alpha_1} = \frac{n_1}{\alpha_1} + \sum_{k=1}^{n_1} \ln(1 - e^{-\lambda_1 t_{k:n}}) - A(\alpha_1, \lambda_1) = 0, \tag{A.8}$$

$$\frac{\partial l_{\text{GE}}}{\partial \lambda_1} = \frac{n_1}{\lambda_1} - \sum_{k=1}^{n_1} t_{k:n} + (\alpha_1 - 1) \sum_{k=1}^{n_1} \frac{t_{k:n} e^{-\lambda_1 t_{k:n}}}{1 - e^{-\lambda_1 t_{k:n}}} - B(\alpha_1, \lambda_1) = 0, \tag{A.9}$$

$$\frac{\partial l_{\text{GE}}}{\partial \alpha_2} = \frac{n_2}{\alpha_2} + \sum_{k=n_1+1}^{n_1+n_2} \ln(1 - e^{-\lambda_2 t_{k:n}}) + C_1(\alpha_2, \lambda_2) - C_2(\alpha_2, \lambda_2) = 0, \tag{A.10}$$

$$\frac{\partial l_{\text{GE}}}{\partial \lambda_2} = \frac{n_2}{\lambda_2} - \sum_{k=n_1+1}^{n_1+n_2} t_{k:n} + (\alpha_2 - 1) \sum_{k=n_1+1}^{n_1+n_2} \frac{t_{k:n} e^{-\lambda_2 t_{k:n}}}{1 - e^{-\lambda_2 t_{k:n}}} + D_1(\alpha_2, \lambda_2)$$
$$- D_2(\alpha_2, \lambda_2) = 0, \tag{A.11}$$

where

$$A(\alpha_1, \lambda_1) = \frac{(n - n_1)\left(1 - e^{-\lambda_1 \tau}\right)^{\alpha_1}}{1 - \left(1 - e^{-\lambda_1 \tau}\right)^{\alpha_1}} \ln\left(1 - e^{-\lambda_1 \tau}\right),$$

$$B(\alpha_1, \lambda_1) = \frac{(n - n_1)\alpha_1 \tau e^{-\lambda_1 \tau}\left(1 - e^{-\lambda_1 \tau}\right)^{\alpha_1 - 1}}{1 - \left(1 - e^{-\lambda_1 \tau}\right)^{\alpha_1}},$$

$$C_1(\alpha_2, \lambda_2) = \frac{(n - n_1)\left(1 - e^{-\lambda_2 \tau}\right)^{\alpha_2}}{1 - \left(1 - e^{-\lambda_2 \tau}\right)^{\alpha_2}} \ln\left(1 - e^{-\lambda_2 \tau}\right),$$

$$C_2(\alpha_2, \lambda_2) = \frac{(n - r)\left(1 - e^{-\lambda_2 t_{r:n}}\right)^{\alpha_2}}{1 - \left(1 - e^{-\lambda_2 t_{r:n}}\right)^{\alpha_2}} \ln\left(1 - e^{-\lambda_2 t_{r:n}}\right),$$

$$D_1(\alpha_2, \lambda_2) = \frac{(n - n_1)\alpha_2 \tau\left(1 - e^{-\lambda_2 \tau}\right)^{\alpha_2 - 1} e^{-\lambda_2 \tau}}{1 - \left(1 - e^{-\lambda_2 \tau}\right)^{\alpha_2}},$$

$$D_2(\alpha_2, \lambda_2) = \frac{(n - r)\alpha_2 t_{r:n}\left(1 - e^{-\lambda_2 t_{r:n}}\right)^{\alpha_2 - 1} e^{-\lambda_2 t_{r:n}}}{1 - \left(1 - e^{-\lambda_2 t_{r:n}}\right)^{\alpha_2}}.$$

Elements of the Fisher Information Matrix

GE Distribution

The Fisher information matrix $I^{\text{GE}}(\alpha_1, \lambda_1, \alpha_2, \lambda_2)$ can be expressed using two block diagonal matrices, viz., $I_1^{\text{GE}}(\alpha_1, \lambda_1)$ and $I_2^{\text{GE}}(\alpha_2, \lambda_2)$. Thus, we have

$$I^{\text{GE}}(\alpha_1, \lambda_1, \alpha_2, \lambda_2) = \begin{bmatrix} I_1^{\text{GE}}(\alpha_1, \lambda_1) & \mathbf{0} \\ \mathbf{0} & I_2^{\text{GE}}(\alpha_2, \lambda_2) \end{bmatrix}$$

The elements of $I_1^{\text{GE}}(\alpha_1, \lambda_1) = \begin{bmatrix} -\dfrac{\partial^2 l^{\text{GE}}}{\partial \alpha_1^2} & -\dfrac{\partial^2 l^{\text{GE}}}{\partial \alpha_1 \partial \lambda_1} \\ -\dfrac{\partial^2 l^{\text{GE}}}{\partial \alpha_1 \partial \lambda_1} & -\dfrac{\partial^2 l^{\text{GE}}}{\partial \lambda_1^2} \end{bmatrix}$ are

$$\frac{\partial^2 l^{\text{GE}}}{\partial \alpha_1^2} = -\left(\frac{n_1}{\alpha_1^2} + \frac{(n-n_1)\left(1-e^{-\lambda_1\tau}\right)^{\alpha_1}\{\ln[1-e^{-\lambda_1\tau}]\}^2}{\{1-\left(1-e^{-\lambda_1\tau}\right)^{\alpha_1}\}^2}\right),$$

$$\frac{\partial^2 l^{\text{GE}}}{\partial \alpha_1 \partial \lambda_1} = \sum_{k=1}^{n_1} \frac{t_{k:n} e^{-\lambda_1 t_{k:n}}}{1-e^{-\lambda_1 t_{k:n}}} - (n-n_1)\tau e^{-\lambda_1\tau} \varrho_1(\alpha_1, \lambda_1),$$

$$\frac{\partial^2 l^{\text{GE}}}{\partial \lambda_1^2} = -\left(\frac{n_1}{\lambda_1^2} - (\alpha_1 - 1)\psi_1(\lambda_1) + (n-n_1)\alpha_1\tau\kappa_1(\alpha_1, \lambda_1, \tau)\right),$$

where

$$\varrho_1(\alpha_1, \lambda_1) = \frac{\{1-r(\lambda_1)^{\alpha_1}\}\left[r(\lambda_1)^{\alpha_1}\{\alpha_1 \ln(r(\lambda_1)+1\}\right] + \alpha_1 r(\lambda_1)^{2\alpha_1}\ln(r(\lambda_1)}{r(\lambda_1)\{1-r(\lambda_1)^{\alpha_1}\}^2},$$

$$\psi_1(\lambda_1) = -\sum_{k=1}^{n_1} \frac{t_{k:n}^2 e^{-\lambda_1 t_{k:n}}}{(1-e^{-\lambda_1 t_{k:n}})^2},$$

$$\kappa_1(\alpha_1, \lambda_1) = \frac{\{1-r(\lambda_1)^{\alpha_1}\}\left[r(\lambda_1)^{\alpha_1-2}\tau e^{-\lambda_1\tau}\{\alpha_1 e^{-\lambda_1\tau} - 1\}\right] + \alpha_1\tau e^{-2\lambda_1\tau} r(\lambda_1)^{2\alpha_1-2}}{\{1-r(\lambda_1)^{\alpha_1}\}^2},$$

$$r_1(\lambda_1) = \left(1-e^{-\lambda_1\tau}\right).$$

The elements of $I_2^{\text{GE}}(\alpha_2, \lambda_2) = \begin{bmatrix} -\dfrac{\partial^2 l^{\text{GE}}}{\partial \alpha_2^2} & -\dfrac{\partial^2 l^{\text{GE}}}{\partial \alpha_2 \partial \lambda_2} \\ -\dfrac{\partial^2 l^{\text{GE}}}{\partial \alpha_1 \partial \lambda_1} & -\dfrac{\partial^2 l^{\text{GE}}}{\partial \lambda_2^2} \end{bmatrix}$ are

$$\frac{\partial^2 l^{GE}}{\partial \alpha_2^2} = -\left(\frac{n_2}{\alpha_2^2} - (n-n_1)\beta_1(\alpha_2,\lambda_2) + (n-r)\eta_1(\alpha_2,\lambda_2)\right),$$

$$\frac{\partial^2 l^{GE}}{\partial \alpha_2 \partial \lambda_2} = \sum_{k=n_1+1}^{n_1+n_2} \frac{t_{k:n} e^{-\lambda_2 t_{k:n}}}{1-e^{-\lambda_2 t_{k:n}}} + (n-n_1)\xi_1(\alpha_2,\lambda_2) - (n-r)\Upsilon_1(\alpha_2,\lambda_2),$$

$$\frac{\partial^2 l^{GE}}{\partial \lambda_2^2} = -\left(\frac{n_2}{\lambda_2^2} - (n-n_1)\sigma_1(\alpha_2,\lambda_2) - (\alpha_2-1)\delta_1(\lambda_2) + (n-r)\zeta_1(\alpha_2,\lambda_2)\right),$$

where

$$\beta_1(\alpha_2,\lambda_2) = \frac{\left(1-e^{-\lambda_2\tau}\right)^{\alpha_2}\{\ln[1-e^{-\lambda_2\tau}]\}^2}{\{1-(1-e^{-\lambda_2\tau})^{\alpha_2}\}^2},$$

$$\eta_1(\alpha_2,\lambda_2) = \frac{\left(1-e^{-\lambda_2 t_{r:n}}\right)^{\alpha_2}\{\ln[1-e^{-\lambda_2 t_{r:n}}]\}^2}{\{1-\left(1-e^{-\lambda_2 t_{r:n}}\right)^{\alpha_2}\}^2},$$

$$\xi_1(\alpha_2,\lambda_2) = \tau e^{-\lambda_2\tau}\frac{\{1-q_1(\lambda_2)^{\alpha_2}\}\left[q_1(\lambda_2)^{\alpha_2}\{\alpha_2\ln(q_1(\lambda_2)+1\}\right]}{q_1(\lambda_2)\{1-q_1(\lambda_2)^{\alpha_2}\}^2}$$

$$+\tau e^{-\lambda_2\tau}\frac{\alpha_2 q_1(\lambda_2)^{2\alpha_2}\ln(q_1(\lambda_2)}{q_1(\lambda_2)\{1-q_1(\lambda_2)^{\alpha_2}\}^2},$$

$$\Upsilon_1(\alpha_2,\lambda_2) = t_{r:n} e^{-\lambda_2 t_{r:n}}\frac{\{1-s_1(\lambda_2)^{\alpha_2}\}\left[s_1(\lambda_2)^{\alpha_2}\{\alpha_2\ln(s_1(\lambda_2)+1\}\right]}{s_1(\lambda_2)\{1-s_1(\lambda_2)^{\alpha_2}\}^2}$$

$$+t_{r:n} e^{-\lambda_2 t_{r:n}}\frac{\alpha_2 s_1(\lambda_2)^{2\alpha_2}\ln(s_1(\lambda_2)}{s_1(\lambda_2)\{1-s_1(\lambda_2)^{\alpha_2}\}^2},$$

$$\sigma_1(\alpha_2,\lambda_2) = \alpha_2\tau\frac{\{1-q_1(\lambda_2)^{\alpha_2}\}\left[q_1(\lambda_2)^{\alpha_2-2}\tau e^{-\lambda_2\tau}\{\alpha_2 e^{-\lambda_2\tau}-1\}\right]}{\{1-q_1(\lambda_2)^{\alpha_2}\}^2}$$

$$+\alpha_2\tau\frac{\alpha_2\tau e^{-2\lambda_2\tau}q_1(\lambda_2)^{2\alpha_2-2}}{\{1-q_1(\lambda_2)^{\alpha_2}\}^2},$$

$$\delta(\lambda_2) = -\sum_{k=n_1+1}^{n_1+n_2}\left[\frac{t_{k:n}^2 e^{-\lambda_2 t_{k:n}}}{\left(1-e^{-\lambda_2 t_{k:n}}\right)^2}\right],$$

$$q_1(\lambda_2) = \left(1-e^{-\lambda_2\tau}\right),\ s_1(\lambda_2) = \left(1-e^{-\lambda_2 t_{r:n}}\right).$$

$$\zeta_1(\alpha_2,\lambda_2) = \alpha_2 t_{r:n}\frac{\{1-s_1(\lambda_2)^{\alpha_2}\}\left[s_1(\lambda_2)^{\alpha_2-2} t_{r:n} e^{-\lambda_2 t_{r:n}}\{\alpha_2 e^{-\lambda_2 t_{r:n}}-1\}\right]}{\{1-s_1(\lambda_2)^{\alpha_2}\}^2}$$

$$+\alpha_2 t_{r:n}\frac{\alpha_2 t_{r:n} e^{-2\lambda_2 t_{r:n}} s_1(\lambda_2)^{2\alpha_2-2}}{\{1-s_1(\lambda_2)^{\alpha_2}\}^2}.$$

GR Distribution with Different Shape and Common Scale Parameter

Let the Fisher information matrix associated with the parameters α_1, λ, α_2, respectively, be

$$I_{\text{sc}}^{\text{GR}}(\alpha_1,\lambda,\alpha_2) = \begin{bmatrix} -\frac{\partial^2 l_{\text{sc}}^{\text{GR}}}{\partial\alpha_1^2} & -\frac{\partial^2 l_{\text{sc}}^{\text{GR}}}{\partial\alpha_1\partial\lambda} & -\frac{\partial^2 l_{\text{sc}}^{\text{GR}}}{\partial\alpha_1\partial\alpha_2} \\ -\frac{\partial^2 l_{\text{sc}}^{\text{GR}}}{\partial\alpha_1\partial\lambda} & -\frac{\partial^2 l_{\text{sc}}^{\text{GR}}}{\partial\lambda^2} & -\frac{\partial^2 l_{\text{sc}}^{\text{GR}}}{\partial\alpha_2\partial\lambda} \\ -\frac{\partial^2 l_{\text{sc}}^{\text{GR}}}{\partial\alpha_1\partial\alpha_2} & -\frac{\partial^2 l_{\text{sc}}^{\text{GR}}}{\partial\alpha_2\partial\lambda} & -\frac{\partial^2 l_{\text{sc}}^{\text{GR}}}{\partial\alpha_2^2} \end{bmatrix}$$

The corresponding elements are

$$\frac{\partial^2 l_{\text{sc}}^{\text{GR}}}{\partial\alpha_1^2} = -\left(\frac{n_1}{\alpha_1^2}+\frac{(n-n_1)\left(1-e^{-\lambda\tau^2}\right)^{\alpha_1}\{\ln[1-e^{-\lambda\tau^2}]\}^2}{\{1-\left(1-e^{-\lambda\tau^2}\right)^{\alpha_1}\}^2}\right),$$

$$\frac{\partial^2 l_{\text{sc}}^{\text{GR}}}{\partial\alpha_1\partial\lambda} = \sum_{k=1}^{n_1}\frac{t_{k:n}^2 e^{-\lambda t_{k:n}^2}}{1-e^{-\lambda t_{k:n}^2}} - (n-n_1)\varrho_3(\alpha_1,\lambda), \quad \frac{\partial^2 l_{\text{sc}}^{\text{GR}}}{\partial\alpha_1\partial\alpha_2} = 0,$$

$$\frac{\partial^2 l^{\text{GR}}}{\partial\lambda^2} = -\left(\frac{n}{\lambda^2} - (\alpha_1-1)\psi_3(\lambda) + (n-n_1)\kappa_3(\alpha_1,\lambda) - (n-n_1)\sigma_3(\alpha_2,\lambda)\right.$$

$$\left. - (\alpha_2-1)\delta_3(\lambda)\right),$$

$$\frac{\partial^2 l_{\mathrm{sc}}^{\mathrm{GR}}}{\partial \alpha_2 \partial \lambda} = \sum_{k=n_1+1}^{n_1+n_2} \frac{t_{k:n}^2 e^{-\lambda t_{k:n}^2}}{1 - e^{-\lambda t_{k:n}^2}} + (n - n_1)\xi_3(\alpha_2, \lambda),$$

$$\frac{\partial^2 l_{\mathrm{sc}}^{\mathrm{GR}}}{\partial \alpha_2^2} = -\left(\frac{n_2}{\alpha_2^2} + \frac{(n - n_1)\left(1 - e^{-\lambda\tau^2}\right)^{\alpha_2}\{\ln[1 - e^{-\lambda\tau^2}]\}^2}{\{1 - (1 - e^{-\lambda\tau^2})^{\alpha_2}\}^2}\right),$$

where

$$\varrho_3(\alpha_1, \lambda) = \tau^2 e^{-\lambda\tau^2} \frac{\{1 - r_3(\lambda)^{\alpha_1}\}\left[r_3(\lambda)^{\alpha_1}\{\alpha_1 \ln(r_3(\lambda) + 1\}\right]}{r(\lambda)\{1 - r_3(\lambda)^{\alpha_1}\}^2} + \tau^2 e^{-\lambda\tau^2} \frac{\alpha_1 r_3(\lambda)^{2\alpha_1} \ln(r_3(\lambda)}{r(\lambda)\{1 - r_3(\lambda)^{\alpha_1}\}^2},$$

$$\psi_3(\lambda) = -\sum_{k=1}^{n_1} \frac{t_{k:n}^4 e^{-\lambda t_{k:n}^2}}{\left(1 - e^{-\lambda t_{k:n}^2}\right)^2},$$

$$\kappa_3(\alpha_1, \lambda_1) = \alpha_1\tau^2 \frac{\{1 - r_3(\lambda)^{\alpha_1}\}\left[r_3(\lambda)^{\alpha_1 - 2}\tau^2 e^{-\lambda\tau^2}\{\alpha_1 e^{-\lambda\tau^2} - 1\}\right]}{\{1 - r_3(\lambda)^{\alpha_1}\}^2} + \alpha_1\tau^2 \frac{\alpha_1\tau^2 e^{-2\lambda\tau^2} r_3(\lambda)^{2\alpha_1 - 2}}{\{1 - r_3(\lambda)^{\alpha_1}\}^2},$$

$$\sigma_3(\alpha_2, \lambda) = \alpha_2\tau^2 \frac{\{1 - r_3(\lambda)^{\alpha_2}\}\left[r_3(\lambda)^{\alpha_2 - 2}\tau^2 e^{-\lambda\tau^2}\{\alpha_2 e^{-\lambda\tau^2} - 1\}\right]}{\{1 - r_3(\lambda)^{\alpha_2}\}^2} + \alpha_2\tau^2 \frac{\alpha_2\tau^2 e^{-2\lambda\tau^2} r_3(\lambda)^{2\alpha_2 - 2}}{\{1 - r_3(\lambda)^{\alpha_2}\}^2},$$

$$\delta_3(\lambda) = -\sum_{k=n_1+1}^{n_1+n_2} \left[\frac{t_{k:n}^4 e^{-\lambda t_{k:n}^2}}{\left(1 - e^{-\lambda t_{k:n}^2}\right)^2}\right],$$

$$\xi_3(\alpha_2, \lambda) = \tau^2 e^{-\lambda\tau^2} \frac{\{1 - r_3(\lambda)^{\alpha_2}\}\left[r_3(\lambda)^{\alpha_2}\{\alpha_2 \ln(r_3(\lambda) + 1\}\right]}{r_3(\lambda)\{1 - r_3(\lambda)^{\alpha_2}\}^2} + \tau^2 e^{-\lambda\tau^2} \frac{\alpha_2 r_3(\lambda)^{2\alpha_2} \ln(r_3(\lambda)}{r_3(\lambda)\{1 - r_3(\lambda)^{\alpha_2}\}^2},$$

$$r_3(\lambda) = \left(1 - e^{-\lambda\tau^2}\right).$$

References

Abdel-Hamid, A. H., Al-Hussaini, E. K. (2009). Estimation in step-stress accelerated life tests for the exponentiated exponential distribution with Type -I censoring. *Computational Statistics & Data Analysis, 53*, 1328–1338.

Al-Hussaini, E. K., Ahsnullah, M. (2015). *Exponentiated distributions*. Atlantis Studies in Probability and Statistics (Vol. 21). Paris, France: Atlantis Press.

Arnold, B. C., Balakrishnan, N., Nagaraja, H. N. (1992). *A first course in order statistics* (Vol. 54). Philadelphia: Society for Industrial and Applied Mathematics.

Bagdonavičius, V. (1978). Testing hypothesis of the linear accumulation of damages. *Probability Theory and Its Applications, 23*, 403–408.

Bhattacharyya, G. K., Soejoeti, Z. (1989). A tampered failure rate model for step-stress accelerated life test. *Communication in Statistics - Theory and Methods, 18*, 1627–1643.

Cox, D. R. (1992). Regression models and life-tables. *Journal of the Royal Statistical Society: Series B(Methodological), 34*, 187–220.

El-Monem, G. A., Jaheen, Z. (2015). Maximum likelihood estimation and bootstrap confidence intervals for a simple step-stress accelerated generalized exponential model with Type -II censored data. *Far East Journal of Theoretical Statistics, 50*, 111–124.

Greven, S., John Bailer, A., Kupper, L. L., Muller, K. E., Craft, J. L. (2004). A parametric model for studying organism fitness using step-stress experiments. *Biometrics, 60*, 793–799.

Gupta, R. C., Gupta, P. L., Gupta, R. D. (1998). Modeling failure time data by Lehman alternatives. *Communications in Statistics-Theory and Methods, 27*, 887–904.

Gupta, R. D., Kundu, D. (1999). Generalized exponential distributions. *Australian & New Zealand Journal of Statistics, 41*, 173–188.

Ismail, A. A. (2014). Estimation under failure-censored step-stress life test for the generalized exponential distribution parameters. *Indian Journal of Pure and Applied Mathematics, 45*, 1003–1015.

Kateri, M., Kamps, U. (2015). Inference in step-stress models based on failure rates. *Statistical Papers, 56*, 639–660.

Kateri, M., Kamps, U. (2017). Hazard rate modeling of step-stress experiments. *Annual Review of Statistics and Its Application, 4*, 147–168.

Khamis, I. H., Higgins, H. H. (1998). A new model for step-stress testing. *IEEE Transactions on Reliability, 47*, 131–134.

Madi, M. T. (1993). Multiple step-stress accelerated life test: the tampered failure rate model. *Communication in Statistics - Theory and Methods, 22*, 2631–2639.

Nadarajah, S. (2011). The Exponentiated exponential distribution. *Advance in Statistical Analysis, 95*, 219–251.

Nelson, W. (1980). Accelerated life testing-step-stress models and data analyses. *IEEE Transactions on Reliability, 29*, 103–108.

Samanta, D., Kundu, D. (2018). Order restricted inference of a multiple step-stress model. *Computational Statistics & Data Analysis, 117*, 62–75.

Sarhan, A. M., Kundu, D. (2009). Generalized linear failure rate distribution. *Communications in Statistics-Theory and Methods, 38*, 642–660.

Sedyakin, N. M. (1966). On one physical principle in reliability theory. *Technical Cybernatics, 3*, 80–87.

Shawky, A. I., Abu-Zinadah, H. H. (2009). Exponentiated Pareto distribution: different method of estimations. *International Journal of Contemporary Mathematical Sciences, 14*, 677–693.

Surles, J. G., Padgett, W. J. (2005). Some properties of a scaled Burr type X distribution. *Journal of Statistical Planning and Inference, 128*, 271–280.

Part VII
Applications

Model-Based Clustering for Cylindrical Data

Ashis SenGupta, Moumita Roy, and Asis Kumar Chattopadhyay

Abstract The objective of this paper is to perform clustering based on data consisting of both linear and circular variables, that is the data that lie on the surface of a cylinder. There are many circular–linear distributions available in the literature. We use the pragmatic approach of specifying the conditional rather than the marginal, which is often easier. Adopting Arnold et al. (Lecture Notes in Statistics: Conditionally Specified Distributions, Springer Verlag Publisher, Berlin Heidelberg, 1992), we provide the conditional distribution of θ given x and that of x given θ. Here, a mixture model approach based on the joint distribution of the linear and the circular variable is proposed. In particular, two types of such mixture models are used. One is based on the joint distribution of the marginal distribution of the linear variable and the conditional distribution of the circular variable given the linear variable and the other vice versa. Convergence property of Expectation Maximization (EM) algorithm for the members of the curved exponential family used for our models is studied. A real-life application on meteorological data is made of the proposed approaches. Comparison of the two models is done based on this example. The distinctive and important feature of preserving the geometry of the cylindrical manifold by our clustering method and its marked deviation from that for data on $\Re^p$ is also revealed by this example.

1 Introduction

Often in real life, we encounter observations not only on linear variables but also on circular ones, i.e., we observe directional data. It is often necessary to group such data as consisting of both linear and circular variables, i.e., data that lie on the

A. SenGupta
Applied Statistics Unit, Indian Statistical Institute, Kolkata, West Bengal, India

M. Roy (✉)
Department of Statistics, Midnapore College (Autonomous), Midnapore, West Bengal, India

A. K. Chattopadhyay
Department of Statistics, University of Calcutta, Kolkata, West Bengal, India

I. Ghosh et al. (eds.), *Advances in Statistics - Theory and Applications*, Emerging Topics in Statistics and Biostatistics, https://doi.org/10.1007/978-3-030-62900-7_17

surface of a cylinder, into several clusters according to similarity of characteristics. There are many circular–linear, to be termed cylindrical, distributions available in the literature. Johnson et al. (1978) have considered angular–linear distributions, viz., generalized von Mises distribution based on the principle of maximum entropy subject to constraints on certain moments and the method of specified marginals. Cylindrical distributions have been constructed also by SenGupta (2004) by generalizing the approach of conditionally specified distributions for linear variables given in Arnold et al. (1992). Kato et al. (2008) considered a maximum entropy distribution through an extension of the distribution by Johnson et al. (1978) and Mardia et al. (1978), which was a conditional of a trivariate normal distribution with some restrictions on the parameters. Abe et al. (2017) proposed a cylindrical distribution by combining von Mises distribution and Weibull distribution. Lagona et al. (2015) has approximated the distribution of cylindrical time series data by the mixture of the distribution proposed by Abe et al. (2017). In this chapter, a mixture model approach based on the joint distribution of the linear and the circular variable is proposed for model-based clustering of such data as on the cylinder. In Sect. 2, the mixture model based on the joint distribution of the marginal distribution of the circular variable and the conditional distribution of the linear variable given the circular variable is used. In Sect. 3, the joint distribution of the marginal distribution of the linear variable and the conditional distribution of the circular variable given the linear variable is used in the mixture model. Expectation Maximization (EM) algorithm is used for estimating the various parameters of the mixture distributions. In Sect. 4, the clustering technique used is described. The methods for determining the optimum number of clusters is given in Sect. 5. A real-life application is made of the above-proposed approaches in Sect. 6. We demonstrate by the plots for the example how clustering using only linear distributions may be misleading. The clustering for the example on environmental data can be helpful to the meteorologists for weather determination and forecasting. Finally, a comparison of the performance of the two models is done in Sect. 7, and some concluding remarks are given in Sect. 8.

2 Model 1

Initially, we consider bivariate data (x_i, θ_i), where x_i and θ_i are observations on the linear and circular variables, respectively, $x_i \in \Re$ and $\theta_i \in (0, 2\pi]$, $i = 1, \dots, n$. Specifically, it is assumed that for $i = 1, \dots, n$, θ_i is distributed as von Mises distribution with mean direction μ_c and concentration parameter κ; that is, the pdf is given by

$$g(\theta_i) = \frac{1}{2\pi I_0(\kappa)} \exp\{\kappa \cos(\theta_i - \mu_c)\}$$

where $I_0(.)$ denotes the Bessel function of the first kind with order zero.

The von Mises or the circular normal distribution is considered here because it belongs to the popular exponential family of distributions rather than the wrapped normal (WN) distribution. The WN distribution as used by, e.g., Modlin et al. (2012), does not belong to the exponential family and also its density is expressed as an infinite series, as a result of which the maximum likelihood estimation of its parameters is difficult. Also it is well known that wrapped normal distribution and circular normal distribution are virtually the same (see SenGupta et al. 2001).

The conditional distribution of x_i given θ_i is $N(\mu_l, \sigma_l^2)$. That is,

$$\mu_l = E(x|\theta) = b_0 + b_1 \cos\theta + b_2 \sin\theta$$

This kind of regression function is popular in the literature. For example, see Ugwuowo et al. (2006).

Then, the joint distribution of x_i and θ_i is given by

$$f(x_i, \theta_i) = \frac{1}{2\pi I_0(\kappa)} \exp\{\kappa \cos(\theta_i - \mu_c)\} \frac{1}{(\sqrt{2\pi})\sigma_l} \exp\left\{-\frac{1}{2\sigma_l^2}(x_i - \mu_l)^2\right\} \quad (1)$$

Now we consider the mixture model to be fitted as

$$f(x, \theta; \psi) = \sum_{j=1}^{p} \pi_j f_j(x_i, \theta_i; \eta_j) \quad (2)$$

where p denotes the number of mixture components,

$$\eta = \left(\mu_{c_1}, \ldots, \mu_{c_p}, \kappa, b_{0_1}, \ldots, b_{0_p}, b_{1_1}, \ldots, b_{1_p}, b_{2_1}, \ldots, b_{2_p}, \sigma_l^2\right)'$$

$\psi = (\eta', \pi_1, \ldots, \pi_{p-1})$ (since $\pi_p = 1 - \sum_{j=1}^{p-1} \pi_j$) denote the parameter vectors of the mixture model, $\eta_j = (\mu_{c_j}, \kappa, b_{0_j}, b_{1_j}, b_{2_j}, \sigma_l^2)'$ $(j = 1, \ldots, p)$ denote the parameter vector of the jth component of the mixture model, and

$$f_j(x_i, \theta_i; \eta_j) = \frac{1}{2\pi I_0(\kappa)\sqrt{2\pi\sigma_l^2}} \exp\left\{\kappa \cos(\theta_i - \mu_{c_j}) - \frac{1}{2\sigma_l^2}(x_{1i} - b_{0_j} - b_{1_j} x_{2i} - b_{2_j} x_{3i})^2\right\} \quad (3)$$

where $x_{1i} = x_i$, $x_{2i} = \cos\theta_i$, $x_{3i} = \sin\theta_i$. It can be shown that (using theorem 2 given in page 143–144 in SenGupta 2004) the above distribution given by (3) is the maximum entropy distribution subject to $E(x_{1i}) = \frac{b_{0j}}{\sigma_l^2}$,

$$E(\cos\theta_i) = -\frac{b_{0_j} b_{1_j}}{\sigma_l^2} + \kappa\cos\mu_{c_j}, \quad E(\sin\theta_i) = -\frac{b_{0_j} b_{2_j}}{\sigma_l^2} + \kappa\sin\mu_{c_j},$$

$$E(x_{1i}\cos\theta_i) = \frac{b_{1_j}}{\sigma_l^2}, \quad E(x_{1i}\sin\theta_i) = \frac{b_{2_j}}{\sigma_l^2}, \quad E\left(\cos^2\theta_i\right) = \frac{b_{1_j}^2}{2\sigma_l^2},$$

$E(\sin^2\theta_i) = \frac{b_{2_j}^2}{2\sigma_l^2}$, $E(x_{1i}^2) = -\frac{1}{2\sigma_l^2}$, and $E(\cos\theta_i\sin\theta_i) = -\frac{b_{1_j} b_{2_j}}{\sigma_l^2}$ taking specified values consistent with the expectations with respect to the specified distributions.

2.1 Estimation of Parameters

We use EM algorithm to estimate the parameters of the mixture model (2). So we introduce an indicator variable z_{ij} as follows:

$$z_{ij} = \begin{cases} 1 \text{ if } (x_i, \theta_i) \text{ comes from the } j\text{th component of the mixture} \\ 0 \text{ otherwise} \end{cases}$$

Using the complete data vector $(z_{ij}, \theta_i, x_{1i}, x_{2i}, x_{3i})'$, the complete data log-likelihood function for ψ is given by

$$L_c(\psi) = \sum_{i=1}^{n}\sum_{j=1}^{p} z_{ij} \ln f_j(x, \theta; \eta_j)$$

$$= -n\ln 2\pi - n\ln I_0(\kappa) - \frac{n}{2}\ln 2\pi - \frac{n}{2}\ln\sigma_l^2 + \sum_{i=1}^{n}\sum_{j=1}^{p} z_{ij}\Big\{\kappa\cos(\theta_i - \mu_{c_j})$$

$$- \frac{1}{2\sigma_l^2}(x_{1i} - b_{0_j} - b_{1_j}x_{2i} - b_{2_j}x_{3i})^2\Big\} \tag{4}$$

If the z_{ij}s are observable, then the MLE of π_j is simply given by

$$\hat{\pi}_j = \sum_{i=1}^{n} z_{ij}/n \tag{5}$$

The likelihood equations for estimating the parameters $\mu_{c_j}, \kappa, b_{0_j}, b_{1_j}, b_{2_j}, (j = 1, \ldots, p)$, and σ_l^2, respectively, are given as

$$\sum_{i=1}^{n} \hat{z}_{ij}\sin\left(\theta_i - \hat{\mu}_{c_j}\right) = 0 \tag{6}$$

$$\sum_{i=1}^{n}\sum_{j=1}^{p}\hat{z}_{ij}\cos\left(\theta_i-\hat{\mu}_{c_j}\right)-\frac{nI_1(\hat{\kappa})}{I_0(\hat{\kappa})}=0 \tag{7}$$

$$\left(I_1(\kappa)=\frac{d}{d\kappa}I_0(\kappa)\right)$$

$$\sum_{i=1}^{n}\hat{z}_{ij}\left(x_{1i}-\hat{b}_{0_j}-\hat{b}_{1_j}x_{2i}-\hat{b}_{2_j}x_{3i}\right)=0 \tag{8}$$

$$\sum_{i=1}^{n}\hat{z}_{ij}x_{2i}\left(x_{1i}-\hat{b}_{0_j}-\hat{b}_{1_j}x_{2i}-\hat{b}_{2_j}x_{3i}\right)=0 \tag{9}$$

$$\sum_{i=1}^{n}\hat{z}_{ij}x_{3i}\left(x_{1i}-\hat{b}_{0_j}-\hat{b}_{1_j}x_{2i}-\hat{b}_{2_j}x_{3i}\right)=0 \tag{10}$$

$$\sum_{i=1}^{n}\sum_{j=1}^{p}\hat{z}_{ij}\left(x_{1i}-\hat{b}_{0_j}-\hat{b}_{1_j}x_{2i}-\hat{b}_{2_j}x_{3i}\right)^2-n\hat{\sigma}_l^2=0 \tag{11}$$

where

$$\hat{z}_{ij}=E_{\psi}(z_{ij}|(x,\theta))=P_{\psi}(z_{ij}=1|(x,\theta))=\frac{\hat{\pi}_j f_j(x_i,\theta_i;\hat{\eta}_j)}{f(x_i,\theta_i;\hat{\psi})}$$

(by Bayes' theorem)

This quantity is the posterior probability that the ith member of the sample with observed value (x_i,θ_i) belongs to the jth component of the mixture.

Hence solving the likelihood equations (6)–(11), the maximum likelihood estimators of the parameters are given by

$$\hat{\mu}_{c_j}=\arctan^*(\bar{\theta}_j)\quad j=1,\ldots,p \tag{12}$$

where

$$\bar{\theta}_j=\frac{\sum_{i=1}^{n}\hat{z}_{ij}\sin\theta_i}{\sum_{i=1}^{n}\hat{z}_{ij}\cos\theta_i}$$

and arctan* is as defined in SenGupta et al. (2001).

$$\hat{\kappa}=A^{-1}(\bar{R}_0) \tag{13}$$

$$\text{where}\quad \bar{R}_0=\frac{\sum_{i=1}^{n}\sum_{j=1}^{p}\hat{z}_{ij}\cos\left(\theta_i-\hat{\mu}_{c_j}\right)}{n}\quad\text{and}\quad A(\kappa)=\frac{I_1(\kappa)}{I_0(\kappa)}.$$

$$\hat{b}_{0_j} = \frac{\sum_{i=1}^{n} \hat{z}_{ij}\left(x_{1i} - \hat{b}_{1_j}x_{2i} - \hat{b}_{2_j}x_{3i}\right)}{\sum_{i=1}^{n} \hat{z}_{ij}}, \tag{14}$$

$$\hat{b}_{1_j} = \frac{\sum_{i=1}^{n} \hat{z}_{ij}x_{2i}\left(x_{1i} - \hat{b}_{0_j} - \hat{b}_{2_j}x_{3i}\right)}{\sum_{i=1}^{n} \hat{z}_{ij}x_{2i}^2}, \tag{15}$$

$$\hat{b}_{2_j} = \frac{\sum_{i=1}^{n} \hat{z}_{ij}x_{3i}\left(x_{1i} - \hat{b}_{0_j} - \hat{b}_{1_j}x_{2i}\right)}{\sum_{i=1}^{n} \hat{z}_{ij}x_{3i}^2} \quad j = 1, \ldots, p \tag{16}$$

$$\text{and} \quad \hat{\sigma}_l^2 = \frac{\sum_{i=1}^{n}\sum_{j=1}^{p} \hat{z}_{ij}(x_{1i} - \hat{b}_{0_j} - \hat{b}_{1_j}x_{2i} - \hat{b}_{2_j}x_{3i})^2}{n} \tag{17}$$

The E-step of the EM algorithm on the $(k+1)$th iteration requires

$$\begin{aligned} E_{\psi^{(k)}}(z_{ij}|(x,\theta)) &= P_{\psi^{(k)}}(z_{ij} = 1|(x,\theta)) = z_{ij}^{(k)} \\ &= \frac{\pi_j^{(k)} f_j\left(x_i, \theta_i; \eta_j^{(k)}\right)}{f\left(x_i, \theta_i; \psi^{(k)}\right)}; \quad j = 1, \ldots, p, \quad i = 1, \ldots, n \end{aligned}$$

The M-step on the $(k+1)$th iteration requires replacing each z_{ij} by $z_{ij}^{(k)}$ in (5) to give $\pi_j^{(k+1)} = \sum_{i=1}^{n} z_{ij}^{(k)}/n, \quad j = 1, \ldots, p.$

The M-step also requires the computation of $\mu_{cj}^{(k)}, b_{0_j}^{(k)}, b_{1_j}^{(k)}, b_{2_j}^{(k)}, (j = 1, \ldots, p)$, $\kappa^{(k)}$, and $\sigma_l^{2(k)}$, which involves replacing z_{ij} by $z_{ij}^{(k)}$ in the estimators in (12)–(17) to give

$$\mu_{cj}^{(k+1)} = \arctan^*\left(\frac{\sum_{i=1}^{n} z_{ij}^{(k)} \sin\theta_i}{\sum_{i=1}^{n} z_{ij}^{(k)} \cos\theta_i}\right) \quad j = 1, \ldots, p$$

$$\kappa^{(k+1)} = A^{-1}\left(\frac{\sum_{i=1}^{n}\sum_{j=1}^{p} z_{ij}^{(k)} \cos(\theta_i - \mu_{c_j}^{(k+1)})}{n}\right)$$

$$b_{0_j}^{(k+1)} = \frac{\sum_{i=1}^{n} z_{ij}^{(k)}\left(x_{1i} - b_{1_j}^{(k)} x_{2i} - b_{2_j}^{(k)} x_{3i}\right)}{\sum_{i=1}^{n} z_{ij}^{(k)}},$$

$$b_{1_j}^{(k+1)} = \frac{\sum_{i=1}^{n} z_{ij}^{(k)} x_{2i}\left(x_{1i} - b_{0_j}^{(k+1)} - b_{2_j}^{(k)} x_{3i}\right)}{\sum_{i=1}^{n} z_{ij}^{(k)} x_{2i}^2},$$

$$b_{2_j}^{(k+1)} = \frac{\sum_{i=1}^{n} z_{ij}^{(k)} x_{3i}\left(x_{1i} - b_{0_j}^{(k+1)} - b_{1_j}^{(k+1)} x_{2i}\right)}{\sum_{i=1}^{n} z_{ij}^{(k)} x_{3i}^2} \qquad j = 1, \ldots, p$$

$$\text{and} \quad \sigma_l^{2(k+1)} = \frac{\sum_{i=1}^{n}\sum_{j=1}^{p} z_{ij}^{(k)}\left(x_{1i} - b_{0_j}^{(k+1)} - b_{1_j}^{(k+1)} x_{2i} - b_{2_j}^{(k+1)} x_{3i}\right)^2}{n}$$

where the parameters with upper suffix k denote the estimators of the parameters at the kth iteration. The E- and M-steps are alternated repeatedly until the difference

$$L_c\left(\psi^{(k+1)}\right) - L_c\left(\psi^{(k)}\right)$$

changes by an arbitrary small amount for convergence of the sequence of the log-likelihood values.

2.2 *Convergence of the EM Algorithm*

We now establish the convergence of the algorithm. First, suppose that SU_1 defines the joint density of $(x_i, \theta_i), i = 1, \ldots, n$, given by (1) for the jth component of Model 1 given by (3). It can be seen that SU_1 is a member of

the curved exponential family $\exp(\gamma' T(x, \theta))$, where $\gamma_1 = \kappa \cos \mu_{c_j}$, $T_1 = \sum_{i=1}^{n} \cos \theta_i$, $\gamma_2 = \kappa \sin \mu_{c_j}$, $T_2 = \sum_{i=1}^{n} \sin \theta_i$,
$\gamma_3 = \frac{1}{\sigma_l^2}$, $T_3 = -\sum_{i=1}^{n} x_{1i}^2/2$, $\gamma_4 = \frac{b_{1j}^2}{\sigma_l^2}$, $T_4 = -\sum_{i=1}^{n} x_{2i}^2$, $\gamma_5 = \frac{b_{2j}^2}{\sigma_l^2}$,
$T_5 = -\sum_{i=1}^{n} x_{3i}^2$, $\gamma_6 = \frac{b_{0j}}{\sigma_l^2}$, $T_6 = \sum_{i=1}^{n} x_{1i}$, $\gamma_7 = \frac{b_{1j}}{\sigma_l^2}$, $T_7 = \sum_{i=1}^{n} x_{1i} x_{2i}$,
$\gamma_8 = \frac{b_{2j}}{\sigma_l^2}$, $T_8 = \sum_{i=1}^{n} x_{1i} x_{3i}$, $\gamma_9 = \frac{b_{0j} b_{1j}}{\sigma_l^2}$, $T_9 = \sum_{i=1}^{n} x_{2i}$, $\gamma_{10} = \frac{b_{0j} b_{2j}}{\sigma_l^2}$,
$T_{10} = \sum_{i=1}^{n} x_{3i}$, $\gamma_{11} = \frac{b_{1j} b_{2j}}{\sigma_l^2}$, and $T_{11} = \sum_{i=1}^{n} x_{2i} x_{3i}$
Hence using property (ii) under section 3 in page 101 of Wu (1983), since SU_1 is a member of the curved exponential family, it follows that $f_j(x_i, \theta_i; \eta_j)$ is continuous in η_j. Further by (i) in that section, the EM parameter vector ψ converges, implying the convergence of $L_c(\psi)$ correspondingly. Thus, the convergence of the EM algorithm is guaranteed theoretically. Numerically also we had no issue with convergence of the EM algorithms above for the examples presented in Sect. 6 below.

3 Model 2

Now consider the situation when the conditional distribution of θ_i given x_i is von Mises with mean direction $\mu(x)$ and concentration parameter $\kappa(x)$, where

$$E(\theta|x) = \mu(x) = \mu + 2\arctan(\beta x)(\text{mod } 2\pi)$$

We assume for simplicity $\kappa(x) = \kappa$ and x_i is distributed as Normal with mean μ_l and variance σ^2; that is, the pdf is given by

$$g(x_i) = \frac{1}{\sqrt{2\pi}\sigma} \exp -\frac{1}{2\sigma^2}(x_i - \mu_l)^2$$

In some cases one may encounter heteroscedastic cylindrical distribution. In such cases one would ideally take $\sigma^2 = \sigma^2(\theta)$ and $\kappa = \kappa(x)$. However this would entail a large number of parameters, as large as the sample size. This would be computationally intensive as the number of parameters to be estimated will increase. One can of course put ad hoc structures on these variance/concentration parameters, but it can be quite complicated. So, for simplicity as also for lack of knowledge regarding such structures, we have taken these as constants. Johnson et al. (1978) and Fisher et al. (1992) have also made this assumption of simplicity. This situation may not universally hold for cylindrical data but is possibly not different from what one also often suggests for bivariate linear data.

Then, the joint distribution of x_i and θ_i is given by

$$f(x_i,\theta_i) = \frac{1}{2\pi I_0(\kappa)} \exp[\kappa \cos\{\theta_i - \mu - 2\arctan(\beta x_i)\}] \times \frac{1}{(\sqrt{2\pi})\sigma} \exp\left\{-\frac{1}{2\sigma^2}(x_i-\mu_l)^2\right\} \tag{18}$$

Here the mixture model to be fitted is

$$f(x,\theta;\psi) = \sum_{j=1}^{p} \pi_j f_j(x_i,\theta_i;\eta_j) \tag{19}$$

where p denotes the number of mixture components,
$\eta = (\mu_1,\ldots,\mu_p,\kappa,\beta_1,\ldots,\beta_p,\mu_{l_1},\ldots,\mu_{l_p},\sigma^2)'$
$\psi = (\eta',\pi_1,\ldots,\pi_{p-1})$ $\left(\text{since } \pi_p = 1 - \sum_{j=1}^{p-1} \pi_j\right)$ denote the parameter vectors of the mixture model, $\eta_j = (\mu_j,\kappa,\beta_j,\mu_{l_j},\sigma^2)', (j=1,\ldots,p)$ denote the parameter vector of the jth component of the mixture model, and

$$f_j(x_i,\theta_i;\eta_j) = \frac{1}{2\pi I_0(\kappa)} \exp[\kappa \cos\{\theta_i - \mu_j - 2\arctan(\beta_j x_i)\}] \times \frac{1}{(\sqrt{2\pi})\sigma} \exp\left\{-\frac{1}{2\sigma^2}(x_i-\mu_{l_j})^2\right\} \tag{20}$$

3.1 Estimation of Parameters

Here also as in Model 1, we use EM algorithm to estimate the parameters of the mixture model (19) and introduce an indicator variable z_{ij} as before.

Hence using the complete data vector $(z_{ij},\theta_i,x_i)'$, the complete data log-likelihood function for ψ is given by

$$\begin{aligned} L_c(\psi) &= \sum_{i=1}^{n}\sum_{j=1}^{p} z_{ij} \ln f_j(x,\theta;\eta_j) \\ &= -n\ln 2\pi - n\ln I_0(\kappa) - \frac{n}{2}\ln 2\pi - \frac{n}{2}\ln\sigma^2 + \sum_{i=1}^{n}\sum_{j=1}^{p} z_{ij}\Big[\kappa\cos\{\theta_i - \mu_j \\ &\quad - 2\arctan(\beta_j x_i)\} - \frac{1}{2\sigma^2}(x_i-\mu_{l_j})^2\Big] \end{aligned} \tag{21}$$

The MLEs of π_j are obtained the same as in case of Model 1.

The maximum likelihood estimators of the other parameters are given by

$$\hat{\mu}_{l_j} = \frac{\sum\limits_{i=1}^{n} \hat{z}_{ij} x_i}{\sum\limits_{i=1}^{n} \hat{z}_{ij}} \quad j = 1, \ldots, p \tag{22}$$

$$\hat{\sigma}^2 = \frac{\sum\limits_{i=1}^{n} \sum\limits_{j=1}^{p} \hat{z}_{ij} (x_i - \hat{\mu}_{l_j})^2}{n} \tag{23}$$

$$\hat{\mu}_j = \arctan^*(\bar{\theta}_1) \quad j = 1, \ldots, p \tag{24}$$

where

$$\bar{\theta}_1 = \frac{\sum\limits_{i=1}^{n} \hat{z}_{ij} \sin\left\{\theta_i - 2\arctan\left(\hat{\beta}_j x_i\right)\right\}}{\sum\limits_{i=1}^{n} \hat{z}_{ij} \cos\left\{\theta_i - 2\arctan\left(\hat{\beta}_j x_i\right)\right\}}$$

and arctan* is as defined in SenGupta et al. (2001).

$$\hat{\kappa} = A^{-1}(\bar{R}_1) \tag{25}$$

where

$$\bar{R}_1 = \frac{\sum\limits_{i=1}^{n} \sum\limits_{j=1}^{p} \hat{z}_{ij} \cos\left\{\theta_i - \hat{\mu}_j - 2\arctan\left(\hat{\beta}_j x_i\right)\right\}}{n} \quad \text{and} \quad A(\kappa) = \frac{I_1(\kappa)}{I_0(\kappa)}$$

The E- and M-steps are alternated repeatedly, as in the case of Model 1, till the convergence of the sequence of the log-likelihood values.

We now establish the convergence of the algorithm in the lines of that for Model 1 above. Let us suppose that SU_2 defines the joint density of (x_i, θ_i), $i = 1, \ldots, n$, given by (18) for the jth component of Model 2 given by (20). It can be seen that (substituting an initial value of β_j) SU_2 is a member of the curved exponential family $\exp(\gamma' T(x, \theta))$ where $\gamma_1 = \kappa \cos \mu_j$, $\gamma_2 = \kappa \sin \mu_j$,

$$T_1 = \sum_{i=1}^{n} \cos\theta_i \cos\{2\arctan(\beta_j x_i)\}, \quad T_2 = \sum_{i=1}^{n} \sin\{\theta_i - 2\arctan(\beta_j x_i)\},$$

$$\gamma_3 = \frac{1}{\sigma^2}, \quad T_3 = -\sum_{i=1}^{n} x_i^2/2 \quad \gamma_4 = \frac{\mu_j}{\sigma^2}, \text{ and } T_4 = \sum_{i=1}^{n} x_i$$

Thus, here also the convergence of the EM algorithm is ensured as in Model 1.

4 Clustering Technique

Suppose that there are n observations on each of which a linear variable and a circular variable are measured, resulting in the bivariate data (x_i, θ_i), $i = 1, \ldots, n$. Our objective is to classify the n observations based on the bivariate data. We assume that each mixture component of the mixture model to be fitted is a cluster. In the E-step of the EM algorithm in Sect. 2.1, a $(n \times p)$ matrix is created whose ith row contains estimates of the conditional (on the current parameter estimates) probabilities that the ith observation (x_i, θ_i) belongs to the jth mixture component or cluster j $(j = 1, \ldots, p)$. So at convergence, the ith observation is assigned to the cluster j for which the conditional probability of membership given by

$$P_{i|j} = \frac{\hat{\pi}_j f_j\left(x_i, \theta_i; \hat{\eta}_j\right)}{\sum_{j=1}^{p} \hat{\pi}_j f_j\left(x_i, \theta_i; \hat{\eta}_j\right)}$$

is the largest.

5 Choice of the Number of Clusters p

One of the important questions that arises is how to decide on a reasonable value for the number of clusters. One of the solutions can be obtained by using Bayesian information criterion (BIC), which is given by

$$\begin{aligned} BIC &= -2 \ln L_{max} + Penalty \\ &= -2 \ln L_{max} + \ln(n) \times \text{number of parameters estimated} \\ &= -2 \ln L_{max} + (5p + 1) \ln(n) \quad \text{in case of Model 1} \\ &= -2 \ln L_{max} + (4p + 1) \ln(n) \quad \text{in case of Model 2} \end{aligned}$$

In order to decide on the number of clusters, we choose that value of p for which the BIC is minimized (McLachlan et al. 1997 and Richard et al. 2007). Another solution can be obtained by using Akaike information criterion (AIC) given by

$$\begin{aligned} AIC &= -2 \ln L_{max} + 2 \times \text{number of parameters estimated} \\ &= -2 \ln L_{max} + 2.(5p + 1) \quad \text{in case of Model 1} \\ &= -2 \ln L_{max} + 2.(4p + 1) \quad \text{in case of Model 2} \end{aligned}$$

The optimum number of clusters is selected as that value of p that minimizes AIC.

6 Example

Twenty-eight observations are available on the January surface wind direction and temperature at 12 h GMT at Kew for the years 1956–1960. This is a popular data set, and we illustrate our methodology through this example. Although the size of the data is small, similar large size data can be visualized in practice for this purpose.

6.1 *Applications of Model 1*

These observations can constitute the bivariate data (x_i, θ_i) for our clustering where x = temperature and θ = wind direction. Here, the objective of clustering is to determine and identify groups corresponding to similar conditions of surface temperature and similar patterns of wind direction. This example of clustering serves to illustrate how meteorologists may be provided with groups of similar overall weather conditions as per the joint variations in surface temperature and wind direction at some specific time (e.g., at 12 h GMT at Kew as in this example). These in turn may be used by them to forecast the weather for some future time period. The values of BIC and AIC are calculated for different values of p in the following table. Here, we restrict the possible number of clusters to 6 due to the size of the data.

It can be observed from Table 1 that the BIC and the AIC criteria are minimum for $p = 4$ clusters. The values in the above table may seem to be an anomaly for nested models. But for small and moderate sample sizes, this anomaly is not quite unexpected as can be seen in Vermunt et al. (2005). Figure 1 also confirms the optimum number of clusters to be 4. The final estimates of the parameters for the optimum number of clusters are shown in Table 2. Then, following the clustering technique as described in Sect. 4, the 28 observations are assigned to the 4 clusters as displayed in Table 3.

It appears from the left plot of Fig. 1 that there are only three clusters due to the structure of the circular variable (wind direction), but actually there are four clusters. We compare the sample means and variances with those based on model as obtained from the EM algorithm. The comparison is shown in Table 4. It can be observed that the means of the circular components of all the clusters almost match with each other. Also Fig. 1 indicates that the four clusters formed are well separated from one another. Thus, the performance of the cluster allocation is quite satisfactory.

Table 1 The values of BIC and AIC

No. of clusters	BIC	AIC
2	249.2102	234.556
3	220.1765	198.8612
4	210.8566	182.8803
5	231.5125	196.8752
6	236.5395	195.2412

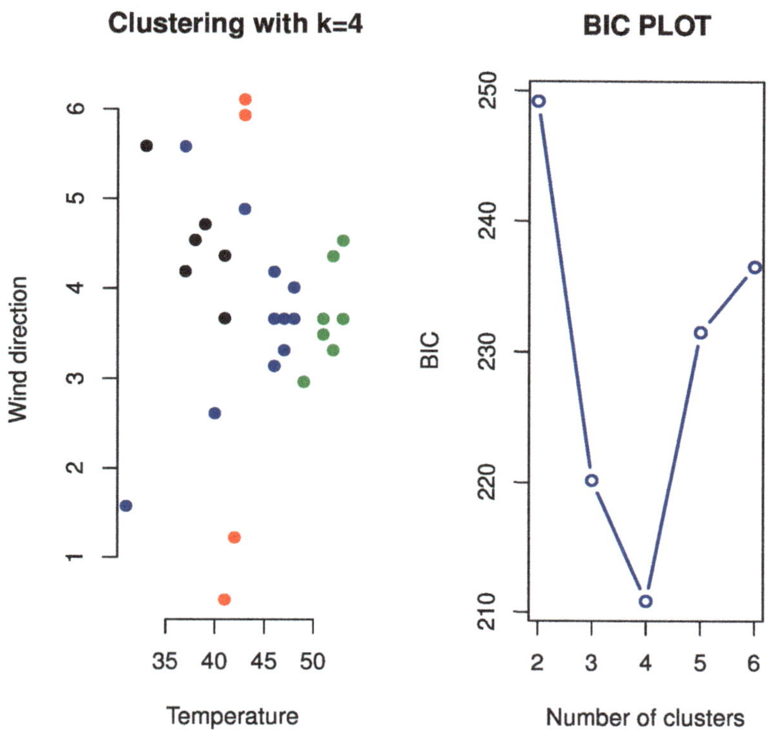

Fig. 1 Plot of BIC and clustering plot for January data based on the variables wind direction and temperature to select the number of clusters under Model 1

Table 2 Results from EM algorithm for the optimum number of clusters

No. of clusters	No. of iterations	$\hat{\mu}_c$	$\hat{\kappa}$	$\hat{b}_0$	$\hat{b}_1$	$\hat{b}_2$	$\hat{\sigma}_l^2$	BIC
4	359	$\begin{pmatrix} -1.801 \\ 0.268 \\ -2.583 \\ -2.573 \end{pmatrix}$	2.300	$\begin{pmatrix} 34.548 \\ 46.246 \\ 47.448 \\ 37.813 \end{pmatrix}$	$\begin{pmatrix} -4.549 \\ -4.213 \\ -2.717 \\ -7.172 \end{pmatrix}$	$\begin{pmatrix} -3.366 \\ -3.008 \\ -4.544 \\ -6.572 \end{pmatrix}$	0.862	210.857

Table 3 Cluster allocation

Cluster number	No. of observations	Observation number
1	6	2–3, 15, 19, 21, 28
2	4	7–9, 24
3	7	1, 5, 12, 17, 23, 25, 27
4	11	4, 6, 10–11, 13–14, 16, 18, 20, 22, 26

Table 4 Cluster means and variances

Cluster number	No. of observations	$\hat{\pi}_j$	Mean of x_i	Variance of x_i	Mean of θ_i after clustering	Mean of θ_i before clustering	Concentration of θ_i
1	6	0.214	38.167	8.967	−1.793	−1.801	0.157
2	4	0.143	42.25	0.917	0.287	0.268	0.184
3	7	0.25	51.571	1.952	−42.577	−2.583	0.128
4	11	0.393	43.545	29.473	−2.596	−2.573	0.399

Table 5 The values of BIC and AIC

No. of clusters	BIC	AIC
2	260.6822	248.6924
3	248.0171	230.6984
4	240.2125	217.5651
5	242.0051	214.0288
6	267.4518	234.1466

6.2 *Applications of Model 2*

Next we are interested in clustering the above 28 observations using Model 2, i.e., (19).

It can be noted from Table 5 and Fig. 2 that the BIC criterion is minimum for $p = 4$ clusters. Thus, the optimum number of clusters is chosen as 4. The final estimates of the parameters of the optimum number of clusters under Model 2 is given in Table 6. Then, following the clustering technique as described in Sect. 4, the 28 observations are assigned to the 4 clusters as displayed in Table 7.

It can be noted that the means of the linear components before and after clustering are quite close to each other for almost all the clusters. Also Fig. 2 indicates that the four clusters formed are well-separated. Hence, the performance of the clustering can be considered to be quite satisfactory.

7 Performance of the Clustering

A comparison of the performance of the optimum cluster allocation is done through the expected misclassification rate (see Dingxi et al. 2007) given by

$$\text{EMCR} = 1 - \sum_{j=1}^{p^*} \hat{\pi}_j P_{i|j}$$

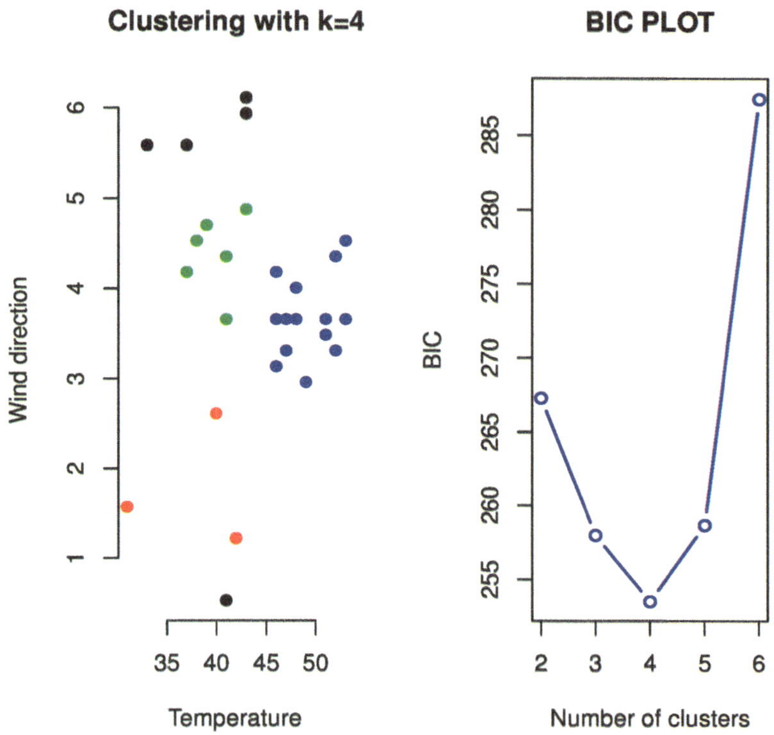

Fig. 2 Plot of BIC and clustering plot for January data based on the variables wind direction and temperature to select the number of clusters under Model 2

Table 6 Results from EM algorithm for the optimum number of clusters

No. of clusters	No. of iterations	$\hat{\mu}$	$\hat{\beta}$	$\hat{\kappa}$	$\hat{\mu}_l$	$\hat{\sigma}^2$	BIC
4	67	$\begin{pmatrix} 2.836 \\ -1.417 \\ 1.310 \\ 0.855 \end{pmatrix}$	$\begin{pmatrix} -2582.458 \\ 500.772 \\ 932.026 \\ 0.127 \end{pmatrix}$	5.150	$\begin{pmatrix} 39.563 \\ 37.587 \\ 39.833 \\ 48.913 \end{pmatrix}$	11.070	253.541

Table 7 Cluster allocation

Cluster number	No. of observations	Observation number
1	5	7–9, 20–21
2	3	4, 16, 24
3	6	2–3, 13, 15, 19, 28
4	14	1, 5–6, 10–12, 14, 17–18, 22–23, 25–27

Table 8 Comparison of cluster means and variances

Cluster number	No. of observations	$\hat{\pi}_j$	Mean of x_i after clustering	Mean of x_i before clustering	Variance of x_i	Mean of θ_i	Concentration of θ_i
1	5	0.179	39.4	39.563	18.8	−0.292	0.097
2	3	0.107	37.667	37.587	34.333	1.782	0.168
3	6	0.214	39.833	39.833	4.967	−1.884	0.076
4	14	0.5	49.214	48.913	7.258	−2.598	0.092

Table 9 Comparison of the performance of clustering under Model 1 and Model 2

Data	p^* under Model 1	EMCR under Model 1	p^* under Model 2	EMCR under Model 2
Jan. wind dir & temp	4	6.362423e–08	4	0.0291549

where p^* denotes the optimum number of clusters and

$$P_{i|j} = \frac{\hat{\pi}_j f_j(x_i, \theta_i; \hat{\eta}_j)}{\sum_{j=1}^{p^*} \hat{\pi}_j f_j(x_i, \theta_i; \hat{\eta}_j)}$$

is the conditional probability of membership of the ith observation to the jth($j = 1, \ldots, p^*$) cluster. Using this measure, the comparison of the two models is shown in Table 9. The results in Table 9 show that the performance of clustering under Model 1 is better than that under Model 2 for our example, since it has a smaller misclassification rate.

Remark In the right figure (of Fig. 1), it appears that there are 3 clusters due to the linear positioning of the circular variable wind direction. However, values at the extremities 0 and 2π rad are, in reality, geometrically in close proximities in the circular scale. So, indeed the 4 clusters are justified. The same is true for Fig. 2. These examples thus reveal yet another unique feature of clustering on the cylindrical manifolds as compared to the R^p case.

8 Conclusion

The results from Tables 4, 8, Figs. 1, and 2 well indicate the satisfactory performance of the clustering methodology enhanced here as the clusters formed clearly exhibit separation from each other. The results in Table 9 show that for the given example, the clustering under Model 1 may be preferred to that under Model 2 since it yields smaller misclassification rate. Finally, as mentioned in Remark above, our model-based clustering methodology enhances and preserves the geometry of the underlying cylindrical manifold.

Acknowledgments The authors greatly appreciate the thorough and scholarly report on the paper by the Referee and express their thanks hereby. The research of the second author of the paper was funded by the Senior Research Fellowship from the University Grants Commission, Government of India. She is also thankful to the Indian Statistical Institute and the University of Calcutta for providing the necessary facilities.

References

Abe, T., Ley, C. (2017). A tractable, parsimonious and highly flexible model for cylindrical data, with applications. *Econometrics and Statistics, 4*, 91–104.

Arnold, B. C., Castillo, E., Sarabia, J. M. (1992). *Conditionally specified distributions*. Lecture Notes in Statistics. Berlin Heidelberg: Springer.

Dingxi, Q., Tamhane, A. (2007). A comparative study of k-means algorithm and the normal mixture model for clustering: Univariate case. *Journal of Statistical Planning and Inference, 137*, 3722–3740.

Fisher, N. I., Lee, A. J. (1992). Regression models for an angular response. *Biometrics, 48*(3), 665–677.

Green, P. J. (1984). Iteratively reweighted least squares for maximum likelihood estimation, and some robust and resistant alternatives. *Journal of the Royal Statistical Society, Series B, 46*, 149–192.

Jammalamadaka, S. R., SenGupta A. (2001). *Topics in circular statistics*. New Jersey: World Scientific Publishers.

Johnson, R. A., Wehrly, T. E. (1978). Some angular-linear distributions and related regression models. *Journal of the American Statistical Association, 73*, 602–606.

Johnson, R. A., Wichern, D. W. (2007). *Applied multivariate statistical analysis*. New Jersey: Pearson Prentice Hall

Kato, S., Shimizu, K. (2008). Dependent models for observations which include angular ones. *Journal of Statistical Planning and Inference, 138*, 3538–3549.

Lagona, F., Picone, M., Maruotti, A. (2015). A Hidden Markov model for the analysis of cylindrical time series. *Environmetrics, 26*, 534–544.

Mardia, K. V., Sutton, T. W. (1978). A model for cylindrical variables with applications. *Journal of the Royal Statistical Society. Series B (Methodological), 40*(2), 229–233.

McLachlan, G. J., Krishnan, T. (1997). *The EM algorithm and extensions*. New York: Wiley.

McLachlan, G. J., Peel, D. (2001). *Finite mixture models*. Wiley Series in Probability and Statistics, United States of America. Hoboken: Wiley.

Modlin, D., Fuentes, M., Reich, B. (2012). Circular conditional autoregressive modeling of vector fields. *Environmetrics, 23*, 46–53.

Seal, B., SenGupta, A. (2012). On the foundations of dependency models and parameters for random variables on cylinder. *Calcutta Statistical Association Bulletin, 64*, 151–165.

SenGupta, A. (2004). On the construction of probability distributions for directional data. *Bulletin of the Calcutta Mathematical Society, 96*(2), 139–154.

SenGupta, A., Ugwuowo, F. (2006). Asymmetric circular-linear multivariate regression models with applications to environmental data. *Environmental and Ecological Statistics, 13*(3), 299–309.

Vermunt, J. K., Magidson, J. (2005). Hierarchical mixture models for nested data structures. In C. Weihs, W. Gaul (Eds.), *Classification – the ubiquitous challenge*. Studies in Classification, Data Analysis, and Knowledge Organization (pp. 240–247). Berlin: Springer.

Wu, J. C. F. (1983). On the convergence properties of the EM algorithm. *Annals of Statistics, 11*(1), 95–103.

Skew-Elliptical Cluster Processes

Ngoc Anh Dao and Marc G. Genton

Abstract This paper introduces skew-elliptical cluster processes. In contrast to the simple Gaussian isotropic structure of the distribution of the "children" events of a Thomas process, we propose an anisotropic structure by allowing the choice of a flexible covariance matrix and incorporating skewness or ellipticity parameters into the structure. Since the theoretical pair correlation functions of these processes are complex and analytically incomplete, and therefore the estimation of the parameters is computationally intensive, we propose reasonable approximations of the theoretical pair correlation functions of these cluster processes, which allow for a simpler parameter estimation. We present the estimation of their parameters using the minimum contrast method. For a data application, we use a fraction of the full redwood dataset. Our analysis shows that an elliptical cluster process can describe this point pattern better than a common Thomas process, since it is able to statistically model the non-circular shapes of the clusters in the data. The skew-elliptical cluster processes can be very meaningful for analyzing complex datasets in the field of spatial point processes since they provide more flexibility to detect interesting characteristics of the data.

1 Introduction

The Thomas process (TP) (Thomas 1949) is very important in the field of spatial point processes because it has the intrinsic statistical ability to model propagation or clustering in nature. In particular, the TP is widely used in astronomy, biology, and forestry, to name a few areas. In this work, we introduce a class of skew-elliptical cluster processes that includes the (traditional) TP and offers the possibility

N. A. Dao
Department of Statistics, Texas A&M University, College Station, TX, USA
e-mail: dao@stat.tamu.edu

M. G. Genton (✉)
Statistics Program, King Abdullah University of Science and Technology, Thuwal, Saudi Arabia
e-mail: marc.genton@kaust.edu.sa

I. Ghosh et al. (eds.), *Advances in Statistics - Theory and Applications*, Emerging Topics in Statistics and Biostatistics, https://doi.org/10.1007/978-3-030-62900-7_18

of modeling the ellipticity, skewness, and, in some situations, information in the tail of the distribution of the "children" events. These characteristics would otherwise remain unknown if the (traditional) TP were used to model the data.

The TP is a special case of the Neyman–Scott cluster point process (Neyman and Scott 1952), which is a specific type of homogeneous, independent clustering applied to a stationary Poisson process. Neyman and Scott (1952, 1958) and Neyman et al. (1953) used this process to model patterns formed by the locations of galaxies in space. Neyman and Scott (1972) gave further examples of such processes to model the distributions of insect larvae in fields and the geometry of bombing patterns. Penttinen et al. (1992) and Tanaka et al. (2008) used Neyman–Scott cluster point processes to model patterns of trees such as pines in natural forests. Similarly, Illian et al. (2008) used the TP to model 207 Phlebocarya filifolia plants, and Diggle (2003, Chap. 6.3) used the TP to model 62 redwood seedlings.

We now look at how Neyman–Scott cluster point processes and the TP are defined. A Neyman–Scott cluster point process is constructed by letting unobservable, the so-called parent events form a stationary Poisson process with intensity κ. The "children" events in a cluster are random in number and scattered independently and with identical distribution around each "parent" event. To construct a TP, a complete spatial randomness (CSR) with intensity κ is generated to obtain the "parent" events. Each "parent" event is replaced by a random cluster of "children" events, the number of which is Poisson distributed with intensity μ. The positions of the "children" events are distributed around the "parent" event according to a bivariate normal distribution with circular covariance matrix $\sigma^2\mathbf{I}_2$, where $\mathbf{I}_2$ is the 2×2 identity matrix (Møller and Waagepetersen 2003; Thomas 1949). Stoyan (2006) introduced a generalized TP with small and large clusters, and Tanaka et al. (2008) proposed a generalized Thomas model of type A, in which the probability density function (pdf) of the distance between the "children" events and their "parent" event corresponds to a mixture of distances from two Gaussian distributions with two different dispersion parameters.

Another generalizing work on TP was done by Castelloe (1998) by extending an isotropic bivariate normal offspring distribution to the case of a general bivariate normal offspring distribution. The extended process is no longer isotropic but anisotropic. The pair correlation function (pcf), a concept borrowed from physics, physical chemistry, and statistical mechanics, is also commonly called a radial distribution function (McQuarrie 1976, Chap. 13), and it describes how the density of points changes with the distance from a reference point. For the aforementioned processes, it is complicated and analytically incomplete. For the estimation, Castelloe (1998) considered a Bayesian approach. Further studies on extension of TP was done by Møller and Toftaker (2014) where anisotropic spatial point processes were introduced. There, Cox, shot noise Cox, and log Gaussian Cox processes having elliptical pcf were studied. In this context, the TP was presented as a limiting case of the Whittle-Matérn shot noise Cox process. Møller and Toftaker (2014) applied a more sophisticated MCMC algorithm to the anisotropic cluster process proposed by Castelloe (1998). However, the estimation still remains complicated and computationally intensive (Møller and Toftaker 2014, p. 426).

Unlike Stoyan (2006) and Tanaka et al. (2008), but like Castelloe (1998) we generalize the TP in our approach not by introducing the pcf first but by presenting the general distribution of the "children" events. In particular, we impose a unified skew-elliptical (SUE) distribution (Arellano-Valle and Genton 2010a) on them. The SUE family is a member of skewed multivariate models (Arnold and Beaver 2000) among which there are some other members with certain characteristics such as skewed multivariate models related to hidden truncation (Arnold and Beaver 2002) and multivariate skew-normal distributions (Azzalini and Dalla Valle 1996) to name a few. Although the SUE family includes a wide range of continuous distributions, we focus on only two representatives of this family here. They are the unified skew-normal (SUN) distribution (Arellano-Valle and Azzalini 2006) and the extended skew-*t* (EST) distribution (Arellano-Valle and Genton 2010b). The reason for our focus on these two distributions is that, in contrast to other continuous distributions in the SUE family, their probabilistic properties have previously been intensively studied. With these results, we can therefore carry out explicit theoretical derivations for approximation. If the "children" events are SUN distributed, then the process would be named a *skew-elliptical-normal* cluster process (CP). If they are EST distributed, then it would be called a *skew-elliptical-t* CP. These two classes of processes together give us *skew-elliptical* CP. It is obvious that a TP is simply a special case of the skew-elliptical-normal CP. Due to its circular shape of the "children" clusters induced by the dispersion matrix $\sigma^2\mathbf{I}_2$ of the bivariate normal distribution, a TP can also be called a circular-normal CP.

The introduction of the skew-elliptical-normal CP and the skew-elliptical-*t* CP is natural because datasets sometimes have non-circular patterns that need to be statistically modeled. If wind or the slope of a location caused the positions of the "children" events to be skew-elliptical distributed, the circular-normal CP (TP) would apparently be inferior to a skew-elliptical-normal or skew-elliptical-*t* CP. Without going into great details about these models, we motivate our approach by showing graphical representations of "children" events of skew-elliptical-normal CPs in Fig. 1 and skew-elliptical-*t* CPs in Fig. 2. The spatial point patterns (SPPs) are generated via R (R Core Team 2019) using the same seed, 999, and all have $\kappa = 5$ and $\mu = 25$. The meanings of the dispersion parameters, σ_1, σ_2, and the skewness parameters, $\boldsymbol{\alpha}$ or $\boldsymbol{\alpha}_{\mathbf{Y}}$, of the skew-elliptical CPs are presented in Sects. 2 and 3. In each of the first rows of Figs. 1 and 2, the patterns of a circular-normal and a circular-*t* CP (left) have clusters in a circular shape induced by the isotropic dispersion matrix, $\sigma^2\mathbf{I}_2$, of the bivariate normal and *t*-distributions of the "children" events. The patterns of an elliptical-normal and an elliptical-*t* CP (middle) have elliptically shaped clusters with the vertical dispersion double the horizontal one induced by the anisotropic dispersion matrix $\text{diag}(\sigma_1^2, \sigma_2^2)$, with $\sigma_2 = 2\sigma_1$, of the bivariate normal and *t*-distribution of the "children" events. Castelloe (1998) dealt with the elliptical-normal CP. The patterns of a skew-normal and a skew-*t* CP (right) have clusters that are relocated further away from the diagonal reference line and skewed toward the upper-right corner. This shape is induced by the isotropic dispersion matrix, $\sigma^2\mathbf{I}_2$, the skewness parameter, $\boldsymbol{\alpha} = \alpha(1, 1)^T$, of the bivariate skew-normal distribution according to Azzalini and Capitanio (1999), and the

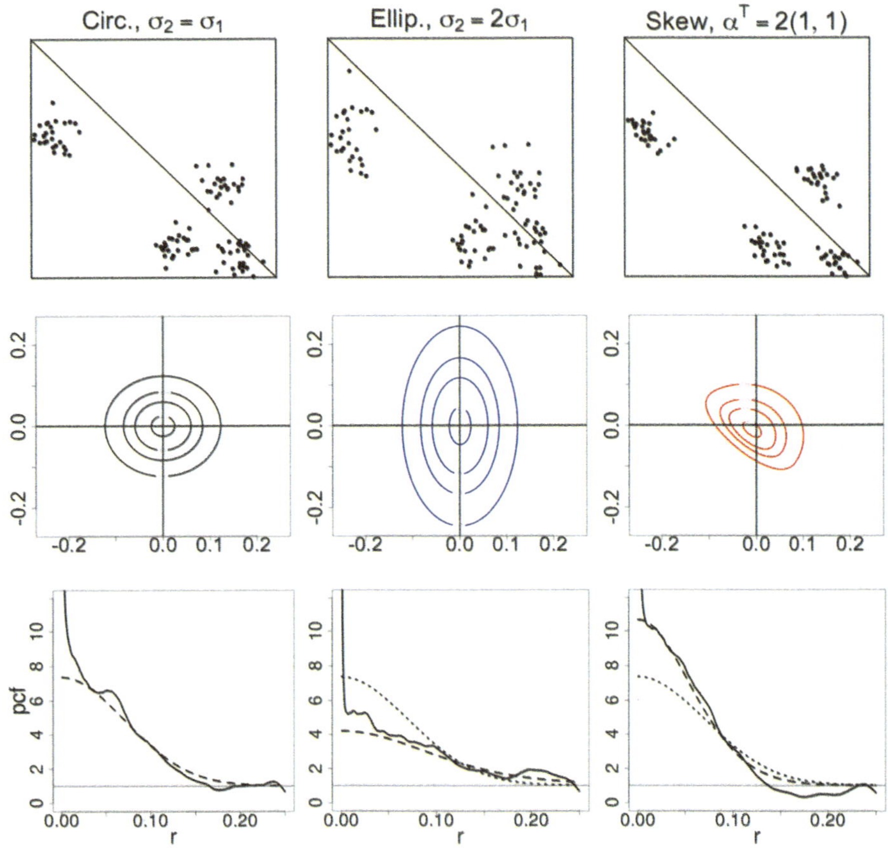

Fig. 1 To generate spatial point patterns (SPPs), $\kappa = 5$, $\mu = 25$, and the same random seed were used. The first row shows a pattern of a circular-normal CP (TP) (left) with "children" events, $\mathbf{Y}$, being bivariate normal distributed with the isotropic dispersion matrix $\sigma^2\mathbf{I}_2$, $\sigma^2 = 0.05^2$; one of an elliptical-normal CP (middle) with $\mathbf{Y}$ being bivariate normal distributed with the anisotropic dispersion matrix with $\sigma_1^2 = 0.05^2$, $\sigma_2^2 = 0.10^2$ in the diagonal; one of a skew-normal CP (right) with $\mathbf{Y}$ being bivariate skew-normal distributed with the isotropic dispersion matrix $\sigma^2\mathbf{I}_2$, $\sigma^2 = 0.05^2$, and skewness parameter $\boldsymbol{\alpha} = 2(1, 1)^T$. The parameters are described in Sect. 2. The diagonal line serves as a reference to better identify the difference in the cluster shape of $\mathbf{Y}$. In the corresponding column, the second row shows the contour plots of the distribution of $\mathbf{Y}$ of the CPs, the SPPs of which are shown in the first row: circular (black), elliptical (blue), and skewed (red). The four contour levels from the most outer to the most inner level correspond to the 95th-, 75th-, 50th-, and 10th-percentile of the distribution of $\mathbf{Y}$. The origin in the second row serves as an unobservable "parent" event. The third row shows the empirical pcf (solid) of the observed SPP from the corresponding first row, the approximating pcf (dashed) of each model, and the theoretical pcf (dotted) of the circular-normal CP (TP) as a reference

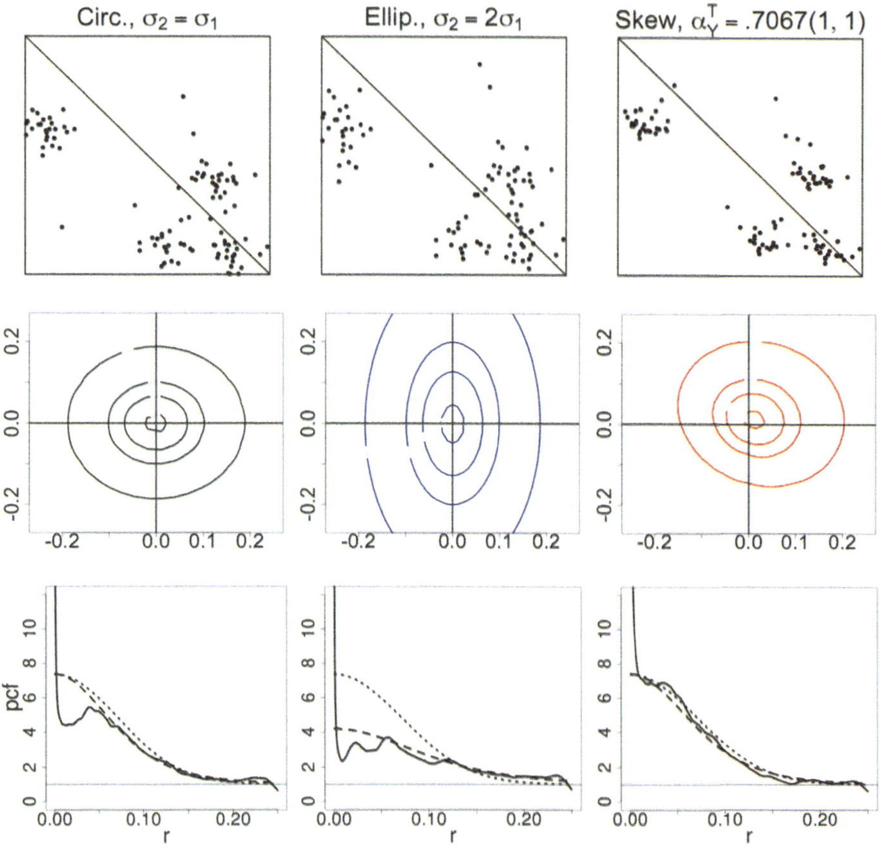

Fig. 2 As in Fig. 1, to generate SPPs of skew-elliptical-t CPs with four df ($\nu = 4$), $\kappa = 5$, $\mu = 25$, and the same random seed were used. The first row shows a pattern of a circular-t CP (left) with "children" events, $\mathbf{Y}$, being bivariate t-distributed with dispersion matrix $\sigma^2 \mathbf{I}_2$ with $\sigma^2 = 0.05^2$, one of an elliptical-t CP (middle) with $\sigma_1^2 = 0.05^2$, $\sigma_2^2 = 0.10^2$, and one of a skew-t CP (right) with $\tau = 1$, $\sigma^2 = 0.05^2$, $\boldsymbol{\alpha}_{\mathbf{Y}}^T = (\alpha_1/\sqrt{1+\alpha_1^2+\alpha_2^2}, \alpha_2/\sqrt{1+\alpha_1^2+\alpha_2^2}) = (0.7067, 0.7067)$, where $\boldsymbol{\alpha}^T = (\alpha_1, \alpha_2) = (20, 20)$. The roles of these parameters are described in Sect. 3. The diagonal line serves as a reference to better identify the difference in the cluster shape of $\mathbf{Y}$. In the corresponding column, the second row shows the contour plots of the distribution of $\mathbf{Y}$ of the CPs, the SPPs of which are shown in the first row: circular (black), elliptical (blue), and skewed (red). The four contour levels from the most outer to the most inner level correspond to the 95th-, 75th-, 50th-, and 10th-percentile of the distribution of $\mathbf{Y}$. The origin in the second row serves as an unobservable "parent" event. The third row shows the empirical pcf (solid) of the observed SPP from the corresponding first row, the approximating pcf (dashed) of each model, and the theoretical pcf (dotted) of the circular-normal CP (TP) as a reference

skewness parameter, $\boldsymbol{\alpha}_{\mathbf{Y}}$ (Sect. 3), of the bivariate EST distribution according to Arellano-Valle and Genton (2010b). The simulated patterns of skew-elliptical-t CPs with four degrees of freedom (df) in the first row of Fig. 2 have more dispersed clusters than do those of the skew-elliptical-normal CPs, in Fig. 1. This distinction is clearer in the second rows where the corresponding contour plots of the distribution of the "children" events are shown. In general, regardless of the df, the "children" events of skew-elliptical-t CPs are more dispersed than those of skew-elliptical-normal CP. The second rows also show the shapes of the clusters: circular (left), elliptical (middle), and skewed or squeezed (right), indicating that the "children" events are not symmetrically distributed around the "parent" event but have fewer events in one particular quarter. In this example, the lower left quarter has fewer events, compared with the number of events in the other three quarters.

The theoretical summary descriptions, in particular pcfs, of the skew-elliptical CPs, except for the TP, are all analytically incomplete. In Castelloe (1998) and Møller and Toftaker (2014), we face the challenge in estimation using the Bayesian approach. However, if we relax the anisotropy condition to the assumption of isotropy, approximation of the pcf is analytically complete. Then, we make use of the minimum contrast method (MCM) for estimation because it is computationally easy, allowing quick exploration of a range of possible models. An estimation via MCM minimizes the discrepancy between the approximating pcf and the empirical pcf of the process. In our case, the minimizer of the discrepancy is the estimator of the parameters of the approximating pcf, but it is also good enough to be considered as the estimator of true parameters.

This paper is organized with the following structure. Sections 2 and 3 present the approximating pcfs of the skew-elliptical-normal and the corresponding skew-elliptical-t CPs. Some analytical derivations were carried out with `Mathematica` (Wolfram Research, Inc. 2020). The intermediate derivation steps are given in the Appendix. Section 4 demonstrates the performance of parameter estimation via the MCM using the function `optim` available in `R` (R Core Team 2019). Section 5 provides a data application of these skew-elliptical CPs on a fraction of the dataset called `fullredwood` available in the `R`-library `spatstat` (Baddeley and Turner 2005; Baddeley et al. 2015). Finally, Sect. 6 introduces alternative probability distributions to extend our work on TP, suggests to generalize a similar clustered spatial point process, and raises a possible exploration for an adjustment of the MCM.

2 Skew-Elliptical-Normal Cluster Processes

2.1 Distributions of "Children" Events

Let $\mathbf{Y}$, the random vector representing the position of the "children" event in a cluster, be bivariate skew-normal distributed with skewness parameter vector $\boldsymbol{\alpha} = (\alpha_1, \alpha_2)^T$, location parameter $-\boldsymbol{\omega}\boldsymbol{\delta}\sqrt{2/\pi}$, where $\boldsymbol{\delta} = \boldsymbol{\alpha}/\sqrt{1+\boldsymbol{\alpha}^T\boldsymbol{\alpha}}$, dispersion matrix $\boldsymbol{\Omega} = \text{diag}(\sigma_1^2, \sigma_2^2)$ with $\sigma_1 > 0$, $\sigma_2 > 0$, and $\boldsymbol{\omega} = \text{diag}(\boldsymbol{\Omega}^{1/2})$. In short, $\mathbf{Y} \sim \mathrm{SN}_2(-\boldsymbol{\omega}\boldsymbol{\delta}\sqrt{2/\pi}, \boldsymbol{\Omega}, \boldsymbol{\alpha})$. In particular, its pdf is $f_{\mathbf{Y}}(\mathbf{y}) = 2\phi_2(\mathbf{y} + \boldsymbol{\omega}\boldsymbol{\delta}\sqrt{2/\pi}; \boldsymbol{\Omega})\ \Phi\{\boldsymbol{\alpha}^T\boldsymbol{\omega}^{-1}(\mathbf{y} + \boldsymbol{\omega}\boldsymbol{\delta}\sqrt{2/\pi})\}$, where $\phi(\cdot)$ and $\Phi(\cdot)$ denote the pdf and cumulative distribution function (cdf) of the univariate standard normal distribution, $\phi_2(\cdot;)$ and $\Phi_2(\cdot;)$ denote the corresponding functions of the bivariate normal distribution and $\mathbf{y} = (y_1, y_2)^T$ (Arellano-Valle and Azzalini 2006; Azzalini and Dalla Valle 1996). Then, $\mathrm{E}(\mathbf{Y}) = \mathbf{0}$ and $\mathrm{Var}(\mathbf{Y}) = \boldsymbol{\Omega} - \frac{2}{\pi}\boldsymbol{\omega}\boldsymbol{\delta}\boldsymbol{\delta}^T\boldsymbol{\omega}$ (Azzalini and Capitanio 1999; Gupta et al. 2013). Then, $\mathbf{Y}$ is also a unified skew-normal (SUN) random vector (Arellano-Valle and Azzalini 2006; Azzalini and Capitanio 2014). It is important to state here that the SUN distribution has the additive property. In general, the SUN distribution introduced by Arellano-Valle and Azzalini (2006) generalizes the parametrization of several variants of the original multivariate skew-normal distribution developed by Azzalini and Dalla Valle (1996). To name a few of these variants, there are the closed skew-normal of González-Farías et al. (2004), the hierarchical skew-normal of Liseo and Loperfido (2003), the fundamental skew-normal of Arellano-Valle and Genton (2005), and the multivariate skew-normal of Gupta et al. (2004).

It is advantageous to use the notation according to Azzalini and Capitanio (2014): $\mathbf{Y}$ has distribution denoted by $\mathrm{SUN}_{2,1}(-\boldsymbol{\omega}\boldsymbol{\delta}\sqrt{2/\pi}, \boldsymbol{\Omega}, \boldsymbol{\delta}, 0, 1)$. For $\mathbf{X} \stackrel{d}{=} \mathbf{Y}_1 - \mathbf{Y}_2$, where $\mathbf{Y}_1$ and $\mathbf{Y}_2$ are two independent "children" events within a cluster, due to the additive property, $\mathbf{X} \sim \mathrm{SUN}_{2,2}(\mathbf{0}, 2\boldsymbol{\Omega}, \boldsymbol{\Delta}, 0, \mathbf{I}_2)$ (Azzalini and Capitanio 2014, Ch. 7), where $\boldsymbol{\Delta} = \boldsymbol{\delta}/\sqrt{2}\,(1, \ -1)$, i.e., the pdf of $\mathbf{X}$ is $f_{\mathbf{X}}(\mathbf{x}) = 4\phi_2\,(\mathbf{x}; 2\boldsymbol{\Omega})$ $\Phi_2(\boldsymbol{\Delta}^T\boldsymbol{\omega}^{-1}\mathbf{x}/\sqrt{2}; \mathbf{I}_2 - \boldsymbol{\Delta}^T\boldsymbol{\Delta})$. Explicitly,

$$f_{\mathbf{X}}(\mathbf{x}) = \frac{\exp\left(-\frac{\sigma_2^2x_1^2+\sigma_1^2x_2^2}{4\sigma_1^2\sigma_2^2}\right)}{\pi\sigma_1\sigma_2}$$
$$\times\ \Phi_2\left\{\frac{\left(\frac{\alpha_1x_1}{\sigma_1}+\frac{\alpha_2x_2}{\sigma_2}\right)\begin{pmatrix}1\\-1\end{pmatrix}}{2\sqrt{1+\alpha_1^2+\alpha_2^2}};\ \frac{\begin{pmatrix}2+\alpha_1^2+\alpha_2^2 & \alpha_1^2+\alpha_2^2\\ \alpha_1^2+\alpha_2^2 & 2+\alpha_1^2+\alpha_2^2\end{pmatrix}}{2(1+\alpha_1^2+\alpha_2^2)}\right\},$$

where $\mathbf{x} = (x_1, x_2)^T$. Note that the distribution of $\mathbf{X}$ shown above is centrally symmetric. The reason for the symmetry is that $\mathbf{Y}_1$ and $\mathbf{Y}_2$ are identically distributed. Hence, $\mathbf{X} = \mathbf{Y}_1 - \mathbf{Y}_2$ and $-\mathbf{X} = \mathbf{Y}_2 - \mathbf{Y}_1 = -(\mathbf{Y}_1 - \mathbf{Y}_2)$ have the same distribution.

2.2 *Approximation of the Pair Correlation Function*

The usual way of defining the pcf of an anisotropic spatial point process is $g(\mathbf{u}, \mathbf{v}) = \lambda^{(2)}(\mathbf{u}, \mathbf{v})/[\lambda(\mathbf{u})\lambda(\mathbf{v})]$, where $\lambda^{(2)}(\mathbf{u}, \mathbf{v})$ is the second-order product density and λ is the intensity function. In our setting, g is anisotropic but translation invariant, $g(\mathbf{u}, \mathbf{v}) = g(\mathbf{v} - \mathbf{u})$, we obtain

$$K(r) = \int_{\mathbb{R}^2} 1_{[\|\mathbf{h}\| \leq r]} g(\mathbf{h}) d\mathbf{h},$$

where $r > 0$ and $1_{[\|\mathbf{h}\| \leq r]}$ is an indicator function. We will then approximate g by g_d, where the subscript d stands for distance and where g_d will be an isotropic function, i.e., $g_d(r)$ with $r = \|\mathbf{h}\|$. Then, $g_d(r) = K_d'(r)/(2\pi r)$, where $K_d'(r) = \partial K_d(r)/\partial r$.

For MCM, the most popular choice for theoretical summary description is the second-order characteristic known as Ripley's K-function (Ripley 1976). The information from Ripley's K-function is the expected number of events found within a distance r from an event of interest, $K(r) = \mathrm{E}[N\{b(\mathbf{o}, r)\}]/\lambda$, where N denotes the number of events within a disc, $b(\mathbf{o}, r)$, of radius $r \geq 0$ at the event of interest $\mathbf{o}$, and λ denotes the global intensity of the process. However, according to Illian et al. (2008, Chap. 4.3.1), the pcf offers the best statistical way to represent the distributional information contained in the point patterns. Additionally, the advantage of using g_d here is that while most approximating pcfs g_d are analytically complete, their corresponding K_d-functions are not. We therefore focus on deriving g_d and provide K_d only if they are analytically complete.

Under the relaxed assumption of isotropy, to derive K_d and g_d, we calculate the distribution of the Euclidean distance, or lag, $R = \sqrt{(\mathbf{Y}_1 - \mathbf{Y}_2)^T(\mathbf{Y}_1 - \mathbf{Y}_2)} = \sqrt{\mathbf{X}^T\mathbf{X}}$, where the $\mathbf{Y}_i$'s represent two independent "children" events within a cluster. They are independently and identically distributed bivariate random vectors, and R is the random variable representing the lag between two randomly distributed "children" events in a cluster under the assumption of isotropy. We first derive its cdf, $F_d(r)$, since $K_d(r) = \pi r^2 + F_d(r)/\kappa$ (Cressie 1993). Then, the pcf is $g_d(r) = 1 + F_d'(r)/(2\pi\kappa r) = 1 + f_d(r)/(2\pi\kappa r)$, where $f_d(r)$ is the pdf of R.

We consider the following transformation with $R \geq 0$, $0 \leq \Theta \leq 2\pi$, $\mathbf{X} = (X_1, X_2)^T$,

$$X_1 = R\cos\Theta, \quad X_2 = R\sin\Theta, \quad \text{and} \tag{1}$$
$$R = \sqrt{\mathbf{X}^T\mathbf{X}} = \sqrt{X_1^2 + X_2^2}, \quad \Theta = \arctan(X_2/X_1).$$

The determinant of the Jacobian matrix is $|\partial(r,\theta)/\partial(x_1,x_2)| = 1/r$. Thus, $f_{R,\Theta}(r,\theta) = r f_{X_1,X_2}(r\cos\theta, r\sin\theta)$, $f_d(r) = \int_0^{2\pi} f_{R,\Theta}(r,\theta)d\theta$, and $F_d(r) = \int_0^r f_d(t)dt$. From (1), the joint distribution, $f_{R,\Theta}(r,\theta)$, is derived in (A.1). The pdf of R follows easily, and from $g_d(r) = 1 + f_d(r)/(2\pi\kappa r)$, the pcf is

$$g_d(r) = 1 + \int_0^{2\pi} \frac{\exp\left(-\frac{\sigma_2^2 r^2\cos^2\theta + \sigma_1^2 r^2 \sin^2\theta}{4\sigma_1^2\sigma_2^2}\right)}{2\pi^2\kappa\sigma_1\sigma_2}$$
$$\times\, \Phi_2\left\{\frac{\left(\frac{\alpha_1 r\cos\theta}{\sigma_1} + \frac{\alpha_2 r\sin\theta}{\sigma_2}\right)\begin{pmatrix}1\\-1\end{pmatrix}}{2\sqrt{1+\alpha_1^2+\alpha_2^2}}; \frac{\begin{pmatrix}2+\alpha_1^2+\alpha_2^2 & \alpha_1^2+\alpha_2^2\\ \alpha_1^2+\alpha_2^2 & 2+\alpha_1^2+\alpha_2^2\end{pmatrix}}{2(1+\alpha_1^2+\alpha_2^2)}\right\} d\theta. \tag{2}$$

For $\boldsymbol{\alpha} \neq \mathbf{0}$, the pcf is analytically incomplete since the integration over the analytically incomplete function, $\Phi_2(\cdot;)$, is analytically incomplete. In particular, the pcf becomes analytically complete if $\alpha_1 = \alpha_2 = 0$, i.e., $\Phi_2(\cdot;) = \Phi_2\left\{(0,0)^T; \mathbf{I}_2\right\} = 1/4$.

2.3 The Elliptical-Normal Cluster Process

Now assume that $\sigma_1 \neq \sigma_2$ and $\boldsymbol{\alpha} = \mathbf{0}$. That is, $\mathbf{Y}$ is bivariate normal distributed, i.e., $\mathbf{Y} \sim N_2(\mathbf{0}, \boldsymbol{\Omega})$. Here, the distribution of the "children" events is elliptical around the "parent" event, and the skewness parameter, $\boldsymbol{\alpha}$, is not present. Then, from (2), the approximating pcf is

$$g_d(r) = 1 + \frac{1}{4\pi\kappa\sigma_1\sigma_2} \exp\left\{-\frac{(\sigma_1^2+\sigma_2^2)r^2}{8\sigma_1^2\sigma_2^2}\right\} \mathrm{BesselI}_0\left\{\frac{(\sigma_1^2-\sigma_2^2)r^2}{8\sigma_1^2\sigma_2^2}\right\},$$

where $\mathrm{BesselI}_0(x) = \sum_{n=0}^{\infty}(x/2)^{2n}/(n!)^2$ is a modified Bessel function of the first kind. A different parametrization, $\sigma_1 \equiv \sigma$ and $\sigma_2 = c_\sigma\sigma$ with $c_\sigma > 0$, can be beneficial in parameter estimation with respect to identifiability because we no longer have two dispersion parameters as above but have one dispersion and its scaling parameter instead,

$$g_d(r) = 1 + \frac{1}{4\pi\kappa c_\sigma\sigma^2} \exp\left\{-\frac{(1+c_\sigma^2)r^2}{8c_\sigma^2\sigma^2}\right\} \mathrm{BesselI}_0\left\{\frac{(1-c_\sigma^2)r^2}{8c_\sigma^2\sigma^2}\right\}.$$

K_d of the elliptical-normal CP is not analytically complete. We estimate κ, σ^2, and c_σ^2 using g_d via the MCM.

As mentioned in Sect. 1, Stoyan (2006) and Tanaka et al. (2008) introduced different models with more than one dispersion parameters to generalize the (traditional) TP. For comparison, we provide the pdf of R of our model in (A.2) and (A.3) in the Appendix.

2.4 The Circular-Normal Cluster Process

Assume that $\boldsymbol{\alpha} = \mathbf{0}$ and $\sigma_1 = \sigma_2 = \sigma$ for the distribution of $\mathbf{Y}$. That is, "children" events are distributed symmetrically circular around their "parent" event. The corresponding process is the traditional TP and is isotropic. For completeness, $f_d(r) = f_R(r)$ is provided in (A.4) in the Appendix. From (2), the true pcf is

$$g(r) = 1 + \frac{\exp\{-r^2/(4\sigma^2)\}}{4\pi\kappa\sigma^2}. \tag{3}$$

The true K-function can be computed as $K(r) = \int_0^r 2\pi t \; g(t) \; dt = \pi r^2 + [1 - \exp\{-r^2/(4\sigma^2)\}]/\kappa$. This formula of the K-function has been widely used prior to this work; for example, it can be found in Cressie (1993). To estimate κ and σ^2, the MCM can use either the pcf or the K-function.

2.5 The Skew-Normal Cluster Process

Let the distribution of $\mathbf{Y}$ be a special case of the SUN distribution mentioned earlier in Sect. 2.1 with $\sigma_1 = \sigma_2 = \sigma$. For a scalar $\sigma > 0$ and a bivariate vector $\boldsymbol{\delta} = \boldsymbol{\alpha}/\sqrt{1 + \boldsymbol{\alpha}^T\boldsymbol{\alpha}}$ with $\boldsymbol{\alpha} = (\alpha_1, \alpha_2)^T$, assume that $\mathbf{Y} = -\boldsymbol{\delta}\sigma\sqrt{2/\pi} + \boldsymbol{\delta}\sigma V_0 + \sigma\mathbf{V}_1$, where V_0 and $\mathbf{V}_1$ are an independent random variable and vector, respectively. Here, V_0 follows the univariate standard normal distribution truncated below 0 with $\mathrm{E}(V_0) = \sqrt{2/\pi}$, $\mathrm{Var}(V_0) = 1 - 2/\pi$, and $\mathbf{V}_1$ is bivariate normal distributed, $\mathrm{N}_2(\mathbf{0}, \boldsymbol{\Psi})$, where

$$\boldsymbol{\Psi} = \mathbf{I}_2 - \boldsymbol{\delta}\boldsymbol{\delta}^T = \mathbf{I}_2 - \boldsymbol{\alpha}\boldsymbol{\alpha}^T/(1 + \boldsymbol{\alpha}^T\boldsymbol{\alpha}) = \begin{pmatrix} 1 + \alpha_2^2 & -\alpha_1\alpha_2 \\ -\alpha_1\alpha_2 & 1 + \alpha_1^2 \end{pmatrix} /(1 + \alpha_1^2 + \alpha_2^2)$$

is a correlation matrix. Under this setting, according to Arellano-Valle and Azzalini (2006, Sect. 2.1.), $\mathbf{Y}$ is bivariate SUN distributed, in particular, $\mathrm{E}(\mathbf{Y}) = \mathbf{0}$, $\mathrm{Var}(\mathbf{Y}) = \sigma^2(\mathbf{I}_2 - 2/\pi\,\boldsymbol{\delta}\boldsymbol{\delta}^T)$. This distribution is purely skewed and does not have any elliptical property. For $\mathbf{Y}_1$ and $\mathbf{Y}_2$ representing two independent positions of the "children" events in a cluster, $\mathbf{X} \stackrel{d}{=} \mathbf{Y}_1 - \mathbf{Y}_2$ has the pdf f_X in Sect. 2.1 with $\sigma_1 = \sigma_2 = \sigma$. Since it is centrally symmetric, we approximate it with a $\mathrm{N}_2\left(\mathbf{0}, 2\sigma^2(\mathbf{I}_2 - 2/\pi\,\boldsymbol{\delta}\boldsymbol{\delta}^T)\right)$ distribution, i.e., bivariate normal with pdf

$$f_{\mathbf{X}}(\mathbf{x}) = \frac{1}{2c_0\sqrt{\pi^2 c_1 c_2 - 4\alpha_1^2\alpha_2^2}} \exp\left[-\frac{\pi\{\pi(c_2 x_1^2 + c_1 x_2^2) + 4\alpha_1\alpha_2 x_1 x_2\}}{2c_0(\pi^2 c_1 c_2 - 4\alpha_1^2\alpha_2^2)}\right],$$

where $c_0 = 2\sigma^2/(1 + \alpha_1^2 + \alpha_2^2)$, $c_1 = 1 + \alpha_1^2(1 - 2/\pi) + \alpha_2^2$, and $c_2 = 1 + \alpha_1^2 + \alpha_2^2(1 - 2/\pi)$. The joint distribution, $f_{R,\Theta}(r, \theta)$, is given in (A.5) in the Appendix. The approximating pcf, $g_d(r)$, is analytically complete only in the following two cases. First, assume that $\alpha_1^2 = \alpha_2^2$, i.e., (i) $\boldsymbol{\alpha} = \alpha(1, 1)^T$, (ii) $\boldsymbol{\alpha} = \alpha(-1, -1)^T$, (iii) $\boldsymbol{\alpha} = \alpha(1, -1)^T$, or (iv) $\boldsymbol{\alpha} = \alpha(-1, 1)^T$, for $\alpha > 0$. Then, $f_d(r)$ is given in (A.6) in the Appendix. Consequently, $g_d(r)$ is

$$g_d(r) = 1 + \frac{\sqrt{1+2\alpha^2}}{4\kappa\sigma^2\sqrt{\pi\{\pi(1+2\alpha^2)-4\alpha^2\}}} \exp\left[-\frac{\{\pi+2\alpha^2(\pi-1)\}r^2}{4\sigma^2\{\pi(1+2\alpha^2)-4\alpha^2\}}\right] \times \mathrm{BesselI}_0\left[\frac{\alpha^2 r^2}{2\sigma^2\{\pi(1+2\alpha^2)-4\alpha^2\}}\right].$$

Second, suppose that (i) $\boldsymbol{\alpha} = (0, \alpha)^T$ or (ii) $\boldsymbol{\alpha} = (\alpha, 0)^T$. Then, $f_d(r)$ is given in (A.7) in the Appendix. Consequently, $g_d(r)$ is

$$g_d(r) = 1 + \frac{r(1+\alpha^2)}{4\pi\kappa\sigma^2\sqrt{(1+\alpha^2)\{1+\alpha^2(1-2/\pi)\}}} \exp\left[-\frac{r^2\{1+\alpha^2(1-1/\pi)\}}{4\sigma^2\{1+\alpha^2(1-2/\pi)\}}\right] \times \mathrm{BesselI}_0\left[\frac{\alpha^2 r^2}{4\pi\sigma^2\{1+\alpha^2(1-2/\pi)\}}\right].$$

K_d of the above scenarios is analytically incomplete. We estimate κ, σ^2, and α^2 via MCM using g_d. The complete determination of $\boldsymbol{\alpha}$ results from choosing the optimal $\hat{\boldsymbol{\alpha}}$ from the above possibilities such that the cluster shape of simulated SPP can illustrate that of the observed SPP as best as possible.

Remark 1 So far we have emphasized on presenting CPs having the approximating pcf g_d as being analytically complete because they are advantageous in MCM. In practice, however, for CP having only analytically incomplete pcfs or K-functions, the parameter estimation can still be carried out, for example, with a Bayesian approach, but the computation is more intensive.

3 Skew-Elliptical-*t* Cluster Processes

3.1 General Scenario and Relaxing Independence

Let $\mathbf{Y}$ be the bivariate random vector representing the position of a "children" event in a cluster, and let $(\mathbf{Y}^T, \mathbf{Y}^{*T})^T$ be four-variate extended skew-t (EST) distributed, i.e., $\mathrm{EST}_4(\mathbf{0}, \mathrm{diag}(\boldsymbol{\Omega}, \boldsymbol{\Omega}), (\boldsymbol{\alpha}^T, \boldsymbol{\alpha}^T)^T, \nu, \tau)$ (Arellano-Valle and Genton 2010b) with a 4×4 dispersion matrix $\mathrm{diag}(\boldsymbol{\Omega}, \boldsymbol{\Omega})$, four-variate shape parameter $(\boldsymbol{\alpha}^T, \boldsymbol{\alpha}^T)^T$, ν df, and extension parameter $\tau \in \mathbb{R}$, where the 2×2 matrix $\boldsymbol{\Omega} = \mathrm{diag}(\sigma_1^2, \sigma_2^2)$ and the bivariate vector $\boldsymbol{\alpha}^T = (\alpha_1, \alpha_2)$. According to Arellano-Valle and Genton (2010b, Prop. 3), the marginal distribution of $\mathbf{Y}$ is also EST distributed: $\mathbf{Y} \sim \mathrm{EST}_2(\mathbf{0}, \boldsymbol{\Omega}, \boldsymbol{\alpha}_\mathbf{Y}, \nu, \tau_\mathbf{Y})$, where $\boldsymbol{\alpha}_\mathbf{Y} = \boldsymbol{\alpha}/\sqrt{1+\boldsymbol{\alpha}^T\boldsymbol{\alpha}}$ is termed as marginal shape parameter, and $\tau_\mathbf{Y} = \tau/\sqrt{1+\boldsymbol{\alpha}^T\boldsymbol{\alpha}}$ is termed as marginal extension parameter. Note that (i) $\boldsymbol{\alpha}_\mathbf{Y}$ is not necessary in the setting of skew-elliptical-normal CPs because there $\boldsymbol{\alpha} = \boldsymbol{\alpha}_\mathbf{Y}$ and (ii) the statistical characteristic of $\boldsymbol{\alpha}_\mathbf{Y}$ of a skew-t CP is equivalent to that of $\boldsymbol{\alpha}$ of a skew-normal CP. Moreover, for simplicity, we have set the location parameter to zero, but it could be adjusted to yield $\mathrm{E}(\mathbf{Y}) = \mathbf{0}$ with the results of

Section 2.3 in Arellano-Valle and Genton (2010b). From Proposition 5 of the same paper, we derive that $\mathbf{X} = \mathbf{Y} - \mathbf{Y}^* \sim \text{EST}_2(\mathbf{0}, 2\boldsymbol{\Omega}, \mathbf{0}, \nu, \tau/\sqrt{1+2\boldsymbol{\alpha}^T\boldsymbol{\alpha}})$.

Although $\boldsymbol{\alpha}$ is neither the shape parameter of the distribution of $(\mathbf{Y}^T, \mathbf{Y}^{*T})^T$ nor of $\mathbf{Y}$, it is important in the setting of skew-elliptical-t CPs. First, it contributes to the shape of the distribution of $(\mathbf{Y}^T, \mathbf{Y}^{*T})^T$ and of $\mathbf{Y}$; thus, we know how the "children" events are distributed and know how the process is constructed. Second, $\boldsymbol{\alpha}$, but not $\boldsymbol{\alpha}_{\mathbf{Y}}$, appears in the formulas of the pcfs of skew-t CPs; hence, we can use the theoretical pcf to estimate the parameter $\boldsymbol{\alpha}$ and then compute $\boldsymbol{\alpha}_{\mathbf{Y}}$. The task of $\boldsymbol{\alpha}_{\mathbf{Y}}$ is to describe the shape of the marginal distribution of $\mathbf{Y}$: the cluster shape of the process.

For independent and identically distributed children $\mathbf{Y}_i, \mathbf{Y}_j$ with $i \neq j$ in a cluster, $\mathbf{X}_{\text{true}} \overset{d}{=} \mathbf{Y}_i - \mathbf{Y}_j$ is not bivariate EST, unified skew-t, or bivariate t distributed. In fact, its distribution is unknown. The only sub-family of the skew-elliptical distributions that has the additive property is the SUN family (Arellano-Valle and Genton 2010a,b; González-Farías et al. 2004). We chose to approximate the distribution of $\mathbf{X}_{\text{true}}$ by $\mathbf{X}$, i.e., $\mathbf{X}_{\text{true}} \overset{d}{\approx} \mathbf{X} \sim \text{EST}_2(\mathbf{0}, 2\boldsymbol{\Omega}, \mathbf{0}, \nu, \tau/\sqrt{1+2\boldsymbol{\alpha}^T\boldsymbol{\alpha}})$. Note that the distribution of $\mathbf{X}$ loses the information about $\boldsymbol{\alpha}$ of the distribution of $\mathbf{Y}$ if $\tau = 0$. The pdf of $\mathbf{X}$ is

$$f_{\mathbf{X}}(\mathbf{x}) = \frac{T_1\left\{\frac{\tau}{\sqrt{1+2\boldsymbol{\alpha}^T\boldsymbol{\alpha}}}\left(\frac{\nu+2}{\nu+\mathbf{x}^T\boldsymbol{\Omega}^{-1}\mathbf{x}/2}\right)^{1/2}; \nu+2\right\}}{2\pi|2\boldsymbol{\Omega}|^{1/2}\left(1+\frac{\mathbf{x}^T\boldsymbol{\Omega}^{-1}\mathbf{x}/2}{\nu}\right)^{(\nu+2)/2} T_1\left(\frac{\tau}{\sqrt{1+2\boldsymbol{\alpha}^T\boldsymbol{\alpha}}}; \nu\right)},$$

where $T_1(\cdot; \nu)$ denotes the cdf of the univariate t-distribution with ν degrees of freedom. The explicit form of $f_{\mathbf{X}}(\mathbf{x})$ is given in (A.8), and under the isotropy assumption, the joint distribution function, $f_{d,R,\Theta}(r, \theta)$, is provided in (A.9). If $\boldsymbol{\alpha} \neq \mathbf{0}$ and $\sigma_1 \neq \sigma_2$, the approximating pcf is analytically incomplete:

$$g_d(r) = 1 + \frac{1}{8\pi^2\kappa\sigma_1\sigma_2 T_1\left\{\frac{\tau}{\sqrt{1+2(\alpha_1^2+\alpha_2^2)}}; \nu\right\}} \times \int_0^{2\pi} \frac{T_1\left[\frac{\tau}{\sqrt{1+2(\alpha_1^2+\alpha_2^2)}}\left\{\frac{\nu+2}{\nu+(r^2\cos^2\theta/\sigma_1^2+r^2\sin^2\theta/\sigma_2^2)/2}\right\}^{1/2}; \nu+2\right]}{\left(1+\frac{r^2\cos^2\theta/\sigma_1^2+r^2\sin^2\theta/\sigma_2^2}{2\nu}\right)^{(\nu+2)/2}} d\theta. \tag{4}$$

For MCM, we use a sequence of ν. For each value of ν, we estimate the other parameters. Then, we choose the set of estimates and the corresponding ν that provide the smallest discrepancy between the approximating and empirical pcfs.

3.2 The Skew-*t* Cluster Process

If $\boldsymbol{\alpha} \neq \mathbf{0}$ and $\sigma_1 = \sigma_2$, i.e., $(\mathbf{Y}^T, \mathbf{Y}^{*T})^T \sim \mathrm{EST}_4(\mathbf{0}, \sigma^2\mathbf{I}_4, (\boldsymbol{\alpha}^T, \boldsymbol{\alpha}^T)^T, \nu, \tau)$ (Arellano-Valle and Genton 2010b) and, hence, $\mathbf{Y} \sim \mathrm{EST}_2(\mathbf{0}, \sigma^2\mathbf{I}_2, \boldsymbol{\alpha}_{\mathbf{Y}}, \nu, \tau_{\mathbf{Y}})$, where $\boldsymbol{\alpha}_{\mathbf{Y}} = \boldsymbol{\alpha}/\sqrt{1+\boldsymbol{\alpha}^T\boldsymbol{\alpha}}$ and $\tau_{\mathbf{Y}} = \tau/\sqrt{1+\boldsymbol{\alpha}^T\boldsymbol{\alpha}}$, we obtain the following approximating pcf under isotropy assumption from (4):

$$g_d(r) = 1 + \frac{T_1\left[\frac{\tau}{\sqrt{1+2(\alpha_1^2+\alpha_2^2)}}\left\{\frac{\nu+2}{\nu+r^2/(2\sigma^2)}\right\}^{1/2}; \nu+2\right]}{4\pi\kappa\sigma^2\, T_1\left\{\frac{\tau}{\sqrt{1+2(\alpha_1^2+\alpha_2^2)}}; \nu\right\}\left(1+\frac{r^2}{2\nu\sigma^2}\right)^{(\nu+2)/2}}.$$

The previous formula has two parameters, α_1 and α_2, of the same role: they both contribute to the skewness of the distribution of $\mathbf{Y}$. A different parametrization, $\alpha_1 = \alpha$ and $\alpha_2 = c_\alpha \alpha$ with c_α being a real constant, can be useful for parameter estimation.

K_d of the skew-*t* CP is analytically incomplete. For the parameter estimation, we estimate κ, σ^2, α^2, and c_α^2 via MCM using the pcf. Then, we can compute the estimates of $\alpha_{\mathbf{Y},1}$ and $\alpha_{\mathbf{Y},2}$ because eventually we are interested in knowing the estimate of the skewness parameter of the skew-*t* CP, which is $\boldsymbol{\alpha}_{\mathbf{Y}}$, not $\boldsymbol{\alpha}$.

Remark 2 Recall that $\alpha_{\mathbf{Y},i} = \alpha_i/\sqrt{1+\alpha_1^2+\alpha_2^2}$, $i = 1, 2$. Thus, they have absolute values less than 1, i.e., $|\alpha_{\mathbf{Y},1}| < 1$, $|\alpha_{\mathbf{Y},2}| < 1$, although the absolute values of α_1 and α_2 can be large. For $|\alpha_{\mathbf{Y},1}| = |\alpha_{\mathbf{Y},2}|$, their absolute values can be at most $1/\sqrt{2} \approx 0.7071$. Consequently, only skew-normal CPs with skewness parameters having absolute values smaller than $1/\sqrt{2}$ can be considered to be approximated by a skew-*t* CP with large df. A demonstration of this statement is given in Sect. 5.

3.3 The Elliptical-*t* Cluster Process

If $\tau = 0$, $\boldsymbol{\alpha} = \mathbf{0}$, but $\sigma_1 \neq \sigma_2$, i.e., $(\mathbf{Y}^T, \mathbf{Y}^{*T})^T \sim \mathrm{t}_\nu((\mathbf{0}^T, \mathbf{0}^T)^T, \mathrm{diag}(\boldsymbol{\Omega}, \boldsymbol{\Omega}))$, where $\boldsymbol{\Omega} = \mathrm{diag}(\sigma_1^2, \sigma_2^2)$ and, hence, $\mathbf{Y} \sim \mathrm{t}_\nu(\mathbf{0}, \boldsymbol{\Omega})$, where t_ν is the multivariate Student *t*-distribution with ν df, then the approximating pcf is

$$g_d(r) = 1 + \frac{1}{8\pi^2\kappa\sigma_1\sigma_2}\int_0^{2\pi}\left(1+\frac{r^2\cos^2\theta/\sigma_1^2 + r^2\sin^2\theta/\sigma_2^2}{2\nu}\right)^{-(\nu+2)/2} d\theta.$$

For $\nu = 1$, $g_d(r) \equiv 1$. Only for $\nu = 2k$, where $k \in \mathbb{N}$, is $g_d(r)$ analytically complete. For each even df, we have to compute the approximating pcf individually since there is no general formula for the pcf. `Mathematica` can compute up to

26 df analytically. For df greater than 6, the formulas of pcfs are very cumbersome and can take several rows to be displayed. We choose to represent the pcfs only for $\nu = 2, 4$, and 6 in the following. For $\nu = 2$,

$$g_d(r) = 1 + \frac{2\{(\sigma_1^2 + \sigma_2^2)r^2 + 8\sigma_1^2\sigma_2^2\}}{\pi\kappa\{(r^2 + 4\sigma_1^2)(r^2 + 4\sigma_2^2)\}^{3/2}},$$

$\nu = 4$,

$$g_d(r) = 1 + \frac{16\left\{512\sigma_1^4\sigma_2^4 + 64\sigma_1^2\sigma_2^2(\sigma_1^2 + \sigma_2^2)r^2 + (3\sigma_1^4 + 2\sigma_1^2\sigma_2^2 + 3\sigma_2^4)r^4\right\}}{\pi\kappa\{(r^2 + 8\sigma_1^2)(r^2 + 8\sigma_2^2)\}^{5/2}},$$

and $\nu = 6$,

$$g_d(r) = 1 + \frac{324\left[\{24\sigma_1^2\sigma_2^2 + (\sigma_1^2 + \sigma_2^2)r^2\}\{1152\sigma_1^4\sigma_2^4 + 96\sigma_1^2\sigma_2^2(\sigma_1^2 + \sigma_2^2)r^2 + (5\sigma_1^4 - 2\sigma_1^2\sigma_2^2 + 5\sigma_2^4)r^4\}\right]}{\pi\kappa\{(r^2 + 12\sigma_1^2)(r^2 + 12\sigma_2^2)\}^{7/2}}.$$

K_d of the elliptical-t CP is analytically incomplete regardless of df. We can estimate κ, $\sigma_1^2 = \sigma^2$, and c_σ^2, where $\sigma_2^2 = c_\sigma^2\sigma^2$, via MCM using the pcf.

3.4 The Circular-t Cluster Process

If $\tau = 0$, $\boldsymbol{\alpha} = \mathbf{0}$, and $\sigma_1 = \sigma_2$, i.e., $(\mathbf{Y}^T, \mathbf{Y}^{*T})^T \sim \mathrm{t}_\nu((\mathbf{0}^T, \mathbf{0}^T)^T, \sigma^2\mathbf{I}_4)$, and, hence, $\mathbf{Y} \sim \mathrm{t}_\nu(\mathbf{0}, \sigma^2\mathbf{I}_2)$, the pcf is

$$g(r) = 1 + \frac{1}{4\pi\kappa\sigma^2}\left(1 + \frac{r^2}{2\nu\sigma^2}\right)^{-(\nu+2)/2}, \tag{5}$$

and the K-function is

$$K(r) = \pi r^2 + \frac{1 - \left\{1 + r^2/(2\sigma^2\nu)\right\}^{-\nu/2}}{\kappa}. \tag{6}$$

We can estimate κ and σ^2. The results presented in Sect. 4 are from an estimation using the pcf; however, the K-function could be employed just as well.

It is important to note that, in this setting, $\tau = 0$, $\boldsymbol{\alpha} = \mathbf{0}$, and $\sigma_1 = \sigma_2$, and the exact distribution of $\mathbf{X}$ is multivariate Behrens–Fisher (Dickey 1966) with pdf (Dickey 1968):

$$f_{\mathbf{X}}(\mathbf{x}) = C\, B\left(\frac{\nu+2}{2}, \frac{\nu+2}{2}\right) F_1\left(\frac{\nu+2}{2}; \nu+1, \nu+1; \nu+2; s_1, s_2\right),$$

where the constant $C = \Gamma(\nu+1)/[\pi\nu\{\Gamma(\nu/2)\}^2]$ for $\Gamma(\cdot)$ denoting the Gamma function, $B\{(\nu+2)/2, (\nu+2)/2\} = \{\Gamma(\nu/2)\}^2/\Gamma(\nu+2)$, and F_1 is the Appell's hypergeometric function. In particular (Erdélyi et al. 1953),

$$
\begin{aligned}
&F_1\left((\nu+2)/2, \nu+1, \nu+1, \nu+2; s_1, s_2\right) \\
&=[B\{(\nu+2)/2, (\nu+2)/2\}]^{-1} \times \int_0^1 \{t(1-t)\}^{\nu/2}\{(1-ts_1)(1-ts_2)\}^{-\nu-1}\, dt,
\end{aligned}
$$

and s_1 and s_2 are the two real roots of the equation $s^2 + (s-1)\mathbf{x}^T\mathbf{x}/(2\sigma^2\nu) = 0$. According to the transformation in (1),

$$
f_d(r) = \frac{2\Gamma(\nu+1)\, r}{\nu\{\Gamma(\nu/2)\}^2} \int_0^1 \frac{\{t(1-t)\}^{\nu/2}}{\{(1-ts_1)(1-ts_2)\}^{\nu+1}}\, dt,
$$

where $s_{1,2} = -r^2/(4\sigma^2\nu) \pm \sqrt{r^2/(2\sigma^2\nu) + \{r^2/(4\sigma^2\nu)\}^2}$. The notation $s_{1,2}$ denotes s_1 and s_2. The pcf, $g(r)$, can be derived from $f_d(r)$. However, the computation of $f_d(r)$ is computationally intensive and does not yield any advantage for the parameter estimation, since $g(r)$ remains analytically incomplete from this approach. This again confirms that using the approximation distribution of $\mathbf{X}_{\text{true}}$ is computationally advantageous.

3.5 *The Case of Orthogonality*

If $\mathbf{Y}_1$ and $\mathbf{Y}_2$ are orthogonal, i.e., E $(\mathbf{Y}_1^T\mathbf{Y}_2) = 0$, and if they are jointly scale mixtures of bivariate normals, i.e., $\mathbf{Y}_i = V^{-1/2}\mathbf{Z}_i$, $i = 1, 2$, where the $\mathbf{Z}_i$'s are independently and identically $\mathrm{N}_2(\mathbf{0}, \mathbf{\Sigma})$ distributed, which are independent of $V \sim G$ and have a cdf with $G(0) = 0$, then $\mathbf{X} = V^{-1/2}\mathbf{Z}$ with $\mathbf{Z} \sim \mathrm{N}_2(\mathbf{0}, 2\mathbf{\Sigma})$ is independent of V. In particular, for $V \sim \text{Gamma}(\nu/2, \nu/2)$, $\mathbf{Y}_i$ follows the bivariate Student t-distribution mentioned above with $\mathbf{\Sigma} = \sigma^2\mathbf{I}_2$, and the exact pcf and K-function are given in (5) and (6).

4 Parameter Estimation by Minimum Contrast

Diggle (2003, Sect. 6) defined the *minimum contrast method* (MCM) using the K-function. MCM minimizes discrepancy between the theoretical K-function, $K(r;\boldsymbol{\theta}) \equiv K(r)$, of the assumed model and the empirical K-function, $\hat{K}(r)$, of the observed pattern. In particular, the discrepancy is defined as $D(\boldsymbol{\theta}) = \int_0^{r_0} w(r)\left[\{\hat{K}(r)\}^{c_{\text{stabil}}} - \{K(r;\boldsymbol{\theta})\}^{c_{\text{stabil}}}\right]^2 dr$, where the constants, r_0 and c_{stabil}, and the weighting function, $w(r)$, are to be chosen. Here, c_{stabil} acts as a variance-stabilizing transformation, and $\boldsymbol{\theta}$ is the vector comprising the parameters of the K-function, $K(r)$, or of the pcf, $g(r)$. The estimator, $\hat{\boldsymbol{\theta}}$, is the minimizer of $D(\boldsymbol{\theta})$.

In our setting, using the approximating pcf $g_d(r;\boldsymbol{\theta})$ and the empirical pcf $\hat{g}(r)$, we redefine the discrepancy,

$$D_{d,g}(\boldsymbol{\theta}) = \int_0^{r_0} w(r)\left[\{\hat{g}(r)\}^{c_{\text{stabil}}} - \{g_d(r;\boldsymbol{\theta})\}^{c_{\text{stabil}}}\right]^2 dr. \tag{7}$$

For the data simulation, we want to work with spatial point patterns (SPPs) having approximately 200 events on a unit square. Consequently, the dispersion parameters σ_1 and σ_2 should not be larger than 0.10; otherwise, the data generation cannot produce enough events because the cluster dispersion is too large. Additionally, we want the number of "parent" and of "children" events to be between 10 and 20, so that the parameter estimation can be stable. Thus, we chose $\kappa = 20$, $\sigma_1 = \sigma = 0.04$, $\mu = 10$. In Table 1, the models of interest are given in the first column and the parameters are given in the second column. For the elliptical-normal CP, $\sigma_2 = 0.08$ or $c_\sigma = 2$ were chosen. For the skew-normal

Table 1 3000 SPPs were generated from each skew-elliptical CP. The first column provides the model specification. The second column gives information about the parameters of the model, and in the second row of each cell in this column, the logarithms of starting values for our estimation are provided. In the third column, the average computational time in seconds is represented by $\bar{T}$. $\overline{\text{Dis}^2_{d,g}(\hat{\boldsymbol{\theta}}_n)}$ denotes the average of $\text{Dis}^2_{d,g}(\hat{\boldsymbol{\theta}}_n)$ according to (8), where $\hat{\boldsymbol{\theta}}_n$ denotes the MCM estimate from the (true) novel (skew-elliptical) CP. $\overline{\text{Dis}^2_{d,g}(\hat{\boldsymbol{\theta}}_t)}$ is the average of $\text{Dis}^2_{d,g}(\hat{\boldsymbol{\theta}}_t)$ according to (8), where $\hat{\boldsymbol{\theta}}_t$ denotes the MCM estimate from the (wrong) traditional TP. In the sixth column, % provides the percentage of how often $\text{Dis}^2_{d,g}(\hat{\boldsymbol{\theta}}_n)$ is smaller than $\text{Dis}^2_{d,g}(\hat{\boldsymbol{\theta}}_t)$

	Parameters/starting values	$\bar{T}$	$\overline{\text{Dis}^2_{d,g}(\hat{\boldsymbol{\theta}}_n)}$	$\overline{\text{Dis}^2_{d,g}(\hat{\boldsymbol{\theta}}_t)}$	%
Elliptical-normal	$(\kappa, \sigma_1, c_\sigma)^T = (20, 0.04, 2)^T$ $\log(\kappa_0, \sigma^2_{1,0}, c^2_{\sigma,0})^T =$ $(0, -4, 3.5)^T$	0.164	0.029	0.031	96.0
Skew-normal	$(\kappa, \sigma, \alpha_1 = \alpha_2 = \alpha)^T =$ $(20, 0.04, 10)^T$ $\log(\kappa_0, \sigma^2_0, \alpha^2_0)^T =$ $(0, -4, 5.5)^T$	0.177	0.176	0.179	83.9
Elliptical-t, df = 6	$(\kappa, \sigma_1, c_\sigma)^T = (20, 0.04, 2)^T$ $\log(\kappa_0, \sigma^2_{1,0}, c^2_{\sigma,0})^T =$ $(0, -4, 3.3)^T$	0.115	0.035	0.038	85.3
Skew-t, df = 6	$(\kappa, \sigma, \alpha_1 = \alpha_2 = \alpha)^T =$ $(20, 0.04, 20)^T$ $\log(\kappa_0, \sigma^2_0, \alpha^2_0)^T =$ $(0, -5, 5)^T$	0.082	0.098	0.101	84.7
Circular-t, df = 6	$(\kappa, \sigma)^T = (20, 0.04)^T$ $\log(\kappa_0, \sigma^2_0)^T = (0, -4)^T$	0.035	0.077	0.085	88.1

CP, $\alpha_1 = \alpha_2 = \alpha = 2$ were chosen. For elliptical-t CP with $\nu = 6$, $\sigma_2 = 0.08$ or $c_\sigma = 2$, and for the skew-t CP with the same df, $\alpha_1 = \alpha_2 = \alpha = 20$, and $\tau = 1$ were selected. Thus, the skewness parameter of the skew-t CP is $\boldsymbol{\alpha}_{\mathbf{Y}}^T = (\alpha_1/\sqrt{1+\alpha_1^2+\alpha_2^2}, \alpha_2/\sqrt{1+\alpha_1^2+\alpha_2^2}) = (0.7067, 0.7067)$.

The R-package `spatstat` computes the empirical pcf with an isotropic-corrected estimator (Ripley 1988) and a translation-corrected estimator (Ohser 1983). Our experience shows that the empirical pcf according to the former sometimes has NA (not-available) values, which can stop the computation of the estimation. Hence, for the parameter estimation in this section as well as for the data application in Sect. 5, we use the empirical pcf according to the translation-corrected estimator. The computation was done on compute nodes that have 8 CPU cores, 32 GB of RAM, and the CPU processors clocked at 2.4 GHz or faster.

Since we generated the SPPs on a unit square, $r_0 = 0.25$ and $c_{\text{stabil}} = 0.25$ were chosen (Diggle 2003, Chap. 6.1) for the parameter estimation. Additionally, $w(r) = 1$ was set due to clustered patterns (Diggle 2003, Chap. 6.3). We used the function `optim` available in `R` to minimize (7).

The logarithms of the starting values needed for the function `optim` are given in the second column of Table 1 since we estimated the logarithms of κ, σ^2, c_σ^2, and α^2. For the parameter estimation, we just need to estimate α^2 since we set $\alpha_1 = \alpha_2 = \alpha$, i.e., $c_\alpha = 1$, for the skew-normal and skew-t CP. Additionally, we set $\nu = 6$ and $\tau = 1$ for a simple computation for the skew-t CP. In practice, however, the parameter estimation is done differently: one sequence of ν and one of τ are considered, and the parameter estimation is done given a pair of (ν, τ). Among these possible combinations, a set of values is chosen as a set of estimates when it delivers the smallest discrepancy between the approximating and empirical pcfs. Table 1 provides the average computational time, $\bar{T}$, in seconds in the third column and provides information to determine whether or not the choice of MCM and the function `optim` makes sense in the last three columns. Let $\overline{\text{Dis}_{d,g}^2}(\hat{\boldsymbol{\theta}})$ denote the average of *bilateral discrepancy*,

$$\text{Dis}_{d,g}^2(\hat{\boldsymbol{\theta}}) = \int \{\hat{g}(r) - g_d(\hat{\boldsymbol{\theta}}, r)\}^2 + \{g_d(\hat{\boldsymbol{\theta}}, r) - g_d(\boldsymbol{\theta}, r)\}^2 dr, \tag{8}$$

where the d, g subscript shows the involvement of the approximating pcf, $g_d(r)$, and $\hat{\boldsymbol{\theta}}$ denotes the estimate. $\overline{\text{Dis}_{d,g}^2}(\hat{\boldsymbol{\theta}}_n)$ is the average of bilateral discrepancy $\text{Dis}_{d,g}^2(\hat{\boldsymbol{\theta}}_n)$, where $\hat{\boldsymbol{\theta}}_n$ denotes the estimate resulting from the assumption of the (true) novel (skew-elliptical) CP. Similarly, $\overline{\text{Dis}_{d,g}^2}(\hat{\boldsymbol{\theta}}_t)$ is the average of bilateral discrepancy $\text{Dis}_{d,g}^2(\hat{\boldsymbol{\theta}}_t)$, where $\hat{\boldsymbol{\theta}}_t$ denotes the estimate resulting from the assumption of the (wrong) traditional TP. For each of 3000 SPPs, we could compute $\text{Dis}_{d,g}^2(\hat{\boldsymbol{\theta}}_n)$ and $\text{Dis}_{d,g}^2(\hat{\boldsymbol{\theta}}_t)$. The percentage in the last column shows how often $\text{Dis}_{d,g}^2(\hat{\boldsymbol{\theta}}_n) < \text{Dis}_{d,g}^2(\hat{\boldsymbol{\theta}}_t)$; i.e., if the correct model is assumed, the MCM using the approximating pcf can provide better estimates than assuming a TP. It shows that in the most cases

$\text{Dis}^2_{d,g}(\hat{\boldsymbol{\theta}}_n) < \text{Dis}^2_{d,g}(\hat{\boldsymbol{\theta}}_t)$. Additional information, $\overline{\text{Dis}^2_{d,g}}(\hat{\boldsymbol{\theta}}_n) < \overline{\text{Dis}^2_{d,g}}(\hat{\boldsymbol{\theta}}_t)$, also supports this statement.

The estimate of the mean number of "children" events, μ, does not come from the MCM directly, since μ does not appear in the pcf and, hence, is not involved in the minimization of $D_{d,g}(\boldsymbol{\theta})$ in (7). The estimator of μ is, in fact, $\hat{\mu} = n/\hat{\kappa}$, where n is the number of events of the observed pattern and $\hat{\kappa}$ denotes the estimate of κ and can be obtained via MCM.

The left column of Table 2 displays the choice of models and statistical information of the estimates. If the hypothesized model is correctly assumed, the MCM estimators of κ and $\sigma = \sigma_1$ outperform the ones under TP, the wrong model, with respect to MSE. The estimators of c_σ or σ_2 of elliptical-normal and -t CP, and of α of skew-normal and skew-t CP seem to be very reasonable since they are relatively unbiased and have tolerable variance. Overall, MCM provided reasonable estimates with respect to minimizing the discrepancy in (7).

5 The Clustered Redwoods Dataset

The `redwoodfull` dataset, available from the library `spatstat` and representing the locations of *195 Californian redwood seedlings and saplings* in a square sampling region, was first described and analyzed by Strauss (1975). Additionally, according to Baddeley and Turner (2005), it has never been subjected to a comprehensive analysis. In fact, only a small subset of it, known as the dataset `redwood` and consisting of only 62 trees, was analyzed in many works of spatial point processes, e.g., Diggle (2003). The `redwoodfull` dataset appears to be interesting because it has many clusters that display non-circular shapes. We plotted `redwoodfull` in Fig. 3 (left) in clustered and inhibitory partitions, represented by circles and triangles, respectively. In our opinion, 73 trees represented by triangles cannot be reasonably described by a clustered spatial point process since they follow an inhibitory pattern. We are interested only in analyzing the *clustered redwoods*, especially in finding out which skew-elliptical CPs can best model the process generating it. Figure 3 (middle) shows the empirical K-function (solid line) of the clustered redwoods and, for reference, the theoretical K-function (dotted line) of a CSR with the same intensity over the polygon. Here, r is the Euclidean distance from the event of interest. Figure 3 (right) displays the empirical F-function (dashed line) and G-function (solid line). For reference, the theoretical F- and G-functions of a CSR of the same intensity over the polygon are shown with a dotted line. Note for CSR, $F \equiv G$. Two facts indicating clustering are given in the following: (i) the empirical F-function lies below the theoretical F-function of a CSR and (ii) the K-function progresses above the theoretical K-function of a CSR. The empirical G-function also suggests clustering although not as clearly as the empirical F- and K-functions do. Sometimes it lies below, indicating inhibition, and sometimes above the reference line (the theoretical G-function of a CSR) over the domain

Table 2 The information about the models is given in Table 1. std = se × $\sqrt{3000}$, where std is the estimate of standard deviation and se is the standard error. 2.5% gives the 2.5-percentile, and 97.5% gives the 97.5-percentile of the distribution of the estimates, respectively. $\text{Bias}^2 = \{E(\hat{\theta}) - \theta\}^2$, where $E(\cdot)$ denotes the expectation and is approximated by average of the 3000 estimates. MSE = $\text{Bias}^2 + \text{Var}(\hat{\theta})$, where $\text{Var}(\hat{\theta})$ is the variance of $\hat{\theta}$ and is approximated by std^2. The four columns under Skew-elliptical Cluster Processes show the estimates and the statistical properties under the true models, and the two columns under Thomas process provide the ones under the (traditional) TP, the wrong model

	Skew-elliptical cluster processes				Thomas process	
	$\hat{\kappa}$	$\hat{\sigma} = \hat{\sigma}_1$	$\hat{\sigma}_2$	$\hat{\alpha} = \hat{\alpha}_1 = \hat{\alpha}_2$	$\hat{\kappa}$	$\hat{\sigma}$
Elliptical-normal	21.854	0.042	0.098		26.485	0.052
Std	12.686	0.013	0.077		12.522	0.011
2.5%	4.711	0.020	0.038		9.374	0.035
97.5%	52.724	0.068	0.313		56.785	0.077
Bias^2	3.436	29×10^{-7}	31×10^{-5}		42.060	14×10^{-5}
MSE	164.366	16×10^{-5}	0.006		198.867	26×10^{-5}
Skew-normal	23.175	0.034		2.355	23.593	0.028
Std	7.486	0.007		4.716	7.611	0.004
2.5%	11.255	0.023		0.066	11.503	0.022
97.5%	40.024	0.049		10.789	40.912	0.037
Bias^2	10.081	4×10^{-5}		20.471	12.907	15×10^{-5}
MSE	66.125	9×10^{-5}		42.711	70.831	16×10^{-5}
Elliptical-*t*, df = 6	20.470	0.046	0.094		26.625	0.053
Std	12.168	0.017	0.064		13.469	0.012
2.5%	4.988	0.018	0.037		9.126	0.035
97.5%	51.158	0.084	0.268		61.441	0.080
Bias^2	0.221	4×10^{-5}	19×10^{-5}		43.897	18×10^{-5}
MSE	148.270	32×10^{-5}	431×10^{-5}		225.319	32×10^{-5}
Skew-*t*	19.596	0.040		19.245	22.244	0.037
Std	7.952	0.010		8.624	8.399	0.007
2.5%	7.174	0.027		6.848	9.108	0.028
97.5%	7.403	0.065		41.041	40.904	0.056
Bias^2	0.163	1×10^{-7}		297.381	5.035	73×10^{-7}
MSE	63.403	5×10^{-5}		371.755	75.584	6×10^{-5}
Circular-*t*	22.030	0.039			22.820	0.039
Std	8.446	0.006			8.703	0.006
2.5%	10.253	0.029			10.538	0.029
97.5%	41.927	0.054			43.340	0.053
Bias^2	4.119	3×10^{-7}			7.952	8×10^{-7}
MSE	75.446	35×10^{-6}			83.702	39×10^{-6}

of r approximately from 0.01 to 0.05, suggesting clustering. Overall, there are graphical hints that the redwoods of interest are clustered. We have, however, to investigate statistically whether this is truly the case. First, we test whether CSR can provide a good fit to the redwoods of interest. For that, the plug-in goodness-of-fit

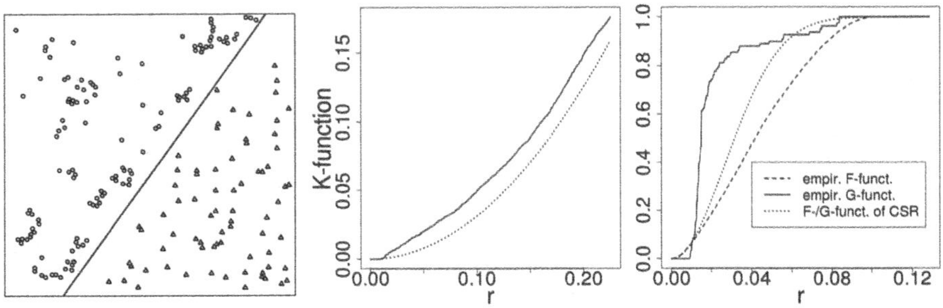

Fig. 3 On the left, the locations of 195 Californian redwood seedlings and saplings in a square sampling region, 130 × 130 feet, are shown. They are displayed in two partitions: circles represent the clustered redwoods and triangles the inhibitory ones, respectively. In the middle, the empirical K-function (solid line) of the clustered redwoods and the theoretical one of a CSR of the same global intensity (dotted line) are shown. Here, the global intensity, λ, over the polygon containing the circles is approximately 221. On the right, the empirical F-function (dashed line) and G-function (solid line) are plotted along with the theoretical F- and G-functions of a CSR of 221 events (dotted line). Note that for a CSR, the theoretical F-function $\equiv$ G-function

test using the G- and F-functions (Diggle 2003, Chap. 1.7) is employed, and the resulting estimated p-values, $\hat{p}$, are all 0. Since the p-values are smaller than the nominal significance level of $\alpha_{\text{GOF}} = 0.05$, we reject that CSR provides a good fit and conclude that the redwoods of interest are clustered. Second, for the circular-, elliptical-, skew-normal CPs, and the corresponding-t CPs with a certain df, we compute the estimates and the corresponding discrepancy between the empirical pcf and the theoretical one of the underlying model. For elliptical-t CPs, we choose 2, 6, 10, 20, and 26 df for simplicity since their pcfs can be computed analytically with `Mathematica`. For skew- and circular-t CPs, we consider all even df up to 30, although we display results only for 2, 10, 20, and 30 df. The estimates such as $\hat{\kappa}$, $\hat{\sigma}^2$, $\hat{c}_{\sigma}^2$, $\hat{\alpha}^2$, and $\hat{c}_{\alpha}^2$ are obtained directly from the MCM (Table 3) except the one of μ, the mean of children number per cluster, which is absent in the pcf and hence irrelevant in this context.

The empirical pcf (solid line, right plot in the first row) in Fig. 4 takes small values for small r, increases over the domain $0.001 < r < 0.0123$, and decreases for $r > 0.0123$. This observation is unlike how the pcf of a cluster process should progress. Illian et al. (2008, Sect. 4.3.1, 4.3.4) state that for a cluster process, the pcf takes large values for small r and decreases as r increases. This empirical pcf is indeed problematic at small r, and we are aware that "the estimation of the pair correlation function is more delicate and complicated than that of K due to the serious issues of bandwidth choice and estimation for small r" (Illian et al. 2008, p. 227, Sect. 4.3.2). We believe that using the complete curve of the empirical pcf would produce misleading estimates of κ, σ^2, c_{σ}^2, α^2, and c_{α}^2. Thus, two estimation possibilities should be investigated. The first data analysis uses the empirical pcf, $\hat{g}(r)$, completely. The second data analysis discards the first 28 pairs from 512 pairs of data (r_i, g_i), $i = 1, \ldots, 512$, where r_i denotes one of 512 grid

Table 3 In the first column, the models applied to the clustered redwoods are shown. The resulting MCM estimates are given in the second and third columns. Here, $\hat{g}(r)$ is the empirical pcf. The discrepancy, $\mathrm{Dis}_g^1(\hat{\boldsymbol{\theta}})$, between the empirical pcf and the theoretical one of certain underlying model is defined in (9). The smallest discrepancy in each column is displayed boldly

	Using $\hat{g}(r)$completely		Using $\hat{g}(r)$ partially	
CP	Estimates	$\mathrm{Dis}_g^1(\hat{\boldsymbol{\theta}})$	Estimates	$\mathrm{Dis}_g^1(\hat{\boldsymbol{\theta}})$
Circular-normal	$\hat{\kappa} = 60.910$, $\hat{\sigma} = 0.022$	0.04824	$\hat{\kappa} = 60.082$, $\hat{\sigma} = 0.018$	0.007080
Elliptical-normal	$\hat{\kappa} = 60.880$, $\hat{\sigma}_1 = 0.022$, $\hat{\sigma}_2 = 0.022$	0.04823	$\hat{\kappa} = 53.098$, $\hat{\sigma}_1 = 0.009$, $\hat{\sigma}_2 = 0.030$	**0.004028**
Skew-normal	$\hat{\kappa} = 60.873$, $\hat{\sigma} = 0.022$, $\hat{\alpha}_1 = -0.185$, $\hat{\alpha}_2 = 0.185$	**0.04822**	$\hat{\kappa} = 58.647$, $\hat{\sigma} = 0.023$ $\hat{\alpha}_1 = -20.254$, $\hat{\alpha}_2 = 20.254$	0.006032
Circular-t, df = 2	$\hat{\kappa} = 47.182$, $\hat{\sigma} = 0.0242$	0.05329	$\hat{\kappa} = 49.164$, $\hat{\sigma} = 0.0172$	0.004481
Circular-t, df = 10	$\hat{\kappa} = 57.988$, $\hat{\sigma} = 0.0223$	0.04899	$\hat{\kappa} = 57.754$, $\hat{\sigma} = 0.0177$	0.005673
Circular-t, df = 20	$\hat{\kappa} = 59.369$, $\hat{\sigma} = 0.0222$	0.04857	$\hat{\kappa} = 58.845$, $\hat{\sigma} = 0.0178$	0.006274
Circular-t, df = 30	$\hat{\kappa} = 59.852$, $\hat{\sigma} = 0.0222$	0.04846	$\hat{\kappa} = 59.283$, $\hat{\sigma} = 0.0179$	0.006513
Elliptical-t, df = 2	$\hat{\kappa} = 47.148$, $\hat{\sigma}_1 = 0.0242$, $\hat{\sigma}_2 = 0.0242$	0.05328	$\hat{\kappa} = 49.158$, $\hat{\sigma}_1 = 0.0172$, $\hat{\sigma}_2 = 0.0172$	0.004481
Elliptical-t, df = 10	$\hat{\kappa} = 57.949$, $\hat{\sigma}_1 = 0.0223$, $\hat{\sigma}_2 = 0.0223$	0.04899	$\hat{\kappa} = 52.712$, $\hat{\sigma}_1 = 0.0095$, $\hat{\sigma}_2 = 0.0282$	0.004154
Elliptical-t, df = 20	$\hat{\kappa} = 59.042$, $\hat{\sigma}_1 = 0.0223$, $\hat{\sigma}_2 = 0.0223$	0.04862	$\hat{\kappa} = 52.845$, $\hat{\sigma}_1 = 0.0092$, $\hat{\sigma}_2 = 0.0292$	0.004112
Elliptical-t, df = 26	$\hat{\kappa} = 59.732$, $\hat{\sigma}_1 = 0.0222$, $\hat{\sigma}_2 = 0.0222$	0.04847	$\hat{\kappa} = 52.959$, $\hat{\sigma}_1 = 0.0091$, $\hat{\sigma}_2 = 0.0296$	0.004078
Skew-t, df = 2	$\hat{\kappa} = 47.174$, $\hat{\sigma} = 0.0243$, $\hat{\alpha}_1 = -5.178$, $\hat{\alpha}_2 = 62.388$ $(\hat{\alpha}_{\mathbf{Y},1} = -0.083$, $\hat{\alpha}_{\mathbf{Y},2} = 0.996)$	0.053	$\hat{\kappa} = 49.180$, $\hat{\sigma} = 0.0172$, $\hat{\alpha}_1 = -12.368$, $\hat{\alpha}_2 = 84.517$ $(\hat{\alpha}_{\mathbf{Y},1} = 0 - 0.145$, $\hat{\alpha}_{\mathbf{Y},2} = 0.989)$	0.004480

(continued)

Table 3 (continued)

CP	Using $\hat{g}(r)$completely		Using $\hat{g}(r)$ partially	
	Estimates	$\mathrm{Dis}_g^1(\hat{\boldsymbol{\theta}})$	Estimates	$\mathrm{Dis}_g^1(\hat{\boldsymbol{\theta}})$
Skew-t, df = 10	$\hat{\kappa} = 57.963$, $\hat{\sigma} = 0.0224$, $\hat{\alpha}_1 = -3.356$, $\hat{\alpha}_2 = 49.077$ ($\hat{\alpha}_{\mathbf{Y},1} = 0 - 0.068$, $\hat{\alpha}_{\mathbf{Y},2} = 0.997$)	0.049	$\hat{\kappa} = 57.732$, $\hat{\sigma} = 0.0177$, $\hat{\alpha}_1 = -2.595$, $\hat{\alpha}_2 = 28.391$ ($\hat{\alpha}_{\mathbf{Y},1} = 0 - 0.091$, $\hat{\alpha}_{\mathbf{Y},2} = 0.995$)	0.005671
Skew-t, df = 20	$\hat{\kappa} = 59.427$, $\hat{\sigma} = 0.0222$, $\hat{\alpha}_1 = -8.095$, $\hat{\alpha}_2 = 51.185$ ($\hat{\alpha}_{\mathbf{Y},1} = 0 - 0.156$, $\hat{\alpha}_{\mathbf{Y},2} = 0.988$)	0.0486	$\hat{\kappa} = 58.890$, $\hat{\sigma} = 0.0178$, $\hat{\alpha}_1 = -4.079$, $\hat{\alpha}_2 = 45.750$ ($\hat{\alpha}_{\mathbf{Y},1} = 0 - 0.089$, $\hat{\alpha}_{\mathbf{Y},2} = 0.996$)	0.006273
Skew-t, df = 30	$\hat{\kappa} = 59.915$, $\hat{\sigma} = 0.0222$, $\hat{\alpha}_1 = -8.646$, $\hat{\alpha}_2 = 18.942$ ($\hat{\alpha}_{\mathbf{Y},1} = 0 - 0.415$, $\hat{\alpha}_{\mathbf{Y},2} = 0.909$)	0.048	$\hat{\kappa} = 59.270$, $\hat{\sigma} = 0.0179$, $\hat{\alpha}_1 = -4.048$, $\hat{\alpha}_2 = 45.369$ ($\hat{\alpha}_{\mathbf{Y},1} = 0 - 0.089$, $\hat{\alpha}_{\mathbf{Y},2} = 0.996$)	0.006519

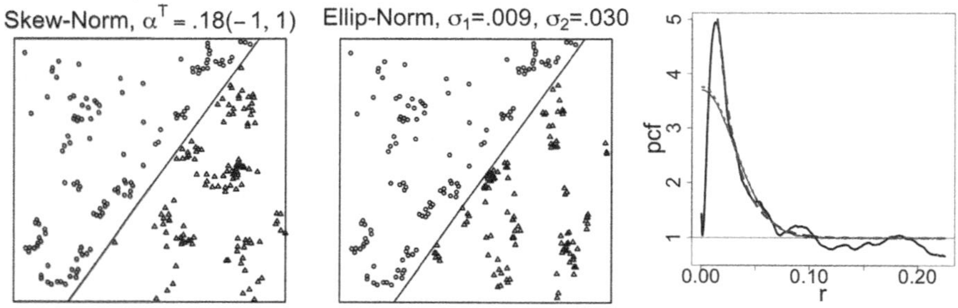

Fig. 4 The 122 clustered redwoods (circles) are displayed in the upper left polygon of the left and middle plots. There, in the lower right polygon, the left plot shows the simulated events (triangles) of the skew-normal CP with parameters $\kappa = 60.873$, $\sigma = 0.022$, $\alpha_1 = -0.185$, $\alpha_2 = 0.185$, and $\mu = 3.632$, and similarly, the middle plot shows the simulated events (triangles) of the elliptical-normal CP with parameters $\kappa = 53.098$, $\sigma_1 = 0.009$, $\sigma_2 = 0.030$, and $\mu = 4.163$. The right plot shows the empirical pcf (solid), the theoretical pcf of the circular-normal CP (TP) (thin), the approximating pcf of skew-normal CP (dotted, red), and the approximating pcf of elliptical-normal CP (dashed, blue). The theoretical pcf of TP and the approximating pcf of skew-normal are very similar due to the negligible estimate, $\hat{\alpha} = 0.185$. Here, these two pcfs overlay each other. For the simulations, the random seed, 999, as in Fig. 1 was used

points representing the domain of r and g_i the value of the empirical pcf at r_i. Estimates and the discrepancies, $\mathrm{Dis}_g^1(\hat{\boldsymbol{\theta}})$ in (9), of the corresponding models from both analyses are listed in Table 3. We define the discrepancy between the empirical and approximating pcfs at $\hat{\boldsymbol{\theta}}$ as follows

$$\mathrm{Dis}_g^1(\hat{\boldsymbol{\theta}}) = \int_0^{r_0} \{\hat{g}(r) - g_d(\hat{\boldsymbol{\theta}}, r)\}^2 \, dr, \tag{9}$$

where $r_0 = 0.25$ is chosen for analysis of datasets on a unit square.

The first analysis using the empirical pcf completely assigns the smallest discrepancy to a skew-normal CP. The second analysis using the empirical pcf partially assigns the smallest discrepancy, however, to an elliptical-normal CP. Before the goodness-of-fit (GOF) of these two models is tested, we want to clarify a point that might appear to be an inconsistency in our calculation. Under the column "Using $\hat{g}(r)$ partially", the discrepancies, $\mathrm{Dis}_g^1(\hat{\boldsymbol{\theta}})$, of the skew-$t$ CPs do not converge to the one (0.006032) of the skew-normal CP when the df increases. The reason for it is the absolute values of the skewness parameters of the skew-normal CP are really large $|\alpha_1| = |\alpha_2| = 20.254$, while the absolute values of the skewness parameters of the skew-t CP are much smaller, $|\alpha_{\mathbf{Y},i}| < 1, i = 1, 2$. On the contrary, under the column "Using $\hat{g}(r)$ completely", the discrepancies, $\mathrm{Dis}_g^1(\hat{\boldsymbol{\theta}})$, of the skew-$t$ CPs do converge to the one (0.04822) of the skew-normal CP when the df increases. The reason for it is the absolute values of the skewness parameters of the skew-normal CP are smaller than 1, in particular $|\alpha_1| = |\alpha_2| = 0.185$, and the absolute values of the skewness parameters of the skew-t CP are also smaller than 1, $|\alpha_{\mathbf{Y},i}| < 1, i = 1, 2$. These phenomena can serve as demonstrations of a statement in Remark 2.

Now, the adjusted goodness-of-fit (AGOF) test (Dao and Genton 2014) is applied since the plug-in GOF test is not appropriate because only one dataset is available. The AGOF test is also termed as the Dao–Genton test in Baddeley et al. (2015) and is made available in the R-library `spatstat`. Diggle (2003, Sect. 6.2.) recommended not to use the GOF test based on the K-function if the K-function was used for parameter estimation. Since we used the empirical pcf (originating from the K-function) for the parameter estimation, we could rely on the GOF conclusion from the AGOF-G or $-F$ test. We expect, however, that the AGOF-G tests would not support the fit of any CP due to the limited support of the clustering of the empirical G-function. Therefore, we decided to rely mainly on the conclusion from the AGOF-F test. For the testing, the nominal significance level is $\alpha_{\text{GOF}} = 0.05$, and $\hat{\alpha}^*_{\text{AGOF}}$ denotes the estimated adjusted level (Dao and Genton 2014). For completeness, we run AGOF-G tests that rejected all the models to be a good fit. This is expected due to the limited support of the clustering of the empirical G-function explained previously. The AGOF-F test, the only test to be relied on, provided (i) $\hat{p} = 0.025$, which is greater than $\hat{\alpha}^*_{\text{AGOF}} = 0.005$ for the skew-normal CP model and (ii) $\hat{p} = 0.035$, which is greater than $\hat{\alpha}^*_{\text{AGOF}} = 0.004$ for the elliptical-normal CP model. For the latter model, we used the empirical pcf partially as described previously for the parameter estimation but used the empirical pcf completely for the computation of the $\hat{p}$-value. The AGOF-F test provided $\hat{p} > \hat{\alpha}^*_{\text{AGOF}}$ for both models. Hence, we conclude that these models provide a good fit, statistically speaking.

Now, we examine these models graphically. The right plot (Fig. 4) shows the empirical pcf (solid), the approximating pcf of the circular-normal CP (TP) (thin), the theoretical skew-normal CP (dotted, red), and the approximating elliptical-normal CP (dashed, blue). The two approximating pcfs of the circular- and the skew-normal are very similar due to the negligible estimate of the skewness parameter, $\hat{\alpha} = 0.185$. The approximating pcf of the skew-normal CP does not represent well the empirical pcf, neither at short nor at middle distance, i.e., $r < 0.066$. The approximating pcf of the elliptical-normal CP, however, does represent the empirical pcf well from the middle distance, $r > 0.0123$. The left plot (Fig. 4) shows that the simulated events (triangles) of the skew-normal CP do not mimic the clustered redwoods (circles) well because while the cluster shape of the clustered redwoods is oblong, that of the simulated data is fairly circular. On the contrary, the middle plot shows that the simulated events (triangles) of the elliptical-normal CP have oblong cluster shape that is similar to the cluster shape of the clustered redwoods. One can see this more clearly if one turns the simulated data by an angle of approximately 40°.

Overall, we think that the elliptical-normal CP represents the data better than does the skew-normal CP. This data application also confirms that the introduction of skew-elliptical CPs is necessary; otherwise; the ellipticity of the cluster shape could not be modeled.

6 Discussion

There are a few robustness problems in estimation. First, the MCM uses the approximating instead of the theoretical pcf. The approximating pcf results from isotropy assumption of the CP to achieve the analytical completeness, easy to be incorporated in MCM. The isotropy leads to a significant loss of information, and therefore the results of estimates need to be carefully verified.

Second, there is sensitivity toward starting values of the empirical pcf under isotropy assumption. It is usually poorly estimated at a short distance, i.e., r close to 0. We encountered this problem in our data application: the empirical pcf does not decrease throughout although it should be strictly decreasing since the assumed model is clustered (Illian et al. 2008, Sect. 4.3.4). It even increases over a short domain close to 0. Using the complete curve of the empirical pcf might produce misleading estimates, but at the same time, ignoring the poorly estimated part of the empirical pcf might cause overfitting. It may be possible to come up with a cut-off point from which data of the pcf can be used.

Third, the more parameters the model has, the more sensitive the estimation can become with respect to the starting values. In general, it is usually difficult to estimate high-dimensional parameters. One can try to improve the robustness by estimating certain parameters at a time. For example, assuming that a few parameters, say $\boldsymbol{\theta}_1$, are given, one estimates the remaining parameters, say $\boldsymbol{\theta}_2$, where $\boldsymbol{\theta}^T = (\boldsymbol{\theta}_1^T, \boldsymbol{\theta}_2^T)$. Then, we plug in the estimates $\boldsymbol{\theta}_2 = \hat{\boldsymbol{\theta}}_2$ in the pcf and estimate

$\boldsymbol{\theta}_1$. The estimation continues until the discrepancy (9) goes below a pre-set limit. According to our limited estimation studies, parameters such as c_α or α could be treated as $\boldsymbol{\theta}_1$, and κ, c_σ, or σ could be treated together as $\boldsymbol{\theta}_2$.

A possible extension of generalizing the TP is to consider enlarging the choice of the distribution that is imposable on $\mathbf{Y}$, which is the location of a "children" event in a cluster. Besides the SUN and EST classes, there may be other distributions of the unified skew-elliptical families. One of the requirements for the distribution of $\mathbf{Y}$ is that it has the additive property because the distribution of $\mathbf{X}$ has to be established where $\mathbf{X} \overset{d}{=} \mathbf{Y}_1 - \mathbf{Y}_2$ and $\mathbf{Y}_i$, $i = 1, 2$, representing two independent positions of the "children" events in a cluster.

In this work, we generalized the TP to some extent. However, we can shift the focus to the Matérn process, the role of which is very similar to that of the TP in the field of spatial point processes. Both are special cases of the Neyman–Scott cluster point process. A Matérn process is constructed similar to a TP except that the positions of the "children" events are distributed independently and uniformly inside a disc with the "parent" event as the center. Similar to this work, it is possible to establish some variations of the Matérn process with respect to the circular, elliptical, and skew properties of the distribution of "children" events.

Acknowledgments The authors would like to thank Professor Reinaldo Arellano-Valle and a reviewer for their useful suggestions and comments. The authors also acknowledge the Texas A&M University Brazos cluster that contributed to the research reported here. The work of the second author was supported by King Abdullah University of Science and Technology (KAUST).

Appendix

Table of Acronyms

Acronym	Complete words
AGOF	Adjusted goodness-of-fit
cdf	Cumulative distribution function
CP	Cluster process
CSR	Complete spatial randomness
df	Degrees of freedom
EST	Extended skew-*t*
GOF	Goodness-of-fit
MCM	Minimum contrast method
pcf	Pair correlation function
pdf	Probability density function
SPP	Spatial point pattern
SUE	Unified skew-elliptical
SUN	Unified skew-normal
TP	Thomas process

Skew-Elliptical-Normal Cluster Processes

According to the transformation in (1), the joint distribution $f_{R,\Theta}(r,\theta)$ of (R,Θ) is

$$f_{R,\Theta}(r,\theta) = \frac{r\exp\left(-\frac{\sigma_2^2 r^2\cos^2\theta+\sigma_1^2 r^2\sin^2\theta}{4\sigma_1^2\sigma_2^2}\right)}{\pi\sigma_1\sigma_2} \quad \text{(A.1)}$$
$$\times\,\Phi_2\left\{\frac{\left(\frac{\alpha_1 r\cos\theta}{\sigma_1}+\frac{\alpha_2 r\sin\theta}{\sigma_2}\right)\begin{pmatrix}1\\-1\end{pmatrix}}{2\sqrt{1+\alpha_1^2+\alpha_2^2}};\frac{\begin{pmatrix}2+\alpha_1^2+\alpha_2^2 & \alpha_1^2+\alpha_2^2\\ \alpha_1^2+\alpha_2^2 & 2+\alpha_1^2+\alpha_2^2\end{pmatrix}}{2(1+\alpha_1^2+\alpha_2^2)}\right\}.$$

Elliptical-Normal Cluster Process

$$f_d(r) = \frac{r}{2\sigma_1\sigma_2}\exp\left\{-\frac{(\sigma_1^2+\sigma_2^2)r^2}{8\sigma_1^2\sigma_2^2}\right\}\text{BesselI}_0\left\{\frac{(\sigma_1^2-\sigma_2^2)r^2}{8\sigma_1^2\sigma_2^2}\right\}. \quad \text{(A.2)}$$

For a different parametrization, $\sigma_1 \equiv \sigma$ and $\sigma_2 = c_\sigma\sigma$ with $c_\sigma > 0$, the pdf $f_d(r)$ can be rewritten as follows:

$$f_d(r) = \frac{1}{2c_\sigma\sigma^2}\exp\left\{-\frac{(1+c_\sigma^2)r^2}{8c_\sigma^2\sigma^2}\right\}\text{BesselI}_0\left\{\frac{(1-c_\sigma^2)r^2}{8c_\sigma^2\sigma^2}\right\}. \quad \text{(A.3)}$$

Circular-Normal Cluster Process

Here, $\sigma_1 = \sigma_2$. We provide the pdf of R, $f_R(r) = f_d(r)$ in the following:

$$f_R(r) = \frac{r}{2\sigma^2}\exp\left(-\frac{r^2}{4\sigma^2}\right). \quad \text{(A.4)}$$

Skew-Normal Cluster Process

Following the transformation defined in (1),

$$f_{R,\Theta}(r,\theta) = \frac{r}{2c_0\sqrt{\pi^2 c_1 c_2 - 4\alpha_1^2\alpha_2^2}} \quad \text{(A.5)}$$
$$\times\,\exp\left(-\frac{\pi r^2[\pi\{\cos^2\theta(c_2-c_1)+c_1\}+4\alpha_1\alpha_2\cos\theta\sin\theta]}{2c_0(\pi^2 c_1 c_2 - 4\alpha_1^2\alpha_1^2)}\right),$$

where $c_0 = 2\sigma^2/(1+\alpha_1^2+\alpha_2^2)$, $c_1 = 1+\alpha_1^2(1-2/\pi)+\alpha_2^2$, and $c_2 = 1+\alpha_1^2+\alpha_2^2(1-2/\pi)$. The pdf, $f_d(r)$, is analytically complete only in the following two cases. First, $\alpha_1^2 = \alpha_2^2$, i.e., (i) $\boldsymbol{\alpha}^T = \alpha(1,1)$, (ii) $\boldsymbol{\alpha}^T = \alpha(-1,-1)$, (iii) $\boldsymbol{\alpha}^T = \alpha(1,-1)$, or (iv) $\boldsymbol{\alpha}^T = \alpha(-1,1)$, assuming that $\alpha > 0$. Consequently, $c_1 = c_2$,

$$f_d(r) = \frac{\pi\sqrt{1+2\alpha^2}r}{2\sigma^2\sqrt{\pi\{\pi(1+2\alpha^2)-4\alpha^2\}}}\exp\left[-\frac{\{\pi+2\alpha^2(\pi-1)\}r^2}{4\sigma^2\{\pi(1+2\alpha^2)-4\alpha^2\}}\right] \quad \text{(A.6)}$$
$$\times \text{BesselI}_0\left[\frac{\alpha^2 r^2}{2\sigma^2\{\pi(1+2\alpha^2)-4\alpha^2\}}\right],$$

where $\text{BesselI}_0(x) = \sum_{n=0}^{\infty}(x/2)^{2n}/(n!)^2$ is a modified Bessel function of the first kind.

Second, suppose that $\boldsymbol{\alpha} = (0,\alpha)^T$ or $\boldsymbol{\alpha} = (\alpha,0)^T$. Then,

$$f_d(r) = \frac{r(1+\alpha^2)}{2\sigma^2\sqrt{(1+\alpha^2)\{1+\alpha^2(1-2/\pi)\}}}\exp\left[-\frac{r^2\{1+\alpha^2(1-1/\pi)\}}{4\sigma^2\{1+\alpha^2(1-2/\pi)\}}\right]$$
$$\times \text{BesselI}_0\left[\frac{\alpha^2 r^2}{4\pi\sigma^2\{1+\alpha^2(1-2/\pi)\}}\right]. \quad \text{(A.7)}$$

Skew-Elliptical-t Cluster Processes

For $\mathbf{x} = (x_1, x_2)^T$,

$$f_{\mathbf{X}}(x_1,x_2) = \frac{T_1\left[\frac{\tau}{\sqrt{1+2(\alpha_1^2+\alpha_2^2)}}\left\{\frac{\nu+2}{\nu+(x_1^2/\sigma_1^2+x_2^2/\sigma_2^2)/2}\right\}^{1/2};\nu+2\right]}{4\pi\sigma_1\sigma_2\left(1+\frac{x_1^2/\sigma_1^2+x_2^2/\sigma_2^2}{2\nu}\right)^{(\nu+2)/2}T_1\left\{\frac{\tau}{\sqrt{1+2(\alpha_1^2+\alpha_2^2)}};\nu\right\}}, \quad \text{(A.8)}$$

where $T_1(\cdot;\nu)$ denotes the cdf of the univariate t-distribution with ν degrees of freedom. According to the transformation in (1), the joint distribution of (R,Θ) is

$$f_{R,\Theta}(r,\theta) \quad \text{(A.9)}$$
$$= \frac{r\,T_1\left[\frac{\tau}{\sqrt{1+2(\alpha_1^2+\alpha_2^2)}}\left\{\frac{\nu+2}{\nu+(r^2\cos^2\theta/\sigma_1^2+r^2\sin^2\theta/\sigma_2^2)/2}\right\}^{1/2};\nu+2\right]}{4\pi\sigma_1\sigma_2\left(1+\frac{r^2\cos^2\theta/\sigma_1^2+r^2\sin^2\theta/\sigma_2^2}{2\nu}\right)^{(\nu+2)/2}T_1\left\{\frac{\tau}{\sqrt{1+2(\alpha_1^2+\alpha_2^2)}};\nu\right\}}.$$

References

Arellano-Valle, R. B., & Azzalini, A. (2006). On the unification of families of skew-normal distributions. *Scandinavian Journal of Statistics, 33*, 561–574.

Arellano-Valle, R. B., & Genton, M. G. (2005). On fundamental skew distributions. *Journal of Multivariate Analysis, 96*, 93–116.

Arellano-Valle, R. B., & Genton, M. G. (2010a). Multivariate unified skew-elliptical distributions. *Chilean Journal of Statistics, 1*, 17–33.

Arellano-Valle, R. B., & Genton, M. G. (2010b). Multivariate extended skew-*t* distributions and related families. *Metron, 68*, 2001–234

Arnold, B. C., & Beaver, R. J. (2000). Some skewed multivariate distributions. *American Journal of Mathematical and Management Sciences, 20*, 27–38.

Arnold, B. C., & Beaver, R. J. (2002). Skewed multivariate models related to hidden truncation and/or selective reporting. *TEST, 11*, 7–54.

Azzalini, A., & Capitanio, A. (1999). Statistical applications of the multivariate skew normal distributions. *Journal of the Royal Statistical Society B, 61*, 579–602.

Azzalini, A., & Capitanio, A. (2014). *The skew-normal and related families*. Cambridge: Cambridge University Press.

Azzalini, A., & Dalla Valle, A. (1996). The multivariate skew-normal distribution. *Biometrika, 83*, 715–726.

Baddeley, A. J., & Turner, R. (2005). SPATSTAT: An R package for analyzing spatial point patterns. *Journal of Statistical Software, 12*, 1–42.

Baddeley, A. J., Rubak, E., & Turner, R. (2015). *Spatial point patterns: Methodology and applications with R*. London: Chapman and Hall/CRC Press.

Castelloe, J. M. (1998). Issues in reversible jump Markov chain Monte Carlo and composite EM analysis, applied to spatial Poisson cluster processes. Ph.D. thesis, University of Iowa (1998)

Cressie, N. A. C. (1993). *Statistics for spatial data*. New York, NY: Wiley (1993)

Dao, N. A., & Genton, M. G. (2014). A Monte Carlo adjusted goodness-of-fit test for parametric models describing spatial point patterns. *Journal of Computational and Graphical Statistics, 23*, 497–517.

Dickey, J. M. (1966). On a multivariate generalization of the Behrens–Fisher distribution. *The Annals of Mathematical Statistics, 37*, 763.

Dickey, J. M. (1968). Three multidimensional-integral identities with Bayesian applications. *The Annals of Mathematical Statistics, 39*, 1615–1627

Diggle, P. J. (2003). *Statistical analysis of spatial point patterns*. London: Arnold.

Erdélyi, A., Magnus, W., Oberhettinger, F., & Tricomi, F. G. (1953). *Higher transcendental functions*. New York, NY: McGraw-Hill.

González-Farías, G., Domíniguez-Molina, J. A., & Gupta, A. K. (2004). The closed skew-normal distribution. In M. G. Genton (Ed.), *Skew-elliptical distributions and their applications: A journey beyond normality* (pp. 25–42). Boca Raton, FL: Chapman & Hall/CRC.

Gupta, A. K., Aziz, M. A., & Ning, W. (2013). On some properties of the unified skew normal distribution. *Journal of Statistical Theory and Practice, 7*, 480–495.

Gupta, A. K., González-Farías, G., & Domíniguez-Molina, J. A. (2004). A multivariate skew normal distribution. *Journal of Multivariate Analysis, 89*, 181–190.

Illian, J., Penttinen, A., Stoyan, H., & Stoyan, D. (2008). Statistical analysis and modelling of spatial point patterns. Wiley, Statistics in Practice.

Liseo, B., & Loperfido, N. (2003). A Bayesian interpretation of the multivariate skew-normal distribution. *Statistics and Probability Letters, 61*, 395–401.

McQuarrie, D. A. (1976). *Statistical mechanics*. New York, NY: Harper & Row.

Møller, J., & Toftaker, H. (2014). Geometric anisotropic spatial point pattern analysis and Cox processes. *Scandinavian Journal of Statistics, 41*, 414–435.

Møller, J., & Waagepetersen, R. P. (2003). *Statistical inference and simulation for spatial point processes*. London: Chapman and Hall/CRC Press.

Neyman, Y., Scott, E. L.: A theory for the spatial distribution of galaxies. *Astrophysics Journal, 116*, 144–163 (1952)

Neyman, Y., & Scott, E. L. (1958). Statistical approach to problems of cosmology. *Journal of the Royal Statistical Society B, 20*, 1–43.

Neyman, Y., Scott, E. L. (1972). Processes of clustering and applications. In P. A. W. Lewis (Ed.), *Stochastic processes* (pp. 646–681). New York, NY: Wiley.

Neyman, Y., Scott, E. L., & Shane, C. D. (1953). On the spatial distribution of galaxies: A specific model. *Astrophysics Journal, 117*, 92–133.

Ohser, J. (1983). On estimators for the reduced second moment measure of point processes. *Statistics: A Journal of Theoretical and Applied Statistics, 14*, 63–71.

Penttinen, A., Stoyan, D., & Henttonen, H. (1992). Marked point processes in forest statistics. *Forest Science, 38*, 806–824.

R Core Team. (2019). R: A language and environment for statistical computing. Vienna: R Foundation for Statistical Computing. https://www.R-project.org/

Ripley, B. D. (1976). The second-order analysis of stationary point processes. *Journal of Applied Probability, 13*, 255–266.

Ripley, B. D. (1988). *Statistical inference for spatial processes*. Australia: Cambridge University Press.

Stoyan, D., & Stoyan, H. (2006). Estimating pair correlation functions of planar cluster processes. *Biometrical Journal, 38*, 259–271.

Strauss, D. J. (1975). A model for clustering. *Biometrika, 63*, 467–475.

Tanaka, U., Ogata, Y., & Stoyan, D. (2008). A model selection and estimation of the Neyman–Scott type spatial cluster models. *Biometrical Journal, 50*, 43–57.

Thomas, M. (1949). A generalization of Poisson's binomial limit for use in ecology. *Biometrika, 36*, 18–25.

Wolfram Research. (2020). *Mathematica version 12.1*. Champaign, IL, USA (2020). https://www.wolfram.com/mathematica

Nonparametric Approximation Methods for the First-Passage Time Distribution for Degradation Data Measured with Unequal Time Intervals

Lochana K. Palayangoda and Hon Keung Tony Ng

Abstract Evaluating the first-passage time (FPT) distribution of a stochastic process is a prominent statistical problem, which has long been studied. This problem has important applications in reliability and degradation data analysis since the time that a degradation process of a product passes a critical level is considered as the failure time of the product. While most of the studies for FPT distribution focus on parametric stochastic process in the past, nonparametric approaches based on empirical saddlepoint approximation (ESA) are proposed recently. An advantage of those nonparametric approaches for evaluating the FPT distribution is that it does not require the specification of the parametric form of the underlying stochastic process. However, those nonparametric approaches based on ESA require the degradation measurements to be measured at equally distanced time points. For this reason, several random imputation methods are proposed by Palayangoda et al. (Appl Stoch Model Bus Ind 36(4):730–753, 2020). To facilitate the ESA method when the degradation data are measured at unequal time intervals, in this chapter, a least-squares modeling approach is proposed as an alternative approach to the random imputation methods. Monte Carlo simulation studies are used to evaluate the performance of the proposed methods for estimating the quantiles of the FPT distribution and for estimating the standard deviation of the FPT. Finally, degradation data analysis of a laser data is used to illustrate the methodologies presented in this chapter.

1 Introduction

In the past, most of the reliability studies are focused on lifetime data analysis in which the statistical analysis is based on data collected from life testing experiments or field failures. Nowadays, due to the significant improvements in product quality

L. K. Palayangoda · H. K. T. Ng (✉)
Department of Statistical Science, Southern Methodist University, Dallas, TX, USA
e-mail: lpalayangoda@mail.smu.edu; ngh@mail.smu.edu

I. Ghosh et al. (eds.), *Advances in Statistics - Theory and Applications*, Emerging Topics in Statistics and Biostatistics, https://doi.org/10.1007/978-3-030-62900-7_19

and reliability, it may be difficult to assess reliability of a product using the traditional lifetime data analysis. Therefore, degradation measures that record the accumulation of damage (e.g., wear, corrosion, crack growth, etc.) of the product over time can contain more important information about the product's performance and reliability. Degradation analysis aims to characterize the underlying failure process by modeling the degradation measures. A prescribed critical level is the level above/below which the product is considered to be failed (or not able to perform its required function). Hence, the failure time distribution based on degradation data is equivalent to the first-passage time (FPT) (also known as the first hitting time) distribution, which is defined as the time when the stochastic degradation process first reaches the critical level.

In different applications, a FPT model usually consists of three underlying components: (1) a parent stochastic process $\{X_t, t \geq 0\}$; (2) a threshold critical level c; and (3) a time scale. In addition to the application in reliability analysis, the problem of determining the FPT distribution frequently occurs in different disciplines such as biology, chemistry, ecology, economics, finance, and physics. Due to the numerous applications of the FPT model, estimating the FPT distribution has long been studied in the literature. However, most of the studies of FPT distribution focus on obtaining the FPT distribution for a specified parametric stochastic process either analytically or numerically, while a few studies considered the nonparametric estimation of the FPT distribution without specifying the parametric form of the underlying stochastic process. Recently, Balakrishnan and Qin (2019) and Palayangoda et al. (2020) developed nonparametric approaches to evaluate the FPT of degradation processes. In addition, Balakrishnan and Qin (2020) discussed the optimal design of degradation tests from a nonparametric perspective, whereas the degradation process is modeled by an empirical Lévy process. In contrast to the parametric approaches, those nonparametric approaches for estimating the FPT distribution of degradation processes require the degradation measurements to be measured at equally distanced time points. For this reason, Palayangoda et al. (2020) proposed several random imputation methods to estimate the FPT distribution nonparametrically based on degradation data measured with unequal time intervals; however, the performance of those imputation methods can be sensitive to the variation in the measurement time points. Moreover, those random imputation methods may give different estimates of FPT in different imputations and lead to different conclusions. To address these issues, in this chapter, we propose a least-square modeling approach as an alternative to the random imputation approach.

The rest of this chapter is organized as follows. In Sect. 2, we briefly review two parametric Lévy process models, the gamma process model and the IG process model. In Sect. 3, the nonparametric approach in estimating the FPT distribution based on empirical saddlepoint approximation (ESA) is presented. In addition, estimation of the moments of FPT distribution, different random imputation methods with ESA, and the issues of these imputation methods are discussed. Then, in Sect. 4, a least-squares modeling approach is proposed as an alternative approach to the imputation methods. In Sect. 5, Monte Carlo simulation studies are used to evaluate the performance of the proposed nonparametric estimation methods for estimating the quantiles of the FPT distribution and for estimating the standard deviation of the FPT. In Sect. 6, an analysis of laser degradation data is used to illustrate the methodologies presented in this chapter.

2 Parametric Lévy Process Models

The Lévy process $\{X_t, t \geq 0\}$ is a right continuous stochastic process, which satisfies stationary and independent increments. In other words, the increment $X_{t+v} - X_t$ has the same distribution $\forall t \geq 0$, $v \geq 0$, and $X_{t_j} - X_{t_{j-1}}$ are independent $\forall t_j \geq 0$ with $t_0 < t_1 < \ldots$, respectively. From the infinitely divisible property, the characteristic function of any Lévy process is defined in Lévy–Khintchine theorem. For any $\theta \in \mathbb{R}$, the characteristics function ψ of an infinitely divisible distribution is given by Bertoin (1996)

$$\log\{\psi(\theta)\} = ia\theta - \frac{1}{2}\sigma^2\theta^2 + \int_{\mathbb{R}} \left(e^{i\theta x} - 1 - i\theta x 1_{|x|<1}\right) \Pi(dx), \tag{1}$$

where $a, \sigma \in \mathbb{R}$, and Π is a measure satisfying $\Pi(\{0\}) = 0$ and $\int_{\mathbb{R}}(1 \wedge x^2)\Pi(dx) < \infty$. From the Lévy-Itō decomposition, $ia\theta$ corresponds to a linear drift, $\frac{1}{2}\sigma^2\theta^2$ is the Brownian motion, and $\int_{\mathbb{R}} \left(e^{i\theta x} - 1 - i\theta x 1_{|x|<1}\right) \Pi(dx)$ represents a Poisson process with jumps. The Wiener process, the gamma process, and the inverse Gaussian (IG) process are some parametric Lévy processes commonly used in the literature with numerous applications. Among the three parametric processes, gamma process and IG process consist of monotonic increments, whereas the Wiener process can support both monotonic and non-monotonic increments. In this chapter, we mainly focus on monotonic degradation processes. Furthermore, we assume that the initial degradation measurement time and the corresponding degradation measurement are $t_0 = 0$ and $X_{t_0} = 0$, respectively. Moreover, suppose $\Delta X_j = X_{t_j} - X_{t_{j-1}}$ and $\Delta t_j = t_j - t_{j-1}$ $(j = 1, 2, \ldots, m)$, where Δt_j is the corresponding time difference between the degradation measurements X_{t_j} and $X_{t_{j-1}}$. We denote the random variable of the first-passage time with threshold c as T_c. A brief introduction for the gamma and IG degradation processes is given in the following subsections.

2.1 *Gamma Process*

The stochastic process $\{X_t, t \geq 0\}$ follows a gamma degradation process if the random increment ΔX_j follows a gamma distribution with shape parameter $\alpha \Delta t_j > 0$ and scale parameter $\beta > 0$ (denoted as $gamma(\alpha t, \beta)$), whereas the probability density function (PDF) and cumulative distribution function (CDF) are, respectively,

$$g_{X_t}(x; \alpha t, \beta) = \frac{1}{\beta^{\alpha t}\Gamma(\alpha t)} x^{\alpha t-1} \exp\left(-\frac{x}{\beta}\right), \ x > 0,$$

and

$$G_{X_t}(x; \alpha t, \beta) = \int_0^x g_{X_t}(w; \alpha t, \beta) dw, \ x > 0,$$

where $\Gamma(a) = \int_0^\infty x^{a-1} \exp(-x)dx$ is the gamma function. We denote the gamma degradation process as Gamma(α, β) process. Suppose the mth degradation measurement taken at time $t = t_m$ is $X_t = \sum_{j=1}^m \Delta X_j$, and thus, the distribution of X_t is $X_t \sim gamma(\alpha t, \beta)$, where $t = \sum_{j=1}^m \Delta t_j$. The cumulant generating function (CGF) of X_t is $\mathscr{K}_{X_t}(s) = \ln[\mathscr{M}_{X_t}(s)] = -\alpha t \ln(1 - \beta s)$ for $s < 1/\beta$. For a given threshold level c, the true FPT distribution of Gamma(α, β) process can be directly obtained by $\Pr(T_c > t) = \Pr(X_t < c) = G_{X_t}(c; \alpha t, \beta)$. As an alternative approach, the Birnbaum–Saunders approximation proposed by Park and Padgett (2005) can be used to estimate the FPT distribution. For more details on the Birnbaum–Saunders distribution, one may refer to Birnbaum and Saunders (1969), Balakrishnan and Kundu (2019).

2.2 *Inverse Gaussian Process*

Let $\{X_t, t \geq 0\}$ be an IG degradation process (Wang and Xu 2010; Ye and Chen 2014), then ΔX_j follows an IG distribution (Chhikara and Folks 1989) with mean parameter $\mu \Delta t_j$ and shape parameter $\lambda(\Delta t_j)^2$, whereas the PDF and CDF are, respectively,

$$\phi_{IG}(x; \mu\Delta t_j, \lambda(\Delta t_j)^2) = \sqrt{\frac{\lambda(\Delta t_j)^2}{2\pi x^3}} \exp\left[-\frac{\lambda(x - \mu\Delta t_j)^2}{2\mu^2 x}\right], x > 0,$$

and

$$\begin{aligned} &\Phi_{IG}(x; \mu\Delta t_j, \lambda(\Delta t_j)^2) \\ &= \Phi\left[\sqrt{\frac{\lambda}{x}}\left(\frac{x}{\mu} - \Delta t_j\right)\right] + \exp\left(\frac{2\lambda\Delta t_j}{\mu}\right)\Phi\left[-\sqrt{\frac{\lambda}{x}}\left(\frac{x}{\mu} - \Delta t_j\right)\right], x > 0, \end{aligned}$$

respectively, where $\Phi(\cdot)$ is the CDF of the standard normal distribution. Let the mth degradation measurement is taken at time t_m, then $X_t = \sum_{j=1}^m \Delta X_j$, and thus, the distribution of X_t is $X_t \sim IG(\mu t, \lambda t^2)$, where $t = \sum_{j=1}^m \Delta t_j$. The CGF of X_t is given by

$$\mathcal{K}_{X_t}(s) = \ln[\mathcal{M}_{X_t}(s)] = (\lambda t/\mu)\left(1 - \sqrt{1 - (2\mu^2 s/\lambda)}\right) \text{ for } s \leq \lambda/(2\mu^2).$$

In this chapter, we denote the IG degradation process as IG(μ, λ) process. If threshold level is c, the true FPT distribution if IG process can be directly obtained by $\Pr(T_c > t) = \Pr(X_t < c) = \Phi_{IG}(c; \mu t, \lambda t^2)$. In addition, Peng (2015) proposed that the FPT distribution of the IG process can be approximated by the Birnbaum–Saunders distribution. For some independence properties and the characterization of the inverse Gaussian distribution, one may refer to Arnold and Seshadri (2009).

3 Empirical Saddlepoint Approximation

Saddlepoint approximation is a well-established procedure for estimating the PDF or CDF of a random variable when the moment generating function (MGF) or the CGF of the random variable is known. For a given dataset, we can obtain the empirical MGF or empirical CGF and then apply the saddlepoint approximation based on the empirical MGF or the empirical CGF. This procedure is named the empirical saddlepoint approximation (ESA). Following the saddlepoint approximation method introduced by Lugannani and Rice (1980), when a degradation process follows a Lévy process, Palayangoda et al. (2020) proposed an ESA method to estimate the FPT distribution of the degradation process. The main advantage of the ESA approach is that it is a nonparametric procedure in which specification of the underlying distribution of the degradation process is not required.

Suppose $\{X_t; t > 0\}$ follows a Lévy process with I units and m measurements, we assume that the measurements are taken at unit time intervals and all units have the same number of measurements. Let the observed values of degradation data are $\mathbf{X} = \{x_{ij}; i = 1, 2, \ldots, I\ , j = 1, 2, \ldots, (m+1)\}$. Furthermore, for a given unit, the difference between two consecutive measurements is $\Delta X_j = X_j - X_{(j-1)}$, and the time interval between two consecutive degradation measurements is $\Delta t_j = t_j - t_{(j-1)} = 1$, $j = 1, 2, \ldots, m$. Therefore, the empirical CGF of this degradation process, this Lévy process, at time t is given by

$$\hat{\mathcal{K}}_{X_t}(s) = t \ln \frac{1}{Im} \left\{ \sum_{i=1}^{I} \sum_{j=1}^{m} \exp(s \Delta x_{ij}) \right\}, \tag{2}$$

where $\Delta x_{ij} = x_{ij} - x_{i(j-1)}$. Using the empirical CGF in Eq. (2) and following the saddlepoint approximation by Lugannani and Rice (1980), Palayangoda et al. (2020) proposed an ESA procedure to estimate the FPT distribution at t for degradation data with threshold level c as follows:

$$\widehat{\Pr}(T_c > t) = \begin{cases} \Phi(\hat{w}) + \phi(\hat{w})(\frac{1}{\hat{w}} - \frac{1}{\hat{u}}), & \text{if } t \neq t_s, \\ \frac{1}{2} + \frac{\hat{\mathscr{K}}'''_{X_t}(0)}{6\sqrt{2\pi}\hat{\mathscr{K}}''_{X_t}(0)^{3/2}}, & \text{if } t = t_s, \end{cases} \tag{3}$$

where $\hat{\mathscr{K}}''_{X_t}$ and $\hat{\mathscr{K}}'''_{X_t}$ are the second and third derivatives of the function $\hat{\mathscr{K}}_{X_t}$, $\hat{w} = sgn(\hat{s})\sqrt{2\{\hat{s}c - \hat{\mathscr{K}}_{X_t}(\hat{s})\}}$, $\hat{u} = \hat{s}\sqrt{\hat{\mathscr{K}}''_{X_t}(\hat{s})}$, and the saddlepoint $\hat{s}$ is obtained by solving $\hat{\mathscr{K}}'_{X_t}(\hat{s}) = c$ such that

$$\hat{\mathscr{K}}'_{X_t}(s) = \frac{\sum_{j=1}^{m}\{\Delta x_j \exp(s\Delta x_i)\}}{\sum_{j=1}^{m}\{\exp(s\Delta x_j)\}} t = c.$$

Furthermore, t_s is the singularity point, which is evaluated by solving $c = \mathbb{E}(X_{t_0})$. Thus, t_s is the solution of $\mathscr{K}'_{X_t}(0) = c$ and is $\hat{t}_s = c/\{\sum_{i=1}^{I}\sum_{j=1}^{m}[\Delta x_{ij}/(Im)]\}$. The empirical CGF, $\hat{\mathscr{K}}_{X_t}(\hat{s})$, can be determined from Eq. (2).

3.1 Estimation of the Moments of FPT Distribution

To find the moments of gamma or IG degradation process, the common practice is to apply the Birnbaum–Saunders approximation (Birnbaum and Saunders 1969; Park and Padgett 2005). Palayangoda (2020) proposed a residue approximate to evaluate the moments of monotone Lévy processes. Suppose X_t follows a Lévy process and Y is a random variable that corresponds to the degradation per unit interval, then the CGF of X_t with respect to the CGF of Y can be obtained as $\mathscr{K}_{X_t}(s) = t\mathscr{K}_Y(s)$. The following result presented in Palayangoda (2020) provides the approximation of the first and second moments of T_c, where T_c is the FPT with threshold level c.

Result 1 *Residue approximations for the MTTF (i.e., the first moment of T_c) and the second moment of T_c are, respectively,*

$$\mathbb{E}(T_c) \simeq \frac{c}{\mathscr{K}'_Y(0)} + \frac{\mathscr{K}''_Y(0)}{2[\mathscr{K}'_Y(0)]^2}, \tag{4}$$

and

$$\mathbb{E}(T_c^2) \simeq \frac{1}{\{\mathscr{K}'_Y(0)\}^2}\left[c\left(2\frac{\mathscr{K}''_Y(0)}{\mathscr{K}'_Y(0)} + c\right) + \frac{3}{2}\left(\frac{\mathscr{K}''_Y(0)}{\mathscr{K}'_Y(0)}\right)^2 - \frac{2}{3}\frac{\mathscr{K}'''_Y(0)}{\mathscr{K}'_Y(0)}\right]. \blacksquare \tag{5}$$

The cumulants $\mathscr{K}'_Y(0)$ and $\mathscr{K}''_Y(0)$ are the mean and variance of Y, respectively, and the first moment of T_c in Eq. (4) is the same as the first moment of the FPT distribution obtained from the Birnbaum–Saunders approximation (Park and

Padgett 2005). In addition, from Eqs. (4) and (5), we can obtain the nonparametric estimates of the first and second moments, denoted as $\widehat{T_{ESA}}^{(1)}$ and $\widehat{T_{ESA}}^{(2)}$, of the FPT distribution as

$$\widehat{T_{ESA}}^{(1)} = \widehat{\mathbb{E}}(T_c) = \frac{c}{\bar{y}} + \frac{s_y^2}{2\bar{y}^2}, \tag{6}$$

$$\widehat{T_{ESA}}^{(2)} = \widehat{\mathbb{E}}(T_c^2) = \frac{1}{\bar{y}^2}\left[c\left\{2\frac{s_y^2}{\bar{y}} + c\right\} + \frac{3}{2}\left\{\frac{s_y^2}{\bar{y}}\right\}^2 - \frac{2}{3}\frac{k_y^3}{\bar{y}}\right], \tag{7}$$

where $\bar{y} = \sum_{j=1}^{m} \Delta x_j$, $s_y^2 = \sum_{j=1}^{m}\{\Delta x_j - \bar{y}\}^2/(m-1)$ and $k_y^3 = \sum_{j=1}^{m}\{\Delta x_j - \bar{y}\}^3/(m-1)$ are the sample mean, the sample variance, and the third sample cumulant of the sample degradation measurements per unit interval (i.e., Y), respectively.

3.2 *ESA for Data with Unequal Time Intervals*

As shown in Palayangoda et al. (2020, Section 3.1), the ESA approach provides promising results on estimating the FPT distribution when the distribution of degradation data is unknown and it is robust under model misspecification. However, the ESA method works only when the degradation data are measured at equal time intervals. To accommodate and make accurate estimation of FPT distribution for the degradation data with unequal time intervals, several imputation techniques are proposed in Palayangoda et al. (2020) to transform the unequal time degradation process to an equal time degradation process. Palayangoda et al. (2020) showed that the random imputation (RImp) and conditional random imputation (CRImp) methods are performing well. In particular, for monotone degradation data, the CRImp method has showed better performance than the RImp method. In addition to the imputation methods proposed by Palayangoda et al. (2020), other imputation methods such as the gamma bridge interpolation suggested by Balakrishnan and Qin (2020, Section 3.2), can also be considered.

To apply these imputation methods, a general assumption is that the degradation process follows a Lévy process. These techniques are developed by setting the unit time interval as the highest common factor (HCF)[1] of the different time intervals (i.e., HCF of Δt_i). Then, imputation techniques are used to impute the missing values at unit time intervals. Therefore, the pseudo-completed degradation data with equal time intervals will be resulted to apply the ESA method to obtain the FPT distribution. Specifically, let the Lévy process $\{X_t : t \geq 0\}$ consist of

[1]The HCF is the largest real number, which when used to divide the time increments leads to all the ratios as positive integers.

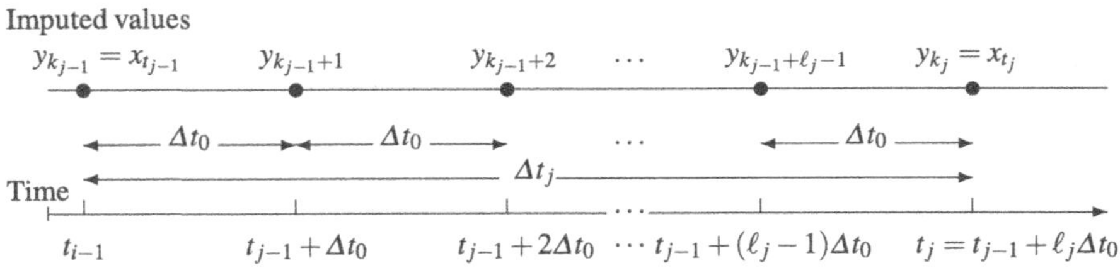

Fig. 1 A schematic diagram for the data imputation method in the jth interval $(t_{j-1}, t_j]$

degradation measurements, $x_t = \{x_{t_0}, x_{t_1}, \ldots, x_{t_m}\}$, which are taken at time points $t = \{t_j; j = 1, 2, \ldots, m\}$. Suppose the jth time interval be $\Delta t_j = t_j - t_{j-1}$ with an initial measurement, $t_0 = 0$. The HCF of Δt (i.e., the pseudo-unit-time interval) $\Delta t_0 = HCF\{\Delta t_j : j = 1, \ldots, m\}$. For example, if the degradation measurements are taken at $t = \{1, 2, 5, 10, 11, 14, 19, \ldots\}$, then $\Delta t_j = \{1, 3, 5, 1, 3, 5, \ldots\}$. Thus, the HCF of Δt_0 is 1 (i.e., $HCF(1, 3, 5) = 1$). Using the imputation techniques, we will fill the missing degradation measurements at time points $t^* = \{3, 4, 6, 7, 8, 9, 12, 13, 15, 16, 17, 18, \ldots\}$.

Suppose that ℓ_j is the number of pseudo-unit-time intervals inside the jth interval $(t_{j-1}, t_j]$ is defined as

$$\ell_j = \frac{t_j - t_{j-1}}{\Delta t_0} = \frac{\Delta t_j}{\Delta t_0},$$

and the total number of pseudo-unit-time intervals up to time t_j (i.e., in $(0, t_j]$) is $k_j = \sum_{l=1}^{j} \ell_l$, for $j = 1, 2, \ldots, m$, with $k_0 = 0$. Thereby, with pseudo-unit-time interval Δt_0, the imputed pseudo-complete degradation data contain $k_m = \sum_{j=1}^{m} \ell_j$ degradation measurements. The imputed pseudo-complete degradation data are denoted as $(y_1, y_2, \ldots, y_m)$, where

$$y_j = (y_{k_j-\ell_j+1}, y_{k_j-\ell_j'+2}, \ldots, y_{k_j-2}, y_{k_j-1}, y_{k_j}),$$

with $y_{k_j} = x_{t_j}$ for $j = 1, 2, \ldots, m$. Therefore, in the jth time interval $(t_{j-1}, t_j]$, we have to impute $\ell_j - 1$ measurements, which are denoted as $(y_{k_j-\ell_j+1}, y_{k_j-\ell_j+2}, \ldots, y_{k_j-2}, y_{k_j-1})$. Figure 1 shows the data imputation scheme in the jth interval.

When $\ell_j \neq 1$, the unit-drift in the jth time interval $(t_{j-1}, t_j]$ is defined as

$$\delta_j = \left(\frac{x_{t_j} - x_{t_{j-1}}}{t_j - t_{j-1}} \right) \Delta t_0, \tag{8}$$

and the set of m unit-drifts is $\delta = \{\delta_1, \delta_2, \ldots, \delta_m\}$ for the m time intervals.

The RImp and CRImp methods for obtaining pseudo-complete degradation data with unit-time interval Δt_0 are discussed in the following subsections. Without loss of generality, we assume that all the I items under the degradation test are measured at the same time points and the increments of the degradation measurements follow the same distribution.

3.2.1 Random Imputation Method (RImp)

In the RImp method, the unit-drift sampling frame for the I items is created as $(\delta_1, \delta_2, \ldots, \delta_I)$, where $\delta_i = \{\delta_{i1}, \delta_{i2}, \ldots, \delta_{im}\}$ is the set of unit-drifts for the ith item ($i = 1, 2, \ldots, I$). After setting $y_{k_j} = x_{t_j}$, for the jth interval $(t_{j-1}, t_j]$, the other values in y_j are imputed by using the following algorithm:

1. Set $L = y_{k_{j-1}}$ and COUNT = 0.
2. Draw a random sample of I values with replacement from the unit-drifts $\{\delta_{1j}, \delta_{2j}, \ldots, \delta_{Ij}\}$ and denote each as δ_j^*.
3. For each item set $y_{k_{j-1}+1} = L + \delta_j^*$, then set $L = y_{k_{j-1}+1}$ and COUNT = COUNT + 1.
4. If COUNT $< \ell_j - 1$, repeat Steps 2 and 3.

The RImp method may provide negative increment at the last imputation of the jth interval (i.e., possibility to have $x_{t_j} - y_{k_j - 1} < 0$). In this situation, the negative imputed value will affect the monotonicity of the degradation process; therefore, the CRImp method is considered to accommodate this issue.

3.2.2 Conditional Random Imputation Method (CRImp)

The CRImp method artificially transforms the unequal time interval degradation data into equal time interval degradation data, while maintaining the monotonicity of the degradation process. By using a constrained sampling frame, the CRImp method ensures that all the increments are positive. In the jth interval $(t_{j-1}, t_j]$, after setting $y_{k_j} = x_{t_j}$, the other values in y_j can be imputed by the following algorithm:

1. Set $L = y_{k_{j-1}}$ and COUNT = 0.
2. Draw a random sample of n values with replacement from the constrained sampling frame $\{\delta_{1j}, \delta_{2j}, \ldots, \delta_{Ij} : \delta_{ij} < x_{t_j} - L, i = 1, 2, \ldots, I\}$, denote each as δ_j^*.
3. Set $y_{k_{j-1}+1} = L + \delta_j^*$, then set $L = y_{k_{j-1}+1}$ and COUNT = COUNT + 1.
4. If COUNT $< \ell_j - 1$, repeat Steps 2 and 3.

3.2.3 Simulated Example for RImp and CRImp

To illustrate the RImp and CRImp methods, a set of simulated degradation data from the Gamma(1, 3) degradation process with threshold level $c = 300$ and 5 degra-

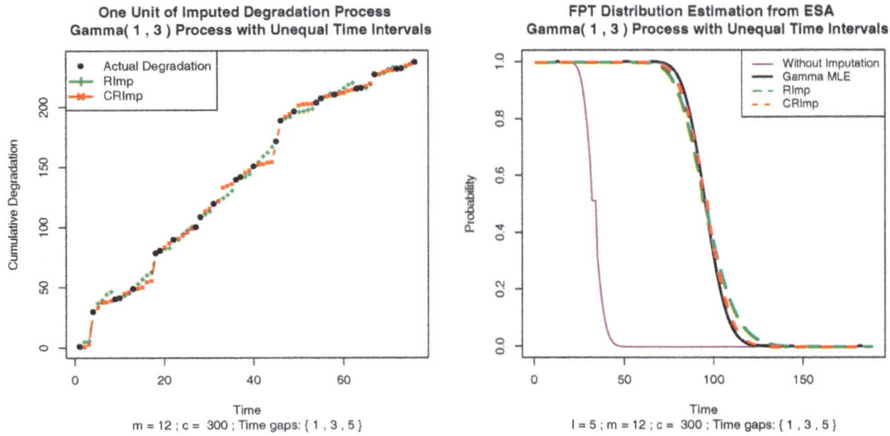

Fig. 2 Imputed degradation (left) and estimated FPT distribution (right) for a simulated Gamma(1, 3) degradation process measured with $\Delta t = \{1, 3, 5\}$ for $I = 5$, total experiment time of 80, and $c = 300$

dation paths (i.e., $I = 5$) measured at $t = \{0, 1, 4, 9, 10, 13, 18, 19, 22, 27, \ldots\}$ (i.e., $\Delta t = \{1, 3, 5, 1, 3, 5, \ldots\}$) up to a total experiment time of each sample $t_m = 80$. Since the degradation process is simulated based on a gamma process, the parameters in the gamma process model are estimated by the maximum likelihood estimation approach, and the FPT distribution based on maximum likelihood estimates (MLEs) with the gamma process assumption is compared to the ESA approach with the RImp and CRImp imputation methods. Note that the ESA approach does not require any distributional assumption about the underlying degradation process, and the parametric form of the underlying degradation process is usually unknown in practice. The imputed values based on the RImp and CRImp methods and the estimates of the FPT distribution based on the parametric approach (i.e., MLEs with gamma process) and based on ESA using RImp, CRImp, and without imputation are presented in Fig. 2.

From Fig. 2, we observe that the estimated FPT distribution based on the ESA approach with CRImp provides a better approximation (closer to the estimated FPT distribution based on the parametric approach) compared to the RImp approach, while the estimated FPT distribution based on ESA without considering the issue of unequal time intervals is problematic.

3.2.4 Issues with the Imputation Methods

As shown in the simulated example in Sect. 3.2.3 (see also, Palayangoda et al. 2020), the imputation methods, RImp and CRImp, provide decent results in estimating the FPT distribution nonparmetrically using ESA; however, when the time intervals between two degradation measurements are large and the HCF of the time intervals

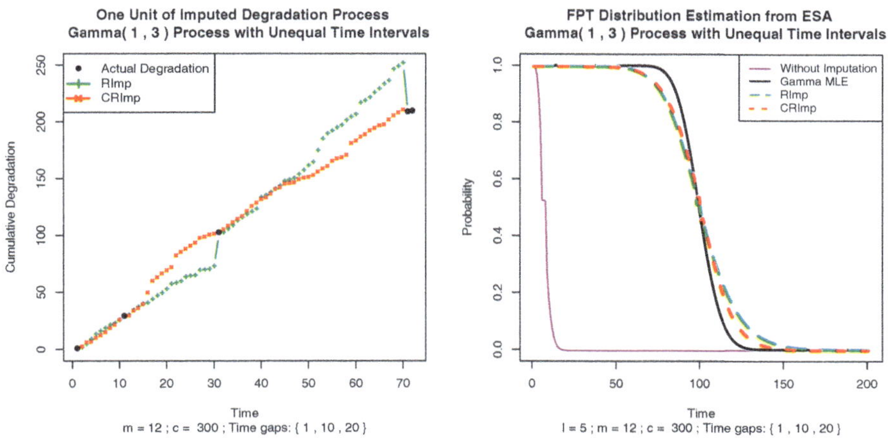

Fig. 3 Imputed degradation (left) and FPT distribution (right) for a sample Gamma(1, 3) degradation process measured at $\Delta t = \{1, 25, 50\}$ for $I = 5$, a total experiment time of 80, and $c = 300$

is relatively small, the performance of the ESA of FPT distribution can be affected. Based on the simulation setting in Sect. 3.2.3, we consider a simulated degradation data measured at time $t = \{0, 1, 26, 76\}$ for each sample, i.e., the time differences of the subsequent measurements are $\Delta t = \{1, 25, 50\}$. The imputed values based on the RImp and CRImp methods and the estimates of the FPT distribution based on the parametric approach (i.e., MLEs with gamma process) and based on ESA using RImp, CRImp and without imputation are presented in Fig. 3. Compared to the results presented in Fig. 2, the estimated FPT distributions based on ESA with the imputation methods are not as close to the parametric estimate of FPT distribution. This illustrates that the performance of the imputation methods, RImp and CRImp, is sensitive to the variations of the time intervals between degradation measurements.

To illustrate this issue with the random imputation methods, Palayangoda et al. (2020) observed that the imputation methods provide nearly unbiased estimate for the mean of FPT distribution (i.e., the mean time to failure (MTTF)). However, the variance of the FPT distribution estimated through these imputation methods can be different from each other. For both the RImp and CRImp methods, we evaluate the degradation per unit time interval for all the degradation measurements (i.e., δ_j in Eq. (8)). Since ΔX_j follows a Lévy process, the mean and variance of ΔX_j are $\mu \Delta t_j$ and $\sigma^2 \Delta t_j$, respectively, and then the mean and variance of δ_j can be obtained as

$$\mathbb{E}(\delta_j) = \mathbb{E}\left(\frac{\Delta X_j}{\Delta t_j} \Delta t_0\right) = \mu \Delta t_0$$

$$\text{and } \mathbb{V}(\delta_j) = \mathbb{V}\left(\frac{\Delta X_j}{\Delta t_j}\Delta t_0\right) = \frac{\sigma^2}{\Delta t_j}(\Delta t_0)^2,$$

respectively. Here, we can see that the mean of δ_j is time independent, yet the variance of δ_j is time dependent. A feasible estimate for the MTTF is $c/\mathbb{E}(\delta_j)$, and thereby, the MTTF is unbiased if we use δ_j ($j = 1, 2, \ldots, m$) as an estimate of the imputed degradation measurements. On the other hand, a feasible estimate of the variance of the FPT distribution is $c^2/\mathbb{V}(\delta_j) = c^2 \Delta t_j / [\sigma^2 (\Delta t_0)^2]$. These results show that when estimating the FPT distribution based on the ESA imputation methods using δ_j, the variance depends on the time differences of the measurements (i.e., Δt_j). Another issue with these imputation methods may give different estimates of FPT in different imputations and lead to different conclusions.

To address these issues about the imputation methods, it is desired to develop an estimation method based on ESA with measurements from unequal time intervals that does not rely on random sampling, and the variance of the estimates is less sensitive to the time differences of the measurements. In the next section, we propose an alternative approach to estimate the FPT distribution using ESA when the degradation data are measured with unequal time intervals.

4 Least-Squares Modeling Approach

As an alternative to imputation methods, in this section, we propose two methods based on a least-squares modeling approach to obtain the FPT distribution for degradation data with unequal time measurements using the ESA method. In the proposed approaches, we transform the degradation data into unit time scale increments to facilitate the ESA approach.

4.1 Transformed Degradation Data with Least-Squares Modeling

From Eq. (1), we observe that the Lévy process can be decomposed into a Wiener process (i.e., linear drift and Brownian motion) and a Poisson process. Considering Donsker's Theorem (Donsker 1951), for sufficiently large sample, we can approximate the decomposition of the Lévy process by a Wiener process. Suppose that $\{X_t; t > 0\}$ follows a Lévy process that consists of I units with m measurements and the time intervals of consecutive measurements are $\{\Delta t_{ij}; i = 1, 2, \ldots, I, j = 1, 2, \ldots, m\}$ and the differences in consecutive measurements are $\{\Delta X_{\Delta t_{ij}}; i = 1, 2, \ldots, I\ ,\ j = 1, 2, \ldots, m\}$. Assuming $\{X_{t_{ij}}\}$ follows a Lévy process and the sample size is sufficiently large, we consider the model

$$X_{t_{ij}} = \mu_Y t_{ij} + \varepsilon_{t_{ij}}, \tag{9}$$

where $\varepsilon_{t_{ij}}$ is a random variable with mean 0 and variance $\sigma_Y^2 t_{ij}$, and μ_Y and σ_Y^2 are the mean and variance of the degradation per unit interval, respectively. For example, if X_t follows Gamma(α, β) process, then $\mu_Y = \alpha\beta$ and $\sigma_Y^2 = \alpha\beta^2$. Here, the variance parameter of the Lévy process is σ_Y. Note that Eq. (9) only captures the mean and variance of $X_{t_{ij}}$ but not the skewness; therefore, an interesting extension for future research is to consider more general models that can capture other features of the Lévy process (see, for example, Tseng and Lee 2016).

Because the Lévy process is infinitely divisible, $\Delta X_{t_{ij}}$ can be written as

$$\Delta X_{\Delta t_{ij}} = \mu_Y \Delta t_{ij} + \varepsilon_{\Delta t_{ij}}, \tag{10}$$

where $\varepsilon_{\Delta t_{ij}}$ is a random variable with mean 0 and variance $\sigma_Y^2 \Delta t_{ij}$.

Suppose the HCF of the time differences $\Delta t_{ij} (i = 1, 2, \ldots, I; j = 1, 2, \ldots, m)$ is Δt_0, the proposed approach is to transform the stochastic process $\Delta X_{\Delta t_{ij}}$ into $\Delta X_{\Delta t_0}$ by estimating μ_Y and σ_Y using a least-squares method. An independent and identically distributed error of the model in Eq. (10) is

$$\varepsilon^*_{\Delta t_{ij}} = \frac{\left(\Delta X_{\Delta t_{ij}} - \mu_Y \Delta t_{ij}\right)}{\sqrt{\Delta t_{ij}}}, \quad i = 1, 2, \ldots, I; \ j = 1, 2, \ldots, m. \tag{11}$$

Then, the sum of squares of the errors is given by

$$\sum_{i=1}^{I}\sum_{j=1}^{m}\left\{\varepsilon^*_{\Delta t_{ij}}\right\}^2 = \sum_{i=1}^{I}\sum_{j=1}^{m}\frac{\left(\Delta X_{\Delta t_{ij}} - \mu_Y \Delta t_{ij}\right)^2}{\Delta t_{ij}}. \tag{12}$$

By minimizing the sum of squares of errors in Eq. (12), we can obtain an estimate of μ_Y as

$$\hat{\mu}_Y = \frac{\sum_{i=1}^{I}\sum_{j=1}^{m}\Delta X_{\Delta t_{ij}}}{\sum_{i=1}^{I}\sum_{j=1}^{m}\Delta t_{ij}}. \tag{13}$$

If the measurements of all units are taken at the same set of time points (i.e., $\Delta t_{ij} = \Delta t_j$), then the estimate in Eq. (13) can be simplified as

$$\hat{\mu}_Y = \frac{\sum_{i=1}^{I}\sum_{j=1}^{m}\Delta X_{\Delta t_j}}{I t_m}, \tag{14}$$

where $t_m = \sum_{j=1}^{m}\Delta t_j$ is the total experiment time. The expected value of the estimate in Eq. (14) is μ_Y; thus, it is unbiased. Furthermore, the variance of the estimate in Eq. (14) is $\sigma_Y^2/(I t_m)$; thereby, $\hat{\mu}_Y$ is consistent as its variance goes to

0 when either $I \to \infty$ (i.e., large sample) or $t_m \to \infty$ (i.e., infinite experimental time). Moreover, the estimate of the random error, $\varepsilon^*_{\Delta t_{ij}}$, can be obtained as

$$\hat{\varepsilon}^*_{\Delta t_j} = \frac{\left(\Delta X_{\Delta t_j} - \hat{\mu}_Y \Delta t_j\right)}{\sqrt{\Delta t_j}}. \tag{15}$$

Thus, the variance of $\hat{\varepsilon}^*_{\Delta t_j}$ is $\sigma_Y^2[1 - \Delta t_j/(I t_m)]$. Using those estimates in Eqs. (14) and (15), the transformed degradation process model for time differences with Δt_0 is estimated by

$$\Delta \tilde{X}_{\Delta t_0|\Delta t_j} = \hat{\mu}_Y \Delta t_0 + \hat{\varepsilon}_{\Delta t_0|\Delta t_j}, \tag{16}$$

where $\hat{\varepsilon}_{\Delta t_0|\Delta t_j} = \sqrt{\Delta t_0}\hat{\varepsilon}^*_{\Delta t_j}$, and $\Delta \tilde{X}_{\Delta t_0|\Delta t_j}$ is the estimated degradation increment for time interval Δt_0 for the jth measurement. The proposed method applies the ESA based on the values $\Delta \tilde{X}_{\Delta t_0|\Delta t_j}$ in Eq. (16), and this method is called the LS method.

The expected value of $\Delta \tilde{X}_{\Delta t_0|\Delta t_j}$ is $\mu_Y \Delta t_0$, which is thereby unbiased. In addition, the variance of $\Delta \tilde{X}_{\Delta t_0|\Delta t_j}$ can be obtained as

$$\mathbb{V}(\Delta \tilde{X}_{\Delta t_0|\Delta t_j}) = \sigma_Y^2 \left[1 - \frac{(\Delta t_j - 1)}{I t_m}\right] \Delta t_0. \tag{17}$$

From Eq. (17), we can see that either $I \to \infty$ (i.e., large sample size) or $t_m \to \infty$ (i.e., infinite experimental time), and the variance of $\Delta \tilde{X}_{\Delta t_0|\Delta t_j}$ reaches $\sigma_Y^2 \Delta t_0$, which is the variance of $\Delta X_{\Delta t_0}$. Therefore, the estimate $\Delta \tilde{X}_{\Delta t_0|\Delta t_j} \to \Delta X_{\Delta t_0}$ as $I \to \infty$ or $t_m \to \infty$ for all Δt_j, $j = 1, 2, \ldots, m$. This shows that the estimate, $\Delta \tilde{X}_{\Delta t_0}$, is asymptotically efficient. From the estimated differences for Δt_0 (i.e., $\Delta \tilde{X}_{\Delta t_0}$), we can apply ESA for a given threshold level.

4.2 CRImp Method Based on Transformed Degradation Data

For the RImp and CRImp methods, we impute the degradation measurements per unit interval based on the estimates presented in Eq. (8). Instead of using the estimates presented in Eq. (8), we propose using the least-squares estimate in Eq. (16) to perform the CRImp algorithm instead of using the estimates presented in Eq. (8). This method is called the CRImp_{LS} method.

5 Monte Carlo Simulation Studies

5.1 Estimating the Quantiles of FPT Distribution

In this simulation study, we generate degradation data from the gamma degradation process and the IG degradation process with time gaps $\{1, 3, 5\}$ (i.e., degradation data are measured at time $t_1 = 1$, $t_2 = 4$, $t_3 = 9$, $t_4 = 10$, $t_5 = 13$, $t_6 = 18$, ...) and with time gaps $\{1, 5, 15\}$ (i.e., degradation data are measured at time $t_1 = 1$, $t_2 = 6$, $t_3 = 21$, $t_4 = 22$, $t_5 = 27$, $t_6 = 42$, ...). The Gamma(1, 2), Gamma(0.5, 4), IG(2,5), and IG(2,10) processes are generated with $I = 5$ or $I = 50$ items with threshold value $c = 200$. Furthermore, we set the termination time of the experiment as $t_m = 75$. In each simulation, the FPT distribution is estimated by using the parametric approach (i.e., obtain the MLEs of the parameters by assuming that the true distribution of the underlying degradation process is known) and the nonparametric ESA approach. For example, when the degradation data are generated from the Gamma(α, β) process, we can obtain the MLEs of the parameters α and β, denoted as $\hat{\alpha}$ and $\hat{\beta}$, respectively, and the parametric estimate of the FPT distribution at time t can be obtained by $\widehat{\Pr}(T_c > t) = G_{X_t}(c; \hat{\alpha}t, \hat{\beta})$. The true values of the FPT distributions at time t are obtained by the procedures provided in Sects. 2.1 and 2.2 for the gamma and inverse Gaussian processes, respectively. Since the simulated degradation data are not measured at equal time intervals, for the nonparametric ESA approach, we consider the RImp, CRImp, LS, and CRImp$_{LS}$ methods to accommodate the unequal time intervals issue. The performance of the estimation methods for FPT distribution is evaluated in terms of the mean squared errors (MSEs) for estimating the 1st, 5th, 10th, 90th, and 99th percentiles. The simulation results based on 10,000 simulations for different settings are presented in Tables 1, 2, 3, and 4.

From Tables 1, 2, 3, and 4, we observe that the CRImp method gives MSEs closest to the MSEs of the parametric MLE approach in many situations. The LS method appears to perform better when the sample size increases. The MSEs of the estimates based on the LS method are smaller than all the other imputation methods except for the CRImp method. On the other hand, the CRImp$_{LS}$ method appears to perform similar to the RImp method.

5.2 Estimating the Standard Deviation of FPT

In this simulation study, the degradation data are generated from gamma and IG degradation processes with different time gaps $\Delta t = \{1, 3, 5\}$ and $\Delta t = \{1, 5, 15\}$ from the Gamma(1, 2), Gamma(0.5, 4), IG(2, 5), and IG(2, 10) degradation processes with $I = 5$ and 50 items, termination time $t_m = 75$, and different threshold values $c = 200$ and 300. For each setting, the standard deviation of the FPT is estimated based on the results for Lévy process model by estimating $\mathbb{E}(T_c)$

Table 1 Simulated MSEs of the estimates of 1st, 5th, 10th, 90th, and 99th percentiles based on MLE, ESA with RImp, CRImp, LS, and CRImp_{LS} methods when the data are generated from the Gamma(1, 2) and Gamma(0.5, 4) processes with $\Delta t = \{1, 3, 5\}$, experiment time $t_m = 75$, and threshold value $c = 200$

		Simulated from Gamma(1, 2)					Simulated from Gamma(0.5, 4)				
Percentile	I	MLE	RImp	CRImp	LS	CRImp_{LS}	MLE	RImp	CRImp	LS	CRImp_{LS}
1st	5	23.9	41.4	26.1	34.1	36.0	42.0	74.1	46.4	62.1	55.3
5th	5	24.3	38.5	26.0	32.4	32.9	45.0	69.2	46.8	60.7	52.6
10th	5	25.4	32.1	25.4	33.4	28.2	46.9	66.3	47.9	61.3	52.0
90th	5	32.7	57.6	34.3	40.9	44.0	67.1	130.7	70.1	83.2	86.1
99th	5	37.7	153.7	41.1	47.3	74.1	79.3	392.7	85.3	101.4	141.5
1st	50	2.7	22.1	4.3	4.2	16.9	4.1	44.8	7.0	7.0	22.4
5th	50	2.5	18.4	4.1	3.2	12.8	4.5	35.0	5.9	6.1	16.0
10th	50	2.6	10.7	2.8	3.5	6.8	4.8	30.2	5.7	6.2	13.3
90th	50	3.3	23.9	4.0	4.1	12.3	6.7	52.7	7.0	8.2	18.8
99th	50	3.8	106.5	5.1	5.0	35.3	7.9	266.3	8.5	10.8	54.6

Table 2 Simulated MSEs of the estimates of 1st, 5th, 10th, 90th, and 99th percentiles based on MLE, ESA with RImp, CRImp, LS, and CRImp_{LS} methods when the data are generated from the Gamma(1, 2) and Gamma(0.5, 4) processes with $\Delta t = \{1, 5, 15\}$, experiment time $t_m = 75$, and threshold value $c = 200$

		Simulated from Gamma(1, 2)					Simulated from Gamma(0.5, 4)				
Percentile	I	MLE	RImp	CRImp	LS	CRImp_{LS}	MLE	RImp	CRImp	LS	CRImp_{LS}
1st	5	27.5	54.6	38.9	63.8	69.2	48.4	98.0	65.3	119.1	104.7
5th	5	26.6	45.6	32.6	61.0	50.0	49.9	83.4	57.4	116.8	80.1
10th	5	27.3	36.5	28.7	62.5	36.8	51.2	77.4	55.4	117.7	70.6
90th	5	34.5	71.6	42.0	77.2	61.3	73.4	163.6	80.2	164.6	122.0
99th	5	41.5	229.1	68.7	91.0	121.2	90.5	478.3	108.4	205.0	246.2
1st	50	2.9	31.3	11.5	7.5	50.0	4.7	59.0	16.1	13.7	69.6
5th	50	2.7	22.2	7.1	6.2	29.4	4.9	40.4	8.8	11.9	39.7
10th	50	2.8	12.5	3.7	6.4	14.9	5.2	32.5	7.1	11.8	28.0
90th	50	3.6	26.8	4.7	7.7	23.6	7.4	62.1	8.0	15.9	42.3
99th	50	4.3	137.0	6.6	9.5	69.0	9.1	353.0	11.2	21.4	131.6

and $\mathbb{E}(T_c^2)$ with Eqs. (4) and (5), respectively, and

$$\widehat{SD}(T_c) = \sqrt{\widehat{\mathbb{E}}(T_c^2) - \left[\widehat{\mathbb{E}}(T_c)\right]^2}. \tag{18}$$

The simulated MSEs of the estimates of standard deviation of FPT based on MLE, ESA with RImp, CRImp, LS, and CRImp_{LS} methods for different settings are presented in Tables 5 and 6. From Tables 5 and 6, we observe that in all the cases considered here, both the CRImp and LS methods give MSEs closest to the MSEs of the MLE method based on the correctly specified degradation process. In addition, the LS method gives the smallest MSEs in estimating the standard deviation of FPT

Table 3 Simulated MSEs of the estimates of 1st, 5th, 10th, 90th, and 99th percentiles based on MLE, ESA with RImp, CRImp, LS, and CRImp$_{LS}$ methods when the data are generated from the IG(2, 5) and IG(2, 10) processes with $\Delta t = \{1, 3, 5\}$, experiment time $t_m = 75$, and threshold value $c = 200$

		Simulated from IG(2, 5)					Simulated from IG(2, 10)				
Percentile	I	MLE	RImp	CRImp	LS	CRImp$_{LS}$	MLE	RImp	CRImp	LS	CRImp$_{LS}$
1st	5	11.9	23.7	15.7	15.8	24.2	6.1	12.0	8.9	7.9	15.9
5th	5	11.6	16.6	12.4	15.1	16.1	5.9	8.6	6.9	7.6	10.3
10th	5	11.3	17.2	13.0	14.3	16.5	5.7	8.4	6.9	7.2	9.5
90th	5	11.2	18.9	13.0	13.9	16.6	5.8	11.0	8.3	7.2	12.1
99th	5	12.0	54.0	21.7	15.1	36.1	6.0	22.0	12.0	7.4	22.7
1st	50	1.2	13.6	5.4	1.8	14.6	0.7	6.9	3.7	1.0	10.4
5th	50	1.3	6.7	2.4	1.8	6.4	0.7	3.6	1.9	0.9	5.1
10th	50	1.3	7.6	3.3	1.6	7.0	0.7	3.5	2.0	0.8	4.5
90th	50	1.2	7.6	2.3	1.5	5.9	0.7	5.4	2.9	0.9	6.2
99th	50	1.4	39.8	8.7	2.0	23.7	0.7	15.3	5.6	0.8	14.7

Table 4 Simulated MSEs of the estimates of 1st, 5th, 10th, 90th, and 99th percentiles based on MLE, ESA with RImp, CRImp, LS, and CRImp$_{LS}$ methods when the data are generated from the IG(2, 5) and IG(2, 10) processes with $\Delta t = \{1, 5, 15\}$, experiment time $t_m = 75$, and threshold value $c = 200$

		Simulated from IG(2, 5)					Simulated from IG(2, 10)				
Percentile	I	MLE	RImp	CRImp	LS	CRImp$_{LS}$	MLE	RImp	CRImp	LS	CRImp$_{LS}$
1st	5	13.6	31.5	25.5	29.5	44.2	7.0	16.4	14.1	21.1	28.4
5th	5	12.8	20.4	17.0	28.0	24.8	6.5	10.7	9.3	19.9	16.0
10th	5	12.2	20.1	16.8	26.6	22.6	6.2	9.8	8.7	19.1	13.4
90th	5	12.3	23.3	17.5	26.2	23.3	6.3	13.0	10.6	17.9	17.3
99th	5	13.7	79.0	45.5	28.4	58.2	6.8	32.1	21.7	18.1	40.4
1st	50	1.4	18.0	11.6	3.3	32.0	0.8	9.2	6.7	1.7	19.9
5th	50	1.5	8.0	4.5	3.2	13.1	0.8	4.3	2.9	1.6	8.7
10th	50	1.4	8.4	5.1	2.9	11.6	0.7	3.9	2.7	1.5	6.7
90th	50	1.3	8.7	3.9	2.8	9.9	0.8	6.1	3.8	1.5	8.7
99th	50	1.6	51.3	20.4	3.5	36.2	0.8	20.1	10.2	1.5	20.6

among all the procedures considered here. Furthermore, when the number of items increases from 5 to 50, the MSEs decrease for all the methods as expected. On the other hand, the MSEs of different estimation methods increase when the time gaps become larger. In addition, it is important to note that when the number of items increases from 5 to 50, the performance of the LS method improved significantly. This indicates an advantage of the LS method over the random imputation methods for large samples. Moreover, the simulation results in Tables 5 and 6 demonstrate the usefulness of the ESA with the CRImp method and the LS method to accommodate the unequal time intervals issue.

Table 5 Simulated MSEs of the estimates of the standard deviation of FPT based on MLE, ESA with RImp, CRImp, LS, and CRImp$_{LS}$ methods when the data are generated from the Gamma(1, 2), Gamma(0.5, 4), IG(2,5), and IG(2,10) processes with $\Delta t = \{1, 3, 5\}$ and experiment time $t_m = 75$

		Simulated from Gamma(1, 2)					Simulated from Gamma(0.5, 4)				
I	c	MLE	RImp	CRImp	LS	CRImp$_{LS}$	MLE	RImp	CRImp	LS	CRImp$_{LS}$
5	200	0.42	11.35	1.17	0.66	5.26	0.92	25.75	2.03	1.80	7.73
5	300	0.63	16.49	1.76	0.98	7.87	1.32	36.75	3.04	2.60	11.66
50	200	0.04	9.87	0.47	0.07	4.59	0.09	21.20	0.38	0.19	6.06
50	300	0.06	14.50	0.73	0.10	6.88	0.13	30.35	0.59	0.28	9.03
		Simulated from IG(2, 5)					Simulated from IG(2, 10)				
I	c	MLE	RImp	CRImp	LS	CRImp$_{LS}$	MLE	RImp	CRImp	LS	CRImp$_{LS}$
5	200	0.16	4.26	1.17	0.24	3.20	0.08	2.07	0.94	0.10	2.62
5	300	0.25	6.32	1.78	0.38	4.81	0.12	3.08	1.42	0.16	3.93
50	200	0.02	3.80	0.86	0.03	2.96	0.01	1.87	0.77	0.01	2.31
50	300	0.02	5.67	1.29	0.04	4.47	0.01	2.80	1.16	0.02	3.48

Table 6 Simulated MSEs of the estimates of the standard deviation of FPT based on MLE, ESA with RImp, CRImp, LS, and CRImp$_{LS}$ methods when the data are generated from the Gamma(1, 2), Gamma(0.5, 4), IG(2,5), and IG(2,10) processes with $\Delta t = \{1, 5, 15\}$ and experiment time $t_m = 75$

		Simulated from Gamma(1, 2)					Simulated from Gamma(0.5, 4)				
I	c	MLE	RImp	CRImp	LS	CRImp$_{LS}$	MLE	RImp	CRImp	LS	CRImp$_{LS}$
5	200	0.88	16.73	4.03	1.34	12.46	1.78	39.52	4.83	3.55	21.45
5	300	1.33	24.75	6.12	2.05	19.10	2.68	54.49	7.31	5.31	31.76
50	200	0.09	12.05	1.02	0.15	10.68	0.18	25.80	0.70	0.38	17.22
50	300	0.13	17.42	1.58	0.22	16.26	0.26	37.26	1.16	0.58	25.78
		Simulated from IG(2, 5)					Simulated from IG(2, 10)				
I	c	MLE	RImp	CRImp	LS	CRImp$_{LS}$	MLE	RImp	CRImp	LS	CRImp$_{LS}$
5	200	0.36	6.27	3.40	0.51	6.71	0.18	2.99	1.98	0.22	5.12
5	300	0.55	9.21	4.97	0.77	10.20	0.27	4.41	2.94	0.34	7.76
50	200	0.04	4.59	1.97	0.06	5.53	0.02	2.24	1.27	0.02	3.64
50	300	0.05	6.83	2.97	0.08	8.43	0.03	3.37	1.92	0.03	5.52

6 Numerical Example: Analysis of Laser Degradation Data

Laser devices are made of light emitting diodes (LEDs), and LEDs are subjected to degradation over time. As a matter of fact, laser devices are designed to maintain constant light output by providing more current to LED; thus, the operating current increases with time. Therefore, the failure time of laser devices is evaluated, which is the time at which the operating current passes a specific threshold level. An experiment is conducted with 15 GaAs laser devices at temperature 80 °C by Meeker and Escobar (1998). In the experiment, for 15 GaAs laser devices, the percent

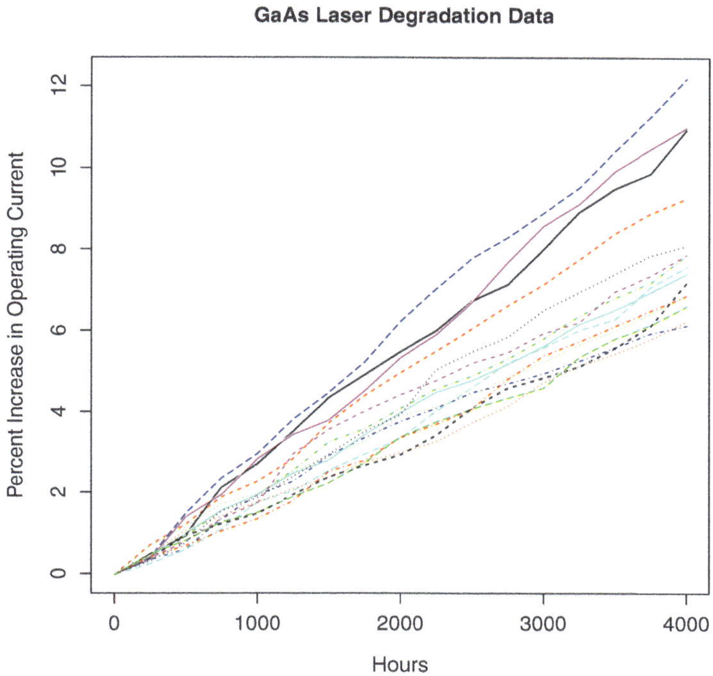

Fig. 4 Degradation paths of the 15 GaAs Laser degradation in an experiment described in Meeker and Escobar (1998)

increase in operating current is recorded for every 250 h up to 4000 h. In Fig. 4, the degradation paths are presented for the corresponding laser devices.

To illustrate the nonparametric approach for handling degradation data measured at unequal time intervals, we artificially remove some data by considering the measurements at time points {250, 500, 1000, 1750, 2000, 2500, 3250, 3500, 4000} with $\Delta t_1 = \Delta t_4 = \Delta t_7 = 250$, $\Delta t_2 = \Delta t_5 = \Delta t_8 = 500$, $\Delta t_3 = \Delta t_6 = 750$, and $\Delta t_0 = HCF(250, 500, 750) = 250$. The FPT distribution is estimated based on the modified data using ESA, and the parametric approach based on the gamma process assumption. To model the data with ESA, we apply the RImp, CRImp, LS, and CRImp$_{LS}$ methods. For the FPT approximation through gamma process, we used the complete data set before the removal to find the MLEs, which can be used as a reference for comparison purposes.

The estimated percentiles of the FPT distribution and the estimates of the standard deviation of FPT based on different estimation approaches are presented in Table 7. Using the estimates based on the parametric method as a reference, the proposed LS method provides estimates closer to the estimates based on the parametric method. It can be seen from Fig. 5 that all the methods considered here, including the proposed LS and CRImp$_{LS}$ methods, are not heavily deviated from the estimates based on the parametric method.

Table 7 Estimates of 1st, 5th, 10th, 50th, 90th, and 99th percentiles of FPT distributions obtained based on Gamma MLE (all data), RImp, CRImp, LS, and CRImp_{LS} methods with threshold levels $c = 10$ and $c = 20$

	$c = 10$					$c = 20$				
Percentile	MLE	RImp	CRImp	LS	CRImp_{LS}	MLE	RImp	CRImp	LS	CRImp_{LS}
1st	3990	3590	3668	3878	3615	8498	7908	8110	8343	7818
5th	4255	3958	4025	4175	3985	8880	8448	8608	8775	8405
10th	4398	4160	4220	4338	4190	9085	8743	8875	9013	8720
50th	4918	4918	4925	4943	4930	9825	9825	9838	9870	9845
90th	5455	5765	5673	5575	5708	10583	10993	10815	10760	10995
99th	5908	6560	6335	6105	6373	11213	12023	11628	11500	11965
$\widehat{SD}(T_c)$	413	633	571	483	594	584	883	758	683	891

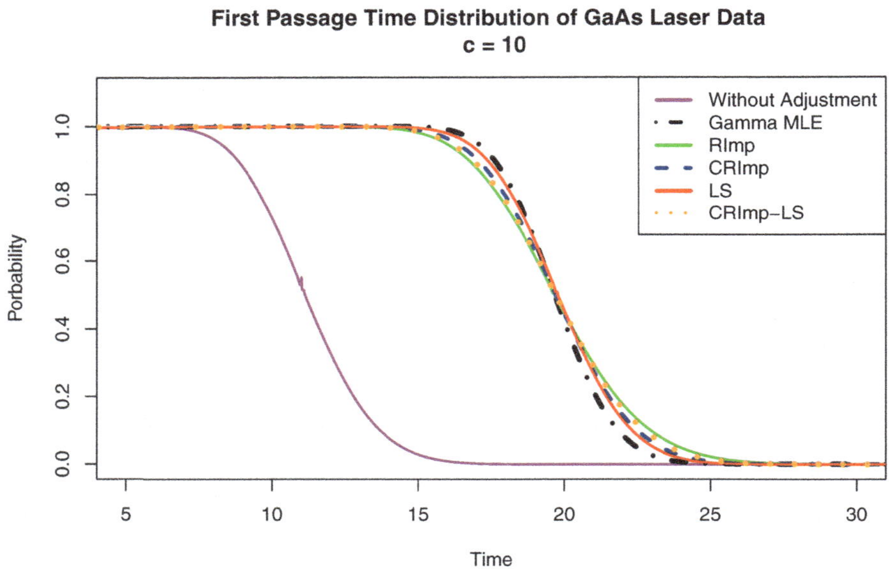

Fig. 5 FPT distribution of GaAs Laser degradation data with threshold $c = 10$ for unequal time intervals

References

Arnold, B. C., & Seshadri, V. (2009). Some new independence properties of the inverse Gaussian law. *Sankhyā: The Indian Journal of Statistics, 71*, 94–108.

Balakrishnan, N., & Kundu, D. (2019). Birnbaum-Saunders distribution: A review of models, analysis, and applications. *Applied Stochastics Models in Business and Industry, 35*, 4–49.

Balakrishnan, N., & Qin, C. (2019). Nonparametric evaluation of the first passage time of degradation processes. *Applied Stochastic Models in Business and Industry, 35*, 571–590.

Balakrishnan, N., Qin, C. (2020). Nonparametric optimal designs for degradation tests. *Journal of Applied Statistics, 47*, 624–641.

Bertoin, J. (1996). *Lévy processes* (Vol. 121). Cambridge, UK: Cambridge University Press.

Birnbaum, Z. W., & Saunders, S. C. (1969). A new family of life distributions. *Journal of Applied Probability, 6*, 319–327.

Chhikara, R. S., & Folks, J. L. (1989). *The inverse Gaussian distribution: Theory, methodology, and applications*. New York, NY: Marcel Dekker.

Donsker, M. D. (1951). An invariance principle for certain probability limit theorems. *Memoirs of the American Mathematical Society, 6*, 12.

Lugannani, R., & Rice, S. (1980). Saddle point approximation for the distribution of the sum of independent random variables. *Advances in Applied Probability, 12*, 475–490.

Meeker, W. Q., & Escobar, L. A. (1998). *Statistical Methods for Reliability Data*. New York, NY: Wiley.

Palayangoda, L. (2020). *Statistical models and analysis of univariate and multivariate degradation data*. Ph.D. thesis, Southern Methodist University, Dallas, Texas, USA.

Palayangoda, L. K., Ng, H. K. T., & Butler, R. W. (2020). Improved techniques for parametric and nonparametric evaluations of the first-passage time for degradation processes. *Applied Stochastic Models in Business and Industry, 36*(4), 730–753.

Park, C., & Padgett, W. (2005). Accelerated degradation models for failure based on geometric Brownian motion and Gamma processes. *Lifetime Data Analysis, 11*, 511–527.

Peng, C.-Y. (2015). Inverse Gaussian processes with random effects and explanatory variables for degradation data. *Technometrics, 57*, 100–111.

Tseng, S. T., & Lee, I.-C. (2016). Optimum allocation rule for accelerated degradation tests with a class of exponential-dispersion degradation models. *Technometrics, 58*, 244–254.

Wang, X., & Xu, D. (2010). An inverse Gaussian process model for degradation data. *Technometrics, 52*, 188–197.

Ye, Z., & Chen, N. (2014). The inverse Gaussian process as a degradation model. *Technometrics, 56*, 302–311.

Index

I. Ghosh et al. (eds.), *Advances in Statistics - Theory and Applications*, Emerging Topics in Statistics and Biostatistics, https://doi.org/10.1007/978-3-030-62900-7

The manufacturer's authorised representative in the EU is Springer Nature Customer Service Centre GmbH, Europaplatz 3, 69115 Heidelberg, Germany. If you have any concerns regarding our products, please contact ProductSafety@springernature.com

Printed and bound by CPI Group (UK) Ltd, Croydon, CR0 4YY

30/09/2026

02225320-0016